Behavioral and Psychopharmacologic Pain Management

Behavioral and Psychopharmacologic Pain Management

Editors

Michael H. Ebert
Associate Dean and Professor of Psychiatry, Yale University School of Medicine, New Haven, CT, USA
Chief of Staff, VA Connecticut Healthcare System, West Haven, CT, USA

Robert D. Kerns
National Program Director for Pain Management, Veterans Health Administration, West Haven, CT, USA
Director, Pain Research, Informatics, Medical comorbidities, and Education (PRIME) Center, West Haven, CT, USA
Professor of Psychiatry, Neurology, and Psychology, Yale University School of Medicine, New Haven, CT, USA

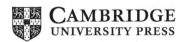

CAMBRIDGE
UNIVERSITY PRESS

CAMBRIDGE
UNIVERSITY PRESS

University Printing House, Cambridge CB2 8BS, United Kingdom

One Liberty Plaza, 20th Floor, New York, NY 10006, USA

477 Williamstown Road, Port Melbourne, VIC 3207, Australia

314-321, 3rd Floor, Plot 3, Splendor Forum, Jasola District Centre, New Delhi - 110025, India

79 Anson Road, #06-04/06, Singapore 079906

Cambridge University Press is part of the University of Cambridge.

It furthers the University's mission by disseminating knowledge in the pursuit of
education, learning and research at the highest international levels of excellence.

www.cambridge.org
Information on this title: www.cambridge.org/9780521884341

© Cambridge University Press 2011

First published 2011

A catalogue record for this publication is available from the British Library

Library of Congress Cataloging in Publication data
Behavioral and psychopharmacologic pain management / [edited by] Michael H. Ebert, Robert D. Kerns.
  p.   ; cm.
  Includes bibliographical references and index.
  ISBN 978-0-521-88434-1 (hardback)
  1. Pain–Treatment. 2. Analgesia.   I. Ebert, Michael H. II. Kerns, Robert D., 1950–
  [DNLM: 1. Pain–therapy. 2. Psychopharmacology. 3. Psychotherapy–methods. 4. Psychotropic
  Drugs–therapeutic use. WL 704]
  RB127.B44 2010
  616′.0472–dc22   2010034897

ISBN 978-0-521-88434-1 Hardback

....

To my father, Richard V. Ebert, M.D., who ignited my interest in medicine.

M.H.E.

To my parents, Robert D. and Altha Kerns, who have always inspired and encouraged me and my career. And to my children, Brandy and Joe, and to my partner, William Broumas, for their gifts of love, patience, and support. I am truly blessed to have you all in my life.

R.D.K.

Contents

Contributors

Charles E. Argoff, M.D.
Professor of Neurology, Albany Medical College;
Director, Comprehensive Pain Program, Albany
Medical Center, Albany, NY, USA

Gerard A. Banez, Ph.D.
Program Director, Pediatric Pain Rehabilitation
Program, Cleveland Clinic Children's Hospital,
Cleveland, OH, USA

Samantha Boris-Karpel, Ph.D., M.P.H., L.M.T.
Research Psychologist, Pain Research, Informatics,
Medical comorbidities, and Education (PRIME)
Center, VA Connecticut Healthcare System, West
Haven, CT, USA

Barbara K. Bruce, Ph.D.
Assistant Professor of Psychology, Department of
Psychiatry and Psychology, Mayo Clinic;
Mayo Clinic Comprehensive Pain Rehabilitation
Center, Rochester, MN, USA

Alexandra S. Bullough, M.B.Ch.B., M.D.
Assistant Professor of Anesthesiology,
University of Michigan Medical School, Ann Arbor,
MI, USA

Annmarie Cano, Ph.D.
Associate Professor, Department of Psychology,
Wayne State University, Detroit, MI, USA

Victor T. Chang, M.D.
Associate Professor of Medicine, University of
Medicine and Dentistry of New Jersey, Newark;
Section Hematology/Oncology, Medical
Service, VA New Jersey Health Care System, East
Orange, NJ, USA

Elizabeth A. Clark, Ph.D.
Postdoctoral Resident in Clinical Health Psychology,
Psychology Service, VA Connecticut Healthcare
System, West Haven, CT, USA

Daniel J. Clauw, M.D.
Professor of Anesthesiology, Medicine, and Psychiatry;
Director, Chronic Pain and Fatigue Research Center,
University of Michigan Medical School, Ann Arbor,
MI, USA

June L. Dahl, Ph.D.
Professor of Pharmacology, University of Wisconsin
School of Medicine and Public Health, Madison,
WI, USA

Tam K. Dao, Ph.D.
Assistant Professor, Department of Educational
Psychology, University of Houston, Houston;
Assistant Professor, Menninger Department of
Psychiatry and Behavioral Sciences, Baylor College of
Medicine, Houston, TX, USA

Amber M. Davis, B.A.
Mental Health Specialist, YWCA Sojourner's Shelter
for Homeless Women and Families, Charleston,
WV, USA

Courtney L. Dixon, B.A.
Department of Psychology, Wayne State University,
Detroit, MI, USA

Michael H. Ebert, M.D.
Associate Dean and Professor of Psychiatry, Yale
University School of Medicine;
Chief of Staff, VA Connecticut Healthcare System,
West Haven, CT, USA

Robin M. Gallagher, M.D., M.P.H.
Clinical Professor of Psychiatry and Anesthesiology,
University of Pennsylvania School of Medicine;
Deputy National Program Director for Pain
Management, Veterans Health Administration;
Director for Pain Policy Research and
Primary Care, Penn Pain Medicine, Philadelphia,
PA, USA

Gerald W. Grass, M.D.
Assistant Professor of Anesthesiology, Yale University
School of Medicine, New Haven;
Chief, Anesthesia Pain Medicine, VA Connecticut
Healthcare System, West Haven, CT, USA

Carmen R. Green, M.D.
Professor, Department of Anesthesiology and
Obstetrics and Gynecology, University of Michigan
Medical School;
Associate Professor of Health Management and
Policy, University of Michigan School of Public
Health, Ann Arbor, MI, USA

Jay Gunkelman
Q-Pro Worldwide, Crockett, CA, USA

Bradford D. Hare, M.D., Ph.D.
Associate Professor and Vice-Chair of Pain, Pain
Research & Management Center, Department
of Anesthesiology, University of Utah School of
Medicine, Salt Lake City, UT, USA

Jennifer A. Haythornthwaite, Ph.D.
Professor, Department of Psychiatry and Behavioral
Sciences, Johns Hopkins University School of
Medicine, Baltimore, MD, USA

Jaclyn Heller Issner, M.A.
Graduate Research Assistant, Department of
Psychology, Wayne State University, Detroit,
MI, USA

W. Michael Hooten, M.D.
Assistant Professor of Anesthesiology, Department
of Anesthesiology, Department of Psychiatry and
Psychology, Mayo Clinic, Rochester, MN, USA
Mayo Clinic Comprehensive Pain Rehabilitation
Center, Rochester,
MN, USA

Mark P. Jensen, Ph.D.
Professor and Vice Chair for Research,
Department of Rehabilitation Medicine, University
of Washington School of Medicine, Seattle,
WA, USA

Mark E. Jones, M.A., Ph.D.
Palliative Care Fellow, VA Interprofessional Palliative
Care Fellowship Program, VISN 3 GRECC,
James J Peters VA Medical Center, Bronx, NY, USA
Staff Psychologist, Home-Based Primary Care, Salem
VA Medical Center, Salem, VA, USA

Robert D. Kerns, Ph.D.
National Program Director for Pain Management,
Veterans Health Administration, West Haven;
Director, Pain Research, Informatics, Medical
comorbidities, and Education (PRIME) Center,
West Haven;
Professor of Psychiatry, Neurology, and Psychology,
Yale University School of Medicine, New Haven,
CT, USA

Raphael J. Leo, M.A., M.D.
Associate Professor of Psychiatry, State University
of New York at Buffalo, School of Medicine and
Biomedical Sciences;
Department of Psychiatry and The Center for
Comprehensive Multidisciplinary Pain
Management, Erie County Medical Center, Buffalo,
NY, USA

Morris Maizels, M.D.
Director, Kaiser Permanente Woodland Hills
Headache Clinic;
Department of Family Medicine, Kaiser Permanente
Medical Center, Woodland Hills, CA, USA

Mary E. Murawski, Ph.D.
Boston University School of Medicine and Harvard
Medical School;
Postdoctoral Resident, VA Boston Healthcare System,
Boston, MA, USA

Brooke Myers-Sorger, Ph.D.
Palliative Care Fellow, VA Interprofessional Palliative
Care Fellowship Program, VISN 3 GRECC, James J.
Peters VA Medical Center, Bronx, NY, USA
Montclair Psychology Associates, Verona,
NJ, USA

Akiko Okifuji, Ph.D.
Professor and Scott M Smith MD Presidential Endowed Chair in Anesthesiology, Pain Research & Management Center, Department of Anesthesiology, University of Utah School of Medicine, Salt Lake City, UT, USA

Renata Okonkwo, Ph.D.
Post-Doctoral Fellow, Department of Psychiatry & Behavioral Sciences, Johns Hopkins University School of Medicine, Baltimore, MD, USA

John D. Otis, Ph.D.
Assistant Professor of Psychiatry and Psychology, Boston University School of Medicine;
Director, Pain Research Program, VA Boston Healthcare System, Boston, MA, USA

Stacy C. Parenteau, Ph.D.
Psychologist, Scott and White Clinic, College Station, TX, USA

Laura E. Pence, Ph.D.
Postdoctoral Fellow, Cancer Prevention Fellowship Program, Cancer Training Center, National Cancer Institute, Bethesda, MD, USA

Donald B. Penzien, Ph.D.
Professor of Psychiatry and Human Behavior, University of Mississippi Medical School;
Director, Head Pain Center, University of Mississippi Medical Center, Jackson, MS, USA

Donna B. Pincus, Ph.D.
Associate Professor;
Director of Research, Child and Adolescent Fear and Anxiety Treatment Program, Center for Anxiety and Related Disorders, Boston University, Boston, MA, USA

Ellyn Poltrock Stein, Ph.D.
Palliative Care Fellow, VA Interprofessional Palliative Care Fellowship Program, VISN 3 GRECC, James J Peters VA Medical Center, Bronx, NY, USA

Wendy J. Quinton, Ph.D.
Adjunct Instructor, State University of New York at Buffalo, Department of Psychology, Buffalo, NY, USA

Jeanetta C. Rains, Ph.D.
Clinical Director, Center for Sleep Evaluation, Elliot Hospital, Manchester, NH, USA

M. Carrington Reid, M.D., Ph.D.
Associate Professor of Medicine, Division of Geriatrics and Gerontology, Weill Cornell Medical Center, New York, NY, USA

Thomas J. Romano, M.D., Ph.D.
Private Practice, Martins Ferry, OH, USA

Jeffrey D. Rome, M.D.
Assistant Professor and Chair Emeritus, Department of Psychiatry and Psychology, Mayo Clinic;
Mayo Clinic Pain Rehabilitation Center, Mayo Clinic, Rochester, MN, USA

Robert L. Ruff, M.D., Ph.D.
Professor, Departments of Neurology and Neurosciences, Case Western Reserve University School of Medicine;
Chief, Neurology Service, Polytrauma Treatment Team, Louis Stokes Cleveland Department of Veterans Affairs Medical Center, Cleveland, OH, USA

Suzanne S. Ruff, Ph.D.
Health Psychologist, Psychology Service, Behavioral Medicine Pain Management, Polytrauma Treatment Team, Louis Stokes Cleveland Department of Veterans Affairs Medical Center, Cleveland, OH, USA

Steven H. Sanders, Ph.D.
Clinical Director, Outpatient Chronic Pain Rehabilitation Program, James A. Haley VA Hospital, Tampa, FL, USA

Ingra Schellenberg, Ph.D.
Assistant Professor of Philosophy and Bioethics and Humanities, University of Washington, Seattle, WA, USA

John J. Sellinger, Ph.D.
Assistant Professor, Department of Psychiatry, Yale University School of Medicine, New Haven;
VA Connecticut Healthcare System, Psychology Service, West Haven, CT, USA

Howard S. Smith, M.D.
Associate Professor, Departments of Anesthesiology, Internal Medicine, and Physical Medicine and Rehabilitation, Albany Medical College, Albany, NY, USA
Academic Director of Pain Management, Department of Anesthesiology, Albany Medical College, Albany, NY, USA

Brenda Stoelb, Ph.D.
Research Scientist, Talaria, Inc., Seattle, WA, USA

Jon Streltzer, M.D.
Professor of Psychiatry, John A. Burns School of Medicine, University of Hawaii;
Director, Queen Emma Pain Center, Queen's Medical Center, Honolulu, HI, USA

Mark D. Sullivan, M.D., Ph.D.
Professor, Department of Psychiatry and Behavioral Sciences, University of Washington School of Medicine;
Adjunct Professor, Department of Bioethics and Humanities, University of Washington, Seattle, WA, USA

Kimberly S. Swanson Ph.D.
Research Interventionist, University of Washington – Scholl of Social Work, Behavioral Medicine Research Group, Seattle WA, USA

Gabriel Tan, Ph.D.
Associate Professor, Departments of Anesthesiology, Psychiatry and Behavioral Science, and Physical Medicine and Rehabilitation, Baylor College of Medicine, Houston, TX, USA
Clinical Health Psychologist, Anesthesiology Pain Program, Michael E. Debakey VA Medical Center, Houston, TX, USA

Stephen Thielke, M.D., M.A.
Assistant Professor, Psychiatry and Behavioral Sciences, University of Washington School of Medicine, Seattle, WA, USA

Beverly E. Thorn, Ph.D.
Professor and Chair, Department of Psychology, University of Alabama, Tuscaloosa, AL, USA

Cynthia O. Townsend, Ph.D.
Assistant Professor of Psychology, Department of Psychiatry and Psychology, Mayo Clinic;
Mayo Clinic Comprehensive Pain Rehabilitation Center, Rochester, MN, USA

Dennis C. Turk, Ph.D.
John and Emma Bonica Professor of Anesthesiology and Pain Research, Department of Anesthesiology and Pain Medicine, University of Washington School of Medicine, Seattle, WA, USA

Stephanie C. Wallio, Ph.D.
VA Connecticut Healthcare System, Psychology Service, West Haven, CT, USA

Lawrence J. Weinberger, Ph.D.
Staff Psychologist, Physical Medicine and Rehabilitation Service, VA New Jersey Health Care System, East Orange, NJ, USA

David A. Williams, Ph.D.
Professor of Anesthesiology, Medicine, Psychiatry, and Psychology, University of Michigan Medical School;
Associate Director, Chronic Pain and Fatigue Research Center, University of Michigan, Ann Arbor, MI, USA

Hilary Wilson, Ph.D.
Research Assistant Professor, Department of Anesthesiology & Pain Medicine, University of Washington School of Medicine, Seattle, WA, USA

Acknowledgments

We wish to express our appreciation to Ellen Levine Ebert for her dedicated editorial assistance. We thank our editors at Cambridge University Press for their help in moving a concept into a manuscript.

M.H.E. and R.D.K.

Introduction

Michael H. Ebert and Robert D. Kerns

This book is focused on the evidence-based practice of behavioral and psychopharmacologic treatment strategies for pain syndromes of various types. A large number and a broad variety of health providers use these therapeutic treatment approaches to treat patients with acute and chronic pain syndromes. These types of providers include primary care physicians and advanced practice nurses, psychologists, psychiatrists, neurologists, physical medicine and rehabilitation physicians, anesthesiologists, surgeons (particularly orthopedic and neurological surgeons), a variety of internal medicine subspecialists including oncologists and rheumatologists, podiatrists, and physicians in occupational medicine. Therefore the text is directed to an interdisciplinary audience, and is intended to be used in a variety of training programs and pain medicine practice groups.

An impetus for developing this text at the present time is the recent reorganization of the training essentials of the subspecialty of pain medicine by the Accreditation Council of Graduate Medical Education (ACGME). A cornerstone of the new pain medicine requirements is that the sponsoring facility must include individuals who are board certified in the fields of anesthesiology, psychiatry, neurology, and physical medicine and rehabilitation by the relevant American Board of Medical Specialties (ABMS). This change reflects the judgment by the ABMS and the ACGME that the successful and competent practice of pain medicine includes evidence-based behavioral and pharmacological interventions as well as the procedural and invasive interventions that are usually performed by anesthesiologists. Dr. Ebert recently concluded a 5-year term on the Residency Review Committee (RRC) of the ACGME, and served during 2004 and 2005 as the chair of the Psychiatry RRC. In this capacity he worked with the chairs of the other three RRCs to complete the final editing and

negotiation of the ACGME pain medicine requirements. These requirements for accredited pain medicine training programs began in July 2007.

The emphasis on interdisciplinary training in the practice of pain medicine is captured in the introductory paragraph of the new ACGME requirements for training in pain medicine. This statement is as follows:

> "Pain medicine is a discipline within the practice of medicine that specializes in the management of patients suffering from acute or chronic pain, or pain in patients who require palliative care. The management of acute and chronic pain syndromes is a complex matter involving many areas of interest and different medical disciplines. Clinical and investigative efforts are vital to the progress of the specialty. Physicians training in pain medicine may originate from different disciplines and approach the field with varying backgrounds and experience. All pain specialists, regardless of their primary specialty, should be competent in pain assessment, formulation, and coordination of a multiple modality treatment plan, integration of pain treatment with primary disease management and palliative care, and interaction with other members of a multidisciplinary team. Therefore, the didactic and clinical curriculum of the multidisciplinary pain program must address attainment of these competencies."

The current text was designed to fill a noted gap by offering a single source volume that provides comprehensive and state of the art consideration of the bio-psychosocial perspective on pain and pain management, and also detailed presentation of the core assessment and intervention strategies informed by that model. Although written with the pain specialist in mind, it is expected that the text will serve as an important resource for a variety of medical specialists, nurses, advanced practice nurses, psychologists, and other associated health professionals.

Section 1 presents a brief history of the treatment of pain, illustrating the fact that psychological approaches to pain management have existed from the early history

Behavioral and Psychopharmacologic Pain Management, ed. Michael H. Ebert and Robert D. Kerns. Published by Cambridge University Press. © Cambridge University Press 2011.

of pain medicine. This section also develops the concept that the physiology of pain, the perception of pain, and the psychological ramifications of the experience of chronic pain are intertwined. A successful therapeutic plan for a given pain condition requires a biopsychosocial approach to the problem.

Section 2 is a detailed presentation of pain assessment techniques and strategies. Chronic pain presents two broad challenges to proper assessment: the inherently subjective nature of pain complaints and the wide-ranging influence of chronic pain on patient functioning. These challenges necessitate a systematic assessment approach that employs standardized assessment of multiple domains of functioning using several assessment techniques, including questionnaires, behavioral observation, psychophysiological measurement, diary data, and reports of significant others. The chapters include a discussion of the clinical goals of psychological and behavioral assessment of the patient with persistent pain, provision of a rationale and context for the use of psychological assessment in the practice of pain medicine, articulation of recommendations for the core domains of assessment, and provision of an overview of the psychological assessment process. Specific information is presented about the most commonly employed psychological and behavioral assessment methods and specific strategies. The final chapter deals with psychiatric and pain comorbidities.

Section 3 presents behavioral, psychopharmacologic, and psychotherapeutic treatment approaches that are evidence-based components of a treatment plan. Psychological interventions have become commonly employed and generally accepted alternatives or adjuncts to traditional medical, surgical, and rehabilitation approaches to the management of persistent pain and pain-related disability. This section begins with a broad discussion of the role of psychological interventions in the context of pain management, including a review of the evidence and a discussion of contemporary practice and policy related to the application of these interventions. General issues such as the incorporation of psychological interventions in the context of multidisciplinary programs, strategies for enhancing motivation to engage in such treatments, and integration of psychological and psychopharmacologic

approaches are reviewed. Subsequent chapters will describe specific treatment approaches and methods (e.g., self-regulatory, behavioral, cognitive-behavioral, supportive) as well as the application of psychological interventions for specific painful conditions.

Many psychotropic drugs have effects on central pain perception. They also have powerful actions on the psychological state of the individual who suffers from chronic pain. Conversely, chronic pain can precipitate a variety of psychiatric disorders, including depressive disorders and anxiety disorders. This section of the book reviews the major classes of psychotropic drugs that have an effect on pain perception and tolerance and the related acute psychiatric syndromes that can result from having a pain disorder. Antidepressant agents and antianxiety agents are a major focus of this section. Opiate and non-opiate analgesics are reviewed, with particular attention to their psychotropic effects and addictive liability. The mechanism of action and evidence-based therapeutic use of these classes of drugs to treat pain syndromes are covered. The management of patients taking these drugs in a way that minimizes the risk of addiction is presented.

Section 4 presents evidence-based psychological and psychopharmacologic interventions for specific pain syndromes. This section develops a series of evidence-based treatment guidelines that combine the therapeutic approaches developed earlier in the book. Specific pain syndromes that are discussed in individual chapters include pain of spinal origin (including radicular pain, zygapophysial joint disease, discogenic pain), myofascial pain, neuropathic pain, headache and orofacial pain, rheumatological aspects of pain, complex regional pain syndromes, visceral pain, cancer pain (including palliative and hospice care), acute pain, and pain in special populations (such as the elderly, pediatric patients, pregnant women, physically disabled, and the cognitively impaired).

The book concludes with chapters on new research directions for the interdisciplinary treatment of pain, policy issues, and ethical issues in pain treatment. Scientifically sound clinical studies of new cognitive and behavioral treatments of pain are a lively area of research at the present time. Double-blind studies of psychopharmacological drugs used in the treatment of pain are also becoming much more frequent.

The process of pain management

June L. Dahl

Introduction

Pain can be a blessing or a curse. It serves as a built-in warning system that alerts us to injury or disease so it is essential for our health and survival [1]. But if pain persists beyond the usual period of healing, it serves no useful purpose, causes untold physical and emotional suffering, and costs the healthcare system and the economy billions of dollars each year [2–4]. In 2003, the American Productivity Audit reported that lost productive time from common pain conditions such as headache, back pain, arthritis, and other musculoskeletal problems alone cost $61.2 billion dollars [5]. Ironically, federal dollars dedicated to pain research do not measure up. In 2003, less than 1% ($26 million) of all funding from the National Institutes of Health (NIH) was allocated to research having a primary emphasis on pain [6]. Although funding increased in 2004, it declined over the next three years. The nation's investment in pain research is "seriously out of scale with the impact of pain on the nation's healthcare burden" [7]. The Patient Protection and Affordable Care Act (often referred to as the healthcare reform bill), which signed into law in March 2010 [8], includes several provisions that should begin to correct this imbalance. It adds a new section to the Public Health Service Act which establishes a Pain Consortium at the NIH that encourages the Director to expand an aggressive program of pain research, to track advances in federally-funded pain research, identify critical research gaps, and coordinate research across NIH and other agencies, e.g., the Veterans Administration and Department of Defense.

One hundred and fifty years ago, surgeons viewed pain as a sign of a patient's vitality and felt it critical to healing [9]. We now know that unrelieved acute post-operative pain delays healing, is a leading cause of delayed discharge and readmission to the hospital, and a risk factor for the development of chronic pain [10–12]. Fear of uncontrolled post-surgical pain is among the primary concerns of many patients about to undergo surgery [11]. Their fears appear to be justified as studies continue to document poor pain control for post-operative and trauma pain. More than 73 million surgeries are performed annually in the USA [13]; 70% of those are performed in the ambulatory care setting. One survey showed that about 80% of adults experienced pain after surgery; 86% of those had moderate, severe, or extreme pain [13].

Pain is also one of the most common and perhaps the most feared symptom of cancer [14]. Almost a million and a half new cases of cancer are diagnosed each year, and more than half a million die of the disease [15]. Persons experience pain from their cancer and also from various surgeries, and diagnostic and treatment procedures. One-third of cancer patients have pain at the time of their diagnosis; 65% of patients with advanced, metastatic, and/or terminal disease report pain [16]; more than one-third of survivors "cured" of their cancer have pain, one-third of those experience moderate to severe pain [17, 18]. As cancer evolves into a chronic illness, pain management challenges in the oncologic patient increase in complexity [19]. Survivors whose disease is in remission may be at special risk for undertreatment and become victims of the increasing debate about the appropriateness of opioid therapy for chronic non-cancer pain [20–22].

Many more millions of Americans are affected by chronic non-cancer pain [2–4, 23]. A 2006 report from the Centers for Disease Control found that 26% of Americans 20 years or older (or an estimated 76.5 million) had experienced a pain problem that persisted for more than 24 hours; 42% of those said the problem persisted for more than a year [24]. A diary-survey

Behavioral and Psychopharmacologic Pain Management, ed. Michael H. Ebert and Robert D. Kerns. Published by Cambridge University Press. © Cambridge University Press 2011.

method used to study pain in a representative sample of the population found more pain and a greater severity of pain in persons with lower incomes [25]. Socioeconomic disadvantage is consistently associated with an increased risk of pain [26]. "The undertreatment of chronic pain is not only a medical issue, but also as detailed above, an economic one that has a tremendous ripple effect as it touches not only those who have pain, but their families, employers and communities" (P. Cowan, Executive Director, American Chronic Pain Association, personal communication).

The good news is that pain management has become a priority in many aspects of healthcare in the USA. In fact, Congress declared this first decade of the twenty-first century to be the Decade of Pain Control and Research [27]. There has been growing recognition that the undertreatment of pain is a major public health problem; this has stimulated the development of numerous clinical practice guidelines [28], countless educational programs, and policy statements that acknowledge the importance of effective pain control [29, 30].

In 1999, the US Department of Veterans Affairs (VA) launched an ambitious program called "Pain as a Fifth Vital Sign" to encourage assessment of pain in all patients in all of its medical facilities [31]. Pain assessment and management standards became part of the Joint Commission's accreditation process in 2001 [32–34], and standards for palliative care were drafted as part of the Commission's Healthcare Services Certification Programs [35] in 2008. The Centers for Medicare and Medicaid Services (CMS) initiated a pain quality improvement program for the nation's long-term care facilities in 2002 [36]. Public reporting on the Nursing Home Compare web site is a cornerstone of CMS's continued efforts to improve the quality of care in long-term care [37]. More recently the VA implemented a stepped care model to provide a single standard of care for veterans as they move through that system [38, 39].

In addition, members of the pain community, state legislators, and federal and state regulators have worked collaboratively to remove uncertainty about the use of opioid analgesics and encourage better pain management. The emphasis has been on promoting balanced policies that prevent diversion and abuse of opioid analgesics while assuring their availability to patients who need them for pain control [40]. The Federation of State Medical Boards released a *Model Guideline* [30] (now a *Model Policy* [41]) *on the Use of Controlled Substances for the Treatment of Pain* to emphasize that treating pain with controlled substances is an integral part of the practice of medicine.

Even though substantial efforts have been made to improve the practice of pain management, multiple challenges continue to impede progress. Sandra Johnson, lawyer and ethicist, has asserted "that the time during which easy changes in policy or education could revolutionize the treatment of patients in pain has passed. We are now operating in what appears to be a complex ecosystem that supports ambivalence, denial, and suspicion of the circumstances of patients in pain and of those who treat them" [42]. This writer takes a more positive view but does believe that the sense of euphoria which pervaded some persons in the pain world a decade ago has been replaced by sobering uncertainties, which must be addressed if we are to ensure that persons obtain relief of their pain.

Knowledge of the basics of pain management strategies is essential for dealing with those uncertainties. This chapter provides an overview of the basic elements underlying effective pain control. It describes the common types of pain and gives a brief review of assessment and treatment strategies, which are subjects discussed in depth in subsequent chapters. There are also references to the medical, legal, and ethical challenges that have arisen as a result of greater demands for better pain control.

Quality pain control is everyone's responsibility

Despite the ubiquity of pain, the evidence for its inadequate treatment, and realization of the devastating physical and psychological impact of poor pain control, clinicians often find pain difficult to diagnose and treat [43]. In many cases, the origin of the pain is complex and not easily understood. Some patients have psychological problems that complicate management. In some cases, clinicians have been hesitant to use the full spectrum of available analgesics because of limited familiarity with the drugs and their effects. Opioids, in particular, may raise concerns about regulatory oversight or undue fears that patients will become addicted.

"High quality pain management requires appropriate assessment: screening for the presence of pain; completion of a comprehensive initial assessment when pain is present; interdisciplinary collaborative care planning, including patient and family input;

and appropriate treatment that is multidisciplinary, evidence-based, rational, safe, and cost effective," [44]. Frequent reassessments of patients' responses to treatment are essential in order to identify the need for adjustments in the plan of care, or the adverse effects or futility of a particular treatment plan.

Every member of the healthcare team needs to become familiar with the characteristics of the most common types of pain, how to perform a multidimensional assessment of pain in order to establish a pain diagnosis (or diagnoses), how to collaborate as a member of an interdisciplinary team and engage the patient in an appropriate goal-oriented plan of care, and when and to whom to refer when specialty care is required. In the words of Deming, the guru of quality improvement: "Quality is everyone's responsibility."

What is pain?

The International Association for the Study of Pain defines pain as: "an unpleasant sensory *and* emotional experience associated with actual or potential tissue damage or described in terms of such damage" [45, 46]. Pain is a conscious experience that results from brain activity in response to a noxious stimulus and engages the sensory, emotional, and cognitive processes of the brain. We can distinguish two dimensions of pain: sensory-discriminative and affective-emotional [47–49]. The former represents the ability to localize a stimulus in space and time and assess its intensity, and the latter consists of evaluation and interpretation of the meaning of the pain experience. Some patients have a dominant affective-emotional component and present with increased pain behaviors, anxiety, and depression that must be treated simultaneously in order to achieve effective pain control.

There is no standard laboratory test or diagnostic procedure that can identify or measure pain . There is no "painometer." All pain is subjective. Furthermore, each person responds individually to a painful stimulus. We learn the meaning of the word through experiences related to injury in early life. Pain is always unpleasant and therefore an emotional experience. Margo McCaffery, nurse educator and advocate, wrote 30 years ago that "pain is whatever the experiencing persons says it is, existing whenever he says it does" [50]. Healthcare professionals must accept the patient's report of pain.

For a variety of reasons, each individual responds differently to pain and to the strategies that are used to provide relief. Emotional factors, cultural and spiritual values and beliefs shape the meaning of the pain experience as well as expectations for pain relief. Previous experiences with pain management shape views about pain. Genetic differences shape our responses to a painful stimulus as well as to drug and non-drug treatments [51]. Assessment and treatment must be tailored to individual needs and responses. Therein lie opportunities and significant challenges.

Although self-report is the single most reliable indicator of pain, there will be times when patients cannot communicate. In those cases, one needs to consider the person's underlying disease state and assume pain is present if those diseases or conditions are likely to cause pain. There may be physical or behavioral changes that suggest pain is present. Some, such as limping or groaning, are obvious indicators; others may be more subtle. Family members or caregivers often know how an individual usually expresses pain and can provide important insights into a patient's pain state.

Classification of pain

There are many ways to categorize pain; the categories may overlap. Pain can be classified in terms of its intensity (mild, moderate, or severe); duration (acute or chronic); pathophysiology (nociceptive, inflammatory, neuropathic, or mixed); or according to type or syndrome (cancer, fibromyalgia, migraine, sickle cell). Classification of pain is essential to guide assessment and treatment approaches, and to establish the goals of therapy. For example, non-opioid analgesics provide relief of mild, but not severe pain. Relief of cancer pain may require a variety of therapies including, but not limited to, surgery, radiotherapy, and analgesics; fibromyalgia is treated with exercise and antidepressants, although some specific drugs for fibromyalgia have been approved recently; an acute migraine headache may be aborted by a triptan, a specific antimigraine drug. Drug and non-drug therapies are used to prevent migraine attacks. Sickle cell pain usually requires aggressive therapy with opioid analgesics. Non-pharmacologic therapies, both physical and behavioral, are essential for the management of most types of pain.

A caution about the classification of pain: some identify pain not due to visible signs of disease or injury as psychogenic pain [52, 53]; this writer believes this term stigmatizes persons and invalidates their report of pain and recommends that it not be used. While psychological factors contribute to the pain experience, particularly when pain is chronic [54], patients should be assured that their pain is real – it is not just a figment of their imagination.

Acute vs. chronic pain

Pain may be classified as acute or chronic on the basis of its temporal characteristics. Many patients have mixed pain problems. Acute pain is associated with strains, sprains, fractures, surgery, diagnostic procedures, or trauma, and has a short time course as it gradually diminishes as healing occurs. Chronic pain may be continuous or intermittent pain and is arbitrarily defined as pain that lasts longer than 3–6 months. Recurrent acute pain, as occurs with migraine headache or sickle cell disease, falls in the category of chronic pain. Some causes of, or types of, chronic pain include cancer, burns, rheumatoid or osteoarthritis, peripheral neuropathies, fibromyalgia, phantom limb pain, low back pain, and complex regional pain syndrome (CRPS). The terms chronic and persistent are often used interchangeably. Many prefer the term persistent pain as it "may foster a more positive attitude" since chronic pain is a pejorative term that is often associated with negative images and stereotypes [54].

Some persons with stable chronic pain experience acute exacerbations of their pain. These are of two types: pain flares which are transient, usually benign, increases in pain that can last for hours to days, or worsening pain due to disease progression. The term "breakthrough pain" was coined to describe a sudden worsening of pain in persons with cancer and stable chronic pain [55, 56]. The term is now used more broadly to describe any increase in pain in a person with underlying stable chronic pain [57]. Whether the term should be used in that context is open to debate as is the approach to treatment [58].

Obviously, there are major differences between acute and chronic pain in terms of timing, causes, and objective signs. Acute pain is useful as a warning sign; its cause is usually known, it diminishes as healing takes place, and there may be changes in vital signs and/or behaviors. Persons with chronic pain may not "look like" they are in pain; however, vegetative or depressive signs may be present. Chronic pain may spread from one site to other parts of the body with diverse physiological and psychological consequences (e.g., CRPS). It results from structural and functional changes in the nervous system. A genetically vulnerable individual who suffers a physical injury such as an ankle sprain may go on to develop chronic pain. Currently one can not predict which patients undergoing surgery or experiencing trauma are at risk to develop persistent pain, although one group of investigators has claimed that they can identify patients at risk by testing their response to experimental pain [59].

Physiological vs. pathophysiological pain

Pain can also be classified as normal (physiological) or abnormal (pathological). Nociceptive (physiological) pain represents a normal response to a noxious stimulus or injury of tissues such as the skin, muscles, visceral organs, joints, tendons, or bones. The sensory experience of acute pain is mediated by a specialized system, called the nociceptive system. It extends from the periphery through the spinal cord, brain stem, and thalamus to the cerebral cortex where the sensation is perceived. Intense noxious stimuli activate a subpopulation of primary sensory neurons called nociceptors. Nociception is the term used to describe the process by which information about a noxious stimulus is conveyed from those nociceptors in the periphery to the brain. It is composed of four processes: transduction, the conversion of noxious stimuli into nerve impulses; transmission, the conduction of nerve impulses from the periphery to the spinal cord and then to the brain; perception, the process by which pain is recognized by a conscious person; and modulation, the process by which the brain dampens or facilitates ascending pain impulses (descending inhibitory or facilitory pathways).

Nociceptive pain is divided into two types: somatic pain arising from the bone, skin, and soft tissues is often described as dull or aching and is well localized, whereas visceral pain caused by obstruction or pressure in hollow organs such as the GI tract or liver capsule is described as pressure-like, deep-aching, or cramping. It is often poorly localized and may be referred to distant dermatomal sites. Nociceptive pain can be acute, such as experienced with a fracture of the femur, or chronic as occurs with arthritis or interstitial cystitis. Continuous activation of nociceptive pathways can lead to complex changes in both the peripheral and central nervous systems. Inflammatory responses to tissue injury can lead to peripheral sensitization (increased excitability of peripheral nociceptors) or central sensitization (increased excitability of spinal cord neurons).

Neuropathic pain is the term applied to pain syndromes that result from pathological changes in the peripheral or central nervous systems. It is described with words such as burning, stabbing, electric shock-like, numbness, or tingling. There may be allodynia (pain due to a non-noxious stimulus) or hyperalgesia (an exaggerated response to a noxious stimulus); there may also be diminished strength and abnormal reflexes. Three symptoms have been found to be significant predictors: tingling, numbness, and increased pain to touch [60]. Post-herpetic neuralgia, diabetic neuropathy, HIV/AIDS, post-thoractomy, post-mastectomy, and chemotherapy-induced neuropathies are examples of neuropathic pain.

Although neuropathic pain may be treated with a variety of drugs including local anesthetics, antidepressants, antiepileptics, and/or opioids [61], there are no treatments that completely, predictably, and specifically control this type of pain. "Despite the best of care and sequential trials of therapy, pain will remain unrelieved or inadequately relieved in 40–60% of patients suffering from neuropathic pain" [62]. This somber assessment has particular poignancy in the context of our belief that patients have the right to relief of pain [63, 64]. It also calls attention to the need to develop measures to prevent neuropathic pain. An exciting development in this area is the finding that a live attenuated vaccine aimed at boosting immunity to varicella zoster virus (VZV) significantly reduces the incidence of both herpes zoster and post-herpetic neuralgia [65]. Herpes zoster, commonly called shingles, is a distinctive syndrome caused by reactivation of VZV. This reactivation occurs when immunity to VZV declines because of aging or immunosuppression.

Positron emission tomography and functional magnetic resonance imaging have been focused on defining the network of brain structures (the pain matrix) involved in normal physiological pain and investigating the neural basis of chronic pathological pain [66, 67]. Imaging studies have shown that chronic pain is accompanied by significant atrophy in certain brain regions. For example, Apkarian and colleagues [68] found that patients with chronic back pain showed 5–11% less neocortical gray matter volume than control subjects and that the loss was more severe in the subgroup of these patients with neuropathic pain. May found decreases in regional gray matter in patients suffering from six different pain syndromes: phantom pain, chronic back pain, irritable bowel syndrome, fibromyalgia, and two types of headache [69]. While the alterations were different for the different syndromes, "they overlapped to an astounding extent."

Principles of assessment

Assessment is the essential first step in pain management [70, Chapter 4]. Without a thorough baseline assessment, it is not possible to develop a rational approach to treatment. Furthermore, frequent reassessments are essential to evaluate the effectiveness of treatment strategies. A thorough pain history should include location, quality, intensity, temporal characteristics; aggravating and alleviating factors; impact of pain on function and quality of life, the meaning of the pain; past treatments and responses; patient fears, expectations and goals; and associated medical and psychological conditions. A history of drug use is essential and should include prescription and non-prescription medications, and herbal remedies. A pain body diagram completed by a chronic pain patient can provide information about the quality and location of the pain. Different colors can be used to identify the different qualities of pain, e.g., blue for burning, black for numbness, red for stabbing, yellow for aches.

Intensity is one of the most important parameters to be determined. Tools to assess intensity are typically one-dimensional and include visual analog, verbal descriptor, and numeric scales. The visual analog scale is a 10 cm line anchored on one end by "no pain" and at the other end by "pain as bad as it could possibly be." The patient makes a mark on the line to correspond to the level of his discomfort and the distance from the low end of the scale to the patient's mark is used as a numerical index of the patient's pain intensity. Verbal descriptor scales with such terms as mild, moderate, or severe may be useful. Some include the word excruciating. A numeric pain rating scale is appropriate in most clinical settings. The most common is an 11-point scale where 0 = no pain and 10 = worst pain imaginable. Since this is an ordinal scale, a score of 8/10 is *not* twice as severe as a score of 4/10. A numeric 6-point scale is often used for children. There is also an observational rating scale for children from 2 months to 7 years. "Faces scales" were first developed for young children; now there are variants that may be useful for the elderly; these scales have from six to eight facial expressions that depict a range of emotions. Herr and colleagues have evaluated a number of pain intensity scales for older adults [71].

Always remember that pain is a subjective experience with a different meaning to each person. The pain rating reflects the patient's interpretation of what that pain means to him/her at that moment; it is a combination of the patient's physical discomfort and emotional response to the discomfort. Changes in pain intensity are valuable when measured for single individuals (e.g., before and after a treatment), but they should not be used to compare pain between different individuals. One person's 4/10 might be another's 8/10.

What is a meaningful reduction in pain intensity? Data from clinical trials suggest that about a 30% reduction in pain intensity is meaningful from a patient's perspective, and this is true for persons with acute as well as chronic pain [72]. However, the change in pain intensity that is meaningful to patients increases as the severity of the baseline pain increases: for patients with moderate pain a 35% reduction corresponds to much improvement; a 45% reduction corresponds to very much improvement. For patients with severe pain, the percentage of pain relief must be larger to obtain meaningful degrees of relief [73].

Non-verbal patients, such as those in coma or with dementia or other cognitive impairments, must be assessed for pain by observing body language, movement, autonomic arousal, and non-verbal pain behaviors. Agitation and disturbing or aggressive behavior in non-verbal older adults may be indicative of pain, but be attributed erroneously to dementia or psychosis leading to treatment with anti-psychotics instead of analgesics. This is a matter for serious concern as half of older persons in long-term care facilities are cognitively impaired. Persistent pain due to degenerative diseases such as osteoarthritis becomes more prevalent as persons age. Not surprisingly, analgesic use is less in those with cognitive impairment and in older subjects having impaired abilities to communicate [74].

Remember that chronic pain is a multidimensional phenomenon that can adversely affect a patient's function, quality of life, emotional state, social and vocational status, and general well-being. Therefore, assessment of chronic pain should also be multidimensional. Focus groups of persons with chronic pain identified a total of 19 important aspects of daily life affected by chronic pain: sleep, sex life, employment, home care, relationships, family life, social and recreational activities, emotional well-being, fatigue, weakness, and cognitive functioning [75]: "These findings emphasize the importance of assessing the *patient* with chronic pain and not just the pain" [76].

Patients need to be reassured that their pain is being taken seriously. A respectful and professional attitude must be maintained. It is always important to believe

patients' reports of pain and distress, particularly in the case of patients with chronic non-cancer pain who may have had difficult encounters with previous healthcare professionals, who may have dismissed them as prevaricators or drug seekers: "Even if psychological issues, including addiction, are present, respectful validation of the patient's suffering is invaluable to assessment and will lead to more effective treatment planning" (MM Backonja, personal communication).

Overview of pain management

Many different strategies are employed in managing pain, but a general approach applies to the treatment of any type of pain: identify and eliminate or minimize the cause (if possible), and treat with a combination of pharmacologic and non-pharmacologic therapies. Combine drug and non-drug modalities in a balanced manner that is tailored to the type of pain and the individual.

A host of resources is available to assist with treatment decisions. The American Pain Society (APS) and other professional organizations have published more than a dozen evidence-based guidelines [28]. The APS first released *Principles of Analgesic Use in the Treatment of Acute Pain and Cancer Pain* in 1987. The 6th edition (fall 2008) provides "updated information on the clinical pharmacology of analgesics and includes a list of nearly 400 resources" [76]. The reader is also encouraged to take advantage of the excellent systematic reviews of various healthcare interventions provided by the Cochrane Collaboration [77]; these are available on their web site at no charge.

Managing acute pain

There have been major advances in the management of acute pain, in particular post-surgical pain, in the past two decades [11, 12, 78–80]. Systemic analgesics (nonopioids, opioids, and adjuvants) are the foundation of multimodal therapy for acute pain, but non-drug methods (patient education, heat/cold, massage, distraction/relaxation, others) are essential as well. Poorly controlled acute pain can result in increased catabolism, increased cardiorespiratory work, immunosuppression, and coagulation disturbances [12]. Ideal management of post-operative pain provides effective pain relief; reduces opioid-related adverse effects (opioids are often a component of treatment), and surgical stress; and decreases morbidity, mortality, and duration of hospital stay. It has been assumed that multimodal analgesia, the use of a combination of analgesics that work by different mechanisms, would improve post-operative pain control. While multimodal analgesia (use of non-steroidal anti-inflammatory drugs or acetaminophen in combination with opioid analgesics) does have an opioid-sparing effect, there are conflicting reports about whether it does or does not reduce the risk of opioid side effects [11, 81].

Programmable infusion pumps that deliver an opioid intravenously have been in use for more than 25 years; patient controlled analgesia (PCA) devices allow patients to self-deliver opioids on an as-needed basis within dosing parameters set by the physician. Patients are highly satisfied with this method of drug delivery, but unfortunately there is not clear evidence of PCA's superiority over nurse-controlled analgesia [11]. Bear in mind that acceptable nurse-controlled analgesia does *not* equate to PRN (as needed) administration of meperidine by the IM route, rigid use of standard doses, or unimodal therapy.

Epidural analgesia using local anesthetics and opioids is widely practiced as a component of multimodal therapy; it reduces cardiac, pulmonary, thromboembolic, and renal complications, and provides superior analgesia. It has been reported that epidural analgesia, regardless of analgesic agent, location of catheter placement, and type and time of pain assessment, provides better post-operative analgesia than parenteral opioids [11, 82].

The management of acute post-operative pain may also involve wound infiltration with local anesthetics, peripheral nerve blocks, and the use of adjuvants such as gabapentin and ketamine. Gabapentin reduces opioid requirements and is thought to reduce central sensitization. Many other non-pharmacologic options have been explored as adjuvants to conventional analgesics: acupuncture, music therapy, hypnosis, and transcutaneous electrical nerve stimulation [83].

A growing challenge is the difficulty of managing acute pain in patients who are being treated chronically with opioid analgesics [11, 84, 85]. They may have developed some level of tolerance to these drugs and are at risk of undertreatment and of experiencing withdrawal if they are dosed inadequately. Chronic pain patients undergoing acute surgical procedures generally report elevated pain scores compared with matched controls and consistently require two- to three-fold more opioid [84]. It is important to maintain baseline opioid therapy and to provide adequate additional analgesia peri-operatively. The addition of non-opioid therapy and the use of peripheral and central blocks may be of benefit. The magnitude of opioid tolerance in persons who have been on chronic opioid therapy is difficult to assess, especially because some who have been on high dose opioid therapy may have developed opioid hyperalgesia [11, 85].

Managing cancer pain

In 1986, the World Health Organization introduced the analgesic ladder and provided guidelines to improve the management of cancer pain worldwide [14]. Opioid analgesics are the drugs of choice for the management of the moderate to severe pain associated with cancer. Numerous other therapies are also available, and a variety of strategies have been used to disseminate the knowledge about how to treat cancer pain effectively [86, 87], and yet, as documented at the beginning of this chapter, inadequate treatment continues [17, 18]. Fears and misunderstandings about tolerance, physical dependence, and addiction continue to be barriers [88]. It is incomprehensible that persons who are dying of cancer may not be getting adequate relief of their pain [89]. Where is our sense of moral outrage?

Managing chronic non-cancer pain

Traditional approaches to the treatment of chronic non-cancer pain are based on a biomedical model: pain results from an identifiable injury or disease process. Identify and treat the underlying problem and pain will be relieved. Unfortunately, chronic pain is not likely to be caused by a single factor that can be eliminated by a single therapeutic modality. In fact, there may be no identifiable cause. In most cases of chronic non-cancer pain, multiple mechanisms are at play and the presentation is complex [90, 91]. Physical, psychological, and social factors affect pain perception and modulation, and pain behaviors. The biopsychosocial model is considered the most appropriate conceptual framework for understanding the clinical course of persistent pain and for developing effective treatment strategies [92, 93].

Complete resolution of chronic pain is rarely achieved in spite of comprehensive multidisciplinary pain management, although as stated earlier, a 30% reduction in pain intensity represents a clinically significant improvement for most persons [72]. The purpose of treatment is to relieve pain and to improve function. Functional improvement goals vary from patient to patient: return to work, live independently, enjoy friends and family. A combination of pharmacologic treatment with educational, behavioral, and physical/rehabilitative therapies provides the most successful approach for patients with chronic non-cancer pain. Physical/rehabilitative therapies may be needed to treat deconditioning and disability, behavioral/psychological treatment to enhance coping and improve mood, and medications to treat underlying mood disorders. Depression and anxiety are common in chronic pain patients and may pre-exist or complicate pain management strategies; their effective treatment may reduce, though not necessarily eliminate, the need for analgesic drugs. It is essential to identify persons with current or past substance abuse disorders or psychiatric issues and refer them to appropriate specialists, to seek a neurology consultation if active/progressive neurological disease is suspected, or a rheumatology consultation if a collagen/vascular disorder or arthritic process is thought to be the source of the pain. Surgical procedures and a variety of interventional approaches may also be critical to the management of chronic pain problems [94, 95].

Multidisciplinary pain centers have been shown to be both therapeutically efficacious and cost-effective relative to conventional medical treatment [2–4]. Yet few such pain centers exist and even if they do, many third-party payers refuse to reimburse such programs. Patients in many healthcare systems and private group practices have limited access to specialty chronic pain services.

Of course, interdisciplinary pain care also occurs in the primary care setting [96]. Several investigators have demonstrated improvements in pain intensity and pain-related function with the use of collaborative approaches [97–99]. A recent study showed that a primary care-based collaborative intervention for chronic pain was significantly more effective than "treatment as usual" and concluded that such an intervention can have positive effects on pain disability and intensity, and on depressive symptoms [100].

This brief overview does not address the multiple challenges that confront the patient with chronic non-cancer pain and the clinician who is dedicated to providing care. Issues of access and payment have been touched on briefly. The reader is strongly encouraged to examine those subjects in greater depth and to review the extensive literature that addresses the role of opioid analgesics in the management of chronic pain as well as the conflicts related to the role of interventional techniques in pain control.

It is critical to understand the basis for the uncertainty and confusion about the role of opioids in the management of chronic non-cancer pain [101]. Their use has increased dramatically in the past 10–15 years in spite of the controversies [102–106]. There is uncertainty about their long-term efficacy and safety with conflicting reports about whether opioid treatment fulfills any of the key outcome goals: pain relief, improved quality of life, and improved function [107]. Concerns have also been raised about their effects on hormonal and immune function, and about the possibility of opioid-induced hyperalgesia [108], which would significantly limit their clinical usefulness. Addiction remains a concern although it is relatively unusual if persons treated with opioids have no history of substance abuse [22]. The APS has recently released *Clinical Guidelines for the Use of Chronic Opioid Therapy in Chronic Noncancer Pain* which concludes that "opioid analgesics can be effective therapy for carefully selected and monitored patients with chronic non-cancer pain" [109].

Unfortunately, there has been a concomitant increase in misuse and abuse of these drugs [110] and in opioid-related mortality [111]. The Food and Drug Administration recently announced that it will require manufacturers of long-acting opioid formulations to develop comprehensive Risk Evaluation Mitigation Strategies [111]. Any such strategies much be crafted very carefully because they may have the unintentional effect of depriving persons with persistent non-cancer pain of a treatment that may be essential to their quality of life. One would hope that these patients would be approached in the same way as any population with a chronic disease. Unfortunately, that is often not the case, and in many instances concerns about the risks of treatment outweigh consideration of the benefits to the patient's quality of life. A prominent advocate with an interest in the ethics of pain has written "that the message that has been sent and clearly received by physicians is that their primary responsibility is to help regulators prevent drug diversion and the excessive prescribing of opioid analgesics, not to effectively manage the pain of their patients" [112].

Pain medicine like many aspects of healthcare is fragmented by competing disciplines. This conflict is illustrated by the difference between the philosophies for treating chronic pain espoused by multidisciplinary pain centers and primary care collaborations and the discipline of medicine referred to as interventional pain management. According to the American Society of Interventionalist Pain Physicians: "An interventionalist perceives comprehensive treatment programs as programs with interventional techniques as the primary treatment modality, with physical therapy, medical therapy, and psychological management, as supplementary" [113]. In contrast, the interdisciplinary approach based on the biopsychosocial model is one in which the patient receives comprehensive rehabilitation that includes multiple therapies provided in a coordinated manner and involves healthcare providers from several disciplines, each of whom specializes in different features of the pain experience [90–93]. Invasive procedures may be useful to relieve painful syndromes to enable functional restoration, but they are used conservatively, not as the core approach to managing chronic pain. This conflict involves significant access and reimbursement issues, which are beyond the scope of this chapter.

Conclusion and conundrums

Pain management advocates had much to celebrate at the beginning of this new century. There was greater awareness of the adverse physiological and psychological consequences of poor pain management and the need for more effective pain control. There were new drugs and new delivery systems, numerous professional and advocacy organizations, and standards from the Joint Commission that meant that accredited facilities could no longer ignore pain. There was increased attention to pain at the end of life, although it was not until 2006 that palliative care was recognized as a subspecialty by the American Board of Medical Specialties. The American Cancer Society made quality of life a major goal of its programs. The Veterans Administration committed to better pain control; there was evidence that opiophobia [114] was on the wane with the resultant greater use of opioid analgesics for control of chronic pain and the general feeling that pain management was improving.

If there was some sense of euphoria a decade ago, it had a very short half-life and was quickly replaced by the somber reality that there were significant risks associated with attempts to introduce changes into the healthcare system, especially when those changes were directed at improving pain management practices. Misunderstandings and controversies emerged related to the treatment of both acute and chronic pain especially when it involved the use of opioid analgesics. Some revolved around the Joint Commission standards. As stated above, others relate to the continuing conundrum about the role of opioid analgesics in the management of chronic non-cancer pain and conflicts about appropriate treatment strategies for chronic pain.

"In our noble efforts to alleviate pain, has safety been compromised?" This provocative question appeared in a 2002 Medication Safety Alert from the Institute for Safe Medication Practices [115] and highlighted the increase in opioid-related sentinel events that occurred after introduction of pain assessment and management standards by the Joint Commission [116]. The standards were intended to provide a framework to guide efforts to make pain management an essential and integral part of patient care. They were met with enthusiasm by patient management advocates because they addressed seemingly intractable barriers in the healthcare system: the failure to assess pain, to hold anyone accountable for poor pain control, to ensure that pain is addressed with patients' transition from one care setting to another, and to provide culturally sensitive information to patients and families. Unfortunately, some misunderstood the intent of the standards and erroneously concluded that they would be forced to prescribe opioids even if they were not appropriate, and that patients would demand to be free of pain. The standards did (and still do) recognize the right of patients to appropriate assessment and management of their pain, but never the right to be free of pain [32, 33].

The introduction of the now familiar "pain as a fifth vital sign" campaign added to the confusion. The VA adopted this slogan as a banner for its quality improvement efforts [31]. The APS embraced this concept as well. It was never intended to make pain intensity a fifth vital sign, but to heighten awareness of the need to assess and record a pain intensity score in a prominent place (which could be the vital signs section of a patient's chart) so as to alert clinicians to the presence of pain and to elicit a clinical response if one was warranted. Unfortunately, some clinicians took this slogan literally and focused on reducing pain scores below an arbitrarily chosen value. Treatment decisions should never be based solely on a number on a 0–10 scale or on one mode of therapy (an opioid) [12, 79, 80]. The anger and frustration were clear from the titles of articles in the anesthesia and surgery literature: "New JCAHO pain standards bigger threat to patient safety than envisioned" [117]; "Has the pendulum swung too far in post-operative pain control?"[118]. Reason has returned to the dialog with a focus on the real uncertainties about the management of post-operative pain [11], but the experience illustrates the care that must be taken when a dramatic change is mandated. It highlights one of the primary reasons for "unfavorable outcomes in the arena of pain management: a lack of education among physicians regarding pain management principles and analgesic pharmacology" [119].

The Institute of Medicine's report "Crossing the Quality Chasm: A New Health System for the 21st Century" highlighted the disturbing absence of real progress toward restructuring healthcare systems to address both quality and cost concerns [120]. The authors wrote that there is not just a gap, but a chasm between the healthcare we have and the care we could have. There is no question that such a chasm exists in pain care. It has been asserted that "pain management presents the most glaring example of a disparity between the current state of medical knowledge and the prevailing custom of medical practice" [121]. "More systematic approaches are needed to analyze and synthesize medical evidence for both clinicians and patients. Far more sophisticated clinical decision support systems will be required to assist clinicians and patients in selecting the best treatment options and delivering safe and effective care" [121]. These words from the Institute of Medicine report provide a charge to all of us who are dedicated to improving the quality of pain care in this nation.

References

1. Woolf CJ. Pain: moving from symptom control toward mechanism-specific pharmacologic management. *Ann Intern Med* 2004; **140**: 441–51.

2. Turk DC. Clinical effectiveness and cost-effectiveness of treatments for patients with chronic pain. *Clin J Pain* 2002; **18**: 355–65.

3. Berger A, Dukes EM, Oxter G. Clinical characteristics and economic costs of patients with painful neuropathic disorders. *J Pain* 2004; **5**: 143–9.

4. Gatchel RJ, Okifuji A. Evidence-based scientific data documenting the treatment and cost-effectiveness of comprehensive pain programs for chronic nonmalignant pain. *J Pain* 2006; **7**: 779–93.

5. Stewart WF, Ricci JA, Chee E, Morganstein D, Lipton R. Lost productive time and cost due to common pain conditions in the US workforce. *JAMA* 2003; **290**: 2443–54.

6. Bradshaw DH, Nakamura Y, Chapman CR. National Institute of Health grant awards for pain, nausea and dyspnea research: An assessment of funding patterns in 2003. *J Pain* 2005; **6**; 277–93.

7. Bradshaw DH, Empy C, Davis P, *et al.* Trends in funding for research on pain: A report on the national Institutes of Health grant awards over the years 2003–2007. *J Pain* 2008; **9**: 1077–87.

8. The Patient Protection and Affordable Care Act (P.L. 111–148) http://dpc.senate.gov/dpcdoc-sen_health_care_bill.cfm

9. Meldrum ML. A capsule history of pain management. *JAMA* 2003; **290**: 2470–5.

10. Woolf CJ, Salter MW. Neuronal plasticity: Increasing gain in pain. *Science* 2000; **288**: 1765–8.

11. Rathmell JP, Wu CL, Sinatra RS, *et al.* Acute post-surgical pain management: A critical appraisal of current practice. *Reg Anesth Pain Med* 2006; **31**: 1–42.

12. Pyati S, Gan TJ. Perioperative pain management. *CNS Drugs* 2007; **21**: 185–211.

13. Apfelbaum JL, Chen C, Mehta SS, Gan TJ. Postoperative pain experience: Results from a national survey suggest postoperative pain continues to be undermanaged. *Anesth Analg* 2003; **97**: 534–40.

14. Breura E, Kim HN. Cancer pain. *JAMA* 2003; **290**: 2476–81.

15. American Cancer Society. Cancer Facts & Figures 2009. Atlanta: American Cancer Society; 2009.

16. Deandrea S, Montanari M, Moja, Apolone G. Prevalence of undertreatment in cancer pain. A review of the published literature. *Ann Oncol* 2008; **19**: 1985–91.

17. Van den Beuken-van Everdingen MHJ, de Rijke JM, Kessels AG, *et al.* Prevalence of pain in patients with cancer: A systematic review of the past 40 years. *Ann Oncol* 2007; **18**: 1437–49.

18. Reid CM, Forbes K. Pain in patients with cancer: Still a long way to go. *Pain* 2007; **132**: 229–30.

19. Burton AW, Fanciullo GJ, Beasley RD, Fisch MJ. Chronic pain in the cancer survivor: A new frontier. *Pain Med* 2007; **8**: 189–98.

20. Simoni-Wastila L. Increases in opioid medication use: Balancing the good with the bad. *Pain* 2008; **38**: 245–6.

21. Ballantyne JL, LaForge KS. Opioid dependence and addiction during opioid treatment of chronic pain. *Pain* 2007; **129**: 235–55.

22. Fields HL. Should we be reluctant to prescribe opioids for chronic non-malignant pain? *Pain* 2007; **129**: 233–4.

23. Clark JD. Chronic pain prevalence and analgesic prescribing in a general population. *J Pain Symp Manage* 2002; **23**: 131–7.

24. National Center for Health Statistics. Chartbook on Trends in the Health of Americans. 2006. http://www.cdc.gov/nchs/data/hus/hus06.pdf

25. Krueger AB, Stone AA. Assessment of pain: a community-based diary survey in the United States. *Lancet* 2008; **371**: 1519–25.

26. Poleshuck EL, Green CR. Socioeconomic disadvantage and pain. *Pain* 2008; **136**: 235–8.

27. Loeser JD. The decade of pain control and research. *APS Bulletin* 2003;**13**:1, 4–5, 8–10.

28. A resource for evidence-based clinical practice guidelines. National Guideline Clearinghouse. www.guideline.gov

29. American Academy of Pain Medicine. The use of opioids for the treatment of chronic pain: a consensus statement from the American Academy of Pain Medicine and the American Pain Society. *Clin J Pain* 1997; **13**: 6–8.

30. Federation of Medical Boards of the United States. Model Guidelines for the use of controlled substances for the treatment of pain. May 1999.

31. 1999 Veterans Health Administration Memorandum: Pain as the Fifth Vital Sign March 1, 1999.

32. Phillips DM. JCAHO pain management standards are unveiled. Joint Commission on Accreditation of Healthcare Organizations. *JAMA* 2000; **284**: 428–9.

33. Dahl JL, Gordon DB. The JCAHO pain standards: a progress report. *APS Bulletin* 2002; **12**: 1, 11–2.

34. http://www.jointcommission.org/AccreditationPrograms/Hospitals/Standards

35. http://www.jointcommission.org/Standards/FieldReviews/

36. The Nursing Home Quality Initiative web site provides consumer and provider information regarding the quality of care in nursing homes. www.cms.hhs.gov/NursingHomeQualityInits/ [accessed June 2010].

37. www.cms.hhs.gov/CertificationandComplianc/Downloads/2008NHActionPlan.pdf

38. Dickinson KC, Sharma R, Duckart JP, *et al.* VA healthcare costs of a collaborative intervention for chronic pain in primary care. *Med Care* 2010; **48**: 38–44.

39. Stepped Care to Optimize Pain Care Effectiveness. www.clinicaltrialssearch.org/stepped-care-to-optimize-pain-care-effectiveness-nct00926588.html

40. Gilson AM, Joranson DE, Mauer MA, Ryan KM, Garthwaite JP. Progress to achieve balanced state policy relevant to pain management and palliative care: 2000–2003. *J Pain Palliat Care Pharmacother* 2003; **19**: 13–26.

41. Federation of State Medical Boards of the United States, Inc. Model Policy for the use of controlled substances for the treatment of pain. www.fsmb.org/pdf/2004_grpol_Controlled_Substances.pdf

42. Johnson SH. Legal and ethical perspectives on pain management. *Anesth Analg* 2007; **105**: 5–7.

43. Breuer B, Cruciani R, Portenoy RK. Pain management by primary care physician, pain physician, chiropractors and acupuncturists: A national survay. *Southern Medical Journal* 2010; **103**: 738–47.

44. Gordon DB, Dahl JL, Miaskowski C, *et al.* American Pain Society recommendations for improving the quality of acute and cancer pain management. American Pain Society Quality of Care Task Force. *Arch Intern Med* 2005; **165**: 1574–80.

45. International Association for the Study of Pain Subcommittee on Taxonomy. *Pain* 1979; **6**: 249.

46. Mersky H, Bogduk N, eds. *Classification of Pain*, 2nd edn. (Seattle: IASP Press, 1994).

47. Julius D, Basbaum AI. Molecular mechanisms of nociception. *Nature* 2001; **413**: 203–10.

48. Willis WD. The somatosensory system, with emphasis on structures important for pain. *Brain Res Rev* 2007; **55**: 297–313.

49. Ladabaum U, Minoshima S, Owyang C. Pathobiology of visceral pain: molecular mechanisms and therapeutic implications. V. Central nervous system processing of somatic and visceral sensory signals. *Am J Physiol Gastrointest Liver Physiol* 2000; **279**: G1–G6.

50. Pasero C, Paice JA, McCaffery M. Basic mechanisms underlying the causes and effects of pain. In *Pain: Clinical Manual*, M McCaffery and C Pasero, eds. (Philadelphia: Mosby, 1999), p. 17.

51. Kim H, Clark D, Dionne RA. Genetic contributions to clinical pain and analgesia: avoiding pitfalls in genetic research. *J Pain* 2009; **10**: 663–9.

52. Zeller JL, Burke AE, Glass RM. Acute pain treatment *JAMA* 2008; **299**: 128.

53. Sullivan M, Ferrell B. Ethical challenges in the management of chronic nonmalignant pain: negotiating through the cloud of doubt. *J Pain* 2005; **6**: 2–9.

54. American Geriatrics Society Panel on Persistent Pain in Older Person. The management of persistent pain in older persons. *J Am Ger Soc* 2002; **50**: S205–S224.

55. Porteny RK, Hagan NA Breakthrough pain: Definition, prevalence and characteristics. *Pain* 1999; **41**: 273–81.

56. Mercadente S, Arcuri E. Breakthrough pain in cancer patients. *Pain Clinical Updates* 2006; **XIV**: 1–4.

57. Swendsen KB, Andersen S, Arnason S, *et al.* Breakthrough pain in malignant and non-malignant diseases: a review of prevalence, characteristics and mechanisms. *Eur J Pain* 2005: **9**: 195–206.

58. Markman JD. Not so fast: The reformulation of fentanyl and breakthrough chronic non-cancer pain. *Pain* 2008: **136**: 227–9.

59. Yarnitsky D, Crispel Y, Eisenberg E, *et al.* Prediction of chronic post-operative pain: Pre-operative DNIC testing identifies patients at risk. *Pain* 2008; **138**: 22–8.

60. Backonja MM, Krause SJ. Neuropathic pain questionnaire-short form. 2003.

61. Dworkin RH, O'Connor AB, Backonja M, *et al.* Pharmacologic management of neuropathic pain: Evidence-based recommendations. *Pain* 2007; **132**: 237–51.

62. Cherny NI. The treatment of neuropathic pain: From hubris to humility. *Pain* 2007: **132**: 225–6.

63. Cousins M. Pain relief as a human right. *Pain Clinical Updates* 2004; **XII**; 1–4.

64. Brennan F, Carr DB, Cousins M. Pain management: A fundamental human right. *Anesth Analg* 2007; **105**: 205–11.

65. Sampathkumar P, Drage LA, Martin DP. Herpes zoster (shingles) and postherpetic neuralgia. *Mayo Clin Proc* 2009; **84**: 274–80.

66. Tracey I. Nociceptive processing in the human brain. *Curr Opin Neurobiol* 2005; **15**: 478–87.

67. Moisset X, Bouhassira D. Brain imaging of neuropathic pain. *Neuroimage* 2007; **37**: S80–S88.

68. Apkarian AV, Sosa Y, Sonty S, *et al.* Chronic back pain is associated with decreased prefrontal and thalamic gray matter density. *J Neurosci* 2004; **24**: 10410–15.

69. May A. Chronic pain may change the structure of the brain. *Pain* 2008; **137**: 7–15.

70. Turk DC, Okifugi A. Pain assessment. *Lancet* 1999; **353**: 1784–8.

71. Bjoro K, Herr K. Assessment of pain in the nonverbal or cognitively impaired older adult. *Clinics in Geriatric Medicine* 2008; **24**: 237–62.

72. Farrar JT, Young Jr JP, LaMoreaux L, Werth PL, Poole RM. Clinical importance of changes in chronic pain intensity measured on an 11-point numerical pain rating scale. *Pain* 2001; **94**: 149–58.

73. Cepeda MS, Africano JM, Rodolfo P, Ramiro A, Carr DB, What decline in pain intensity is meaningful to patients with acute pain? *Pain* 2003; **105**: 151–7.

74. Mantyselka P. Balancing act with geriatric pain treatment. *Pain* 2008; **138**: 1–2.

75. Turk DC, Dworkin RH, Revicki D, *et al.* Identifying important outcome domains for chronic pain clinical trials: An IMMPACT survey of people with pain. *Pain* 2008; **137**: 276–85.

76. American Pain Society. *Principles of Analgesic Use in the Treatment of Acute Pain and Cancer Pain.* 6th edn. 2008.

77. The Cochrane Collaboration. Working together to promote the best evidence for health care. www.cochrane.org/cochrane-reviews [accessed June 2010].

78. Carr DB, Goudas LC . Acute pain. *Lancet* 1999; **353**: 2051–8.

79. American Society of Anesthesiologists Task Force on Acute Pain Management. Practice guidelines for acute pain management in the perioperative setting: an updated report by the American Society of Anesthesiologists Task Force on Acute Pain Management. *Anesthesiology* 2004; **100**: 1573–81.

80. Institute for Clinical Systems Improvement. Health Care Guideline: Assessment and Management of Acute Pain. Sixth Edition, March 2008. www.icsi.org/pain_acute/pain__acute__assessment_and_management_of__3.html

81. Buvanendran A, Kroin JS, Tuman KJ, *et al.* Effects of perioperative administration of a selective cycloxygenase 2 inhibitor on pain management and recovery of function after knee replacement. *JAMA* 2003; **290**: 2411–8.

82. Block BM, Liu SS, Rowlingson AJ, *et al.* Efficacy of postoperative epidural analgesia: A meta-analysis. *JAMA* 2003; **290**: 2455–63.

83. McQuay HJ, Poon KH, Derry S, Moore RA. Acute pain: Combination treatments and how we measure their efficacy. *Br J Anaesth* 2008; **101**: 69–76.

84. Mitra S, Sintra RS. Perioperative management of acute pain in the opioid-dependent patient. *Anesthesiology* 2004; **101**: 212–27.

85. Mehta V, Langford RM. Acute pain management for opioid dependent patients. *Anesthesia* 2006; **61**: 269–76.

86. Cancer Pain Management Guideline Panel (Miaskowski C, Cleary J, Co-Chairs). Guideline for the Management of Cancer Pain in Adults and Children. American Pain Society. 2004.

87. Dy SM, Asch SM, Nacim A, *et al.* Evidence-based standards for cancer pain management. *J Clin Oncol* 2008; **26**: 3879–85.

88. Gunnarsdottir S, Donovan HS, Serlin RC, Voge C, Ward S. Patient-related barriers to pain management: the Barriers Questionnaire II (BQ-II). *Pain* 2002; **99**: 385–96.

89. Institute of Medicine and National Research Council. *Improving Palliative Care for Cancer* (Washington, DC: National Academy Press, 2001).

90. Ashburn MA, Staats PS. Management of chronic pain. *Lancet* 1999; **353**: 1865–9.

91. Gallagher RM. Rational integration of pharmacologic, behavioral and rehabilitation strategies in the treatment of chronic pain. *Am J Phys Med Rehab* 2005; **84**: S64–S76.

92. Borrell-Carrio F, Suchman AL, Epstein RM. The biopsychosocial model 25 years later: principles, practice, and scientific inquiry. *Ann Fam Med* 2004; **2**: 576–82.

93. Lakhan S. The biopsychosocial model of health and illness. [Connexions web site]August 3, 2006. http://cnx.org/content/m13589/1.2/

94. Boyajian SS. Interventional pain management: an overview for primary care physicians. *JAOA* 2005; **4**: 1–6.

95. Manchikanti L, Singh V, Pampati V, *et al*. Interventional techniques in the management of chronic pain: part 2.0. *Pain Physician* 2001; **4**: 24–96.

96. Jackman RP, Purvis JM, Mallett B. Chronic nonmalignant pain in primary care. *Am Fam Physician* 2008; **78**: 1155–62.

97. Bodenheimer T, Wagner EH, Grumbach K. Improving primary care for patients with chronic illness: The chronic care model. Part 2. *JAMA* 2002; **288**: 1909–14.

98. Ahles TA, Wasson JH, Seville JL, *et al*. A controlled trial of methods for managing pain in primary care patients with or without co-occurring psychosocial problems. *Ann Fam Med* 2006; **4**: 341–50.

99. Chelminski PR, Ives TJ, Felix KM, *et al*. A primary care, multi-disciplinary disease management program for opioid-treated patients with chronic non-cancer pain and a high burden of psychiatric comorbidity. *BMC Health Serv Res* 2005; **5**: 3.

100. Dobscha SK, Corson K, Perrin NA, *et al*. Collaborative care for chronic pain in primary care. *JAMA* 2009; **301**: 1242–52.

101. Rosenblum A, Marsch LA, Joseph H, Portenoy RK. Opioids and the treatment of chronic pain: controversies, current status, and future directions. *Exp Clin Psychopharmacol* 2008; **16**: 405–16.

102. Noble M, Tregear SJ, Treadwell JR, Schoelles K. Long-term opioid therapy for chronic noncancer pain: A systematic review and meta-analysis of efficacy and safety. *Journal of Pain and Symptom Management* 2008; **35**: 214–28.

103. Edlund MJ. Steffick D, Hudson T, Harris KM, Sullivan M. Risk factors for clinically recognized opioid abuse and dependence among veterans using opioids for chronic non-cancer pain. *Pain* 2007; **129**: 514–9.

104. Portenoy RK, Farrar JT, Backonja M-M, *et al*. Long-term use of controlled-release oxycodone for noncancer pain: Results of a 3-year registry study. *Clin J Pain* 2007; **23**: 287–99.

105. Pletcher MJ, Kertesz SG, Sidney S, Kiefe CI, Hulley SB. Incidence and antecedents of nonmedical prescription opioid use in four US communities. The Coronary Artery Risk Development in Young Adults (CARDIA) prospective cohort study. *Drug Alcohol Depend* 2006; **85**: 171–6.

106. Fleming MF, Balousek SL, Klessig CL, Mundt MP. Substance use disorders in a primary care sample receiving daily opioid therapy. *J Pain* 2007; **8**: 573–82.

107. Eriksen J, Sjogren P, Bruera E, Ekholm O, Rasmussen NK. Critical issues on opioids in chronic non-cancer pain: An epidemiological study. *Pain* 2006; **125**: 172–9.

108. Ballantyne JC, Mao J. Opioid therapy for chronic pain. *N Engl J Med* 2003; **349**: 1943–53.

109. Chou R, Fanciullo GJ, Fine PG, *et al*. Clinical guidelines for the use of chronic opioid therapy in chronic noncancer pain. *J Pain* 2009; **10**: 113–30.

110. Kuehn BM. Opioid prescriptions soar: Increase in legitimate use as well as abuse. *JAMA* 2007; **297**: 249–51.

111. Kuehn BM. Efforts aim to curb opioid deaths, injuries. *JAMA* 2009; **301**: 1213–1215.

112. Rich BA. Ethics of opioid analgesia for chronic noncancer pain. *Pain Clinical Updates*. 2007; **XV**: 1–4.

113. Trescot AM, Boswell MV, Atluri SL, *et al*. Opioid guidelines in the management of chronic non-cancer pain. *Pain Physician* 2006; **9**: 1–40.

114. Morgan JP. American opiophobia: customary underutilization of opioid analgesics. In *Advances in Pain Research and Therapy, Drug Treatment of Cancer Pain in a Drug-Oriented Society*, CS Hill, Jr. and WS Fields, eds. (New York, Raven Press, 1989), pp. 181–9.

115. Smetzer JL. Cohen MR. Pain scales don't weigh every risk. *J Pharmaceut Care Pain Symptom Control* 2003; **17**: 67–70.

116. The Joint Commission. Helping health care organizations help patients. www.jointcommission.org/ [accessed June 2010].

117. Vila H, Downs JB . New JCAHO pain standards bigger threat to patient safety than envisioned. *Anesth Analg* 2006; **102**: 1596–7.

118. Taylor S, Voytovich AE, Kozol RA. Has the pendulum swung too far in postoperative pain control? *Am J Surg* 2003; **186**: 472–5.

119. Rosseau P. Pain as the fifth vital sign. *Arch Surg* 2008: **143**: 98.

120. Richardson W, Berwick D, Bisgard J. *Crossing the Quality Chasm. A New Health System for the 21st Century*. Institute of Medicine, (Washington, DC, 2001).

121. Rich BA. An ethical analysis of the barriers to effective pain management. *Camb Q Healthc Ethics* 2000; **9**: 54–70.

3 The biopsychosocial model of pain and pain management

Dennis C. Turk, Hilary Wilson and Kimberly S. Swanson

Pain is a part of existence; it is used as a means of torture, as a rite of passage, and is a source of inspiration for artists. The human experience of pain is personal, influenced by cultural norms, individual history, as well as genetics and neurophysiology. Accordingly, treatments aimed at alleviating pain are influenced by societal and political views and the accepted theoretical understanding of pain processing and experience.

The theoretical view of pain has changed dramatically over the past century although vestiges of early thinking remain. The traditional biomedical model of medicine viewed pain as a dichotomy: it was either of physiological origin (somatogenic) or due to psychological issues (psychogenic). Thus, pain severity that was not linearly related to the amount of pathological abnormality was considered "all in the patients head" or psychogenic. The current view of pain experience is multidimensional and dynamic rather than linear. Psychological, social, cognitive, physiological, and behavioral factors are hypothesized to interact and result in individual pain experience [1–3].

Despite radical changes in the theoretical concept of pain, advances in knowledge of the physical mechanisms, development of sophisticated diagnostic procedures, and development of innovative treatments, there is currently no treatment available that consistently and permanently alleviates pain for all those afflicted. Our intention in this chapter is to examine how a biopsychosocial framework integrating psychological, social, and physical factors can be applied in a treatment setting to improve the quality of life of people with chronic pain. After a brief description of the biopsychosocial perspective, we will review research focusing specifically on the role of psychological, behavioral, and social factors in pain, and we will discuss the implications of these contributors for treatment and rehabilitation.

The biopsychosocial perspective: a basic description

The distinction between "disease" and "illness" is crucial to understanding chronic pain. Disease is generally characterized by an "objective biological event" that involves disruption of specific body structures or organ systems caused by pathological, anatomical, or physiological changes. In contrast to this customary view of physical disease, illness can be conceptualized as a "subjective experience or self-attribution" that a disease is present; it yields physical discomfort, emotional distress, behavioral limitations, and psychosocial disruption. In other words, illness refers to how the sick person and members of his or her family and wider social network receive, live with, and respond to symptoms and disability.

The distinction between disease and illness is analogous to the distinction between "pain" and "nociception." Nociception entails stimulation of nerves that convey information *about* tissue damage to the brain. Pain is a subjective perception that results from the transduction, transmission, and modulation of sensory input filtered through a person's genetic composition, prior learning history, and modulated further by their current physiological status, idiosyncratic appraisals, expectations, current mood state, and sociocultural environment [4]. In contrast to the biomedical model's emphasis on disease, the biopsychosocial model focuses on illness, the result of a complex interaction of biological, psychological, and social variables. From this perspective, diversity in illness expression (which includes its severity, duration, and consequences for the individual) is accounted for by the interrelationships among biological changes, psychological status, and the social and cultural contexts; all of these variables shape the person's perception and response to illness.

Behavioral and Psychopharmacologic Pain Management, ed. Michael H. Ebert and Robert D. Kerns. Published by Cambridge University Press. © Cambridge University Press 2011.

The biopsychosocial way of thinking about the differing responses of people to symptoms and the presence of chronic conditions are based on an understanding of the dynamic nature of these conditions. That is, by definition, chronic syndromes extend over time. Therefore these conditions need to be viewed longitudinally as ongoing, multifactorial processes in which there is a dynamic and reciprocal interplay among biological, psychological, and social factors that shapes the experience and responses of patients. Biological factors may initiate, maintain, and modulate physical perturbations; while psychological variables influence appraisals and perception of internal physiological signs; and social factors shape patients' behavioral responses to the perceptions of their physical perturbations.

Conversely, psychological factors may influence biology by affecting hormone production [5], brain structure and processes [6, 7], and the autonomic nervous system [8, 9]. Behavioral responses may also affect biological contributors, as when a person avoids engaging in certain activities in order to reduce his or her symptoms. Although avoidance may initially reduce symptoms, in the long run it will lead to further physical deconditioning, which can exacerbate nociceptive stimulation.

The picture is not complete unless we consider the direct effects of disease factors and treatment upon cognitive and behavioral factors. Biological influences and medications (e.g., steroids, opioids) may affect the ability to concentrate, cause fatigue, and modulate peoples' interpretation of their state as well as of their ability to engage in certain activities.

At different points during the evolution of a disease or impairment, the relative weighting of physical, psychological, and social factors may vary. For example, during the acute phase of a disease biological factors may predominate, but over time psychological and social factors may assume a disproportionate role in accounting for symptoms and disability. Moreover, there is considerable discrepancy in behavioral and psychological manifestations of dysfunction, both across persons with comparable symptoms and within the same person over time [10].

To understand the diverse responses of people to chronic conditions, it is essential that biological, psychological, and social factors all be considered. Moreover, a longitudinal perspective is essential. A cross-sectional approach will only permit consideration of these factors at a specific point in time, and

chronic conditions continually evolve. What is observed at any one point in time is a person's adaptation to interacting biological, personal, and environmental factors. However, people have prior learning histories that serve as filters through which pathology and symptoms will be appraised, the ways in which they are responded to, and subsequent adaptation. In sum, the hallmarks of the biopsychosocial perspective are (1) integrated action, (2) reciprocal determinism, and (3) development and evolution. No single factor in isolation – pathophysiological, psychological, or social – will adequately explain chronic pain status. This can be contrasted with the traditional biomedical model, whose emphasis on the somatogenic-psychogenic dichotomy is too narrow in scope to accommodate the complexity of chronic pain. It is not that the traditional model is wrong, rather it is inadequate and incomplete.

Support for the importance of non-physiological factors

The history of medicine is replete with descriptions of interventions believed to be appropriate for alleviating pain, many of which are now known to have little therapeutic merit and some of which may actually have been harmful to patients [3]. Prior to the second half of the nineteenth century and the advent of research on sensory physiology, much of the pain treatment arsenal consisted of interventions that had no direct mode of action upon organic mechanisms associated with the source of the pain: descriptions of the treatments of Charles II of England and George Washington provide particularly dramatic illustrations [11, 12]. Despite the absence of an adequate physiological basis, these treatments proved to have some therapeutic merit, at least for some patients. The effects were despairingly referred to as "placebo effects" or "psychological cures," with the implicit message being that alleviated symptoms must be psychological (i.e., imaginary) [13].

Although some of many sophisticated treatment regimens are based on specific knowledge of physiology, the mode of action may be unrelated to modification of physiological processes [14]. For example, in a study of headache patients treated with pharmacological preparations, Fitzpatrick et al. [15] concluded that although a large number of patients benefited from drug treatment, most improvements appeared to be unrelated to the pharmacological action per se.

Similarly, although biofeedback is beneficial for several disorders (e.g., headache, back pain) the actual effects of biofeedback may be unrelated to modification of physiological activity [16, 17].

Deyo *et al.* [18] studied patients who had experienced intractable low back pain for a mean duration of over 4 years. Given the long duration of symptoms, few improvements would be expected in the absence of an efficacious treatment. However, following treatment with transcutaneous electrical nerve stimulation (TENS) and/or exercise, patients experienced statistically significant and substantial improvements in overall functioning, physical functioning, and pain severity. Remarkably, however, the same results were produced with *sham* TENS, suggesting that the treatment effects were not related to the physiological mechanism on which treatment was based. There is also a history of sham surgery producing dramatic beneficial effects [19, 20].

Some pain syndromes seem responsive to almost any treatment. For example, in reviewing the treatments for fibromyalgia, Turk [21] noted that there were published studies reporting on the efficacy of more than 35 pharmacological treatments ranging from non-steroidal anti-inflammatory agents to antidepressants along with more than 29 non-phamacological treatments as varied as musically fluctuating muscle vibration, whole body cryotherapy, exercise, and stress management, and the diversity and numbers continue to grow. The curious observation is that such diverse treatments produced roughly the same benefits, namely, 30–35% reported up to 50% reduction in some symptoms. These treatments were all given in combination with reassurances, explanation for self-management, and a "general attitude of sympathetic understanding."

The placebo effect has been well documented, and modern day imaging techniques provide insight into the higher-order mechanisms involved in placebo-induced analgesia. Craggs and colleagues provide evidence that a network of brain regions involved in cognitive and affective pain processing, including the anterior cingulate cortex and the dorsolateral prefrontal cortex, are activated in patients experiencing placebo analgesia [22].

The common factors for the diverse set of successful treatments appear to be non-specific features. Should this, along with physiological evidence of central affective and cognitive mechanisms in placebo analgesia be taken as an indication that fibromyalgia is psychological having no physical basis? Absolutely not: rather, it highlights the important role of non-physiological factors in the maintenance of these symptoms and responses to treatment. A more in-depth discussion of specific non-physiological factors that are addressed in the biopsychosocial model of pain is given below.

Sociocultural factors

Common sense beliefs about illness and healthcare providers are based both on prior experience and on social and cultural transmission of beliefs and expectations. Ethnic group membership influences how one perceives, labels, responds to, and communicates various symptoms, as well as from whom one elects to obtain care when it is sought, and the types of treatments received [23]. Several authors have specifically noted the importance of sociocultural factors [24, 25], and sex differences [26] in beliefs about and responses to pain. Social factors influence how families and local groups respond to and interact with patients (see discussion of operant conditioning below). Furthermore, ethnic expectations and sex and age stereotypes may influence the practitioner–patient relationship [26–28].

Social learning mechanisms

The role of social learning has received some attention in the development and maintenance of chronic pain states. From this perspective, pain behaviors (i.e., overt expressions of pain, distress, and suffering) may be acquired through observational learning and modeling processes. That is, people can learn responses that were not previously in their behavioral repertoire by observing others who respond in these ways [29].

Children acquire attitudes about health and healthcare, perceptions and interpretations of symptoms, and appropriate responses to injury and disease from their parents, cultural stereotypes, and the social environment [30, 31]. Based on their experiences, children develop strategies to help them avoid pain and learn "appropriate" (expected) ways to react. Children are exposed to many minor injuries daily [32]. How adults address these experiences provides ample learning opportunities. Children's learning influences whether they will ignore, how they will respond, or over-respond to symptoms. The observation of others in pain is an event that captivates attention as witness the arts and media.

There is a large amount of experimental evidence of the role of social learning from controlled studies in the laboratory [33, 34] and observations of patients' behavior in clinical settings [35]. For example, Vaughan and Lanzetta demonstrated that physiological responses to pain stimuli may be conditioned simply by observation of others in pain [36, 37]. Richard found that children whose parents had chronic pain chose more pain-related responses to scenarios presented to them and were more external in their health locus of control than were children with healthy or diabetic parents [38]. Moreover, teachers rated the pain patients' children as displaying more illness behaviors (e.g., complaining, days absent, visits to school nurse) than children of healthy controls.

Operant learning mechanisms

Early in the twentieth century, Collie discussed the effects of environmental factors in shaping the experience of people suffering with pain [39]. However, a new era in thinking about pain was initiated with Fordyce's description of the role of operant factors in chronic pain [40]. The operant approach stands in marked contrast to the disease model of pain described earlier.

In the operant formulation, behavioral manifestations of pain rather than pain per se are central. When a person is exposed to a stimulus that causes tissue damage, their immediate response is withdrawal or an attempt to escape from the noxious sensations. Their behaviors are observable, and consequently are subject to the principles of learning.

The operant view proposes that through external contingencies of reinforcement, acute pain behaviors, such as limping to protect a wounded limb from producing additional nociceptive input can evolve into chronic pain problems. Pain behaviors may be positively reinforced directly, for example, by attention from a spouse or healthcare provider. They may also be maintained by negative reinforcement through the escape from noxious stimulation by using drugs, resting, or avoiding undesirable activities such as work or exercise.

In addition, "well behaviors" (e.g., activity, working, exercising) may not be sufficiently reinforced. This allows more rewarding pain behaviors to be maintained. Pain behaviors originally elicited by organic factors may respond to reinforcement from environmental events. Because of this, Fordyce proposed that pain behaviors might persist long after the initial cause of the pain is resolved or greatly reduced [40]. The operant conditioning model does not concern itself with the initial cause of pain. Rather, it considers pain an internal subjective experience that may be maintained even after its initial physical basis is resolved.

Several studies have provided evidence that supports the underlying assumptions of the operant conditioning model [41, 42]. Interestingly, Block et al. demonstrated that pain patients reported differential levels of pain in an experimental situation, depending upon whether they knew they were being observed by their spouses or by ward clerks [43]. Pain patients with non-solicitous spouses reported more pain when neutral observers were present than when the spouses were present, and patients with solicitous spouses reported more pain when their spouses were present than when neutral-observers were present. On the other hand, patients with solicitous spouses reported more pain when their spouses were present than when observed in the presence of more neutral ward clerks.

Romano et al. videotaped patients and their spouse engaged in a series of cooperative household activities, and recorded patients' pain behaviors and spouses' responses [44]. Sequential analyses revealed that spouses' solicitous behaviors were more likely to precede and follow pain behaviors in pain patients than in healthy controls. Several additional studies observed that chronic pain patients reported more intense pain and less activity when they indicated that their spouses were solicitous [42, 45, 46]. Taken together, these studies suggest that spouses can serve as important discriminative stimuli for the display of pain behaviors, including their reports of pain severity.

Treatment from the operant perspective focuses on extinction of pain behaviors and increasing well behaviors by positive reinforcement. This treatment has proven to be effective for select samples of chronic pain patients [47–49]. Although operant factors undoubtedly play a role in the maintenance of pain and disability, the operant conditioning model of pain has been criticized for its exclusive focus on motor pain behaviors, failure to consider the emotional and cognitive aspects of pain [50–53], and failure to treat the subjective experience of pain [54]. Moreover, Turk and Okifuji demonstrated that patients' appraisals were better predictors of pain behavior than environmental factors including responses from significant others [55].

Respondent learning mechanisms

Factors contributing to chronicity that have previously been conceptualized in terms of operant learning may also be initiated and maintained by respondent conditioning [56]. Fordyce et al. hypothesized intermittent sensory stimulation from the site of bodily damage, environmental reinforcement, or successful avoidance of aversive social activity is not necessarily required to account for the maintenance of avoidance behavior or protective movements [57]. Linton, among others showed that avoidance of activities was related more to anxiety about pain than to actual pain [58].

Once an acute pain problem is established the patient may fear motor activities that he or she expects to result in pain, and this fear results in avoidance of activity [59, 60]. Non-occurrence of pain is a powerful reinforcer for future reduction of activity. In this way, the original respondent conditioning may be followed by an operant learning process whereby the nociceptive stimuli and the associated responses need no longer be present for the avoidance behavior to occur. In acute pain states it may be useful to reduce movement, and consequently to avoid pain in order to accelerate the healing process. Over time, however, anticipatory anxiety related to activity may develop and act as a conditioned stimulus for sympathetic activation (the conditioned response), which may be maintained after the original unconditioned stimulus (injury) and unconditioned response (pain and sympathetic activation) have subsided [59, 61].

Sympathetic activation and increases in muscle tension may be viewed as unconditioned responses that can elicit more pain. Even when no injury is present, pain related to sustained muscle contractions may also be conceptualized as an unconditioned stimulus, and conditioning may proceed in the same fashion as outlined above. Although an original association between pain and pain-related stimuli may result in anxiety regarding these stimuli, with time the expectation of pain related to activity may lead to avoidance of adaptive behaviors even if the nociceptive stimuli and the related sympathetic activation are no longer present.

In acute pain, many activities that are otherwise neutral or pleasurable may elicit or exacerbate pain, and are thus experienced as aversive and avoided. Over time, more and more activities may be seen as eliciting or exacerbating pain, and may be feared and avoided (stimulus generalization). Avoided activities may involve simple motor behaviors, but also work, leisure, and sexual activity [61]. In addition to avoidance learning, pain may be exacerbated and maintained in an expanding number of situations. For example, anxiety-related sympathetic activation and accompanying muscle tension may occur both in anticipation and also as a consequence of pain; cf. [1]. Thus, psychological factors may directly affect nociceptive stimulation and

need not be viewed as only reactions to pain. We will return to this point later in the chapter.

Persistent avoidance of specific activities reduces disconfirmations that are followed by corrected predictions [62]. Prediction of pain promotes pain avoidance behavior and over prediction of pain promotes excessive avoidance behavior [49, 50]. Insofar as pain avoidance succeeds in preserving the over predictions from repeated disconfirmation, they will continue unchanged [63]. By contrast, people who repeatedly engage in behavior that produces significantly less pain than they *predicted* will likely make adjustments in subsequent expectations, which will subsequently become more accurate. Increasingly accurate predictions will be followed by reduction of avoidance behavior [64]. These observations add support to the importance of physical therapy and exercise quota, with patients progressively increasing their activity levels despite their fears of injury and discomfort associated with renewed use of deconditioned muscles.

From the respondent conditioning perspective, the people with pain may have learned to associate increases in pain with all kinds of stimuli that were originally associated with nociceptive stimulation (i.e., stimulus generalization). As the pain symptoms persist, more and more situations may elicit anxiety and anticipatory pain and depression because of the low rate of reinforcement obtained when behavior is greatly reduced; cf. [59]. Sitting, walking, cognitively demanding work or social interaction, sexual activity, or even thoughts about these activities may increase anticipatory anxiety and concomitant physiological and biochemical changes [61]. Subsequently, patients may respond inappropriately to several stimuli reducing the frequency of many activities in addition to those that initially induced nociception. Physical abnormalities often observed in chronic pain patients (e.g., distorted gait, decreased range of motion, muscular fatigue) may actually result from secondary changes initiated in behavior through learning rather than continuing nociception. With chronic pain, the anticipation of suffering or prevention of suffering may be sufficient for the long-term maintenance of avoidance behaviors.

Cognitive factors

As noted previously, people are not passive responders to physical sensation; rather, they actively seek to make sense of their experience. They appraise their conditions by matching sensations to some pre-existing implicit model and determine whether a particular sensation is a symptom of a particular physical disorder that requires attention or can be ignored. In this way, to some extent, each person functions with a uniquely constructed reality. When information is ambiguous, people rely on general attitudes and beliefs based on experience and prior learning history. These beliefs determine the meaning and significance of the problems, as well as the perceptions of appropriate treatment. If we accept the premise that pain is a complex, subjective phenomenon that is uniquely experienced by each person, then knowledge about idiosyncratic beliefs, appraisals, and coping repertoires becomes critical for optimal treatment planning and for accurately evaluating treatment outcome [65, 66].

A great deal of research has been directed toward identifying cognitive factors that contribute to pain and disability [67, 68]. These studies have consistently demonstrated that patients' attitudes, beliefs, and expectancies about their plight, themselves, their coping resources, and their healthcare system affect their reports of pain, activity, disability, and response to treatment [69–71].

Beliefs about pain

Clinicians working with chronic pain patients are aware that patients having similar pain histories and reports of pain may differ greatly in their beliefs about their pain. Certain beliefs may lead to maladaptive coping, exacerbation of pain, increased suffering, and greater disability. For example, if pain is interpreted as signifying ongoing tissue damage rather than viewed as being the result of a stable problem that may improve, it is likely to produce considerably more suffering and behavioral dysfunction even though the amount of nociceptive input in the two cases may be equivalent [72]. People who believe that their pain is likely to persist may be quite passive in their coping efforts and fail to use cognitive or behavioral strategies to cope with pain. People with chronic pain who consider their pain an unexplainable mystery may minimize their own abilities to control or decrease pain, and be less likely to rate their coping strategies as effective in controlling and decreasing pain [73, 74].

Moreover, people with chronic pain's beliefs about the implications of a disease can affect their perception of symptoms [66, 75]. For example, Cassell cited the case of a patient whose pain could easily be controlled with codeine when he attributed it to sciatica, but required significantly greater amounts of opioids to achieve the same degree of relief when he attributed it to metastatic

cancer [76]. Cassell's observation was confirmed in a study published by Spiegel and Bloom who found that the pain severity ratings of cancer patients could be predicted by the use of analgesics and by the patients' affective state, but also by their *interpretations of pain* [72]. Patients who attributed their pain to a worsening of their underlying disease experienced more pain than did patients with more benign interpretations, despite the same level of disease progression.

A person's cognitions (beliefs, appraisals, expectancies) regarding the consequences of an event and his or her ability to deal with it, are hypothesized to affect functioning in two ways – by directly influencing mood and indirectly influencing coping efforts. Both influences may affect physiological activity associated with pain such as muscle tension [77] and production of endogenous opioids [5].

The presence of pain may change the way people process pain-related and other information. For example, chronic pain may focus attention on all types of bodily signals. Arntz and Schmidt [78] suggested that the processing of internal information may become disturbed in chronic pain patients. It is possible that pain patients become preoccupied with and over emphasize physical symptoms and interpret them as painful stimulation. In fact, studies of patients with diverse conditions, e.g., irritable bowel syndrome [79], fibromyalgia [80], angina pectoris [81], headaches [82], support the presence of what appears to be a hypersensitivity characterized by a lowered threshold for labeling stimuli as noxious. Patients may interpret pain symptoms as indicative of an underlying disease, and they may do everything to avoid pain exacerbation, most often by resorting to inactivity [60, 83]. For example, in acute pain states, bed rest is often prescribed to relieve pressure on the spine. People with chronic pain may subsequently subscribe to a belief that any movement of the back may worsen their condition, and they may still maintain this belief in the chronic state, when inaction is not only unnecessary but also detrimental.

In a set of studies, Schmidt found that patients with low back pain demonstrated poor behavioral persistence in various exercise tasks, and that their performance on these tasks was independent of physical exertion or actual self-reports of pain [50, 51]. Instead, these patients' exercise behaviors were related to their previous pain reports suggesting that having a negative view of their abilities and expecting increased pain influenced their behavior more than actual events or sensations. In another study, Council et al. noted that 83% of patients with low back pain reported that they were unable to complete a movement sequence including leg lifts and lateral bends because of *anticipated* pain; yet, only 5% were unable to perform the activities because of actual lack of ability [84]. Thus, the rationale for their avoidance of exercise was not the presence of pain, but their *learned expectation* of heightened pain and accompanying physical arousal, factors which might further exacerbate pain and reinforce the patients' beliefs regarding the pervasiveness of their disability [66, 75]. These results are consistent with the respondent learning factors described above. Patients' negative perceptions of their capabilities for physical performance form a vicious circle, with the failure to perform activities reinforcing the perception of helplessness and incapacity [50, 51].

Most recently, there has been a shift in focus from patients' negative perceptions about their abilities, to their healthcare providers' beliefs. Linton *et al.* evaluated healthcare providers' beliefs regarding chronic pain, and reported that two-thirds of healthcare providers reported they would advise avoidance of pain-inducing activities, and more than 25% reported the belief that sick leave was beneficial in the recuperation from back pain [85]. Further, patients that were treated by doctors that recommended bed rest and analgesics as needed experienced more disability at follow-up as compared to patients that were treated by doctors that recommended self-care strategies [86]. This interaction among providers and patients highlights the importance of social factors in pain experience.

Jensen *et al.* demonstrated that patient beliefs that emotions affected their pain, that others should be solicitous when they experienced pain, and that they were disabled by pain were positively associated with psychosocial dysfunction [70]. For example, patients who believed that they were disabled by pain and that they should avoid activity because pain signified damage were more likely to reveal physical disability than were patients who did not hold these beliefs.

Once cognitive structures (based on memories and meaning) about a disease are formed, they become stable and are very difficult to modify. Patients tend to avoid experiences that could invalidate their beliefs, and they guide their behavior in accordance with these beliefs even in situations where the beliefs are no longer valid. Consequently, as noted above in describing respondent conditioning, they do not receive corrective feedback.

In addition to beliefs about the ability to function despite pain, beliefs about pain per se appear to be of importance in understanding patients' adherence to treatment, response to treatment, and disability. For example, Schwartz *et al.* presented patients with information about the role of cognitive, affective, and behavioral factors and their own role in the rehabilitation process [87]. Following treatment, patients who rated the information as applicable to their pain condition had much better outcomes. Those who disagreed with the concepts presented were found at follow-up to have higher levels of pain, lower levels of activity, and a high degree of dissatisfaction.

The results of several studies suggest that when successful rehabilitation occurs, there appears to be an important cognitive shift – a shift from beliefs about helplessness and passivity to resourcefulness and ability to function regardless of pain. For example, Williams and Thorn [74] found that chronic pain patients who believed that their pain was an "unexplained mystery" reported high levels of psychological distress and pain, and also showed poorer treatment compliance than patients who believed that they understood their pain.

In a process study designed to evaluate the direct association between patients' beliefs and symptoms, a thought-sampling procedure was used to evaluate the nature of patients' cognitions during and immediately following headache, both prior to and following treatment [88]. Results indicated that there were significant changes in certain aspects of headache-related thinking in treated groups compared to a control group. Treated patients made significantly fewer negative appraisal (e.g., "It's getting worse," "There is nothing I can do") and significantly more positive appraisals than untreated patients. Treated patients learned to evaluate headaches in a more positive fashion. Importantly, patients who had the largest positive shifts in appraisal reported the greatest reduction in headache intensity. Remarkably, treated patients also reported significantly fewer headache days per week and lower intensity of pain than untreated controls.

The results of Newton and Barbaree's study support the argument that changes in cognitive reactions to headache may underlie headache improvement [88]; see also [16, 89]. Many additional pain treatment outcome studies support the idea that reducing negative appraisals is one way to reduce pain and associated suffering. In considering the efficacy of biofeedback for back pain patients, Nouwen and Solinger concluded that "simultaneous accomplishment of muscle tension reduction and lowering reported pain convinced patients that muscle tension, and subsequently pain, could be controlled [90]. As self-control could not be demonstrated in most patients, it seems plausible that the feeling of self-control, rather than actual control of physiological functions or events is crucial for further reductions." In other words, it appears that the extent to which patients believe that voluntary control over muscles has been achieved dictates the outcome, even when their beliefs are not accompanied by lasting reductions in muscular reactivity.

Similar to Nouwen and Solinger's interpretation [90], Blanchard speculated that for headache patients the maintenance of treatment effects endures in spite of almost universal cessation of regular home practice of biofeedback, because the self-perpetuating cycle of chronic headache has been broken [16]. The experience of headache serves as a stressor, which can contribute to future headaches. By the end of biofeedback treatment, when patients have experienced noticeable headache relief, it is as if they have redefined themselves as able to cope with headaches. Removing one source of stress appears to help patients to cope with recurrences more adaptively.

Clearly, it appears essential for people with chronic pain to develop adaptive beliefs about the relation among impairment, pain, suffering, and disability, and to de-emphasize the role of experienced pain in their regulation of functioning. In fact, results from numerous treatment outcome studies have shown that changes in pain level do not parallel changes in other variables of interest, including activity level, medication use, return to work, rated ability to cope with pain, and pursuit of further treatment [91, 92].

Beliefs about controllability

There are many laboratory studies demonstrating that controllability of aversive stimulation reduces its impact [93, 94]. Conversely, there is evidence that the explicit expectation of uncontrollable pain stimulation may cause subsequent nociceptive input to be perceived as more intense [95].

People with chronic pain typically perceive a lack of personal control, which probably relates to their ongoing but unsuccessful efforts to control their pain. A large proportion of chronic pain patients appear to believe that they have limited ability to exert control over their pain [96]. Such negative, maladaptive appraisals about the situation and their personal efficacy may reinforce the experience of demoralization, inactivity, and over-reaction to nociceptive stimulation commonly observed in chronic pain patients [97].

Mizener *et al.* demonstrated that among successfully treated migraine headache patients increases in

perceived control over physiological activity and general health was significantly correlated with reduction in headache activity [98]. Flor and Turk examined the relationship among general and situation-specific pain-related thoughts, conceptions of personal control, pain severity, and disability levels in people with low back pain and rheumatoid arthritis (RA) [69]. General and situation-specific convictions of uncontrollability and helplessness were more highly related to pain and disability than were disease-related variables for both samples. The combination of both situation-specific and general cognitive variables explained 32% and 60% of the variance in pain and disability, respectively. The addition of disease-related variables improved the predictions only marginally. People' beliefs about the extent to which they can control their pain are associated with various other outcome variables including medication use, activity levels, and psychological functioning [93].

Self-efficacy

Closely related to the sense of control over aversive stimulation is the concept of "self-efficacy." A self-efficacy expectation is defined as a personal conviction that one can successfully execute a course of action (i.e., perform required behaviors) to produce a desired outcome in a given situation. This construct appears to be a major mediator of therapeutic change.

Bandura suggested that if a person has sufficient motivation to engage in a behavior, the person's self-efficacy beliefs are what determine which activities to initiate, the amount of effort expended, and extent of persistence in the face of obstacles and aversive experiences [99, 100]. Efficacy judgments are based on the following four sources of information regarding one's capabilities, in descending order of impact:

1. one's own past performance at the task or similar tasks;
2. the performance accomplishments of others who are perceived to be similar to oneself;
3. verbal persuasion by others that one is capable; and
4. perception of one's own state of physiological arousal, which is in turn partly determined by prior efficacy estimation.

Encouraging patients to undertake subtasks that are increasingly difficult, or close to the desired behavioral repertoire, can create performance mastery experience. From this perspective, the occurrence of coping behaviors is conceptualized as being mediated by the individual's beliefs that situational demands do not exceed his or her coping resources.

Dolce *et al.* [101], and Litt [102] reported that low self-efficacy ratings regarding pain control are related to low pain tolerance, and that they are better predictors of tolerance than are objective levels of noxious stimuli. The relationship between pain patients' self-efficacy ratings of perceived ability to control pain has been replicated in several studies. For example, Manning and Wright obtained self-efficacy ratings from women expecting their first child concerning their ability to have a medication-free childbirth [103]. These ratings were good predictors of medication use and time in labor without medication. Similarly, Council *et al.* had patients rate their self-efficacy as well as expectancy of pain related to the performance of movement tasks [84]. Patients' performance levels were highly related to their self-efficacy expectations, which in turn appeared to be determined by their expectancy of pain levels.

Converging lines of evidence from investigations of both laboratory and clinical pain indicate that perceived self-efficacy operates as an important cognitive factor in pain control, adaptive psychological functioning, disability, impairment, and treatment outcome [104]. What are the mechanisms that account for the association between self-efficacy and behavioral outcome? Cioffi has suggested that at least four psychological processes may be responsible[105]:

1. as perceived self-efficacy decreases anxiety and its concomitant physiological arousal, the person may approach the task with less potentially distressing physical information to begin with;
2. the efficacious person is able to willfully distract attention from potentially threatening physiological sensations;
3. the efficacious person perceives and is distressed by physical sensations, but simply persists in the face of them (stoicism); and
4. physical sensations are neither ignored nor necessarily distressing, but rather are relatively free to take on a broad distribution of meanings (change interpretations).

Bandura [99, 100] suggested that those techniques that most enhance mastery experiences would be the most powerful tools for bringing about behavior change. He proposed that cognitive variables are the primary determinants of behavior, but that these variables are most affected by performance accomplishments. The studies on headache, back pain,

and RA cited above appear to support Bandura's proposal.

Cognitive errors

In addition to specific self-efficacy beliefs, a number of investigators have suggested that a common set of "cognitive errors" affect perceptions of pain, affective distress, and disability [106–108]. A cognitive error is a negatively distorted belief about oneself or one's situation.

As is the case with self-efficacy, specific cognitive errors and distortions have been linked consistently to depression, self-reported pain severity, and disability in chronic pain patients [109]. Such negative thoughts (1) appear to predict long-term adjustment to chronic pain; (2) may mediate a portion of the relationship between disease severity and adjustment; and (3) uniquely contribute (over and above other cognitive factors) to the prediction of adjustment [108].

Catastrophizing appears to be a particularly potent cognitive error that greatly influences pain and disability [110, 111]. Several lines of research, including experimental laboratory studies of acute pain with normal volunteers and field studies with patients suffering clinical pain, show that catastrophizing and adaptive coping strategies (see below) are important in determining the reaction to pain.

People who spontaneously utilized fewer catastrophizing self-statements and more adaptive coping strategies rated experimentally induced pain as lower, and tolerate nociceptive stimuli longer than did those who reported more catastrophizing thoughts; moreover, people who spontaneously utilize more catastrophizing self-statements reported more pain, distress and disability in several acute and chronic pain studies, as reviewed by various authors [112, 113].

Butler *et al.* demonstrated that in the case of post-surgical pain, cognitive coping strategies and catastrophizing thoughts correlated significantly with medication use, pain reports, and nurses' judgments of peoples' pain tolerance [114]. Turner and Clancy showed that during cognitive-behavioral treatment, reductions in catastrophizing were significantly related to increases in pain tolerance and reductions in physical and psychosocial impairment [115].

Following treatment, reductions in catastrophizing were related to reduction in pain intensity and physical impairment. In a cognitive behavioral treatment study specifically designed to decrease catastrophic thinking for people with chronic headache, participants reported significant reductions in catastrophic thinking as compared to wait-list controls, and approximately 50% of those treated reported meaningful changes in health indices as well [116]. As noted earlier, Flor and Turk [69] found that in low back pain patients and people with RA, significant percentages of the variance in pain and disability were accounted for by cognitive factors that were labeled catastrophizing, helplessness, adaptive coping, and resourcefulness. In both the low back pain and the RA groups, the cognitive variables of catastrophizing and adaptive coping had substantially more explanatory power than did disease-related variables or impairment. Finally, Keefe *et al.* found that RA patients who reported high levels of pain, physical disability, and depression had reported excessive catastrophizing ideation on questionnaires administered 6 months earlier [117].

In an effort to explore the combined predictive capacity of catastrophizing measures and physiological measures, Wolff and colleagues evaluated lower paraspinal muscle tension and cardiac reactivity to emotional arousal, and found that high catastrophizers who had high resting muscle tension reported the highest pain levels [118]. Additionally, high catastrophizers with low cardiovascular reactivity to emotional arousal, reported the greatest pain levels. This experiment highlights the important interaction among physiological and cognitive factors in pain experience.

Coping

Self-regulation of pain and its impact depend on peoples' specific ways of dealing with pain, adjusting to pain, and reducing or minimizing distress caused by pain – in other words, their coping strategies. Coping is assumed to involve spontaneously employed purposeful and intentional acts, and it can be assessed in terms of overt and covert behaviors. Overt behavioral coping strategies include rest, use of relaxation techniques, or medication. Covert coping strategies include various means of distracting oneself from pain, reassuring oneself that the pain will diminish, seeking information, and problem solving. Coping strategies are thought to act to alter both the perception of pain intensity and the ability to manage or tolerate pain and to continue everyday activities [3, 108].

Studies have found active coping strategies (efforts to function in spite of pain or to distract oneself from pain, such as engaging in activity or ignoring pain) to be associated with adaptive functioning, and passive coping strategies (such as depending on others for help in pain control and restricting one's activities)

to be related to greater pain and depression [71, 119]. However, beyond this, there is no evidence supporting the greater effectiveness of any one active coping strategy compared to any other [120]. It seems more likely that different strategies will be more effective than others for some people at some times, but not necessarily for all people all of the time.

A number of studies have demonstrated that if individuals are instructed in the use of adaptive coping strategies, their ratings of pain intensity decrease and tolerance for pain increases, as reviewed by Fernandez and Turk [120]. The most important factor in poor coping appears to be the presence of catastrophizing, rather than differences in the nature of specific adaptive coping strategies [121]. Turk *et al.* concluded that "what appears to distinguish low from high pain tolerant individuals are their cognitive processing, catastrophizing thoughts and feelings that precede, accompany, and follow aversive stimulation" [3].

Affective factors

Pain is ultimately a subjective, private experience, but it is invariably described in terms of sensory and affective properties. As defined by the International Association for the Study of Pain: "(Pain) is unquestionably a sensation in a part or parts of the body but it is also always unpleasant and therefore also an emotional experience" [122]. The central and interactive roles of sensory information and affective state are supported by an overwhelming amount of evidence [123].

The affective components of pain include many different emotions, but they are primarily negative in quality. Anxiety and depression have received the greatest amount of attention in chronic pain patients.

Depression

After reviewing a large body of literature, Banks and Kerns concluded that from 30% to 50% of chronic pain patients suffer from depression [124]. In the majority of cases, depression appears to be patients' reaction to their plight. Some have suggested that chronic pain is a form of masked depression; although this may be true in a small number of cases, there is no empirical support for the hypothesis that depression precedes the development of chronic pain [125].

Given our description of the plight of people with chronic pain, it is not surprising that a large number of chronic pain patients are depressed. It is interesting to ponder the other side of the coin. How is it that all people with chronic pain disorders are *not* depressed?

Turk and colleagues examined this question and determined that patients' appraisals of the impact of the pain on their lives and of their ability to exert any control over their pain and lives mediated the pain–depression relationship [27, 28, 94, 126]. That is, those patients who believed that they could continue to function despite their pain, and that they could maintain some control despite their pain, did not become depressed.

Anxiety

Anxiety is commonplace in chronic pain. Pain-related fear, and concerns about harm-avoidance appear to exacerbate symptoms [49]. Anxiety is an affective state that is influenced by appraisal processes, to cite the stoic philosopher Epictetus, "There is nothing either bad or good but thinking makes it so." There is a reciprocal relationship between affective state and cognitive-interpretive processes whereby thinking affects mood and mood influences appraisals and ultimately the experience of pain.

Threat of intense pain captures attention and is difficult to disengage from. Continual vigilance and monitoring of noxious stimulation and the belief that it signifies disease progression may render even low intensity nociception less bearable. As we noted in our discussion of respondent conditioning, the experience of pain may initiate a set of extremely negative thoughts and arouse fears – fears of inciting more pain, injury, and the future impact [127]. Fear of pain and anticipation of pain are cognitive-perceptual processes that are not driven exclusively by the actual sensory experience of pain and can exert a significant impact on the level of function and pain tolerance [128, 129]. Several investigators have suggested that fear of pain, driven by the anticipation of pain rather than the sensory experience of pain, is a strong negative reinforcement for the persistence of avoidance behavior and the functional disability [49, 59, 60].

Avoidance behavior is reinforced in the short-term, through the reduction of suffering associated with nociception [130]. Avoidance, however, can be a maladaptive response if it persists and leads to increased fear, limited activity, and other physical and psychological consequences that contribute to disability and persistence of pain. Studies have demonstrated that fear of movement and fear of (re)injury are better predictors of functional limitations than biomedical parameters [49, 130, 131]. For example, Crombez *et al.* showed that pain-related fear was the best predictor of behavioral performance in trunk-extension, flexion, and weight-lifting tasks, even after statistically controlling for the effects of pain intensity. Moreover, Vlaeyen *et al.* found that fear of movement/(re)injury was the best predictor of the patient's self-reported disability among chronic back pain patients and that physiological sensory perception of pain and biomedical findings did not add any predictive value [60]. Approximately two-thirds of chronic non-specific low back pain sufferers avoid back straining activities because of fear of (re)injury [132]. Interestingly, reduction in pain-related anxiety predicts improvement in functioning, affective distress, pain, and pain-related interference with activity [133]. Clearly, fear, pain-related anxiety, and concerns about harm-avoidance all play an important role in chronic pain and need to be assessed and addressed in treatment.

Enduring psychological and functional limitation following a traumatic event is frequently indicative of "post-traumatic stress disorder" (PTSD). Traumatic events have been associated with a set of symptoms including nightmares, recurrent and intrusive recollections about the trauma, avoidance of thoughts or activities associated with the traumatic event, and symptoms of increased arousal such as insomnia and hyperarousal. When this set of symptoms closely follows a known traumatic event over an extended period of time, they are labeled PTSD. Significant minorities of chronic pain sufferers attribute the onset of their symptoms to a specific trauma such as a motor vehicle accident. Results of research suggest an exceedingly high prevalence of PTSD in patients presenting to chronic pain clinics [134, 135].

In a preliminary study, Sherman *et al.* found that over 50% of a sample of 93 treatment-seeking fibromyalgia syndrome (FMS) patients reported symptoms of PTSD [136]. Those who experienced these anxiety-related symptoms reported significantly greater levels of pain, life interference, emotional distress, and greater inactivity than did the patients who did not report PTSD-like symptoms. Over 85% of the sample with significant PTSD symptoms compared to 50% of the patients without significant PTSD symptoms demonstrated significant disability. Geisser, *et al.* reported similar results for a heterogeneous sample of chronic pain patients [137]. Sherman *et al.* suggest that based on these results, clinicians should assess the presence of these symptoms, as the failure to attend to them in treatment may undermine successful outcomes [136].

Anger

Anger has been widely observed in patients with chronic pain [138, 139]. Summers *et al.* examined patients with spinal cord injuries and found that anger and hostility explained 33% of the variance in pain severity [140]. Kerns *et al.* found that the internalization of angry feelings accounted for a significant proportion of variances in measures of pain intensity, perceived interference, and reported frequency of pain behaviors [141].

Frustrations related to persistence of symptoms, limited information on etiology, and repeated treatment failures along with anger toward employers, insurance companies, the healthcare system, family members, and themselves, all contribute to the general dysphoric mood of patients [142, 143]. Kerns *et al.* noted that internalization of angry feelings was strongly related to measures of pain intensity, perceived interference, and reported frequency of pain behaviors [141].

The precise mechanisms by which anger and frustration exacerbate pain are not known. One reasonable possibility is that anger exacerbates pain by increasing autonomic arousal [144]. Anger may also block motivation for and acceptance of treatments oriented toward rehabilitation and disability management rather than cure. Yet rehabilitation and disability management are often the only treatments available for these patients.

Personality factors

The search for specific personality factors that predispose people to develop chronic pain has been a major emphasis of psychosomatic medicine. Studies have attempted to identify a specific "migraine-personality," an "RA" personality, and a more general "pain-prone personality" [145]. By and large, these efforts have received little support and have been challenged [125]. However, on the basis of their prior experiences, people develop idiosyncratic ways of interpreting information and coping with stress. Avoidance and the resulting failure to experience disconfirmation prevent the extinction or modification of these interpretations and expectations. There is no question that these unique patterns will have an effect on their perceptions of and responses to the presence of pain [146].

Pain is essential for survival. Thus, attention may be primed to process painful stimuli ahead of other attentional demands. People with high levels of anxiety sensitivity (AS) may be especially hypervigilant to pain as well as other noxious sensations. Selective attention directed towards threatening information like bodily sensations leads to greater arousal. Because of this attentional process those with high AS may be primed such that minor painful stimuli may be amplified [83].

Anxiety sensitivity refers to the fear of anxiety symptoms based on the belief that they will have harmful consequence [147]. Asmundson *et al.* have demonstrated that AS is correlated with exaggerated fear responses [148]. The unpleasantness of this exaggerated fear response can lead people with high AS to behave in ways that reduce fear and anxiety-related bodily sensations. Such behavior often takes the form of avoidance to prevent exacerbation of symptoms and further injury.

Preliminary studies that demonstrate the importance of anxiety sensitivity as a predispositional factor in chronic pain have been reported. Asmundson and Norton [149] found a positive association between AS and pain-related anxiety, escape/avoidant behaviors, fear of negative consequences of pain, and negative affect. Not only were patients with high AS more likely to experience greater cognitive disturbance as a result of their pain, they were likely to use greater amounts of analgesic medication to control equal amounts of pain compared to those with low or medium AS. Further, Asmundson and Taylor demonstrated that AS directly exacerbates fear of pain and indirectly exacerbates pain-specific avoidance behavior even after controlling for the direct influences of pain severity on these variables [150]. For a more extensive review see Asmundson *et al.* [148].

General fearful appraisals of bodily sensations may sensitize predisposed people and cause high awareness of bodily sensations. Thus, AS is only one individual difference characteristic that might predispose people to develop and maintain chronic pain and disability. For example, somatization, negative affectivity, bodily preoccupation, and catastrophic thinking also may be involved [151, 152]. Vlaeyen *et al.* argue that a style of catastrophic thinking about pain may be a risk factor for the emergence of pain-related fear [60]. Many studies have attempted to use different measures of psychopathology to predict pain patients' responses to conservative and surgical interventions, but discussion of this topic is beyond the scope of this chapter [153].

The effect of psychological and social factors on pain

Psychological and social factors may act indirectly on pain and disability by reducing physical activity, and consequently reducing muscle flexibility, muscle tone, strength, and physical endurance. Fear of reinjury, fear of loss of disability compensation, and job dissatisfaction can also influence the return to work. Several studies have suggested that psychological factors may also have a direct effect on physiological parameters associated more directly with the production or exacerbation of nociception. Cognitive interpretations and affective arousal may directly affect physiology by increasing sympathetic nervous system arousal [154], endogenous opioid (endorphin) production, and elevated levels of muscle tension [77, 155].

Effect of thoughts on sympathetic arousal and muscle tension

Circumstances that are appraised as potentially threatening to safety or comfort are likely to generate strong physiological reactions. For example, Rimm and Litvak demonstrated that subjects exhibited physiological arousal by simply thinking about a painful stimulus [156]. In an early study, Barber and Hahn showed that subjects' self-reported discomfort and physiological responses [frontalis electromyographic (EMG) activity, heart rate, skin conductance] were similar whether they imagined taking part in a cold-pressor test or actually participated in it [157]. In patients with recurrent migraine headaches simply processing words describing migraine headaches can increase skin conductance [158].

Chronic increases in sympathetic nervous system activation, known as increased skeletal muscle tone, may set the stage for hyperactive muscle contraction and possibly for the persistence of a contraction following conscious muscle activation. Excessive sympathetic arousal and maladaptive behaviors can be immediate precursors of muscle hypertonicity, hyperactivity, and persistence. These in turn may be the proximate causes of chronic muscle spasm and pain. It is common for persons in pain to exaggerate or amplify the significance of their problem and needlessly "turn on" their sympathetic nervous systems [159]. In this way, cognitive processes may influence sympathetic arousal and thereby predispose individuals to further injury or otherwise complicate the process of recovery.

Several studies support the direct effect of cognitive factors on muscle tension. For example, Flor et al. demonstrated that discussing stressful events and pain produced elevated levels of EMG activity localized to the site of back pain patients' pain [77]. The extent of abnormal muscular reactivity was better predicted by depression and cognitive coping style than by pain demographic variables (e.g., number of surgeries or duration of pain). Flor et al. replicated these results and extended them to patients with temporomandibular disorders (TMDs) [155]. For this group, imagery reconstruction of pain episodes produced elevated tension in facial muscles.

The natural evolution and course of many chronic pain syndromes are unknown. At the present time, it is probably more appropriate to refer to abnormal psychophysiological patterns as antecedents of chronic pain states or to view them as consequences of chronic pain that subsequently maintain or exacerbate the symptoms, rather than to assign them any direct etiological significance [160].

Implications for treatment

We have emphasized that pain is a subjective perceptual event that is not solely dependent on the extent of tissue damage or organic dysfunction. The intensity of pain reported and the responses to the perception of pain are influenced by a wide range of factors, such as meaning of the situation, attentional focus, mood, prior learning history, cultural background, environmental contingencies, social supports, and financial resources, among others. The research we reviewed supports the importance of these in the etiology, severity, exacerbation, and maintenance of pain, suffering, and disability.

Treatment based on the biopsychosocial perspective must not only address the biological basis of symptoms; it must incorporate the full range of social and psychological factors that have been shown to affect pain, distress, and disability. Therefore, treatment should be designed not only to alter physical contributors but also to change the patient's behaviors regardless of the patient's specific pathophysiology and without necessarily controlling pain per se [3, 40]. Treatment from the biopsychosocial perspective focuses on providing the patient with techniques to gain a sense of control over the effects of pain on his or her life, by modifying the affective, behavioral, cognitive, and sensory facets of the experience. Behavioral experiences help to show patients that they are capable of more than they assumed they were, thus increasing their sense of personal competence.

Treatment

There are a number of different approaches to facilitate adaptation and self-management of symptoms.

The most common treatment approaches include insight-oriented therapies, behavioral treatments, and cognitive-behavioral therapy (CBT). In addition several techniques based on these models have been efficacious (i.e., motivational interviewing, biofeedback, relaxation, guided imagery, hypnosis, and meditation) independently or as part of comprehensive rehabilitation. In this review, we provide an overview of psychological approaches and techniques for the treatment of patients with chronic pain. We emphasize the cognitive-behavioral perspective for conceptualization and treatment within an interdisciplinary framework because it has the greatest empirical support [3, 92, 161].

Insight-oriented approaches

Insight-oriented approaches are predicated on the belief that chronic physical pain may be somatic presentations of emotional distress, and non-conscious factors will influence both the onset and maintenance of symptoms. As one set of evidence to support this assumption, insight-oriented practitioners often cite the data on the prevalence of childhood physical and sexual abuse acknowledged by people reporting chronic pain [85, 162].

Psychodynamically oriented therapy and insight-oriented approaches primarily focus on early relationship experiences that are reconstructed within the therapeutic relationship. The therapeutic relationship reintegrates emotions into symbolic and available mental processes, resulting in improved emotional regulation [163]. Although insight-oriented psychotherapy may be useful with selected individuals to our knowledge, no randomized controlled trials have been published demonstrating its efficacy for people with chronic pain problems [163].

The role of reinforcement in maintenance of pain behavior

Pain is subjective, the only way we know about someone's pain is to ask, observe, and make inferences about their behavior. When patients are asked about their pain, they may provide a number of descriptors that convey information; however, there is no objective criterion. Observation of behavior, for example, limping or grimacing, may indicate something about subjective states. However this inference can only be confirmed by self-report since the association between objective evidence of pathology is only weakly associated with reported pain [164]. Self-report or other behaviors are merely surrogates for the subjective experience of pain. Furthermore persistent noxious symptoms will take a toll on those others living with or in close contact with the patients [165].

Behavior is communication that elicits responses from observers. Consider a woman who is rubbing her neck and moaning. Her husband observes these behaviors and *infers* his wife's neck pain is flaring up. If he acknowledges her pain, brings her medication, then rubs her neck, and spends time talking with her, assuming these are desired responses, they will serve as positive reinforcement. What the patient has learned is that her "pain-related" behaviors communicated a message to her husband. This learning process may increase the likelihood that she will increase these behaviors as a way of obtaining desired responses from others in the future.

Behavioral principles work in another way. Avoidance of undesirable activity and or behaviors that reduce distress is negatively reinforcing. Negative reinforcement strengthens a behavior because the negative condition is terminated or avoided as a consequence of the behavior. Consider a patient in physical therapy who reports that whenever he performs certain exercises his pain increases. The physical therapist may tell him to stop the activity ("if it hurts, don't do it"). Assuming his pain is reduced by termination of the activity, the patient will learn that avoidance of activity has a positive effect. Avoidance is a positive outcome and may negatively reinforce similar behaviors when the circumstance arises again. This has the unintended consequence of increasing physical deconditioning. Although this may be an appropriate response for acute pain, it may not be in the context of chronic pain and the attainment of corrective feedback – activity may not increase pain. Corrective feedback is necessary in order to learn that "hurt" and "harm" are not the same thing.

Physicians and patients also demonstrate a potent reciprocal relationship of reinforcement influencing each others' behaviors. Studies have shown that physicians prescribe treatment for pain patients based on observations of patients' behaviors including emotional distress, vs. physical pathology or pain severity [55, 166]. Conversely, patients observe the responses of their physicians. If they note (learning may not be a conscious process) that either the physician increases their analgesic medication when they are more demonstrative – "pain behaviors", complain more, appear more distressed, the next time they visit the physician they may present as more extreme to obtain attention and further treatment.

Failure to positively reinforce "well-behaviors" such as activity will influence behavior. Behavior that is not positively reinforced will be reduced or even extinguished.

Two treatment approaches have been developed based on the behavioral principles of reinforcement and conditioning, as discussed above. These are described briefly in the next section.

Respondent conditioning

If a nociceptive stimulus is repeatedly paired with a neutral stimulus in close temporal proximity, the neutral stimulus will elicit a pain response. This is referred to as classical or respondent conditioning. In chronic pain, many neutral or pleasurable activities may elicit or exacerbate pain. Thus, over time, a number of stimuli (e.g., activities) may be expected to elicit or exacerbate pain and will be avoided (i.e., stimulus generalization). The anticipatory fear of pain and restriction of activity, and not just the actual nociception, may contribute to disability. Anticipatory fear can also elicit physiological reactivity that may aggravate pain. Thus, conditioning may directly increase nociceptive stimulation and pain.

The longer inactivity prevails the more difficult it is to modify people's convictions and behaviors. Treatment of pain from the respondent conditioning model includes repeatedly engaging in behaviors that produce progressively less pain than was predicted (corrective feedback) – exposure, which is then followed by reductions in anticipatory fear and anxiety associated with the activity. Such transformations lend support to the importance of quota-based exercise programs, with participants progressively increasing their activity despite fear of injury and discomfort associated with use of deconditioned muscles.

Operant conditioning

Operant approaches focus on the extinction of pain behaviors. Therapists withdraw positive attention for pain behaviors while increasing reinforcement of well behaviors. The operant paradigm does not seek to uncover the etiology of symptoms but focuses on the maintenance of pain behaviors and deficiency of well behaviors. Pain behaviors are identified, as are their controlling antecedents and consequent reinforcers or punishments [161], such as overly solicitous behaviors by a spouse [167].

Reduction and ultimately elimination of the connection between pain behaviors and their positive or negative consequences is used to increase and maintain desired behaviors and decrease pain-compatible behaviors. With operant behavioral treatment, persons are expected to be active in setting treatment goals and follow through with recommendations [3]. The efficacy of operant treatment has been demonstrated in several studies of persons with various chronic pain disorders, including low pain [49] and fibromyalgia syndrome [168].

Cognitive-behavioral perspective and therapies

Perhaps the most commonly adopted treatment approach for chronic pain patients is CBT [92]. It is important to make a distinction between the cognitive-behavioral *perspective* and cognitive and behavioral *techniques* [169]. The cognitive-behavioral perspective is predicated on the assumption that people hold beliefs that they are unable to function because of their pain, and that they are helpless to improve their situation. Treatment goals focus on helping people with pain to realize that they can, in fact, manage their problems, and provide them with skills to respond in more adaptive ways that can be maintained after treatment is terminated. Cognitive-behavior therapy typically involves a combination of stress management, problem-solving, goal-setting, pacing of activities, and assertiveness. These skills can be integrated within a rehabilitation approach. Cognitive and behavioral techniques are woven into the fabric of treatment in an effort to enhance patients' sense of self-control. Biofeedback, relaxation, mediation, guided imagery, and hypnosis (described below) can all be incorporated within CBT to facilitate perceptions of self-control. The objective is to help patients acquire a sense of hopefulness, resourcefulness, and action to replace their more typical feelings of hopelessness, stress reactivity, and passivity.

Four key components of CBT have been described [169]: "education", "skills acquisition", "skills consolidation", and "generalization and maintenance". The "education" component focuses on helping patients challenge their negative perceptions regarding their abilities, and to manage pain by making them aware of the role that thoughts and emotions play in potentiating and maintaining stress and physical symptoms – "cognitive restructuring." Cognitive restructuring includes identifying maladaptive thoughts during problematic situations (e.g., during pain exacerbations, stressful events), introduction and practice of coping thoughts and behaviors, shifting from self-defeating to coping thoughts, practice of positive thoughts, and home practice and follow-up. The therapist encourages patients to test the adaptiveness of their thoughts, beliefs, expectations, and predictions. The crucial element is bringing about a shift in the patient's repertoire from well-established, habitual, and automatic but ineffective responses toward systematic problem-solving and planning, control of affect, behavioral persistence, or disengagement from self-defeating situations when appropriate [168].

The goal of "skills acquisition" and "consolidation" is to help people learn and, importantly, practice new pain management behaviors and cognitions, including relaxation, problem solving, distraction methods, activity pacing, and communication. Therapists use education, didactic instruction, Socratic questioning, and role-playing techniques among others. The techniques, however, are less important than the general message of self-management that is derived from experience using various techniques (some of which are described below). Patients may learn best from observing the outcomes of their own efforts rather than by instruction alone. Often CBT is carried out in a group context where the therapist can use the support of other patients and also have patients interact with each other to assist in providing alternative ways of thinking and behaving.

Finally, "generalization and maintenance" is geared toward solidifying skills and preventing relapse. Homework is an essential ingredient of CBT. Once patients have been taught and have practiced self-management skills within the therapeutic context, it is essential that they practice these in their home environment where the therapist is not present to guide and support them. The difficulties that will inevitably arise when attempts are made at patients' homes become important topics for discussion and further problem solving during therapeutic encounters. Problems that arise during home practice are viewed as opportunities to assist patients to learn how to handle setbacks and lapses that will likely occur following treatment. In this phase, therapists assist patients to anticipate future problems and high-risk situations so that they can think about and practice the behavioral responses that may be necessary for adaptive coping.

The goal during the latter phase, then, is to enable patients to develop a problem-solving perspective where they believe that they have the skills and competencies to respond in appropriate ways to problems as they arise. In this manner, attempts are made to help patients learn to anticipate future difficulties, develop plans for adaptive responding, and adjust their behavior accordingly.

An important implication of the biopsychosocial perspective is the need first to identify the relevant physical, psychological, and social characteristics of patients, and then to develop treatments matched to patients' characteristics and to evaluate their efficacy. The ultimate aim is the prescription of treatment components that have been shown to maximize outcome for different subsets of patients [170].

The efficacy of CBT in treating various chronic pain disorders has been demonstrated in a large number of studies and has been reviewed in a number of reviews and meta-analyses [92, 171–173]. There is a wealth of evidence that CBT can help to restore function as well as reduce pain and disability-related behaviors [92, 168]. Although CBT has been found to be helpful for a number of individuals, there are some for whom CBT is not beneficial. Investigators are just beginning to explore different aspects of CBT to answer the question "what works for whom?" [170, 174, 175].

With this overview of the cognitive-behavioral perspective, we now discuss specific techniques that can be incorporated with CBT when treating chronic pain patients. The primary objective of these techniques is enhancement of patients' sense of self-efficacy by increasing a sense of control to combat the feelings of helplessness and demoralization often felt by people with chronic pain.

Motivational interviewing

Motivational interviewing was initially developed for substance abusers [176]; however, it has been adapted to chronic pain patients [177]. In the "contemplation" stage people with chronic pain acknowledge the risks associated with inactivity and passivity. The clinical goal at this stage is to assist the patient to realize that the risks of inactivity outweigh the perceived benefits.

When the patient is ready to become more active ("preparation" stage), the clinician helps the patient outline appropriate structured physical activities in which the person is willing to participate. Finally, in the "action" the stage clinician helps the person increase activity. This is followed by the "maintenance stage," which is geared towards the person's ongoing motivation and commitment [176].

Clinicians can encourage transition to different stages by providing motivational statements, listening with empathy, asking open-ended questions, providing feedback and affirmation, and handling resistance [176]. Motivational interviewing should be thought of not as a treatment itself but as a general framework for preparing persons for treatment and for adhering within the cognitive-behavioral perspective and can be readily used with CBT. Motivational interviewing is one means of fostering motivation for self-control. Success using various techniques will directly reinforce feelings of self-efficacy [100, 178]. Thus, it is of central importance to direct practice and attention to the usefulness of these methods in improving quality of life in people with chronic pain despite the presence of noxious symptoms that cannot be totally eliminated. The assessment process [179] should help the therapist determine the person's motivation for the use of biomedical approaches.

Relaxation

There are a large number of relaxation techniques. The literature is inconsistent as to which techniques are the most effective. Moreover the different components may be synergistic. The important message to the patient is that there is a broad spectrum of approaches available and no one method is more efficacious. It is most important to help patients learn which technique(s) are most helpful for them by trying a variety. Clinicians may also note that no one technique is effective for all people all of the time: hence, knowledge of a range of methods may be the best approach. It is important to acknowledge that these methods are skills that require practice to become more proficient. In this section, we provide a brief overview of some of the most popular methods.

Meditation

Meditation is defined as the "intentional self-regulation of attention", a systematic inner focus on particular aspects of inner and outer experience [180, 181]. Meditation was originally developed within a religious or spiritual context and held as the ultimate goal of spiritual growth, ending suffering, personal transformation, or transcendental experience [182]. However, as a healthcare intervention, it has been taught effectively regardless of patients' cultural or religious backgrounds [183, 184].

There are many forms of meditation. We will describe two extensively researched general approaches; transcendental meditation and Zen or mindfulness meditation [185].

Transcendental meditation requires concentration; it involves focus on any one of the senses, like a zoom lens, on a specific object. For example, the individual repeats a silent word or phrase ("mantra") with the goal of transcending the ordinary stream of thought [182, 186]. Mindfulness meditation is the opposite of transcendental meditation in that its goal is attempting awareness of the whole perceptual field, like a wide angle lens. Thus, it incorporates focused attention and whole field awareness in the present moment. For example, the individual observes without judgment, thoughts, emotions, sensations, and perceptions as they arise moment by moment [183, 187]. Bonadonna proposed that individuals with chronic illness have an altered ability to concentrate: therefore, transcendental meditation may be less useful than mindfulness meditation when one is sick [188].

Mindfulness meditation reframes the experience of discomfort in that physical pain or suffering becomes the object of meditation. Attention and awareness of discomfort or suffering is another part of human experience: rather than be avoided it is to be experienced and explored [188]. Studies have found that mindfulness based interventions have decreased pain symptoms, increased healing speed, improved mood, decreased stress, contained healthcare costs, and decreased visits to primary care [182, 189].

Meditation has captured the attention of medicine, psychology, and neurocognitive sciences. This is in part due to experienced meditators demonstrating reduced arousal to daily stress, better performance of tasks that require focused attention, and other health benefits [190, 191]. Lazar *et al.* found that long-term meditation in Western practitioners showed increased cortical thickness in areas related to somatosensory, auditory, visual, and interoceptive processing [190]. They found thickening in right Brodmann's areas 9/10, which has been shown to be involved in the integration of cognition and emotion. Meditation may be useful for chronic pain patients due to the reciprocal relationship between stress and pain symptoms. Higher alpha brain wave activity has been found to have beneficial health effects as well as promote a general sense of well-being [192]. Furthermore, gamma wave activity is the synchrony of areas of the brain communicating with each other, and research on the effects of meditation on gamma wave activity demonstrates meditation may be beneficial for people with chronic pain due to dysregulation within the hypothalamic pituitary adrenal axis and autonomic nervous system [191].

Biofeedback

Biofeedback is a self-regulatory technique. The assumption with regard to biofeedback treatment is that the level of pain is maintained or exacerbated by autonomic nervous system dysregulation believed to be associated with the production of nociceptive stimulation. The objective of biofeedback is to teach people to exert control over their physiological processes to assist in re-regulating the autonomic nervous system. When people are treated with biofeedback, they are attached by surface electrodes to equipment that is linked to a computer that transforms and records physiological responses. These monitored physiological processes may include skin conductance, respiration, heart rate, heart rate variability, skin temperature, brain wave activity, and muscle tension. The biofeedback equipment conveys physiological responses as visual or auditory signals that the person can observe on a computer monitor. In this way, the physiological information is "fed back". With practice, individuals learn to control and change their physiological responses by learning to manipulate the auditory or visual signals by their own efforts. In addition to the physiological changes accompanying biofeedback, patients are provided with a sense of control over their bodies. Given the high levels of helplessness observed in people with chronic pain problems, the perception of control may be as important as the actual physiological changes observed.

Biofeedback has been used successfully to treat a number of chronic pain states such as headaches, back pain, chronic myofascial pain, TMDs, irritable bowel syndrome, and fibromyalgia, either as primary treatment or within the broader context of CBT integrated within rehabilitation programs [182, 193]. Examples of prominent forms of biofeedback include electromyographic biofeedback, in which patients, for example with tension headaches, are provided with information feedback to them from the physiological recordings and taught to manipulate the tension in their frontalis muscle (or other muscles, for example splenius captitis). Patients with migraine are provided with thermal

feedback. They are instructed to warm their hands using visual or auditory temperature biofeedback cues. Also, heart rate variability biofeedback demonstrated some preliminary results in relieving depression and pain and improving functioning in fibromyalgia patients [194].

Recently, "real-time" functional MRI (rtfMRI) has been used as a sophisticated source of biofeedback to train participants to control activation in the rostral anterior cingulate cortex (rACC). This brain region is reputedly involved in pain perception and regulation. When the participants deliberately induced changes in the rACC, there was a corresponding change in the perception of pain [195].

The actual mechanisms involved in the success of biofeedback are still unknown; however, a general sense of relaxation is an important feature of biofeedback. It is not clear whether the alteration of specific physiological parameters putatively associated with pain is the most important ingredient of biofeedback compared to the broader relaxation and sense of control created.

Guided imagery

Guided imagery can be a useful method for helping people with pain to relax, achieve a sense of control, and distract themselves from pain and accompanying symptoms. This modality involves the generation of different mental images, evoked either by oneself or with the help of the practitioner. It overlaps with different relaxation techniques and hypnosis. Although guided imagery has been advocated as a stand-alone intervention to reduce pre-surgical anxiety and post-surgical pain, and to accelerate healing [196], it is most often used in conjunction with other treatment interventions such as relaxation and within the context of CBT.

With guided imagery, using the capacities of visualization or imagination, people are asked to evoke specific images that they find pleasant and engaging. In this way, a detailed representation that is tailored to the person can then be created. When patients with chronic pain are feeling pain or are experiencing pain exacerbation, they can use imagery with the goals to redirect their attention away from their pain and achieve a psychophysiological state of relaxation.

The most successful images involve all of the senses (vision, sound, touch, smell, and taste). Some people, however, may have difficulty generating images and may find it helpful to listen to a taped description or purchase a poster that they can focus their attention upon as a way of assisting their imagination.

Hypnosis

Hypnosis has been defined as a natural state of aroused attentive focal concentration coupled with a relative suspension of peripheral awareness. There are three central components in hypnosis: (1) absorption, or the intense involvement in the central object of concentration; (2) dissociation, where experiences that would commonly be experienced consciously occur outside of conscious awareness; (3) suggestibility, in which persons are more likely to accept outside input without cognitive censoring or criticism [197].

Hypnosis has been used as a treatment intervention for pain control at least since the 1850s. It has been shown to be beneficial in relieving pain for people with headache, burn injury, arthritis, cancer, and chronic back pain [198–200]. As with relaxation techniques, imagery, and biofeedback, hypnosis is rarely used alone in chronic pain although it has been used as a solo psychological model with some success with cancer patients [201]: practitioners often use it concurrently with other treatment interventions.

A meta-analysis suggests an overall benefit of the addition of hypnosis to non-hypnotic pain management strategies, although this may be mediated by a person's level of hypnotic suggestibility [199]. Furthermore, there are discrepancies in the literature with regard to the methods used to induce hypnosis, making it difficult to accurately evaluate the efficacy of this intervention [201]. Based on systematic reviews, Patterson and Jensen suggested that hypnosis has more utility in the treatment of acute pain than chronic pain [198, 200]. Thus, the degree to which hypnosis is effective above and beyond other interventions and for which populations is yet to be determined.

The techniques and modalities described can be readily integrated with more comprehensive rehabilitation programs. They can be useful complements to physical therapy, medication management, and rehabilitation by providing patients with something that they can do when pain flares up as well as being a routine part of a self-management program. They convey a sense of hopefulness as an antidote to the more common feelings of helplessness and dependency.

Efficacy of psychological approaches

The first reported trial of behavioral treatment for chronic pain was published by Fordyce, Fowler, Lehmann, and deLateur in 1968 [202]. Since that initial publication, there have been a large number of clinical trials evaluating the efficacy of various psychological treatment approaches and modalities (e.g., cognitive-behavioral therapy, biofeedback, hypnosis) for chronic pain. Psychoeducational and multidisciplinary pain management approaches often incorporate some combination of psychological treatments based on behavioral principles within comprehensive rehabilitation programs.

In early studies, the questions that most interested researchers and practitioners were whether behavioral approaches was effective, and if the efficacy of these treatments was comparable to other therapeutic options. Although there was at first a lack of well-controlled randomized clinical trials (RCTs) or dismantling studies, and the meta-analytic techniques used needed refinement, the clinical outcomes always tended to support the utility of psychological approaches and treatment modalities [155, 203]. Although only modest improvements in pain-related outcomes were observed, analgesic medication use, physical incapacity, and healthcare utilization, and disability rates showed marked reductions [204–206].

With the basic questions of efficacy addressed, increased availability of RCTs, and refined meta-analytic techniques, research began focusing on variables that influence outcomes or that change with treatment. Several meta-analyses [207, 208]; Campbell *et al.* reviewed the evidence of the effectiveness of the psychological treatments with samples of chronic pain patients with diverse patient samples [92, 204, 205]. The results of these meta-analyses with adult patients came to somewhat similar conclusions – as a group, psychological treatments have modest benefits on improving pain, physical, and emotional functioning. For example, van Tulder *et al.* concluded that behavioral treatments, as compared to placebo or wait-list control, were moderately effective for low back pain intensity in over half of the studies they reviewed [209]; however, the evidence was inconclusive regarding which behavioral technique was more effective as compared to another, and there was weak evidence that they were more effective when compared to usual care.

In the case of migraines, Campbell *et al.* concluded that all behavioral treatments (except hypnosis) were effective in the prevention of migraines and if used concomitantly with medications to augment relief [208]. The authors concluded that the evidence for hypnosis was incomplete. Nestoruic and Martin also found that all biofeedback methods were effective for chronic headaches [210]. Moderators (factors that affect outcome but are not part of the treatment process) for follow-up outcomes included headache years, study validity and treatment setting. Based on the outcomes of published studies of treatment of children and adolescents with chronic headache, Eccleston, *et al.* determined that there was strong evidence that behavioral treatments were effective in reducing severity and frequency of chronic headache pain [211]; however, the data was insufficient regarding mood, function, or disability, and there was a non-significant trend in favor of behavioral treatments used for abdominal pain.

Recently, Turner *et al.* found that the mediators of improvement in pain and activity 1 year following CBT were cognitive variables including patients' perceptions of control, disability, self-efficacy, harm, and catastrophizing, and rumination [212]. They also found moderators that predicted therapeutic change were number of pain sites, depression, somatization, rumination, catastrophizing, and stress existing before treatment. These data confirm the need to address psychosocial as well as physical aspects of the chronic pain experience, to obtain positive results, even in the absence of cure.

It is important to acknowledge that the modest reduction in pain severity obtained with psychological interventions and with comprehensive rehabilitation studies observed in the various meta-analyses were comparable to those observed with more traditional pharmacological and procedural treatment modalities [213]. This observation suggests that none of the most commonly prescribed treatment regimens, by themselves, are sufficient to eliminate pain and to have a major impact on physical and emotional functioning. This is hardly surprising given the complexity of chronic pain. A more realistic approach will likely be one that combines pharmacologic, physical, and psychological components, with the balance among these being tailored to individual patients' needs. As one author opined in an editorial regarding combinations of treatment for chronic pain, "Sometimes 1 + 1 does = 3" [214].

Novel treatment techniques are being proposed that target the central mechanisms involved in pain processing. deCharms *et al.* recently demonstrated in a clinical experiment that in a similar fashion to biofeedback, individuals could learn to voluntarily control the activation of various brain regions involved in pain processing, following real-time imaging feedback [195]. The ability to impact the activation of these brain regions was positively related to reported pain reductions, suggesting this could be a useful tool in helping train chronic pain patients to manage their pain.

Although we have described a number of cognitive and behavioral techniques as if they are "stand alone" treatments, and they may be for problems such as headache, many of these are combined within multidisciplinary rehabilitation programs that include physical and occupational therapy, medication management, and education along with the psychological approaches described. The efficacy of these rehabilitation programs have been well established in numerous meta-analyses [92, 155, 207].

Summary and conclusion

The variability of patients' responses to nociceptive stimuli and treatment is somewhat more understandable when we consider that pain is a personal experience influenced by attention, meaning of the situation, and prior learning history as well as physical pathology. In the majority of cases, biomedical factors appear to instigate the initial report of pain. Over time, however, secondary problems associated with deconditioning may exacerbate and serve to maintain the problem. Inactivity leads to increased focus on and preoccupation with the body and pain, and these cognitive-attentional changes increase the likelihood of misinterpreting symptoms, the overemphasis on symptoms, and the patient's self-perception as disabled. Reduction of activity, anger, fear of reinjury, pain, loss of compensation, and an environment that perhaps unwittingly supports the *pain patient role* can impede alleviation of pain, successful rehabilitation, reduction of disability, and improvement in adjustment.

Pain that persists over time should not be viewed as either solely physical or solely psychological. Rather, the experience of pain is a complex amalgam maintained by an interdependent set of biomedical, psychosocial, and behavioral factors, whose relationships are not static but evolve and change over time. The various interacting factors that affect a person with chronic pain suggest that the phenomenon is quite complex and requires a biopsychosocial perspective.

From the biopsychosocial perspective, each of these factors contributes to the experience of pain and the response to treatment. The interaction among the various factors is what produces the subjective experience of pain. There is a synergistic relationship whereby psychological and socio-environmental factors can modulate nociceptive stimulation and the response to treatment. In turn, nociceptive stimulation can influence patients' appraisals of their situation and the treatment, their mood states, and the ways they interact with significant others, including medical practitioners. An integrative, biopsychosocial model of chronic pain needs to incorporate the mutual interrelationships among physical, psychological, and social factors and the changes that occur among these relationships over time [1, 215]. A model and treatment approach that focuses on only one of these three core sets of factors will inevitably be incomplete.

References

1. Flor H, Birbaumer N, Turk DC. The psychobiology of chronic pain. *Adv Behav Res Ther* 1990; **12**: 47–84.

2. Melzack R. Casey KL. Sensory, motivational and central control determinants of pain: A new conceptual model. In *The Skin Senses*, ed. D Kenshalo. (Springfield, IL: Thomas, 1968), pp. 423–43.

3. Turk DC, Meichenbaum D, Genest M. *Pain and Behavioral Medicine: A cognitive-behavioral perspective* (New York: Guilford Press, 1983), p. 197.

4. Turk DC, Flor H. Chronic pain: A biobehavioral perspective. In *Psychosocial Factors in Pain. Critical perspectives*, eds. RJ Gatchel and DC Turk. (New York: Guilford Press, 1999), pp. 18–34.

5. Bandura A, O'Leary A, Taylor CB, Gauthier J, Gossard D. Perceived self-efficacy and pain control: Opioid and nonopioid mechanisms. *J Pers Soc Psychol* 1987; **53**: 563–71.

6. Flor H, Elbert T, Muhlnickel W, *et al.* Cortical reorganization and phantom phenomena in congenital and traumatic upper extremity amputees. *Exp Brain Res* 1998; **119**: 205–12.

7. Knost B, Flor H, Braun C, Birbaumer N. Cerebral processing of words and the development of chronic pain. *Psychophysiology* 1997; **34**: 474–81.

8. Bansevicius D, Westgaard RH, Jensen C. Mental stress of long duration: EMG activity, perceived tension, fatigue, and pain development in pain-free subjects. *Headache* 1997; **37**: 499–510.

9. Rainville P, Bao QVH, Chretien P. Pain-related emotions modulate experimental pain perception and autonomic responses. *Pain* 2005; **228**: 306–18.

10. Crook J, Weir R, Tunks E. An epidemiologic follow-up survey of persistent pain sufferers in a group family practice and specialty pain clinic. *Pain* 1989; **36**: 49–61.

11. Haggard H. *Devils, Drugs, and Doctors* (New York: Harper, 1929).

12. Power L. Placebos and medical research. *San Francisco Chronicle*, March 15, 1978, p. 24.

13. Price DD, Finniss DG, Benedetti F. A comprehensive review of the placebo effect: Recent advances and current thought. *Annu Rev Psychol* 2008; **59**: 565–90.

14. Benedetti F. How the doctor's words affect the patient's brain. *Eval Health Prof* 2002; **25**: 369–86.

15. Fitzpatrick RM, Hopkins AP, Harvard-Watts O. Social dimensions of healing: A longitudinal study of outcomes of medical management of headaches. *Soc Sci Med* 1983; **17**: 501–510.

16. Blanchard EB. Long-term effects of behavioral treatment of chronic headache. *Behav Ther* 1987; **18**: 375–85.

17. Holroyd KA, Penzien DB, Hursey KG, *et al.* Change mechanisms in EMG biofeedback training: Cognitive changes underlying improvements in tension headache. *J Consult Clin Psychol* 1984; **52**: 1039–53.

18. Deyo RA, Walsh NE, Martin D. A controlled trial of transcutaneous electrical nerve stimulation (TENS) and exercise for chronic low back pain. *N Engl J Med* 1990; **322**: 1627–34.

19. Beecher HK. Surgery as placebo: Quantitative study of bias. *JAMA* 1961, **176**; 1102–07.

20. Van Wijk RMAW, Geurts JWM, Wynne JJ, *et al.* Radiofrequency denervation of lumbar facet joints in the treatment of chronic low back pain. A randomized, double-blind, sham lesion-controlled trial. *Clin J Pain* 2005; **21**: 335–44.

21. Turk DC. Fibromyalgia: A patient-oriented perspective. In *Psychosocial Aspects of Pain: A handbook for health care providers*, eds. RD Dworkin and WS Breitbart. (Seattle, WA: IASP Press, 2004), pp. 309–38.

22. Craggs JG, Price DD, Verne GN, Perlstein WM, Robinson MM. Functional brain interactions that serve cognitive-affective processing during pain and placebo analgesia. *NeuroImage* 2007; **38**: 720–29.

23. Mechanic D. Effects of psychological distress on perceptions of physical health and use of medical and psychiatric facilities. *J Hum Stress* 1978; **4**: 26–32.

24. Nerenz DR, Leventhal H. Self regulation theory in chronic illness. In *Coping with Chronic Illness*, eds. T Burish and LA Bradley. (Orlando: Academic Press, 1983), p. 1337.

25. Zborowski, M. *People in Pain* (San Francisco: Jossey-Bass, 1969).

26. Unruh AM. Gender variations in clinical pain experience. *Pain* 1996; **65**: 123–67.

27. Turk DC, Okifuji A, Scharff L. Assessment of older women with chronic pain. *J Women Aging* 1994; **6**: 25–42.

28. Turk DC, Okifuji A, Scharff L. Chronic pain and depression: Role of perceived impact and perceived control in different age cohorts. *Pain* 1995; **61**: 93–102.

29. Bandura A. *Principles of Behavior Modification* (New York: Holt, Rinehart, and Winston, 1969).

30. Bachanas PJ, Roberts MD. Factors affecting children's attitudes toward health care and responses to stressful medical procedures. *J Pediatr Psychol* 1995; **20**: 261–75.

31. McGrath PA, Hillier LM. A practical cognitive-behavioral approach for treating children's pain. In *Psychological Approaches to Pain Management. A practitioner's handbook*, 2nd edn, eds. DC Turk and RJ Gatchel. (New York: Guilford Press, 2002), pp. 534–52.

32. Fearon I, McGrath PJ, Achat H. 'Booboos': The study of everyday pain among young children. *Pain* 1996; **68**: 55–62.

33. Craig KD. Social modeling influences: Pain in context. In *The Psychology of Pain*, 2nd edn, ed. RA Sternbach. (New York: Raven Press, 1986), pp. 67–95.

34. Craig KD. Consequences of caring: Pain in human context. *Can Psychol* 1988; **28**: 311–21.

35. Schanberg LE, Keefe FJ, Lefebvre JC, Kredich DW, Gil KM. Social context of pain in children with juvenile primary fibromyalgia syndrome: Parental pain history and family environment. *Clin J Pain* 1998; **14**: 107–15.

36. Vaughan KB, Lanzetta JT. Vicarious instigation and conditioning of facial expressive and autonomic responses to a model's expressive display of pain. *J Pers Soc Psychol* 1980; **38**: 909–23.

37. Vaughan KB, Lanzetta JT. The effect of modification of expressive displays on vicarious emotional arousal. *J Exp Soc Psychol* 1981; **17**: 16–30.

38. Richard K. The occurrence of maladaptive health related behaviors and teacher related conduct problems in children of chronic low back pain patients. *J Behav Med* 1988; **11**: 107–16.

39. Collie J. *Malingering and Feigned Sickness* (London: Edward Arnold, 1913).

40. Fordyce WE. *Behavioral Methods for Chronic Pain and Illness* (St. Louis, MO: C.V. Mosby, 1976).

41. Doleys DM, Crocker M, Patton D. Response of patients with chronic pain to exercise quotas. *Phys Ther* 1982; **62**: 1112–15.

42. Thieme K, Spies C, Sinha P, Turk DC, Flor H. Predictors of pain behaviors in fibromyalgia syndrome patients. *Arthritis Care Res* 2005; **53**: 343–50.

43. Block AR, Kremer EF, Gaylor M. Behavioral treatment of chronic pain: Variables affecting treatment efficacy. *Pain* 1980; **8**: 367–75.

44. Romano JM, Turner JA, Friedman LS, *et al*. Sequential analysis of chronic pain behaviors and spouse responses. *J Consult Clin Psychol* 1992; **60**: 777–82.

45. Flor H, Kerns RD, Turk DC. The role of spouse reinforcement, perceived pain, and activity levels of chronic pain patients. *J Psychosom Res* 1987; **31**: 251–9.

46. Turk DC, Kerns RD, Rosenberg R. Effects of marital interaction on chronic pain and disability: Examining the down-side of social support. *Rehabil Psychol* 1992; **37**: 259–74.

47. Nicholas MK, Wilson PH, Goyen J. Operant-behavioural and cognitive-behavioral and cognitive-behavioral treatment for chronic back pain. *Behav Res Ther* 1991; **29**: 225–38.

48. Thieme K, Flor H, Turk DC. Psychological treatment in fibromyalgia syndrome: efficacy of operant behavioural and cognitive behavioural treatments. *Arthritis Res Ther* 2006; **8**: R121.

49. Vlaeyen JWS, Haazen IWCJ, Schuerman JA, *et al*. Behavioral rehabilitation of chronic low back pain – comparison of an operant, and operant cognitive treatment and an operant respondent treatment. *Br J Clin Psychol* 1995; **34**: 95–118.

50. Schmidt AJM. Cognitive factors in the performance of chronic low back pain patients. *J Psychosom Res* 1985a; **29**: 183–89.

51. Schmidt AJM. Performance level of chronic low back pain patients in different treadmill test conditions. *J Psychosom Res* 1985; **29**: 639–46.

52. Schmidt AJM, Gierlings REH, Peters ML. Environment and interoceptive influences on chronic low back pain behavior. *Pain* 1989; **38**: 137–43.

53. Turk DC, Flor H. Pain greater than pain behaviors: The utility and limitations of the pain behavior construct. *Pain* 1987; **31**: 277–95.

54. Kotarba JA. *Chronic Pain: Its social dimensions* (Beverly Hills, CA: Sage, 1983).

55. Turk DC, Okifuji A. Evaluating the role of physical, operant, cognitive, and affective factors in pain behavior in chronic pain patients. *Behav Modif* 1997; **21**: 259–80.

56. Gentry WD, Bernal GAA. Chronic pain. In *Behavioral Approaches to Medical Treatment*, eds. R Williams, WD

Gentry. (Cambridge, MA: Ballinger, 1977), pp. 171–82.

57. Fordyce WE, Shelton J, Dundore D. The modification of avoidance learning pain behaviors. *J Behav Med* 1982; **4**: 405–14.

58. Linton S. The relationship between activity and chronic back pain. *Pain* 1985; **21**: 289–94.

59. Lenthem J, Slade PO, Troup JPG, Bentley G. Outline of a fear-avoidance model of exaggerated pain perception. *Behav Res Ther* 1983; **21**: 401–8.

60. Vlaeyen JWS, Kole-Snijders AM, Boeren RGB, van Eek H. Fear of movement/(re)injury in chronic low back pain and its relation to behavioral performance. *Pain* 1995; **62**: 363–72.

61. Philips HC. Avoidance behaviour and its role in sustaining chronic pain. *Behav Res Ther* 1987; **25**: 273–9.

62. Rachman S, Arntz A. The overprediction and underprediction of pain. *Clin Psychol Rev* 1991; **11**: 339–56.

63. Rachman S, Lopatka C. Accurate and inaccurate predictions of pain. *Behav Res Ther* 1988; **26**: 291–6.

64. Vlaeyen JWS, de Jong J, Geilen M, Heuts PHTG, van Breukelen G. Graded exposure in vivo in the treatment of pain-related fear: A replicated single-case experimental design in four patients with chronic low back pain. *Behav Res Ther* 2001; **39**: 151–66.

65. Reesor KA, Craig K. Medically incongruent chronic pain: Physical limitations, suffering and ineffective coping. *Pain* 1988; **32**: 35–45.

66. Turk DC, Okifuji A. Perception of traumatic onset and compensation status: Impact on pain severity, emotional distress, and disability in chronic pain patients. *J Behav Med* 1996; **9**: 435–53.

67. Jensen MP, Turner JA, Romano JM, Karoly P. Coping with chronic pain: A critical review of the literature. *Pain* 1991; **47**: 249–83.

68. Turk DC, Rudy TE. Cognitive factors and persistent pain: A glimpse into Pandora's box. *Cognit Ther Res* 1992; **16**: 99–112.

69. Flor H, Turk DC. Chronic back pain and rheumatoid arthritis: Predicting pain and disability from cognitive variables. *J Behav Med* 1988; **11**: 251–65.

70. Jensen MP, Turner JA, Romano JM, Lawler BK. Relationship of pain-specific beliefs to chronic pain adjustment. *Pain* 1994; **57**: 301–9.

71. Tota-Faucette ME, Gil KM, Williams FJ, Goli V. Predictors of response to pain management treatment. The role of family environment and changes in cognitive processes. *Clin J Pain* 1993; **9**: 115–23.

72. Spiegel D, Bloom JR. Pain in metastatic breast cancer. *Cancer* 1983; **52**: 341–5.

73. Williams DA, Keefe FJ. Pain beliefs and the use of cognitive-behavioral coping strategies. *Pain* 1991, **46**: 185–90.

74. Williams DA, Thorn BE. An empirical assessment of pain beliefs. *Pain* 1989; **36**: 251–8.

75. Turk DC, Okifuji A, Starz TW, Sinclair JD. Effects of type of symptom onset on psychological distress and disability in fibromyalgia syndrome patients. *Pain* 1996; **68**: 423–30.

76. Cassell EJ. The nature of suffering and the goals of medicine. *N Engl J Med* 1982; **396**: 639–45.

77. Flor H, Turk DC, Birbaumer N. Assessment of stress-related psychophysiological responses in chronic pain patients. *J Consult Clin Psychol* 1985; **35**: 354–64.

78. Arntz A., Schmidt AJM. Perceived control and the experience of pain. In *Stress, Personal Control and Health,* eds. A Steptoe and A Appels. (Brussels-Luxembourg: Wiley, 1989), pp. 131–62.

79. Whitehead WE. Interoception. In *Psychophysiology of the Gastrointestinal Tract,* eds. R Holzl and WE Whitehead. (New York: Plenum, 1980), pp. 145–61.

80. Tunks E, Crook J, Norman G, Kalasher S. Tenderpoints in fibromyalgia. *Pain* 1988; **34**: 11–19.

81. Droste C, Roskamm H. Experimental pain measurement inpatients with asymptomatic myocardial ischemia. *J Am Coll Cardiol* 1983; **1**: 940–45.

82. Borgeat F, Hade B, Elie R, Larouche LM. Effects of voluntary muscle tension increases in tension headache. *Headache* 1984; **24**: 199–202.

83. Okifuji A, Turk DC. Fibromyalgia: Search for mechanisms and effective treatment. In *Psychosocial Factors in Pain: Critical perspectives,* eds. RJ Gatchel and DC Turk. (New York: Guilford Press, 1999), pp. 227–46.

84. Council JR, Ahern DK, Follick MJ, Kline CL. Expectancies and functional impairment in chronic low back pain. *Pain* 1988; **33**: 323–31.

85. Linton S J, Vlaeyen J W, Ostello R W. The back pain beliefs of health care providers: Are we fear-avoidant? *J Occup Rehabil* 2002; **12**: 223–32.

86. Von Korff M, Barlow W, Cherkin D, Deyo R A. Effects of practice style in managing back pain. *Ann Intern Med.* 1994; **121**, 187–95.

87. Schwartz DP, DeGood DE, Shutty MS. Direct assessment of beliefs and attitudes of chronic pain patients. *Arch Phys Med Rehabil* 1985; **66**: 806–9.

88. Newton CR, Barbaree HE. Cognitive changes accompanying headache treatment: The use of a thought-sampling procedure. *Cognit Ther Res* 1987; **11**, 635–52.

89. Holroyd KA, Andrasik F. Do the effects of cognitive therapy endure? A two-year follow-up of tension headache sufferers treated with cognitive therapy or biofeedback. *Cognit Ther Res* 1982; **6**: 325–33.

90. Nouwen A, Solinger JW. The effectiveness of EMG biofeedback training in low back pain. *Biofeedback Self-Regul* 1979; **4**: 103–11.

91. Flor H, Fydrich T, Turk DC. Efficacy of multidisciplinary pain treatment centers: A meta-analytic review. *Pain* 1992; **49**: 221–30.

92. Morley S, Eccleston C, Williams A. Systematic review and meta-analysis of randomized controlled trials of cognitive behaviour therapy and behaviour therapy for chronic pain in adults, excluding headache. *Pain* 1999; **80**: 1–13.

93. Jensen MP, Karoly P. Control beliefs, coping effort, and adjustment to chronic pain. *J Consult Clin Psychol* 1991; **59**: 431–8.

94. Wells N. Perceived control over pain: Relation to distress and disability. *Res Nursing Health* 1994; **17**: 295–302.

95. Leventhal H, Everhart D. Emotion, pain and physical illness. In *Emotion and Psychopathology,* ed. CE Izard. (New York: Plenum Press, 1979), pp. 263–99.

96. Turk DC, Rudy TE. Toward an empirically derived taxonomy of chronic pain patients: Integration of psychological assessment data. *J Consult Clin Psychol* 1988; **56**: 233–8.

97. Biedermann HJ, McGhie A, Monga TN, Shanks GL. Perceived and actual control in EMG treatment of back pain. *Behav Res Ther* 1987; **25**: 137–47.

98. Mizener D, Thomas M, Billings R. Cognitive changes of migraineurs receiving biofeedback training. *Headache* 1988; **28**: 339–43.

99. Bandura A. Self-efficacy: Toward a unifying theory of behavior change. *Psychological Review* 1977; **84**: 191–215.

100. Bandura A. Self-efficacy: Toward a unifying theory of behavioral change. *Psychol Rev* 1997; **84**: 191–215.

101. Dolce JJ, Crocker MF, Moletteire C, Doleys DM. Exercise quotas, anticipatory concern and self-efficacy expectancies in chronic pain: A preliminary report. *Pain* 1986; **24**: 365–75.

102. Litt MD. Self-efficacy and perceived control: cognitive mediators of pain tolerance. *J Pers Soc Psychol* 1988; **54**: 149–60.

103. Manning MM, Wright TL. Self-efficacy expectancies, outcome expectancies, and the persistence of pain control in childbirth. *J Pers Soc Psychol* 1983; **45**: 421–31.

104. Turner JA, Ersek M, Kemp C. Self-efficacy for managing pain is associated with disability, depression, and pain coping among retirement community residents with chronic pain. *J Pain* 2005; **6**: 471–9.

105. Cioffi D. Beyond attentional strategies: A cognitive-perceptual model of somatic interpretation. *Psychol Bull* 1991; **109**: 25–41.

106. Smith TW, Aberger EW, Follick MJ, Ahern DL. Cognitive distortion and psychological distress in chronic low back pain. *J Consult Clin Psychol* 1986a; **54**: 573–5.

107. Smith TW, Follick MJ, Ahern DL, Adams A. Cognitive distortion and disability in chronic low back pain. *Cognit Ther Res* 1986b; **10**: 201–10.

108. Smith TW, Peck JR, Milano RA, Ward JR. Helplessness and depression in rheumatoid arthritis. *Health Psychol* 1990; **9**: 377–89.

109. DeGood DE, Tait RC. Assessment of pain beliefs and pain coping. In *Handbook of Pain Assessment,* 2nd edn, eds. DC Turk and R Melzack. (New York: Guilford Press, 2001), pp. 320–45.

110. Keefe FJ, Caldwell DS, Williams DA, *et al.* Pain coping skills training in the management of osteoarthritis knee pain: A comparative approach. *Behav Ther* 1990; **21**: 49–62.

111. Keefe RJ, Caldwell DS, Williams DA, *et al.* Pain coping skills training in the management of osteoarthritis knee pain II. Follow-up results. *Behav Ther* 1990b; **21**: 435–47.

112. Sullivan MJL, Thorn B, Hatyhornthwaite JA, *et al.* Theoretical perspectives on the relationship between catastrophizing and pain. *Clin J Pain* 2001; **17**: 52–64.

113. Turner JA, Aaron LA. Pain-related catastrophizing: What is it? *Clin J Pain* 2001; **17**: 65–71.

114. Butler R, Damarin F, Beaulieu C, Schwebel A, Thorn BE. Assessing cognitive coping strategies for acute post-surgical pain. *Psychol Assess* 1989; **1**: 41–5.

115. Turner JA, Clancy S. Strategies for coping with chronic low back pain: Relationship to pain and disability. *Pain* 1986; **24**: 355–63.

116. Thorn BE, Pence LB, Ward LC, *et al.* A randomized clinical trial of targeted cognitive behavioral treatment to reduce catastrophizing in chronic headache sufferers. *J Pain* 2007; **8**: 938–49.

117. Keefe FJ, Brown GK, Wallston KS, Caldwell DS. Coping with rheumatoid arthritis pain. Catastrophizing as a maladaptive strategy. *Pain* 1989; **37**: 51–6.

118. Wolff B, Burns JW, Quartana PJ, *et al.* Pain catastrophizing, physiological indexes, and chronic

pain severity: tests of mediation and moderations models. *J Behav Med* 2008; **31**: 105–14.

119. Lawson K, Reesor KA, Keefe FJ, Turner JA. Dimensions of pain-related cognitive coping: Cross validation of the factor structure of the Coping Strategies Questionnaire. *Pain* 1990; **43**: 195–204.

120. Fernandez E, Turk DC. The utility of cognitive coping strategies for altering perception of pain: A meta-analysis. *Pain* 1989; **38**: 123–35.

121. Heyneman NE, Fremouw WJ, Gano D, Kirkland F, Heiden L. Individual differences in the effectiveness of different coping strategies. *Cognit Ther Res* 1990; **14**: 63–77.

122. Merskey H, Bogduk N. Classification of chronic pain. Description of chronic pain syndromes and definitions of pain terms. *Pain* 1986; Suppl. **3**: S1–S225.

123. Fernandez E, Turk DC. Sensory and affective components of pain: Separation and synthesis. *Psychol Bull* 1992; **112**: 205–17.

124. Banks SM, Kerns RD. Explaining high rates of depression in chronic pain: A diathesis-stress framework. *Psychol Bull* 1996; **119**: 95–110.

125. Turk DC, Salovey P. "Chronic pain as a variant of depressive disease": A critical reappraisal. *J Nerv Ment Dis* 1984; **172**: 398–404.

126. Okifuji A, Turk DC, Sherman JJ. Evaluation of the relationship between depression and fibromyalgia syndrome: Why aren't all patients depressed? *J Rheumatol* 2000; **27**: 212–9.

127. Vlaeyen JWS, Linton SJ. Fear-avoidance and its consequences in chronic musculoskeletal pain: A state of the art. *Pain* 2000; **85**: 317–32.

128. Feuerstein M, Beattie P. Biobehavioral factors affecting pain and disability in low back pain: Mechanisms and assessment. *Phys Ther* 1995; **75**: 267–9.

129. Vlaeyen JWS, Seelen HAM, Peters M, *et al.* Fear of movement/(re)injury and muscular reactivity in chronic low back pain patients: An experimental investigation. *Pain* 1999; **82**: 297–304.

130. McCracken LM, Gross RT, Sorg PJ, Edmands TA. Prediction of pain in patients with chronic low back pain: Effects of inaccurate prediction and pain-related anxiety. *Behav Res Ther* 1993; **31**: 647–52.

131. Crombez G, Vlaeyen JW, Heuts PH. Pain-related fear is more disabling than pain itself: Evidence on the role of pain-related fear in chronic back pain disability. *Pain* 1999; **80**: 329–39.

132. Crombez G, Vervaet L, Lysens R, Eelen P, Baeyerns F. Avoidance and confrontation of painful, back straining movements in chronic back pain patients. *Behav Modif* 1998; **22**: 62–77.

133. McCracken LM, Gross R T. The role of pain-related anxiety reduction in the outcome of multidisciplinary treatment for chronic low back pain: Preliminary results. *J Occup Rehabil* 1998; **8**: 179–89.

134. Aghabeigi B., Feinmann C., Harris M. Prevalence of post-traumatic stress disorder in Patients with chronic idiopathic facial pain. *Br J Oral Maxillofac Surg* 1992; **30**: 360–4.

135. Sherman J, Carlson C, Cordova M, Mager W, Studts J, Moesko M, Okeson J. Identification of posttraumatic stress disorder in orofacial pain patients. *J Dent Res* 1988; **77**: 111–7.

136. Sherman JJ, Turk DC, Okifuji A. Prevalence and impact of posttraumatic stress disorder (PTSD) symptoms on patients with fibromyalgia syndrome. *Clin J Pain* 2000; **16**: 212–9.

137. Geisser ME, Roth RS, Bachman JE, Eckert TA. The relationship between symptoms of post-traumatic stress disorder and pain, affective disturbance and disability among patients with accident and non-accident related pain *Pain* 1996; **66**: 207–14.

138. Schwartz L, Slater M, Birchler G, Atkinson JH. Depression in spouses of chronic pain patients: The role of pain and anger, and marital satisfaction. *Pain* 1991; **44**: 61–7.

139. Fernandez E, Turk DC. The scope and significance of anger in the experience of chronic pain. *Pain* 1995; **61**: 165–75.

140. Summers JD, Rapoff MA, Varghese G, Porter K, Palmer K. Psychological factors in chronic spinal cord injury pain. *Pain* 1992; **47**: 183–9.

141. Kerns RD, Rosenberg R, Jacob MC. Anger expression and chronic pain. *J Behav Med* 1994; **17**: 57–68.

142. Burns JW, Quartana PJ, Bruell S. Anger inhibition and pain conceptualizations, evidence, and new directions. *J Behav Med* 2008; **31**: 259–79.

143. Okifuji A, Turk DC, Curran SL. Anger in chronic pain: Investigation of anger targets and intensity. *J Psychosom Res* 1999; **61**: 771–80.

144. Burns JW. Anger management style and hostility: Predicting symptom-specific physiological reactivity among chronic low back pain patients. *J Behav Med* 1997; **20**: 505–22.

145. Blumer D, Heilbronn M. Chronic pain as a variant of depressive disease: The pain-prone disorder. *J Nerv Ment Dis* 1982; **170**: 381–406.

146. Weisberg JN, Keefe FJ. Personality, individual differences, and psychopthology in chronic pain. In *Psychosocial Factors in Pain: Critical perspectives,* eds.

RJ Gatchel and DC Turk. (New York: Guilford Press, 1999), pp. 56–73.

147. Reiss S, McNally RJ. The expectancy model of fear. In *Theoretical Issues in Behavior Therapy*, eds. S Reiss and RR Bootzin. (New York: Academic Press, 1985), pp. 107–21.

148. Asmundson GJG, Norton PJ, Norton GR. Beyond pain: The role of fear and avoidance in chronicity. *Clin Psychol Rev* 1999; **19**: 97–119.

149. Asmundson GJG, Norton GR. Anxiety sensitivity in patients with physically unexplained chronic back pain: A preliminary report. *Behav Res Ther* 1995; **33**: 771–7.

150. Asmundson GJG, Taylor S. Role of anxiety sensitivity in pain-related fear and avoidance. *J Behav Med* 1996; **19**: 577–86.

151. Linton SJ, Buer N, Vlaeyen JWS, Hellsing A-L. Are fear-avoidance beliefs related to the inception of an episode of back pain: A prospective study. *Psychol Health* 2000; **14**: 1051–9.

152. Turk DC. Combining somatic psychological treatments for chronic pain patients: Perhaps 1 +1 does = 3. [Editorial]. *Clin J Pain* 2001; **17**: 281–3.

153. Bradley LA, McKendree-Smith NL. Assessment of psychological status using interviews and self-report instruments. In *Handbook of Pain Assessment*, 2nd edn, eds. DC Turk and R Melzack. (New York: Guilford Press, 2001), pp. 292–319.

154. Bandura A, Taylor CB, Williams SL, Mefford IN, Barchas JD. Catecholamine secretion as a function of perceived coping self-efficacy. *J Consult Clin Psychol* 1985; **53**: 406–14.

155. Flor H, Birbaumer N, Schugens MM, Lutzenberger W. Symptom-specific psychophysiological responses in chronic pain patients. *Psychophysiology* 1992; **29**: 452–60.

156. Rimm DC, Litvak SB. Self-verbalizations and emotional arousal. *J Abnorm Psychol* 1969; **74**: 181–7.

157. Barber T, Hahn KW. Physiological and subjective responses to pain producing stimulation under hypnotically-suggested and waking-imagined "analgesia." *J Abnorm Soc Psychol* 1962; **65**: 411–8.

158. Jamner LD, Tursky B. Syndrome-specific descriptor profiling: A psychophysiological and psychophysical approach. *Health Psychol* 1987; **6**: 417–30.

159. Ciccone DS, Grzesiak RC. Cognitive dimensions of chronic pain. *Soc Sci Med* 1984; **19**: 1339–45.

160. Hatch JP, Prihoda TJ, Moore PJ, *et al.* A naturalistic study of the relationship among electromyographic activity, psychological stress, and pain in ambulatory tension-type headache patients and headache-free controls. *Psychosom Med* 1991; **53**: 576–84.

161. Novy DM. Psychological approaches for managing chronic pain. *J Psychopathol and Behav Assess* 2004; **26**: 279–88.

162. Toomey TC, Seville JL, Mann JD, Abashian SW, Grant JR. Relationship of sexual and physical abuse to pain description, coping, psychological distress, and health-care utilization in a chronic pain sample. *Clin J Pain* 1995; **11**: 307–15.

163. Frischenschlager O, Pucher I. Psychological management of pain. *Disabil Rehabil* 2002; **24**: 416–22.

164. Waddell G. A new clinical model for the treatment for low back pain. *Spine* 1987; **12**: 632–44.

165. Flor H, Turk DC, Scholz OB. Impact of chronic pain on the spouse: Marital, emotional and physical consequences. *J Psychosom Res* 1987; **31**: 63–71.

166. Martell BA, O'Connor PG, Kerns RD, *et al.* Systematic review: Opioid treatment for chronic back pain: Prevalence, efficacy, and association with addiction. *Ann Intern Med* 2007; **146**: 116–127.

167. Romano JM, Turner JA, Jensen MP, *et al.* Chronic pain patient-spouse behavioral interactions predict patient disability. *Pain* 1995; **63**: 353–60.

168. Thieme K, Gromnica-Ihle E, Flor H. Operant behavioral treatment of fibromyalgia: A controlled study. *Arthritis Rheum* 2003; **49**: 314–20.

169. Turk DC. Cognitive-behavioral approach to the treatment of chronic pain patients. *Regional Anesthesia Pain Med* 2003; **28**: 573–9.

170. Turk DC. Customizing treatment for chronic pain patients. Who, what and why. *Clin J Pain* 1990; **6**: 255–70.

171. McCracken LM, Turk DC. Behavioral and cognitive-behavioral treatment for chronic pain: Outcome, predictors of outcome, and treatment process. *Spine* 2002; **27**: 2564–73.

172. Turner-Stokes L, Erkeller-Yuksel F, Miler A, *et al.* Outpatient cognitive behavioral pain management programs: A randomized comparison of a group-based multidisciplinary versus an individual therapy model. *Arch Phys Med* Rehabil 2003; **84**: 781–8.

173. van Tulder MW, Koes B, Seitsalo S, Malmivaara A. Outcome of invasive treatment modalities on back pain and sciatica: An evidence-based review. *Eur Spine J* 2006; **15** Suppl 1: S82–92.

174. Turk DC. The potential of treatment matching for subgroups of patients with chronic pain: Lumping versus splitting. *Clin J Pain* 2005; **21**: 44–55; discussion 69–72.

175. Vlaeyen JW, Morley S. Cognitive-behavioral treatments for chronic pain: What works for whom? *Clin J Pain* 2005; **21**: 1–8.

176. Jensen MP, Nielson WR, Kerns RD. Toward the development of a motivational model of pain self-management. *J Pain* 2003; **4**: 477–92.

177. Kerns RD, Habib S. A critical review of the pain readiness to change model. *J Pain* 2004; **5**: 357–67.

178. Bandura A. *Self-efficacy: The exercise of control* (New York: W.H. Freeman, 1997).

179. Turk DC, Okifuji A, Skinner M. Assessment of the persons with persistent pain In *A Guide to Assessments that Work*, eds. K Hunsley and E Mash. (New York: Oxford Press, 2008), pp. 576–592.

180. Goleman DJ, Schwartz GE. Meditation as an intervention in stress reactivity. *J Consult Clin Psychol* 1976; **44**: 456–66.

181. Shapiro SL, Schwartz GE, Bonner G. Effects of mindfulness-based stress reduction on medical and premedical students. *J Behav Med* 1998; **21**: 581–99.

182. Astin JA, Shapiro SL, Eisenberg DM, Forys KL. Mind-body medicine: State of the science, implications for practice. *J Am Board Fam Pract* 2003; **16**: 131–47.

183. Kabat-Zinn J. An outpatient program in behavioral medicine for chronic pain patients based on the practice of mindfulness meditation: Theoretical considerations and preliminary results. *Gen Hosp Psychiatry* 1982; **4**: 33–47.

184. Kabat-Zinn J, Lipworth L, Burney R. The clinical use of mindfulness meditation for the self-regulation of chronic pain. *J Behav Med* 1985; **8**: 163–90.

185. Alexander CN, Robinson P, Orme-Johnson DW. The effects of transcendental meditation compared to other methods of relaxation and meditation in reducing risk factors, morbidity, and mortality. In *CIANS-ISBM Satellite Conference Symposium: Lifestyle changes in the prevention and treatment of disease.* (Hanover, Germany, 1992), pp. 243–63.

186. Astin JA. Stress reduction through mindfulness meditation. Effects on psychological asymptomatology, sense of control, and spiritual experiences. *Psychother Psychosom* 1997; **66**: 97–106.

187. Kabat-Zinn J. *Full Catastrophe Living* (New York: Delacorte Press, 1990).

188. Bonadonna R. Meditation's impact on chronic illness. *Holist Nurs Pract* 2003; **17**: 309–19.

189. Grossman P, Niemann L, Schmidt S, Wallch H. Mindfulness-based stress reduction and health benefits. A meta-analysis. *J Psychosom Res* 2004; **57**: 35–43.

190. Lazar SW, Kerr CE, Wasserman RH, *et al.* Meditation experience is associated with increased cortical thickness. *Neuroreport* 2005; **16**: 1893–97.

191. Lutz A, Greischar LL, Rawlings NB, Matthieu R, Davidson RJ. Long-term meditators self-induced high-amplitude gamma synchrony during mental practice. *Proc Natl Acad Sci U S A* 2004; **101**: 16369–73.

192. Adelman, EM. Mind-body intelligence: A new perspective integrating eastern and Western healing traditions. *Holist Nurs Pract* 2006; **20**: 147–51.

193. Seers K, Carroll D. Relaxation techniques for acute pain management: A systematic review. *J Adv Nursing* 1998; **27**: 466–75.

194. Hassett AL, Radvanski DC, Vaschillo EG, *et al.* A pilot study of the efficacy of heart rate variability (HRV) biofeedback in patients with fibromyalgia. *Appl Psychophysiol Biofeedback* 2007; **32**: 1–10.

195. deCharms RC, Maeda F, Glover GH, *et al.* Control over brain activation and pain learned by using real-time functional MRI. *Proc Natl Acad Sci USA* 2005; **102**: 1826–31.

196. Halpin LS, Speir AM, CapoBianco P, Barnett SD. Guided imagery in cardiac surgery. *Outcomes Manag* 2002; **6**: 132–37.

197. Spiegel D, Moore R. Imagery and hypnosis in the treatment of cancer patients. *Oncology (Williston Park)* 1997; **11**: 1179–89; discussion 1189–95.

198. Jensen MP, Patterson DR. Hypnotic treatment of chronic pain. *J Behav Med* 2006; **29**: 95–124.

199. Montgomery GH, DuHamel KN, Redd WH. A meta-analysis of hypnotically induced analgesia: How effective is hypnosis? *Int J Clin Exp Hypnosis* 2000; **48**: 138–53.

200. Patterson DR, Jensen MP. Hypnosis and clinical pain. *Psychol Bull* 2003; **129**: 495–521.

201. Pinnell CM, Covino NA. Empirical findings on the use of hypnosis in medicine: A critical review. *Int J Clin Exp Hypnosis* 2000; **48**: 170–194.

202. Fordyce W, Fowler R, Lehmann J, deLateur B. Some implications of learning in problems of chronic pain. *J Chron Dis* 1968; **21**: 179–90.

203. Fishbain DA, Cutler RB, Rosomoff HL, Steele-Rosomoff R. Pain facilities: A review of their effectiveness and selection criteria. *Curr Revi Pain* 1997; **1**: 107–15.

204. Holroyd KA, Penzien DB. Client variables and the behavioral treatment of recurrent tension headache: a meta-analytic review. *J Behav Med* 1986; **9**: 515–36.

205. Malone MD, Strube MJ. Meta-analysis of non-medical treatments for chronic pain. *Pain* 1988; **34**: 231–44.

206. Scheer SJ, Watanabe TK, Radack KL. Randomized controlled trials in industrial low back pain. Part 3. Subacute/chronic pain interventions. *Arch Phys Med Rehabil* 1997; **78**: 414–23.

207. Guzman J, Esmail R, Karjalainen K, *et al.* Multi-disciplinary rehabilitation for chronic low back pain: Systematic review. *BMJ* 2001; **322**: 1511–16.

208. Campbell JK, Penzien DB, Wall EM. Evidence-based guidelines for migraine headache: Behavioral and physical treatments. (The US Headache Consortium, 2002). www.aan.com.

209. van Tulder MW, Ostelo RWJG, Vlaeyen JWS, *et al.* Behavioral treatment for chronic low back pain (Cochrane review). In: The Cochrane Library, issue 3. Oxford: Update Software, 2002.

210. Nestoruic Y, Martin A. Efficacy of biofeedback for migraine: A meta-analysis. *Pain* 2007; **128**: 111–27.

211. Eccleston C, Morley S, Williams A, Yorke L, Mastroyannopoulou K. Systematic review of randomized controlled trials of psychological therapy for chronic pain in children and adolescents, with a subset meta-analysis of pain relief. *Pain* 2002; **99**: 157–65.

212. Turner J, Holtzman S, Mancl L. Mediators, moderators, and predictors of therapeutic change in cognitive-behavioral therapy for chronic pain. *Pain* 2007; **127**: 276–86.

213. Turk DC. Clinical effectiveness and cost effectiveness of treatments for chronic pain patients. *Clin J Pain* 2002; **18**: 355–65.

214. Turk DC. Physiological and psychological bases of pain. In *Handbook of Health Psychology,* eds. A Baum, T Revenson, and J Singer. (Hillsdale, NJ: Erlbaum, 2001), pp. 117–38.

215. Turk DC, Rudy TE. Persistent pain and the injured worker: Integrating biomedical, psychosocial, and behavioral factors. *J Occup Rehabil* 1991; **1**: 159–79.

4

Comprehensive pain assessment: the integration of biopsychosocial principles

John J. Sellinger, Stephanie C. Wallio, Elizabeth A. Clark and Robert D. Kerns

Pain is a complex subjective experience. Influential in its effects on many aspects of an individual's physical, psychological, and social functioning, the experience of pain is also subject to the influence of these same factors. Therefore, seeking to understand the experience of pain from a patient's perspective is not only central to understanding this subjective experience, but is also paramount to developing an adequate treatment plan that can address pain both directly and indirectly through interventions focused on these related areas of functioning. Among the key aspects of pain-related functioning that are typically cited in the scientific literature are psychological and emotional functioning, physical disability, quality of life, and social functioning. Inherent in these various domains is the need to employ a multidisciplinary approach to pain treatment, and from a comprehensive pain assessment emerges the guidance needed to tailor pain treatment in a way that will meet the unique needs of each patient.

This chapter will present a rationale for adopting and utilizing a multidisciplinary assessment of pain. Information will be provided to assist in the assessment of pain in special populations, and a variety of assessment instruments for use in multidisciplinary assessment will be reviewed. The use of these assessment strategies and approaches to enact effective treatment planning will be woven throughout the chapter, and suggestions for overcoming the challenges inherent in performing comprehensive pain assessment will be discussed.

Guiding principles in pain assessment

The inherent subjectivity of pain perception and reporting, coupled with a wide variety of biological,

psychological, and social factors that can contribute to the subjectivity of this experience, make it imperative that healthcare providers conduct a comprehensive assessment of not just the pain in isolation, but of the "person with pain." Inadequate pain assessment has been identified by physicians as the greatest obstacle to effective pain management [1], and adequate pain assessment requires sufficient focus on the biopsychosocial aspects of each patient's pain experience. To ensure adequate follow-up assessment of treatment effectiveness, documentation of pain evaluations in the medical record is also of great importance, though often not completed adequately [2].

One contemporary model of pain assessment grows out of the work of Melzack and Wall [3], and their delineation of the gate control theory of pain. This theory gives credence to the role of both efferent and afferent messages within the central nervous system, and more specifically, the ability of biological, psychological (i.e., cognitive, affective), and social factors to influence the flow of these messages to and from the pain processing centers in the brain. Earlier pain models were more mechanistic, suggesting that the experience of pain was perfectly correlated with the size and severity of physical damage to the body. These early theories failed to recognize the complexity of the mind-body interaction, and the manner in which the social context can impact this interaction to alter pain perception (for better or worse) [4]. By contrast, the gate control theory offers explanation for how two individuals with similar objective clinical findings can present with very different qualitative reports of pain severity and perceived disability. It is now recognized that pain has two component parts – somatic damage and perception of that damage. It is the perceptual aspect that is most susceptible to the influence of psychosocial variables, and it is often these variables that account for the diversity of

Behavioral and Psychopharmacologic Pain Management, ed. Michael H. Ebert and Robert D. Kerns. Published by Cambridge University Press. © Cambridge University Press 2011.

pain presentations in the presence or absence of comparable objective findings.

Use of the biopsychosocial perspective in pain assessment can help to highlight the sometimes conflicting relationship between the very components of this model. It is these discrepancies which can provide insight into potential strengths and weaknesses for pain coping. For example, some patients who present with significant clinical pathology may also present with stability in the psychosocial domains, while at the same time a patient with limited objective findings may present with elevated pain scores and significant deficits in psychosocial functioning. To treat the pain in both of these individuals, it is necessary to have an understanding of all three elements that make-up the "person with pain," as this knowledge will highlight the avenue(s) of treatment that will likely yield the most meaningful results.

Objectives of a comprehensive pain assessment

As many as 80% of healthcare visits are precipitated by pain [5], and the obvious objectives include reducing the patient's experience of pain and discomfort and improving functional capacity. It can be argued that comprehensive pain assessment is the cornerstone of effective pain care, and some have found that the routine use of comprehensive pain management strategies with difficult patient populations (e.g., patients with dementia) actually translates into improved pain intervention [6]. To guide your assessment of pain, it is important to keep in mind some important assessment objectives. First, a comprehensive pain assessment is best when it is multi-source. Although the patient's self-report is most important, additional information from family members, nurses, and other involved providers can only help to further clarify the pain presentation and inform the treatment plan. A second important objective in pain assessment is to remain vigilant of the emerging relationships between the biological, psychological, and social aspects of a patient's pain presentation. Sometimes these relationships will be obvious, such as when a patient makes a comment such as, "I have been much more irritable since this pain in my lower back started." This message provides insight into the patient's current ability to cope, but also into his emotional reactions that could be worsening the pain through added stress placed on the musculoskeletal system by resulting increases in muscle tension. However, keep in mind that sometimes the relationships are not as obvious, such as the cases of individuals who present as stoic and

not wanting to let on about the difficulties that they are having in various aspects of their life due to their pain. It is in clinical interactions such as this that input from a significant other or close family member can help to inform the pain assessment.

A third important objective of pain assessment involves treatment planning. By using a broad scope in the evaluation process, clinicians can develop a treatment plan that involves many levels. In the example above, the patient may benefit from opiate therapy, physical therapy, and assistance with relaxation training to help control the anger which may be further exacerbating his pain problem. A treatment plan that fails to incorporate any one of these options may run the risk of increasing patient and provider frustrations, and lead to a series of mid-treatment adjustments that may not get at the source of the problem. After all, a patient who has come to associate his anger with his pain may still continue to experience "pain" if his anger persists beyond the effective use of opiate therapy. It is imperative that clinicians involve the patient in treatment planning so as to help the patient to feel ownership over the plan, which increases the likelihood of the patient adhering to such a plan.

A fourth objective of a pain assessment is the identification of appropriate outcome assessment criterion. The Initiative on Methods, Measurement, and Pain Assessment in Clinical Trials (IMMPACT) group, which is composed of leading experts in the fields of pain assessment, treatment, and outcome measurement, has worked to develop a list of pain treatment outcome domains and clinical measures to assess each domain. The work of the IMMPACT group has focused on clinical trial outcomes, but their work can also assisted in the development of appropriate treatment outcomes for clinical practice [7]. It is important for patients to understand the outcome criteria that will be assessed, as the patient's input on those criteria will help to ensure that the goals and objectives of treatment are relevant to the patient. This can often be effectively achieved by simply asking the patient, "What are your goals for pain treatment?" In the case of chronic pain, patients quite often acknowledge that their pain will never completely disappear, and instead, they may have a goal of simply doing more than they currently feel capable of doing. Such a goal may not necessitate medication as a form of intervention, but rather, a trial of physical therapy or cognitive-behavioral therapy focused on coping skill development may be in order.

One final objective of a comprehensive pain assessment is patient education. This should involve educating patients about treatment options, all appropriate treatment recommendations, and about the inter-relatedness of the biopsychosocial components of pain. Patients become confused about why providers are asking about areas of their life that seem unrelated to pain, and this confusion an carry over to the subsequent treatment recommendations that are made to address their pain. Further, a set of comprehensive recommendations for pain treatment may include components that the patient does not understand. For example, the patient described above may not understand the relationship between a recommendation for relaxation training and his pain management. It is through educating the patient about the biopsychosocial model of pain management that a clinician can enhance a patient's willingness to engage in comprehensive pain treatment. It is also through education that clinicians can engage patients in the process of self-help that will carry the patient far beyond the short-term benefits of acute medical intervention.

Challenges to comprehensive pain assessment

A review of comprehensive pain assessment would be remiss without discussion of some of the challenges and barriers that are present in clinical practice. The roots of these challenges stem from several sources, including the clinician, the patient, the clinical environment, and the interaction of these factors. For clinicians, it is important to have an awareness of one's own attitudes and biases related to patients who present with chronic pain, as these attitudes and biases can influence the process of pain assessment and intervention. For example, frustration with the ongoing reports of pain from a patient who has no objective clinical findings suggestive of pain may lead a clinician to conclude that attending to the pain is only encouraging pain reports and medication seeking on the part of the patient. If a clinician does not remain mindful of the biopsychosocial model of pain, these types of thoughts and frustrations are likely to develop and subsequently impact pain care in a negative way. Other clinician barriers can include inadequate knowledge and experience with pain assessment and treatment, and failure to routinely assess and document changes in pain over time. To overcome these barriers, clinicians are encouraged to seek continuing education on pain assessment and treatment, consultation with colleagues, and implementation of a standardized assessment protocol that

incorporates a review of biological, psychological, and social factors germane to pain management.

On the other side of the clinical interaction, the patient may also present challenges to comprehensive pain assessment. Because of the subjective nature of pain, clinicians are forced to rely on self-reports of the pain experience provided by patients. This can be challenging when patients describe their pain using language that is unfamiliar to the clinician. For example, a patient may describe his or her pain using words and phrases that do not clearly indicate whether they are referring to right leg pain or to a pain that radiates into the right leg in a sequence that would suggest pathology in the lower back. To overcome this challenge, clinicians must exercise patience and ensure to ask appropriate questions to further tease apart the nature and quality of the pain that the patient is describing. It is also important to keep in mind the differences in the frames of reference that clinicians and patients use when managing pain, as these differences can present challenges and contribute to different expectations for treatment and outcome. For example, a new pain complaint may seem overwhelming for a patient, thus contributing to exaggerated reports and unrealistic expectations for treatment. For the clinician, this patient's pain presentation may appear routine in the context of the clinician's busy clinical schedule. If the clinician does not appreciate these different frames of reference, he or she will be challenged in effectively assessing and managing pain.

Other patient issues that may present challenges to comprehensive and accurate pain assessment include chemical dependency, diversion of pain medications, complex medical and psychiatric backgrounds, and language or cultural barriers. One additional challenge that can be easily overlooked is the tendency for patients to underreport the presence or severity of pain. This may be motivated by a wish to avoid acknowledging the possibility of a more serious medical condition, or out of concern for being perceived as a complainer or a "bad" patient. Many patients report fear of taking pain medications, and so underreporting the severity of pain may serve to avoid such medications. Some of these challenges can be overcome by using multisource assessment procedures, particularly from individuals who are familiar with the patient and who will be a source of support for them as they undergo treatment.

Finally, there are healthcare system issues that can present challenges to comprehensive pain assessment. Perhaps most significant is the brevity of the average clinical visit, coupled with the growing number of "clinical items" that must be covered during these visits. A recent study found that the average number of clinical items per visit has increased at a greater rate than the average duration of visits [8]. This is a growing challenge for comprehensive assessment of any condition, and pain is no exception. One strategy for addressing this issue is to incorporate assessment strategies that can be completed outside of the clinical encounter, such as questionnaires and clinical measures (described later). These instruments can inform the clinician about areas of functioning that should become the focus of the more comprehensive clinical interaction. The use of support staff (i.e., nurses, health technicians, and clerical staff) to administer and score these measures is a way of increasing efficiency. Another systems issue that can present challenges is limited resources, such as the lack of an interdisciplinary team or specialty care service relevant to pain assessment and treatment. If unable to advocate for additional services within their facility (i.e., psychologist, physical therapist, pharmacist), clinicians are encouraged to identify close relationships with providers in the local community who can provide consultation services that can contribute to a better understanding of complex patients with pain.

Components of comprehensive pain assessment

As previously stated, the essence of a comprehensive pain assessment involves the evaluation of the person with pain, and not the pain alone. To conduct this type of assessment, it is necessary for clinicians to examine the psychosocial context of the person who presents with pain, and to use this information to supplement the physical evaluation. One common fault in the application of the biopsychosocial perspective is the tendency for clinicians to assume that in the absence of physical pathology, a patient's pain must therefore be rooted in psychological factors [9]. This dichotomous interpretation does not represent the spirit of the biopsychosocial model of pain, and if allowed to persist, such an approach will likely result in failed interventions, patient dissatisfaction, and clinician frustration. The following sections offer guidance to clinicians in methods and instruments that can help in the development of a multimodal pain assessment protocol.

Biological/medical assessment

A comprehensive pain assessment should always be preceded by a pain screening, which should be a part of all healthcare visits. In the mid-1990s, the American Pain Society (APS) launched a campaign to establish pain as the "Fifth Vital Sign" to increase awareness of pain management among healthcare providers. This campaign led to adoption of pain as the fifth vital sign in pain management initiatives on the national, state, and local level. These initiatives direct that pain should be assessed each time the other vital signs (pulse, blood pressure, core temperature, and respiration) are measured. Assessing pain as a vital sign serves as a screening mechanism for the detection of unrelieved pain; it also ensures that pain can be assessed quickly and routinely during medical care. As healthcare providers are accustomed to responding to abnormal vital signs, assessing pain within this frame prompts the same quick response when the assessment is positive. Pain is distinctly different from the other vital signs in that patient self-report is the gold standard, and must be respected as valid. Physicians have reported that inadequate pain assessment is a significant barrier to effective pain management, and assessing pain as the fifth vital sign is the first step towards the goals of increasing pain detection and improving pain assessment and intervention.

The APS has also partnered with the Joint Commission on Accreditation of Healthcare Organizations (JCAHO) in developing new standards for pain assessment and treatment. These standards went into effect in 2001 and apply to ambulatory care facilities, behavioral healthcare facilities, healthcare networks, home care, hospitals, long-term care organizations, long-term care pharmacies, and managed behavioral healthcare organizations. In brief, JCAHO requires that healthcare organizations comply with the following pain-related standards [10]:

- Patients have the right to appropriate assessment and management of pain.
- Pain is assessed in all patients and a comprehensive assessment is completed when warranted.
- When identified, pain is treated or appropriate referrals for care are made.
- Pain is recorded in a way that facilitates repeated assessment and follow-up according to organizational criteria.
- Pain assessment and management is addressed during orientation for new staff, and staff competency in these areas is monitored.
- Policies and procedures are developed to support appropriate prescription or ordering of pain medications.

- Patients are provided with education about pain and pain management.
- Continuing care is provided based on assessment of the patient's needs at the time of discharge.
- Data are collected to monitor and improve pain management performance.

A complete and accurate assessment of pain through patient interview is one of the first actions following a positive report of pain. Because pain is a subjective experience, a thorough interview is necessary to understand each patient's unique experience of pain. Evaluating the patient's pain history and self-report of the impact and intensity of pain are components of the current major models of pain assessment and treatment as proposed by the APS, World Health Organization (WHO), and the Agency for Health Care Policy and Research (AHCPR). The following are key areas that should be addressed during a pain interview, along with specific questions to guide the assessment:

Location: Clearly identify the specific physical area(s) where the patient experiences pain. Is there more than one area? Are those areas separate or related? Does the pain radiate or extend to other areas?

Onset and pattern: Assess when and how the pain started, if it has changed over time, and the current frequency of pain. Was there a precipitating injury or event? How often does the pain occur and how long does it last?

Intensity of the pain: Use a rating scale appropriate to the patient's cognitive abilities and one that can be repeated by multiple healthcare providers interacting with the patient to assess the intensity of pain. Most commonly, a 0 to 10 numeric rating scale (NRS) (0 = no pain, 5 = moderate pain, 10 = worst pain possible) will be appropriate and feasible. Ask the patient to rate pain currently, at its worst, at its best, and on average. Other useful pain intensity measures include the visual analog scale (VAS), which is composed of a 10-cm line with the anchors "no pain" and "pain as bad as it could be." The patient places a mark on the line in a position that best reflects his or her pain intensity. A score is derived by measuring the distance from the "no pain" end of the line. This measure is slightly more cumbersome than the NRS, but it can be an effective tool for use with patients who have a difficult time providing a numerical rating for their pain. Another alternative is the verbal rating scale (VRS), which includes a list of pain description words ordered by level of intensity. Patients are asked to pick the word that best indicates their pain, and the corresponding score indicates pain intensity. This measure is easy to administer and score, but it can be difficult for people with language difficulties. One additional drawback is that the VRS may not include a descriptor that matches the patient's pain experience. The NRS, VAS, and the VRS are all valid measures of pain intensity, and each has demonstrated sensitivity to change in the context of pain treatment [11].

Description of pain: Ask the patient to describe how the pain feels and any other associated symptoms. If the patient is unable to provide descriptors, suggest possibilities such as "shooting," "throbbing," "burning," "tingling," or "tender." Does the pain feel superficial or deep? Is the pain constant or intermittent? Does it fluctuate in intensity? Assess associated symptoms which may result from pain including nausea, vomiting, weakness, or confusion.

Aggravating and relieving factors: Assess the factors that increase or decrease the patient's experience of pain. Offer possibilities such as sitting, lying down, standing, heat, cold, exercises, or movement.

Previous interventions: Patients may have tried numerous treatments or management techniques not reflected in the medical record. Assess for previous medical diagnostics and treatments such as imaging, medications, surgeries, or injections. Non-medical interventions might include physical therapy, occupational therapy, biofeedback, chiropractic care, massage therapy, psychological treatment, or use of equipment such as a transcutaneous electrical nerve stimulation unit. In addition, patients may have tried home intervention including the application of heat, cold, distraction through engagement in activities, exercises or stretching, over-the-counter medications, herbal supplements, or relaxation techniques. Assess the effectiveness of each intervention and any barriers to prior interventions (e.g., side effects from medication). This discussion allows for assessment of the patient's willingness to engage and expectations for effectiveness of future interventions as the pain management plan is developed and implemented.

Effects of pain: Pain can impact every facet of a patient's life. Therefore, it is important that clinicians assess the effect of pain on the patient's physical, psychological, and social functioning. Sleep and appetite are important, and often overlooked components of physical functioning. Psychological functioning includes concentration, motivation, or energy, and emotions such as depression or anxiety. Social functioning is a broad category encompassing lifestyle and activities (e.g., exercise and hobbies), personal relationships, work or school, activities of daily living (ADLs) including dressing, bathing, and toileting, and instrumental activities of daily living (IADLs) such as cleaning, cooking, and yard work. Also, assess the economic impact of pain including the patient's ability to work, the need for financial support such as Social Security Disability, or litigation or compensation related to their pain.

Patient's pain goals: Assessing the patient's goals related to pain will necessarily help guide the pain management plan. Areas for improvement may be comfortable and consistent sleep, comfortable movement, or a return to specific activities. In addition, use a rating scale to assess the level of pain the patient would find tolerable, which helps set a frame for assessing improvement or reduction in pain in the absence of total pain. At times, the patient's goals may differ from the provider's goals for treatment; if the patient's goals are not identified and addressed, decreased adherence and lack of treatment success may result. Such differences are important to address, as they will directly impact the criterion that will be selected for the purpose of assessing treatment effectiveness.

In conjunction with a patient interview, clinicians should perform a routine physical examination and diagnostic evaluation of the patient's signs and symptoms. Particular emphasis should be placed on the neurologic examination, especially in the context of head, neck, back, and leg pain. Attempts should be made to obtain medical records from other healthcare providers who have treated or performed diagnostic work-ups of the patient's pain. New diagnostic tests and imaging should be ordered to further assist in the process of differential diagnosis, and comparison of these findings to previous outcomes can inform conclusions about the progression of any organic pathology. Also important in the context of pain assessment is a review of other co-existing diseases or conditions. Certain conditions can serve to exacerbate pain, such as in the cases of obesity and musculoskeletal pain, or diabetes and peripheral neuropathy. However, it should be noted that the presence of chronic pain has also been shown to interfere with self-care and exacerbation of these same conditions [12, 13]. If such patterns become evident during the course of a pain assessment, they should be addressed with the patient and included in the pain care plan.

Behavioral assessment

Pain can negatively impact upon many important behaviors in which patients engage daily. The limitations in these behaviors can be traced back to several key factors, including the underlying organic pathology (e.g., bulging disc in lower back), the pain resulting from that pathology, and the patient's perception of his or her abilities and limitations (e.g., "I don't have the ability to perform any type of exercise"). It is often the case that patients will limit their behavior in the face of pain as a means of protecting themselves from further physical damage. Although this can be adaptive in the acute phase of pain, this approach becomes detrimental in the face of chronic pain. A comprehensive pain evaluation requires the assessment of current behaviors and physical disability. The following paper-and-pencil measures can assist with this assessment, and provide insight into a patient's perceptions of ability as it relates to his or her pain. More details on these and other related measures of functioning are also provided in the following chapter.

Pain Disability Index

The Pain Disability Index (PDI) is designed to assess pain-related interference in seven key areas of role functioning, including: life-support activity, self-care, occupation, social activity, family/home responsibilities, recreation, and sexual behaviour [14]. This is a brief and simple measure to complete and score. Patients are asked to respond to seven questions via Likert scale ranging from 0 (no disability) to 10 (total disability). The PDI is a psychometrically sound instrument with good internal consistency, test-retest reliability, and concurrent validity [15, 16].

Roland Morris Disability Questionnaire

The Roland Morris Disability Questionnaire (RMDQ) is a measure of physical disability that is specific to back pain [17]. Respondents are asked to read a set of 24 statements about their experience of back pain and select the items that are reflective of their experience (e.g., "I walk more slowly than usual because of pain"). The number of endorsed items is tallied, with scores ranging from 0 to 24. Higher scores indicate higher degrees of disability. The RMDQ has demonstrated good psychometric properties, including test-retest reliability, and concurrent validity when correlated with physician assessments of pain and physical disability [17]. Strengths of this measure include ease of administration and scoring, as well as ease of interpretation and incorporation of endorsed items into the evaluation that clinicians perform. One drawback may be the reduced reliability of this measure with patients who have limited reading ability.

The Brief Pain Inventory

The Brief Pain Inventory (BPI) is designed to measure pain intensity and interference [18]. The measure was originally developed for assessment of cancer pain, but it has subsequently been used to assess non-cancer pain as well. A short-form containing 15 items is available, and has been shown to be a reliable and valid measure for use with non-cancer pain samples, including those with low back pain and arthritis [19]. The BPI is responsive to change in the context of pain treatment, thus making it a good measure for assessment of treatment effectiveness. Additional benefits include the ease of administration and the limited amount of time needed to score and interpret the patient's responses.

Tampa Scale for Kinesiophobia

The Tampa Scale for Kinesiophobia (TSK) is utilized to assess fear of injury or re-injury due to physical movement or activity [20]. Fear is believed to be a significant contributor to perceived disability among patients suffering from painful conditions. The TSK provides 17 statements about a patient's behavior in the context of pain, to which they respond on a four-point scale ranging from "strongly disagree" to "strongly agree". Four items are negatively worded, and require reverse scoring. Psychometric work on the TSK has strongly supported a two-factor structure, including *activity avoidance* and *pathologic somatic focus*. The reliability of the TSK has been established (Cronbach's alpha = 0.84), and the validity of the measure has been established through significant correlations with measures of related constructs including pain catastrophizing, subjective disability, and fear-avoidance behavior [21]. Overall, the TSK is an easy measure to administer, score, and interpret, and the information gathered can

help to inform the clinical presentation and the establishment of a multimodal treatment plan.

Emotional functioning

Living in the context of a painful condition, be it acute or chronic, can have a dramatic impact on an individual's emotional functioning. Especially in the context of chronic pain, negative changes in emotional functioning can have a detrimental effect on one's use of effective pain coping mechanisms (i.e., staying active, engaging in pleasant and distracting activities). Negative mood can also contribute to negative thoughts about oneself (e.g., "I'm useless"), as well as to negative thought patterns (e.g., catastrophizing – "This pain will never get any better"). Studies that have experimentally induced negative mood have found that compared to subjects in whom a positive mood was induced, subjects in the negative mood induction condition had lower pain tolerance, higher ratings of pain intensity, and increased catastrophic thinking about pain. Similar findings have been found in studies focused on pain-related anxiety [22–24]. These findings, coupled with data which suggest higher incidence of depression in patients who have chronic pain, highlight the importance of assessing and treating mood changes in the context of pain treatment. The following paper-and-pencil measures are recommended for the assessment of mood in the context of a medical care setting. Additional details of these measures are provided in Chapter 7.

Beck Depression Inventory

The Beck Depression Inventory (BDI) and the BDI-II are widely used tools to assess the cognitive and behavioral aspects of depression [25]. Originally developed in 1961, the BDI underwent revisions in 1978 and 1996. The revisions involved refinement of items to limit redundancy, and a change to the time frame from which respondents were asked to reflect – from "right now" in the original version, to "during the last week, including today" in the later versions. The most recent revision (BDI-II) was designed to increase the consistency between the measure and the criteria for depression set forth by the Diagnostic and Statistical Manual for Mental Disorders (DSM-IV). The BDI consists of 21 items, which contain four statements about a particular symptom of depression (e.g., sleep). Each statement reflects increasing severity of that symptom, and they are scored from 0 (no symptom present) to 3 (highest level of that symptom). The BDI is easily scored, and a clear set of criteria are provided to translate the scores into a depression severity rating, ranging from *minimal* to *severe*. The BDI is appropriate for patients aged 13 and over, and it has been widely used in clinical and research settings. A compilation of psychometric investigations of this measure has revealed good reliability metrics of internal consistency and stability, as well as concurrent validity. The BDI has also been shown to be sensitive to change in the context of depression treatment [26]. Due to the BDI's assessment of several physical symptoms of depression (e.g., fatigue), there is a risk that elevated scores from patients who suffer from physical illness may inappropriately be interpreted as indicative of depression. However, the elevated score may simply be a reflection of the symptoms of the physical illness. Therefore, it is recommended that the BDI be interpreted in the context of the patient's medical conditions, and that items for which high scores were endorsed be followed-up with questioning to further elicit the nature of the symptoms (depression vs. physical illness, or both).

Geriatric Depression Scale

Assessment of depression in the context of a comprehensive pain assessment is appropriate for all patients, regardless of age. For this reason, alternatives to common measures such as the BDI need to be considered for older adults for whom physical health problems and declining cognitive function can serve to cloud the diagnostic picture for depression. The Geriatric Depression Scale (GDS) contains 30 items about various components of depression, and respondents indicate with a *yes* or *no* whether that statement reflects the way that they have felt over the past week [27]. A briefer 15-item version of the measure is also available. Compared to the BDI, the GDS is less focused on the somatic symptoms of depression that can often be the result of medial illness in a geriatric population, and not depression. At the time of release, the GDS was shown to have sound psychometric properties, including internal consistency (0.94) and split-half reliability (0.94). Validity was also established through correlation with other measures of depression, while discriminant validity has been demonstrated by the GDS's ability to discriminate between depressed and non-depressed individuals, including a group of elderly subjects with arthritis [27, 28].

Pain Anxiety Symptom Scale

The Pain Anxiety Symptom Scale (PASS) is a 53-item measure which assesses the cognitive, behavioral, and physiological aspects of pain-relevant fear [29]. Respondents rate the frequency of each symptom descriptor using a seven-point Likert scale ranging from 0 (never) to 6 (always). The PASS is composed of four subscales, including Fear of Pain, Cognitive Anxiety, Somatic Anxiety, and Escape Avoidance. The PASS has been found to have good internal consistency, with ratings from 0.81 to 0.94 for the subscales and the total score. The measure's predictive validity has also been demonstrated through its ability to predict nonspecific physical complaints in patients suffering from chronic pain [30]. Results of this measure can guide the patient-provider interaction by providing clinicians with insight into a patient's fears and anxieties which may be impacting his or her behavior in the context of chronic pain and pain self-management. A reassuring word from a clinician can often be helpful to alleviate fears and irrational thoughts that develop in response to chronic pain, and this measure can be helpful for eliciting such thoughts and related behaviors.

Spielberger State-Trait Anxiety Inventory

Anxious reactions in the context of pain are not uncommon, and can often lead to exaggerated responses and adverse reactions that can serve to increase the perception of pain. However, anxiety can also be a pre-existing condition in some patients. Distinguishing between a patient's anxious reactions to pain (state) and their baseline level of anxiety (trait) will be important when assessing pain, when interpreting a patient's reactions to pain and diagnostic feedback, and when planning a course for intervention. The Spielberger State-Trait Anxiety Inventory (STAI) is a useful measure to assess both state and trait anxiety [31]. It contains two 20-item self-report measures that ask respondents to indicate how much they agree or disagree with statements related to anxiety (e.g., "I feel calm"). The items are rated using a four-point scale of agreement, ranging from "not at all" to "very much so". One form of the measure asks respondents about their current state (state measure) and the other relates to frequency of such states (trait measure). The STAI is widely used in the context of pain research and clinical practice, it has good reliability and validity [32], and it has been shown to be sensitive to change in anxiety within the context of pain intervention [33].

McGill Pain Questionnaire (MPQ)

The full McGill Pain Questionnaire (MPQ) assesses pain quality, including the sensory, affective, evaluative, and miscellaneous components of pain [34]. The measure includes 78 pain adjectives, divided into 20 sets of related words to describe the pain experience. Each set is listed in order of intensity from lowest to highest, and the patient is asked to select one word from each set that best describes his or her pain, with the option of not selecting any words if none of the options match his or her pain experience. Scores for each domain are derived by adding the numerical values assigned to each of the selected descriptor words. This measure is widely used in research settings, and the validity of the scales from the MPQ has been established through correlations with related factors such as quality of life, pain medication use, and pain reduction in the context of treatment. Often used as a measure of pain intensity, the MPQ has been found to have greater utility as a measure of pain-related affect. The MPQ Affective subscale score has been shown to have strong correlations with other measures of psychological distress, thus lending validity to this component of the MPQ [35]. Due to its strength in measuring pain-related affect (vs. pain intensity), it is recommended that the MPQ be used in conjunction with other measures of pain intensity, such as the NRS or the VRS, in order to provide a more complete evaluation of both pain intensity and the affective component of pain.

Pain Discomfort Scale

The Pain Discomfort Scale (PDS) was designed to measure the negative affect that often occurs in the context of pain [36]. This is a brief 10-item questionnaire that asks respondents to rate statements about their pain and affect using a five-point Likert scale ranging from 0 ("this is very untrue for me") to 4 ("this is very true for me"). The PDS includes positively and negatively worded statements (e.g., "I never let the pain in my body affect my outlook on life" and "I am scared about the pain I feel", respectively). The positively worded items are reverse scored such that higher scores on the measure reflect higher levels of affective distress. The PDS has demonstrated good psychometric properties, including reliability in the form of internal consistency (coefficient alpha = 0.77) and test-retest reliability (correlation coefficients of 0.64 and 0.76 at 1-month and 4-month follow-ups, respectively). The validity of the PDS has been established through significant correlations with other measures of pain affect, including the BDI and the affective subscale of the MPQ. Investigation has also revealed that the PDS distinguishes pain-related affect from pain intensity, as demonstrated by non-significant correlations with pain intensity measures. The primary benefits of the PDS include the ease of administration and scoring, and the fact that it assesses a broader scope of

pain-related affect than other measures (e.g., annoyance, fear, helplessness, distress). A potential drawback is that the PDS has only been validated in the context of chronic pain, and therefore its suitability for use with acute pain is unknown [36].

Psychosocial functioning

Beyond emotional functioning lies the broader social context in which patients live, work, and play. An assessment of the impact of pain and related emotional status on these various domains of function is central to a comprehensive pain assessment. The cyclical relationship between pain, mood, and social/occupational functioning is central to a complete understanding of a patient. Without understanding the impact of a patient's pain on his or her ability to socialize, work, or maintain a reasonable quality of life, clinicians will set themselves up for failure as they seek to intervene to address that patient's pain – especially when that pain is chronic. Clinicians must seek to fit pain interventions into the patient's existing world, and so to understand that world and the patient's functioning within it will help to target appropriate areas for intervention in an effort to improve the patient's pain and their quality of life. The following measures are designed to assess the psychosocial functioning of patients who live with pain.

West Haven-Yale Multidimensional Pain Inventory

As its name implies, the West Haven-Yale Multidimensional Pain Inventory (WHYMPI) is a multidimensional inventory that is divided into three main sections which assess broad aspects of functioning – pain intensity and interference, social support, and daily activity [37]. Each of these sections contains scales that measure more specific constructs. For example, the first section of the WHYMPI is composed of scales which assess pain severity, pain interference across domains (work, family, social function), perceived support, self-control, and negative affect. The second section more closely assesses patient perceptions of support received from significant others, such as a spouse or close friend or relative. Specific scales in this section include perceptions of punishing responses (e.g., "expresses irritation at me"), solicitous responses (e.g., "takes over my chores"), or distracting responses (e.g., "tries to involve me in some activities"). The third section assesses the frequency with which a patient engages in common activities, including the broad categories of household chores, outdoor work, activities away from home, and social activities.

The WHYMPI is composed of 52 items, and for each item the respondent is asked to rate the relevance of the statement to his or her experience using a seven-point Likert scale. Scores are derived for each of the 12 subscales itemized above by dividing the relevant item scores by the total number of items. Higher scores reflect a greater strength of presence for each construct assessed, be it positive (e.g., life control) or negative (e.g., affective distress). In the section that assesses frequency of common activities, higher scores are indicative of higher engagement in each category of activity. The WHYMPI has demonstrated good reliability, with internal consistency estimates for all of the subscales ranging from 0.70 to 0.90. Test-retest reliability coefficients for the scales range from 0.62 to 0.91. The construct validity of the WHYMPI was established through correlation of the 12 subscales with related scales from other validated measures [37]. In addition to its strong psychometric properties, the WHYMPI is a straightforward and comprehensive measure that is easy to administer, score, and interpret. It is estimated to take 10–15 minutes to complete the WHYMPI, and so patients can be sent this measure in advance of their healthcare visit, or asked to complete the measure in the waiting room. The information gathered from this multidimensional measure will add tremendous depth to the clinical assessment of pain, and can help the clinician to focus the clinical interview on the strengths and weaknesses of a patient's psychosocial functioning.

The Medical Outcomes Study Short Form Health Survey (SF-36)

The Medical Outcomes Study Short Form Health Survey (SF-36) has been utilized extensively as a measure of both health status and health-related quality of life [38]. This is a self-report 36-item questionnaire that is composed of eight subscales that tap various psychosocial constructs, including General Health, Physical Function, Bodily Pain, Role Limitations – Physical, Role Limitations – Emotional, Social Functioning, Vitality, and Mental Health. Respondents indicate on a Likert scale the extent to which the question reflects their experience in terms of severity or frequency (e.g., "during the past 4 weeks, how much did pain interfere with your work?"). Each subscale yields a score ranging from 0 to 100, with higher scores reflecting better functioning. The eight subscales can be utilized to calculate a Physical and Mental composite score. The composite scores have been standardized to the US population with a mean score of 50 and a standard deviation of 10.

The subscales of the SF-36 have demonstrated reliability, with internal consistency estimates ranging from 0.62 to 0.94 and test-retest reliability coefficients ranging from 0.60 to 0.81 over a 2-week period [39]. The validity of the SF-36 has been demonstrated through correlations with other measures of similar constructs (i.e., Sickness Impact Profile, Duke Health Profile) [40]. Some concern has been raised about the sensitivity to change over time among the SF-36 subscales, but a recent investigation comparing the SF-36 to similar measures found the Physical Function, Social Functioning, and Bodily Pain subscales to be sensitive to change among patients with chronic pain [41]. The ease of administration, scoring, and interpretation, along with the established psychometrics and broad range of psychosocial assessment make the SF-36 a valuable tool to incorporate as part of a comprehensive pain assessment.

Millon Behavioral Health Inventory

The Millon Behavioral Health Inventory (MBHI) was designed to assess the psychological functioning of medically ill individuals, and to predict response and adherence to medical intervention given the individual's behavior style [42]. The measure consists of 150 true/false items, which make-up numerous scales under the following broad headings: style of interaction with medical staff, response to illness, and psychosocial stressors (e.g., social isolation). The normative sample for this measure is comprised of medically ill individuals, which makes the MBHI an attractive alternative to other measures which are normed on healthy individuals, or on individuals who are psychiatrically ill. The MBHI has demonstrated good reliability and validity, and though its use with pain samples is growing, there is evidence to support this measure's predictive validity in a rehabilitation pain setting [43].

Pain coping and beliefs

Two important constructs that are necessarily part of any comprehensive pain assessment are the patient's current pain coping strategies, and their beliefs about the pain they are experiencing. The process of pain coping can be quickly assessed through interview questions, such as, "What have you been able to do to reduce your pain?" Answers to such questions will often elicit common responses such as "rest" or "apply heat." But on occasion, responses will include imaginative and unique responses that will speak directly to the lengths to which a patient has gone to be proactive in his or her attempts to try and control their pain. On occasion, the question will elicit responses such as, "There is nothing I can do to relieve my pain." Such a response reflects the patient's current coping abilities, as well as their beliefs about the pain (e.g., "There's nothing I can do"). In such situations, the emotional reaction of hopelessness can be overcome by asking more pointed questions about possible coping mechanisms the patient may be using. Further guidance in this regard can be offered by the Chronic Pain Coping Inventory (CPCI) [44].

The CPCI contains 64 items that are designed to assess the extent to which an individual utilizes behavioral pain coping strategies. The measure is composed of three general categories of coping, and each contains several relevant subscales. The general categories include wellness-focused strategies (e.g., Exercise), illness-focused strategies (e.g., Guarding), and neutral strategies (e.g., Seeking Social Support). Respondents read about various coping strategies under each of these categories, and they are asked to indicate how many days over the past week that they utilized each strategy. The reliability of the scales of this measure has been demonstrated by internal consistency coefficients ranging from 0.74 to 0.91. The validity of the CPCI in the original publication of the measure was demonstrated through significant correlations between a patient version of the measure and a significant-other version, as well as through comparable trends in the correlation of both of these measures with related measures of activity, disability, and pain discomfort. Furthermore, the relationships between the CPCI and these other measures were in the predicted directions (e.g., illness-focused coping was positively correlated with dysfunction and negatively correlated with activity level) [44]. Further validation of the CPCI was demonstrated through correlations in the predicted directions with measures of depression, pain interference, activity level, disability, and pain severity [45]. As previously mentioned, there is a corresponding version of the CPCI for spouses or significant others, which can prove helpful for gathering a true picture of a patient's level of coping, or lack thereof, which may be inaccessible with self-report due to a patient's defensiveness or need to please the clinician.

The use of pain coping skills, such as the ones measured by the CPCI, are often heavily influenced by a patient's beliefs and attitudes about the pain they are experiencing. Likewise, pain beliefs will motivate treatment seeking, influence adherence to treatment recommendations (or lack thereof), and impact patient reports of treatment effectiveness. Therefore, it is important to incorporate an assessment of pain attitudes and beliefs into a comprehensive assessment, particularly if there is concern about the patient's attitudes or beliefs interfering with treatment outcome. To aid this assessment, the Survey of Pain Attitudes (SOPA) was developed [46]. The original SOPA was composed of five subscales, including beliefs about medical cure for pain (Medical Cure), belief in one's ability to control pain (Control), belief in appropriateness of solicitous responses from significant others (Solicitude), belief that one is disabled because of pain (Disability), and belief that a medical intervention exists to cure one's pain (Medical Cure). Two additional subscales were added to the measure, and include the belief in the relationship between pain and emotion (Emotion), and belief that pain indicates bodily damage that should be responded to with decreased physical activity to avoid further harm (Harm) [47]. The final scale is composed of 57 statements about the pain experience, and the patient is asked to indicate the extent to which the statement is true of their personal experience. Responses are provided on a five-point scale ranging from 0 ("this is very untrue for me") to 4 ("this is very true for me").

The internal consistency of the seven subscales of the SOPA is adequate, as evidenced by alpha coefficients ranging from 0.71 to 0.81. In addition, test-retest reliability of the subscales ranged from 0.63 to 0.68 over an average of 6 weeks [47]. The validity of the original SOPA was demonstrated via correlation with self-report measures of pain behavior and pain coping strategies. The test developers report that the majority (72%) of the hypothesized relationships between the SOPA and the self-report of pain behaviors and use of pain coping strategies were confirmed [46]. Subsequent work has also demonstrated strong correlations between the SOPA and treatment outcomes measures such as physical disability and emotional functioning. Given the ease of administration and scoring, the SOPA stands to offer good insight into a patient's pain beliefs and attitudes, and such information can readily inform the pain assessment and treatment planning process. A highly correlated 30-item short form of the SOPA is also available, which can reduce administration time without jeopardizing the validity or clinical utility of the original measure.

Readiness to engage in pain treatment

Pain treatment is conceptualized by many patients as involving primarily medication or other medically focused intervention. However, the widely accepted biopsychosocial conceptualization of pain prescribes that pain treatment take numerous forms, including patient-driven self-management. Because this is not always consistent with patient expectations for treatment, it is imperative that clinicians educate their patients about this multifaceted approach to pain management and address any questions or concerns that they might have. As clinicians move beyond assessment and into the development of a multi-step treatment plan, it is important that they have a sense of how ready a patient is to engage in pain treatment beyond just medication or medical intervention. For example, a clinician will want to know how inclined a patient is to adopt recommendations for pain self-management (i.e., relaxation training, behavior pacing).

The Multidimensional Pain Readiness to Change Questionnaire

Reflective of the complex matrix of factors that contribute to pain and its treatment, the Multidimensional Pain Readiness to Change Questionnaire (MPRCQ) assesses an individual's readiness to adopt nine specific pain coping strategies [48]. The specific strategies assessed include exercise, task persistence, relaxation, cognitive control, pacing, avoiding contingent rest, avoid asking for assistance, assertive communication, and proper body mechanics. The measure is composed of 46 items, which ask the patient to respond by indicating their readiness to change their current level of the stated activity. Responses are given using a six-point scale, ranging from 1 ("I don't plan to do this") to 6 ("I have been doing this for at least 6 months"). The initial validation of this measure yielded a two-factor structure, including Active Coping and Perseverance. The psychometric properties of the MPRCQ are strong. Alpha coefficients ranging from 0.70 to 0.93 reflect good internal consistency among the various subscales of the MPRCQ, and test-retest reliabilities were good to very good, ranging from 0.56 to 0.76. The validity of the MPRCQ was established through significant correlations between the subscales and related scales from the SOPA, which ranged from -0.55 to 0.51. The primary advantage of this measure is the breadth of coping skills that is assessed.

The Pain Stages of Change Questionnaire (PSOCQ) [49] is a related measure that assesses readiness to change. The PSOCQ predated the MPRCQ, and one limitation that was found with the PSOCQ is the fact that it offers a more global assessment of an individual's readiness to change. The PSOCQ rates an individuals' readiness to change according to four change stages dictated by the transtheoretical model of behavior change (precontemplation, contemplation, action, maintenance). The PSOCQ has been found to show appropriate change following intervention to increase self-management, but it was not shown to be a good predictor of such change pre-treatment. It has been argued that because pain management is so multifaceted, an individual could potentially be at different stages of change for different coping strategies (e.g., cognitive coping vs. increased physical activity). Because the PSOCQ is not designed to capture such differences across domains, the MPRCQ furthered the work of the PSOCQ by incorporating specific coping behaviors for which motivation could be separately assessed [50].

Summary of domain-specific assessment

The measures reviewed in the previous sections are not designed to be a full account of all of the measures available to assess the constructs discussed. Instead, these sections were designed to highlight the important elements of a comprehensive pain assessment, and to provide a sampling of some of the more widely used measures of these constructs. Many of the measures discussed, as well as others that can be found in the literature, are appropriate for use at various stages of the assessment and treatment process. The reader should consider pain evaluation as an ongoing process, and during that process new insights may develop as you work with a patient. These insights may be new ideas or new questions, and the measures discussed will help to provide further assessment that can address your ongoing questions, concerns, or working hypotheses. Therefore, if it is not practical to administer these various measures at the outset of your work with a patient, be familiar with the measures and the important constructs that they assess so that you can utilize them throughout the treatment process to inform your work as new questions and challenges arise.

Pain assessment in special populations

The difficult work of assessing and treating pain is further complicated when dealing with special populations. For example, many of the pain assessment strategies previously discussed require a certain degree of sophistication and cognitive capacity on the part of the patient. Thus, many of the measures described are not appropriate for use with children, the elderly, those with severe cognitive impairments, or non-verbal patients. However, despite these limitations, there exists an ethical obligation to assess and treat pain in all patients. It is this obligation that has motivated researchers and clinicians to develop pain assessment strategies for use with these special populations. The following sections will focus on some of the tools and techniques developed for pain assessment in each of these patient populations.

Assessment in children

There has been increasing focus on the assessment of pain in children. However, compared to adults, pain in children is generally not adequately recognized or treated, and many assessment tools lack sufficient evidence to determine effectiveness. Like adults, children are the best sources of information about their pain. Self-report should be used to assess pain in children whenever possible and appropriate. However, children present unique challenges in pain assessment including limited communication skills and assessment behavior such as a tendency to be drawn to the extreme ends of self-report scales. Assessment of pain in children ages three and older is addressed in this section; measurement of pain in infants presents unique needs and challenges and the reader is referred to the specific literature for recommendations (see the work of Herr and colleagues for a brief review and clinical practice recommendations [51]).

Self-report measures for acute pain

There are currently more than 30 pediatric self-report measures of pain intensity, however, only six have well-established reliability and validity. The majority of self-report and observational measures of pain in children were developed for acute post-operative or procedural pain due to the low prevalence of chronic pain in children. Appropriateness of a measurement instrument depends on the age and developmental stage of the child and individual child preference. Assessment of pain is most difficult in pre-school age children who lack the communication skills to appropriately describe their pain and use measurement instruments. The measures described here have adequate reliability and validity, generally for children 3 years of age or older (the reader is referred to the work of Stinson and colleagues for detailed information [52]).

Pieces of Hurt Tool

The Pieces of Hurt Tool (or Poker Chip Tool) consists of four red plastic poker chips representing "a little hurt" (1) to "the most hurt you could ever have" (4) [53]. Children are asked to select "how many pieces of hurt"

they have. The *Pieces of Hurt Tool* is most appropriate for pre-school aged children (3 and 4 years of age).

Faces Pain Scale – Revised

The Faces Pain Scale – Revised (FPS-R) uses six gender-neutral faces to depict pain on a scale from 0 to 10 [54]. It is recommended for acute or disease-related pain in children ages 4 to 12. For school-aged children (ages 8 to 12), the FPS-R or other face-based tools may be used in conjunction with a VAS, described below.

Wong-Baker FACES Pain Rating Scale

This six-point scale (0–5) provides verbal descriptions of pain from "no hurt" (0) to "hurts worst" (5) with corresponding facial expressions [55].

Oucher

This measure consists of two scales: a photographic faces scale and a 0–100 mm vertical numeric rating scale [56]. The six photographic faces are culturally appropriate (Caucasian, African American, and Hispanic) and scored 0 to 5. The numeric rating scale is scored 0 to 100.

Visual analog scales

Visual analog scales consist of a pre-measured vertical or horizontal line where the end-points represent the extreme limits of pain intensity. The child points to or marks a place on the line to represent their level of pain. A 100 mm scale is most commonly used with a score of 0 to 100. A VAS is most appropriate for school-aged children and adolescents (8 years of age and older). It should be noted that the 0 to 10 NRS commonly used with adults currently lacks psychometric studies for use with children and may be prone to bias or poor validity because of the lack of criteria for rating. Thus this type of scale is not recommended for use with children.

Behavioral observation measures for acute pain

Behavioral observation measurement of pain can be used to supplement self-report measures, particularly in young children (under age seven). Behavioral observation may be used exclusively with children who are under 5 years of age, too distressed to use a self-report measure, impaired in their cognitive or communication abilities, restricted due to procedural or treatment features (e.g., ventilation, bandages), or believed to be providing exaggerated or minimized self-report rating due to a variety of possible factors. The measures described below have been adequately researched and most have extensive reliability and validity data for children 1 year of age and older [57].

Face, Legs, Activity, Cry, Consolability

The Face, Legs, Activity, Cry, Consolability (FLACC) scale assesses pain behavior on a three-point scale (0–2) through observation of behaviors on five dimensions (face, legs, activity, crying, and consolability) [58]. This measure is appropriate for observation of pain while the child is in the hospital.

Children's Hospital of Eastern Ontario Pain Scale

The Children's Hospital of Eastern Ontario Pain Scale (CHEOPS) assesses pain through six behaviors (crying, facial expression, verbal expression, torso position, touch, and leg position) [59]. A score is generated by selecting from multiple descriptive criteria for each of these six behaviors.

Parent's Post-operative Pain Measure

The Parent's Post-operative Pain Measure (PPPM) questionnaire asks parents to report on changes to their child's usual behavior on a yes/no (0 or 1) scale [60]. This 15-item measure allows for observation of pain by the parents in the home and is the only measure recommended to be completed by parents.

COMFORT Scale

This scale measures six behavioral (facial tension, alertness, muscle tone, physical movement, respiration, calmness/agitation) and two physiological (heart rate and blood pressure change) dimensions on a five-point (1–5) scale [61]. This measure is appropriate for children on a ventilator or in critical care.

Measures of affective response to pain

Adolescent Pediatric Pain Tool

This instrument is similar to the McGill Pain Questionnaire (previously described), but is appropriate for children 8 years of age and older [62].

Procedure Behavior Checklist

The Procedure Behavior Checklist (PBCL) is an observational tool used to assess operationally-defined behavioral distress indicating pain and anxiety during procedure pain in children ages 1 year and older [63]. The PBCL has eight items measured on a five-point (1 to 5) scale indicating both occurrence and intensity.

Measures for chronic pain

Chronic or recurrent pain is much less common among children compared to adults. As a result, nearly all research examining this type of pain has been conducted with adolescents. Conditions resulting in chronic or recurrent pain in children include chronic headaches and sickle cell disease. The self-report measures previously described are appropriate for measuring chronic pain in children, although behavioral measures of pain are not recommended for assessing chronic pain intensity. There is also a need to measure pain over time by assessing information such as the number of pain-free days or days in which the pain does not reach a specified level. In addition, increased importance is placed on measuring facets of functioning affected by pain including physical, emotional, role functioning, and sleep (the reader is referred to the work of McGrath and colleagues [64] for specific instrument recommendations).

A pain diary is a useful tool for assessing chronic or recurrent pain and response to treatment in children and adolescents. Pain diaries assess pain using a VAS, NRS, or face-based scale, such as the previously described Wong-Baker FACES Pain Rating Scale, prospectively or retrospectively. Prospective completion and use of electronic recording formats when possible may improve reporting accuracy.

Scales for specific pain experiences (e.g., headache) are available. In addition, numerous measures exist to assess the many areas of functioning (e.g., emotional, social, school, sleep) impacted by chronic or recurrent pain in children and adolescents. Description of all available instruments is beyond the scope of this chapter. Readers are encouraged to identify and use these specific measures if applicable to their patient population (see McGrath and colleagues [64]).

Assessment in the elderly

The assessment of pain in the elderly is of both high importance and complexity. The percentage of adults over age 65 is growing, thus increasing the need for providers who are trained to work with this population. Compared to children and younger adults, older adults are at increased risk for chronic pain, often due to multiple clinical diagnoses such as musculoskeletal and neurological conditions. In addition, older adults are more likely to undergo medical tests or procedures which result in acute pain [65]. Sensory and cognitive impairments which may develop during later adulthood serve as a barrier to traditional assessment methods for pain. Consequently, older adults with cognitive impairment may be less likely to have their pain evaluated and treated compared to their cognitively intact peers. To compound this problem, pain can present itself as or exacerbate existing cognitive impairment through symptoms such as social withdrawal, confusion, or aggression.

Regardless of the measurement tactic, provider behavior can help result in an accurate assessment of pain. The provider should position his or her face in view of the patient, speak in a slow and normal tone of voice, aim to reduce extraneous noise and distractions, and allow adequate time for a response. In addition, written directions should be provided in an easy-to-read format with necessary adaptations for visual impairments. The provider should also ensure the patient has their usual aids (e.g., eyeglasses, hearing aids) to maximize comprehension [65]. Questions about current pain as opposed to past or average pain may also increase an elderly patient's ability to report accurately. Ideally, a provider will have information about a patient's baseline level of pain to better assess any acute or chronic changes. In addition, pain measurements should be made in consistent situations to reduce variations due to circumstances such as movement or position. Pain assessments completed while the patient is at rest are likely to be inaccurate as pain levels and indicators will increase during movement and providers are encouraged to ensure pain assessments are not taken solely while the patient is at rest.

Self-report measures of pain

As with children and adults, self-report of pain is the single best source of information about both acute and chronic pain in older adults, including adults with mild to moderate cognitive impairment. Self-report should be attempted with older adults with severe cognitive impairments, but clinical judgment about the validity of the report should be used. Many of the pain assessment guidelines and measures previously discussed are appropriate for the older adult population. In particular, a thorough pain interview, as described, should be conducted whenever possible, with input from family or caregivers as appropriate. In addition, the pain assessment measures recommended for use with the general adult population are appropriate for use with elderly adults who are cognitively intact.

Older adults tend to underreport pain due to a variety of factors including expectation that pain is a part of growing older or the fear that pain is an indication of serious illness. Elderly patients may also think of pain in alternative terms such as "hurt," "uncomfortable," or "sore." Providers should ask questions including these alternative terms and then the patient's preferred term should be used consistently in pain assessments [65]. In addition, providers should ask patients about recent changes in behavior or functional status that may signal the presence of pain.

Many of the unidimensional pain assessment measures previously described are appropriate for use with older adults, including VAS and NRS:

Faces Pain Scales (FPS), like the *Wong-Baker FACES Pain Rating Scale* [55] previously described, pairs facial expressions with corresponding verbal and numerical ratings of pain. Faces pain scales have been adapted to include older faces for the elderly patient population.

The Verbal Rating Scales (VRS) or *Verbal Descriptor Scales (VDS)* consists of verbal descriptions of pain for the patient to select. Examples include "no pain," "slight pain," "severe pain," or "pain as bad as it could be". Words may correspond to numerical ratings for recording and comparison purposes. Providers should be conscious of the patient's vocabulary and reading ability with using a VRS.

No single unidimensional self-report tool is appropriate for all older adults. The 0–10 numeric rating scale commonly used in medical settings is generally most familiar to older adults; however, elderly adults may also have a harder time completing this type of scale due to reduced abstract thinking ability. A verbal rating scale is generally well understood and preferred in this population resulting in a more sensitive and reliable assessment. Whichever tool is selected based on patient preferences and abilities, it should be used consistently across time and providers.

A pain diary is also a useful tool in this population for assessing pain intensity (using a self-report measure), mood, adherence and response to treatment, and impact on activities over time. Retrospective reporting should generally be avoided.

The American Geriatrics Society (AGS) has offered specific recommendations for pain assessment in older adults, including a suggestion to use a multidimensional tool when possible. Multidimensional tools provide the advantage of generally incorporating a unidimensional self-report pain assessment, components of a pain interview, and a brief assessment of functioning. The following brief multidimensional tools have adequate reliability and validity for use with older adults:

Brief Pain Inventory (BPI) [18]: As described earlier in this chapter, the BPI assesses severity of pain, impact of pain on daily functioning, location of pain, pain medications, and amount of pain relief in the past 24 hours or the past week through a variety of question formats and over 20 items. The BPI is also available in a short form with nine items.

Geriatric Pain Measure (GPM) [66]: This is a 24-item tool assessing pain intensity, pain with activity, and interference of pain. Most items are answered on a two-point (Yes/No) scale and two NRS items assessing current and average pain are included.

Pain Disability Index (PDI) [15]: As previously described in this chapter, this measure includes seven items rated on an 11-point scale (0 = no disability, 10 = worst disability). Items measure daily functioning such as recreation, social activity, and family/home responsibilities.

As in younger adults, correlates of pain and facets of psychosocial functioning such as depression and anxiety should be assessed in older adult patients with chronic pain. One scale specific to the geriatric population is the Geriatric Depression Scale (GDS) [27]. This scale measures depression through 30 items scored on a yes/no scale. It is also available in a 15-item short version. Numerous other measures are available to assess functioning, disability, coping, self-efficacy, pain beliefs, or disease-specific issues; a full review of these measures is beyond the scope of this chapter, though some appropriate for the general adult population, including older adults who can provide accurate self-report, were reviewed previously.

Behavioral observation measures of pain

Behavioral observation is the current primary source of information about pain in non-communicative or severely demented older adults. Some common pain behaviors in older adults have been identified by the AGS, and are listed in Table 4.1. In older adults, the inability to verbally report pain may result from dementia, delirium, or episodes of critical illness. While informative, these measures present challenges including the fact that behavioral changes may stem from many sources other than pain. In addition, physical limitations or changes in older adults may limit behavioral expressions of pain such as guarding, rubbing, or facial expressions. Research has suggested

Table 4.1 Common pain behaviors in cognitively impaired elderly patients

Facial expressions
Slight frown; sad, frightened face
Grimacing, wrinkled forehead, closed or tightened eyes
Any distorted expression
Rapid blinking
Verbalizations, vocalizations
Sighing, moaning, groaning
Grunting, chanting, calling out
Noisy breathing
Asking for help
Verbally abusive
Body movements
Rigid, tense body posture, guarding
Fidgeting
Increased pacing, rocking
Restricted movement
Gait or mobility changes
Changes in interpersonal interactions
Aggressive, combative, resisting care
Decreased social interactions
Socially inappropriate, disruptive
Withdrawn
Changes in activity patterns or routines
Refusing food, appetite change
Increase in rest periods
Sleep, rest pattern changes
Sudden cessation of common routines
Increased wandering
Mental status changes
Crying or tears
Increased confusion
Irritability or distress

Source: Ref. [67]

the behavioral observation tools can underestimate pain compared to patient self-report when available. Physiological changes (e.g., blood pressure, pulse rate, respiratory rate) may be useful for identifying acute pain but should not be used to assess chronic pain as these factors often remain stable in patient's experiencing long-lasting pain; however, the absence of these changes does not mean the absence of pain. Finally, these tools are most accurate compared to patient self-report when administered by providers trained to use the specific instrument.

Behavioral observation measures should be used as part of a larger pain assessment that includes evaluating the nature and underlying causes of pain, the impact of pain on the patient's functioning (e.g., sleep, mood, activities of daily living), and inclusion of the family and multidisciplinary providers in the completion of an assessment and treatment plan (see 'Pain assessment in the non-verbal patient' below).

Tremendous growth in this area of research has recently occurred and many behavioral measurement tools are still in the early stages of development and testing. All of these tools have some issues related to reliability and validity, and further revision and testing is recommended for each. Despite growing evidence to support a few measures, there is currently no standardized measure that is recommended for broad use. Behavioral observation tools with promising reliability and validity for use with older adults are described below. In addition, these measures are relatively brief and practical for use in clinical settings (see the work of Herr and colleagues [51] for a brief review).

Pain Assessment Checklist for Seniors with Limited Ability to Communicate

The Pain Assessment Checklist for Seniors with Limited Ability to Communicate (PACSLAC) instrument provides a checklist with 60 items in the domains of facial expressions, activity/body movement, social/personality mood, and other (e.g., physiological, eating, or sleeping changes, vocal behaviors) scored on a present/absent scale [68].

DOLUPLUS-2

This measure consists of ten items across the domains of somatic, psychomotor, and psychosocial reactions scored on a four-point (0–3) scale with behavioral descriptions for each level to assess pain intensity [69].

Pain Assessment in Advanced Dementia

Pain Assessment in Advanced Dementia (PAINAD) assesses pain intensity through five items (breathing, negative vocalizations, facial expression, body language, and consolability) on an 11-point (0–10) scale [81].

Checklist of Non-Verbal Pain Indicators

The Checklist of Non-Verbal Pain Indicators (CNPI) provides six items (vocalizations, facial grimacing or wincing, bracing, rubbing, restlessness, and vocal complaints), which are scored as present or absent at rest and with movement [70]. The CNPI is most appropriate in an acute care setting.

Non-Communicative Patient's Pain Assessment Instrument [71]

The Non-Communicative Patient's Pain Assessment Instrument (NOPPAIN) is completed by a caregiver while completing daily care activities with the patient [71]. Pain presence and intensity is assessed based on observation of pain (yes/no scale) during nine potential care activities, ratings of six pain behaviors each on a six-point numeric rating scale, identification of the location of pain, rating of the patient's highest level of pain on a six-point verbal rating scale, and self-report, if possible.

In summary, having multiple self-report and behavioral observation measures available provides the benefits of being able to accommodate patient preference, unique patient factors, and provider confidence to increase the frequency and accuracy of pain assessments. Overall, pain assessment in elderly adults requires time, patience, and creativity to adequately meet this important need.

Assessment in the non-verbal and cognitively impaired

The subjective response to pain is mediated by developmental and cognitive factors. Self-report measures are the "gold standard" to assess pain and require cognitive capacity. Most of the existing scales are designed for use with patients who can respond verbally to assessment commands, but the use of pointing may be an effective manner to solicit direct pain information when using scales such as the VAS, NRS, or FPS. Other ways to obtain feedback from non-verbal patients include asking them to move a specific body part (e.g., head, eyes, fingers, hand, arm, leg) or squeeze the health provider's hand to signal the presence of pain. With those unable to self-report, objective pain measures are utilized. These instruments evaluate a person's response to pain on one aspect (e.g., facial expression) or in multiple domains (e.g., facial expression and body movements) [72]. In any case, there is evidence that non-verbal expressions of pain as well as knowledge of baseline functioning without pain are critical components in assessment for non-verbal and cognitively impaired populations. That healthcare providers are sometimes unable to recognize pain in the non-verbal population portends the need for unique assessment encompassing multiple sources of information.

The American Society of Pain Management Nursing (ASPMN) has published recommendations for pain assessment in non-verbal patients [51]. These general recommendations are appropriate for patients who are non-communicative or have reduced verbal abilities due to advanced dementia, intubation, or unconsciousness.

The sequential recommendations begin with the use of the Hierarchy of Pain Assessment Techniques [73] as follows: obtain self-report if at all possible, investigate possible pathologies that could produce pain, observe for behaviors that may indicate pain, solicit report(s) from surrogate(s) (e.g., family or caregivers/medical staff who are familiar with the patient), and use analgesics to evaluate whether reductions in the behavioral indicators thought to be related to pain can be observed. A trial of analgesics is advised based on the theory that a change in behavior following initiation of the trial is related to improved pain control. An appropriate medication and dosage should be determined through estimating the anticipated level of pain based on the other components of the assessment. Attempting a trial before adjusting other medications may result in faster improvement and, if effective, may eliminate the need for other changes.

Competent professionals should use appropriate, reliable, and valid behavioral pain assessment tools to elicit the patient's pain experience. While the tools mentioned herein provide clinically relevant pain information, broad adoption of a specific measure has not yet been recommended. This area continues to undergo development including research on the potential impact of various environmental settings on samples of non-verbal and cognitively impaired patients.

With behavioral assessment tools, it is important to consider that the scores are providing evidence of pain presence, and they are not appropriate to compare with pain intensity or severity ratings. Worthy of note is that changes in physiologic measures (e.g., blood pressure, heart rate) are generally not specific enough to indicate the presence of pain vs. other sources of distress and, therefore, should not be used as primary resource information. Finally, pain assessment should be ongoing and recurring at regular intervals, and it should be individualized by using measures and indicators that are specific and appropriate. Physical conditions or common problems or procedures known to cause

pain should initiate an assessment and preventative intervention. In addition, the presence of pain should be attended to before a potentially exacerbating procedure, movement or transfers. These evaluations should be recorded and accessible to all providers.

Behavioral observation tools are generally not appropriate for use with patients who are unconscious, sedated, or paralyzed and cannot behaviorally respond to pain. In these situations, an assumption should be made that pain is present, rather than absent, depending on other components of the assessment (e.g., existing medical condition; observation of grimacing, rubbing a body part, moaning; physiological changes). If behavioral measures are appropriate, they must be suitable for the patient population and setting. The capacity to appropriately use a tool depends on several factors including the patient's ability to provide input, the provider's familiarity with the patient, the time and range of circumstances available for observation, and the specific questions of interest related to pain.

Factors to consider when selecting a behavioral observation tool include:

- Measurement of specific (e.g., vocalizations) vs. subtle (e.g., change in interpersonal interactions) behaviors – *Are individuals who would recognize subtle changes in the patient participating in the assessment?*
- Direct observation vs. surrogate report – *Are the providers who are completing the assessment able to directly observe the patient?*
- Pain presence vs. severity – *Are the providers interested in whether the patient is in pain or how much pain they are experiencing?*
- Sensitivity vs. specificity – *Are the providers concerned about over- or under-identifying pain in patients?*
- Screening vs. diagnostic certainty – *Are the providers interested in screening for the presence of pain or establishing the exact nature and cause of pain?*

Behavioral observation measures for use with pediatric or geriatric populations have been reviewed in previous sections. For adults who are non-verbal due to disease (e.g., cerebrovascular disease) or health procedures, cognitive impairment, or mental retardation, the measures described below are appropriate for use.

Behavioral Pain Scale

The Behavioral Pain Scale (BPS) consists of three items (facial expression, movements in upper limbs, and compliance with ventilation) scored on a four-point scale with behavioral descriptions for each level [74]. The scale, indicating pain presence and severity, is appropriate for critically ill patients who are sedated and on mechanical ventilation. The BPS has been shown to be internally consistent, with a reliability coefficient of 0.72. Validity was demonstrated by the change in BPS scores, and by the principal components factor analysis, which revealed a large first-factor accounting for 65% of the variance in pain expression. The BPS also exhibits excellent responsiveness to change in the context of intervention.

Critical-Care Pain Observation Tool

The Critical-Care Pain Observation Tool (CPOT) contains four items (facial expression, body movements, muscle tension, and compliance to ventilator or vocalizations) scored on a three-point (0–2) scale to record behavioral reactions [75]. This instrument reports pain presence and severity. Inter-rater reliability of the CPOT is shown with high intra-class correlation coefficients (0.80 to 0.93). Discriminant validity was supported with increases of the CPOT and physiologic indicators during turning, but stability of these during a non-painful medical procedure.

Behavioral Pain Rating Scale

The Behavioral Pain Rating Scale (BPRS) assesses four behavioral domains (restlessness, tense muscles, frowning/grimacing, and verbal response) on a scale from 0 to 3 indicating progressive increases in pain severity [76]. This instrument requires vocalization and distinct movements by the patient, which may limit its utility for certain non-communicative populations. The BPRS assesses for the presence and severity of pain.

PAIN algorithm

This measure establishes the rate of pain severity by evaluating the presence or absence of pain on six behavioral dimensions (facial expression, movement, posture, vocal sounds, pallor, and perspiration) and three physiological elements (heart rate, blood pressure, respiration) [77].

Pain Behavior Assessment Tool

The Pain Behavior Assessment Tool (PBAT) contains multiple descriptors on three domains (facial expressions, body movement, verbal responses) [78]. This instrument is based on the absence or presence of these pain descriptors relative to common hospital procedures which often cause pain. If the patient is physically limited (e.g., in a state of decreased consciousness or intubated), the health professional may need to make appropriate modifications in the assessment of verbal and movement responses.

The assessment measures for the non-verbal patient included heretofore are also appropriate for those with cognitive impairment, as they are not reliant on high levels of intellectual capacity. Self-report pain scales are preferred with cognitively impaired patients, although verbal or other interactive reports need to be interpreted within the idiosyncratic context. In addition to possible communication limitations, cognitively impaired individuals may inaccurately transform outgoing or incoming information about pain. Some may mimic pain behavior that they have seen demonstrated even when they are not in pain. There is also evidence for the severely cognitively impaired to have an excessively high threshold for pain. Others have shown a tendency toward slower and less accurate expression of pain. However, pain reliably leads to similar kinds of non-verbal sensory pain expression demonstrated by people without mental impairment (e.g., grimacing, moaning, rubbing the affected area).

Chronic pain is often a complication of traumatic brain injury, and alterations in the experience and expression of pain may result from associated cognitive impairment [79]. Due to resulting communication limitations, behavioral pain measures are often utilized. As discussed previously, pain assessed with observational scales necessarily focuses on affective aspects rather than sensory characteristics of pain. This dictates an emphasis on pain presence rather than quality or intensity.

Non-verbal expressions of pain may lead to misinterpretations particularly in the cognitively impaired patient. For example, two features of Parkinson's Disease, akathesia and facial rigidity, could be interpreted as more or less pain respectively. Therefore, in a cognitively impaired patient with Parkinson's Disease, these observable behaviors may not be specific to pain, and it may be difficult to determine the origin of the behavior due to the patient's intellectual ability. To further specify the observed behaviors as ones associated with pain, a noxious event may be introduced to compare observable change correlations with the timing of the episode [80], in essence controlling for the cognitive impairment.

Summary

It is the hope of these authors that the scope of this chapter is enough to convince the reader of the complexities of pain assessment. From the widely accepted gate control theory of pain comes the responsibility to incorporate the biological, psychological, and social components of a patient's experiences into the assessment of his or her pain. The old metaphor "we don't live in a bubble" could be just as easily applied to pain, which certainly does not occur in a bubble. Therefore, to assess and treat pain effectively clinicians must be aware of the many factors that both impact pain and are impacted by it. The challenges are real, and the resources for the average clinician are often limited. However, this chapter has hopefully helped the reader to realize that assessment of "the person with pain" can be achieved even with limited resources, particularly with the use of paper-and-pencil measures that do not have to take away from the efficiency of a clinical visit and do not take many resources to administer.

The field of pain care has come a long way in recognizing the multidimensional make-up of the pain experience. It is the responsibility of each clinician to continue this movement by avoiding the temptation to view pain as one-dimensional (physical), or as a dichotomous experience (physical or psychological). Instead, clinicians must recognize the intimate relationship between pain and factors such as mood, activity, social relations, quality of life, pain beliefs, and motivation for self-care. Once a clinician works these dimensions into the assessment process, it will become easier to understand why objective clinical findings are not the gold standard for assessing the presence or absence of pain. Clinicians must trust patient's self-reports, and seek to utilize many of the instruments described in this chapter to corroborate these reports and identify the avenues that are most appropriate for treatment. The subsequent chapters of this book will guide the reader through various approaches to pain treatment, and adherence to the assessment techniques and strategies advocated in this chapter will help to guide the clinician in selecting from these alternatives.

References

1. Von Roenn JH, Cleeland CS, Gonin R, Hatfield AK, Pandya KJ. Physician attitudes and practice in cancer pain management. A survey from the Eastern Cooperative Oncology Group. *Ann Intern Med* 1993; **119**: 121–6.

2. Chisholm CD, Weaver CS, Whenmouth LF, Giles B, Brizendine EJ. A comparison of observed versus documented physician assessment and treatment of pain: the physician record does not reflect the reality. *Ann Emerg Med* 2008; **52**: 383–9.

3. Melzack R, Wall PD. Pain mechanisms: a new theory. *Science* 1965; **150**: 971–9.

4. Melzack, R. Pain: past, present and future. *Can J Exp Psychol* 1993; **47**: 615–29.

5. Gatchel, RJ, Turk, DC. *Psychological Approaches to Pain Management: A practitioner's handbook* (New York: Guilford Press, 1996).

6. Fuchs-Lacelle S, Hadjistavropoulos T, Lix L. Pain assessment as intervention: A study of older adults with severe dementia. *Clin J Pain* 2008; **24**: 697–707.

7. Dworkin RH, *et al*. Interpreting the clinical importance of treatment outcomes in chronic pain clinical trials: IMMPACT recommendations. *J Pain* 2008; **9**: 105–21.

8. Abbo ED, Zhang Q, Zelder M, Huang ES. The increasing number of clinical items addressed during the time of adult primary care visits. *J Gen Intern Med* 2008; **23**: 2058–65.

9. Turk, DC, Okifuji A. Assessment of patients' reporting of pain: an integrated perspective. *Lancet* 1999; **353**: 1784–8.

10. Chapman, CR, New Joint Commission standards for pain management: Carpe diem. *APS Bulletin* 2000; **10**: 3.

11. Jensen, MP, Karoly, P. Self-report scales and procedures for assessing pain in adults. In *Handbook of Pain Assessment*, 2nd edn, eds. DC Turk and R Melzack. (New York: Guilford Press, 2001).

12. Verbunt JA, Seelen HA, Vlaeyen JW, *et al*. The effect of chronic pain on diabetes patients' self-management. *Diabetes Care* 2005; **28**: 65–70.

13. Verbunt JA, Seelen HA, Vlaeyen JW, *et al*. Disuse and deconditioning in chronic low back pain: Concepts and hypotheses on contributing mechanisms. *Eur J Pain* 2003: 7: 9–21.

14. Pollard, CA. Preliminary validity study of the pain disability index. *Percept Mot Skills* 1984; **59**: 974.

15. Tait, RC, Chibnall, JT, Krause, S. The Pain Disability Index: Psychometric properties. *Pain* 1990; **40**: 171–82.

16. Grönblad M, Järvinen E, Hurri H, Hupli M, Karaharju EO. Relationship of the Pain Disability Index (PDI) and the Oswestry Disability Questionnaire (ODQ) with three dynamic physical tests in a group of patients with chronic low-back and leg pain. *Clin J Pain* 1994; **10**: 197–203.

17. Roland, M, Morris, R. A study of the natural history of back pain. Part I: development of a reliable and sensitive measure of disability in low-back pain. *Spine*; 1983; **8**: 141–4.

18. Cleeland, CS, Ryan, KM. Pain assessment: Global use of the Brief Pain Inventory. *Ann Acad Med Singapore* 1994; **23**: 129–38.

19. Keller S, Bann CM, Dodd SL, *et al*. Validity of the brief pain inventory for use in documenting the outcomes of patients with noncancer pain. *Clin J Pain* 2004; **20**: 309–18.

20. Kori KS, Miller RP, Todd DD. Kinesiophobia: A new view of chronic pain behavior. *Pain Management* 1990; **3**: 35–43.

21. French DJ, France CR, Vigneau F, French JA, Evans RT. Fear of movement/(re)injury in chronic pain: A psychometric assessment of the original English version of the Tampa scale for kinesiophobia (TSK). *Pain* 2007; **127**: 42–51.

22. Willoughby SG, Hailey BJ, Mulkana S, Rowe J. The effect of laboratory-induced depressed mood state on responses to pain. *Behav Med* 2002; **28**: 23–31.

23. Alden AL, Dale JA, DeGood DE. Interactive effects of the affect quality and directional focus of mental imagery on pain analgesia. *Appl Psychophysiol Biofeedback* 2001; **26**: 117–26.

24. al Absi M, Rokke PD. Can anxiety help us tolerate pain? *Pain* 1991; **46**: 43–51.

25. Beck AT, Ward CH, Mendelson M, Mock J, Erbaugh J. An inventory for measuring depression. *Arch Gen Psychiatry* 1961; **4**: 561–71.

26. Beck AT, Steer, RA, Garbin, MG. Psychometric properties of the Beck Depression Inventory: Twenty-five years of evaluation. *Clin Psychol Rev* 1988; **8**: 77–100.

27. Yesavage JA, Brink TL, Rose TL, *et al*. Development and validation of a geriatric depression screening scale: a preliminary report. *J Psychiatr Res* 1982; **17**: 37–49.

28. Brink, TA, Yesavage, JA, Lum, O, *et al*. Screening tests for geriatric depression. *Clin Gerontologist* 1982; **1**: 37–43.

29. McCracken, LM, Zayfert C, Gross RT. The Pain Anxiety Symptoms Scale: development and validation of a scale to measure fear of pain. *Pain* 1992; **50**: 67–73.

30. McCracken, LM, Faber SD, Janeck AS. Pain-related anxiety predicts non-specific physical complaints in persons with chronic pain. *Behav Res Ther* 1998; **36**: 621–30.

31. Spielberger CD, Gorsuch, RL, Lushene R. *Manual for the State-Trait Anxiety Inventory* (Palo Alto: Consulting Psychologists Press, 1970).

32. Speilberger CD, Gorsuch, RL, Lushene R, Vagg PR, Jacobs, GA, *Manual for the State-Trait Anxiety Inventory (Form Y)* (Palo Alto: Consulting Psychologists Press, 1983).

33. Bradley LA, Young LD, Anderson KO, *et al*. Effects of psychological therapy on pain behavior of rheumatoid arthritis patients. Treatment outcome and six-month followup. *Arthritis Rheum* 1987; **30**: 1105–14.

34. Melzack R. The McGill Pain Questionnaire: Major properties and scoring methods. *Pain* 1975; **1**: 277–99.

35. Jensen MP. The validity and reliability of pain measures for use in clinical trials in adults. In *Initiative on Methods, Measurement, and Pain Assessment in Clincal Trials (IMMPACT)*. 2003.

36. Jensen MP, Karoly P, Harris P. Assessing the affective component of chronic pain: Development of the Pain Discomfort Scale. *J Psychosom Res* 1991; **35**: 149–54.

37. Kerns RD, Turk DC, Rudy TE. The West Haven-Yale Multidimensional Pain Inventory (WHYMPI). *Pain* 1985; **23**: 345–56.

38. Ware JE, Jr, Sherbourne CD. The MOS 36-item short-form health survey (SF-36). I. Conceptual framework and item selection. *Med Care* 1992; **30**: 473–83.

39. McHorney CA, Ware JE Jr, Lu JF, Sherbourne CD. The MOS 36-item Short-Form Health Survey (SF-36): III. Tests of data quality, scaling assumptions, and reliability across diverse patient groups. *Med Care* 1994; **32**: 40–66.

40. McHorney CA, Ware, JE Jr, Raczek AE. The MOS 36-Item Short-Form Health Survey (SF-36): II. Psychometric and clinical tests of validity in measuring physical and mental health constructs. *Med Care* 1993; **31**: 247–63.

41. Wittink H, Turk DC, Carr DB, Sukiennik A, Rogers W. Comparison of the redundancy, reliability, and responsiveness to change among SF-36, Oswestry Disability Index, and Multidimensional Pain Inventory. *Clin J Pain* 2004; **20**: 133–42.

42. Millon T, Green, CJ, Meagher R. *Millon Behavioral Health Inventory Manual*. 3rd edn. (Minneapolis: National Computer Systems, 1983).

43. Gatchel RJ, Mayer TG, Capra P, Barnett J, Diamond P. Millon Behavioral Health Inventory: Its utility in predicting physical function in patients with low back pain. *Arch Phys Med Rehabil* 1986; **67**: 878–82.

44. Jensen MP, Turner JA, Romano JM, Strom SE. The Chronic Pain Coping Inventory: Development and preliminary validation. *Pain* 1995; **60**: 203–16.

45. Tan G, Nguyen Q, Anderson KO, Jensen M, Thornby J. Further validation of the chronic pain coping inventory. *J Pain* 2005; **6**: 29–40.

46. Jensen MP, Karoly P, Huger R. The development and preliminary validation of an instrument to assess patients' attitudes toward pain. *J Psychosom Res* 1987; **31**: 393–400.

47. Jensen MP, Turner JA, Romano JM, Lawler BK. Relationship of pain-specific beliefs to chronic pain adjustment. *Pain* 1994; **57**: 301–9.

48. Nielson, WR, Jensen MP, Kerns RD. Initial development and validation of a multidimensional pain readiness to change questionnaire. *J Pain* 2003; **4**: 148–58.

49. Kerns RD, Rosenberg R, Jamison RN, Caudill MA, Haythornthwaite J. Readiness to adopt a self-management approach to chronic pain: The Pain Stages of Change Questionnaire (PSOCQ). *Pain* 1997; **72**: 227–34.

50. Kerns RD, Habib S. A critical review of the pain readiness to change model. *J Pain* 2004; **5**: 357–67.

51. Herr K, Coyne PJ, Key T, *et al.* Pain assessment in the nonverbal patient: Position statement with clinical practice recommendations. *Pain Manag Nurs* 2006; **7**: 44–52.

52. Stinson JN, Kavanagh T, Yamada J, Gill N, Stevens B. Systematic review of the psychometric properties, interpretability and feasibility of self-report pain intensity measures for use in clinical trials in children and adolescents. *Pain* 2006; **125**: 143–57.

53. Hester NK. The preoperational child's reaction to immunization. *Nurs Res* 1979; **28**: 250–5.

54. Hicks CL, von Baeyer CL, Spafford PA, van Korlaar I, Goodenough B. The Faces Pain Scale-Revised: Toward a common metric in pediatric pain measurement. *Pain* 2001; **93**: 173–83.

55. Wong DL, Baker CM. Pain in children: Comparison of assessment scales. *Okla Nurse* 1988; **33**: 8.

56. Beyer JE, Aradine CR. Content validity of an instrument to measure young children's perceptions of the intensity of their pain. *J Pediatr Nurs* 1986; **1**: 386–95.

57. von Baeyer, CL, Spagrud LJ. Systematic review of observational (behavioral) measures of pain for children and adolescents aged 3 to 18 years. *Pain* 2007; **127**: 140–50.

58. Merkel SI, Voepel-Lewis T, Shayevitz JR, Malviya S. The FLACC: A behavioral scale for scoring postoperative pain in young children. *Pediatr Nurs* 1997; **23**: 293–7.

59. McGrath PJ, Johnson G, Goodman JT, *et al.* CHEOPS: A behavioral scale for rating postoperative pain in children. *In Advances in Pain Research and Therapy, Vol. 9*, eds. HL Fields, R Dubner and F Cervero (New York: Raven Press, 1985) pp. 395–402.

60. Chambers CT, Reid GJ, McGrath PJ, Finley GA Development and preliminary validation of a postoperative pain measure for parents. *Pain* 1996; **68**: 307–13.

61. Ambuel B, Hamlett KW, Marx CM, Blumer JL. Assessing distress in pediatric intensive care environments: The COMFORT scale. *J Pediatr Psychol* 1992; **17**: 95–109.

62. Savedra MC, Holzemer WL, Tesler MD, Wilkie DJ. Assessment of postoperation pain in children and adolescents using the adolescent pediatric pain tool. *Nurs Res* 1993; **42**: 5–9.

63. LeBaron S, Zeltzer L. Assessment of acute pain and anxiety in children and adolescents by self-reports, observer reports, and a behavior checklist. *J Consult Clin Psychol* 1984; **52**: 729–38.

64. McGrath PJ, Walco GA, Turk DC, *et al.* Core outcome domains and measures for pediatric acute and chronic/recurrent pain clinical trials: PedIMMPACT recommendations. *J Pain* 2008; **9**: 771–83.

65. Ardery G, Herr KA, Titler MG, Sorofman BA, Schmitt MB. Assessing and managing acute pain in older adults: A research base to guide practice. *Medsurg Nurs* 2003; **12**: 7–18; quiz 19.

66. Ferrell BA, Stein W, Beck JC. The Geriatric Pain Measure: Validity, reliability and factor analysis. *J Am Geriatr Soc* 2000; **48**: 1669–73.

67. American Geriatrics Society. The management of persistent pain in older persons. *J Am Geriatr Soc* 2002; **50**(6 Suppl): S205–24.

68. Fuchs-Lacelle S, Hadjistavropoulos T. Development and preliminary validation of the pain assessment checklist for seniors with limited ability to communicate (PACSLAC). *Pain Manag Nurs* 2004; **5**: 37–49.

69. Lefebvre-Chapiro, S. The Dolophus group. The Dolophus 2 scale: Evaluating pain in the elderly. *Eur J Pall Care* 2001; **8**: 191–4.

70. Feldt KS. The checklist of nonverbal pain indicators (CNPI). *Pain Manag Nurs* 2000; **1**: 13–21.

71. Snow AL, Weber JB, O'Malley KJ, *et al.* NOPPAIN: A nursing assistant-administered pain assessment instrument for use in dementia. *Dement Geriatr Cogn Disord* 2004; **17**: 240–6.

72. Li D, Puntillo K, Miaskowski C. A review of objective pain measures for use with critical care adult patients unable to self-report. *J Pain* 2008; **9**: 2–10.

73. McCaffery M, Pasero C, eds. *Assessment: Underlying complexities, misconceptions, and practical tools.* Pain: Clinical manual 2nd edn. (Mosby: St. Louis, 1999).

74. Payen JF, Bru O, Bosson JL. *et al.* Assessing pain in critically ill sedated patients by using a behavioral pain scale. *Crit Care Med* 2001; **29**: 2258–63.

75. Gélinas C, Fillion L, Puntillo KA, Viens C, Fortier M. Validation of the critical-care pain observation tool in adult patients. *Am J Crit Care* 2006; **15**: 420–7.

76. Mateo OM, Krenzischek DA. A pilot study to assess the relationship between behavioral manifestations and

self-report of pain in postanesthesia care unit patients. *J Post Anesth Nurs* 1992; **7**: 15–21.

77. Puntillo KA, Miaskowski C, Kehrle K, *et al.* Relationship between behavioral and physiological indicators of pain, critical care patients' self-reports of pain, and opioid administration. *Crit Care Med* 1997; **25**: 1159–66.

78. Puntillo KA, Miaskowski C, Kehrle K, *et al.* Pain behaviors observed during six common procedures: Results from Thunder Project II. *Crit Care Med* 2004; **32**: 421–7.

79. Nampiaparampil DE. Prevalence of chronic pain after traumatic brain injury: A systematic review. *JAMA* 2008; **300**: 711–9.

80. Scherder E, Wolters E, Polman C, Sergeant J, Swaab D. Pain in Parkinson's disease and multiple sclerosis: Its relation to the medial and lateral pain systems. *Neurosci Biobehav Rev* 2005; **29**: 1047–56.

81. Warden V, Hurley AC, Volicer L. Development and psychometric evaluation of the Pain Assessment in Advanced Dementia (PAIN – AD) Scale. *J Am Med Dir Assoc* 2003; **4**: 9–15.

5

Assessment of functioning and disability in pain syndromes

Stacy C. Parenteau and Jennifer A. Haythornthwaite

Introduction

This chapter will address three important and related dimensions of pain-related physical function. The first dimension, *perceived interference*, is typically measured using global ratings of the extent to which pain interferes with various key activities. Individuals make ratings in which they are typically asked to isolate the impact of pain from other aspects of their illness or lifestyle that interfere with daily activities. Not surprisingly, these ratings not only correlate with pain, but also with other psychological factors such as depression. The second dimension, *activity level*, is typically measured using ratings of what specific activities the individual participates in on a regular basis. These ratings are not tied to pain and do not take into account, in general, whether the activity is appropriate for the individual. And finally, the third dimension is *sleep*. Sleep is measured either with diaries or summary scales, and often ratings are made regarding the extent to which pain interferes with sleep.

Challenges in selecting a scale

There are a number of challenges that need to be considered before selecting a measure of pain-related physical function. First, most measures of pain-related physical function are correlated with ratings of pain intensity. Although correlated, the relationship has been shown to be non-linear [1], and a number of factor analyses that have combined measures of pain with measures of physical function often identify distinct factors [2]. There is some indication from the literature reviewed below that ratings of interference made within specific domains – sleep, recreation, etc. – are easier for people to make and show more independence from ratings of pain intensity than more global ratings, such as "daily activities"[3].

The second challenge pertains to the inherent limitations of self-report. The potential for response biases need to be considered whenever using self-report measures. Some of the measures reviewed have been examined for the influence of response biases, such as social desirability, the tendency to present oneself in a positive or more socially acceptable light [4]. Similarly when disability determinations are being made or litigation is a factor, measures of physical function may be particularly vulnerable to response biases. While self-report measures have limitations, the value of self-reported function is well established and should not be discarded for observer reports, since providers' ratings of function do not correlate well with patients' self-reports [5], a finding that is common with ratings of pain severity.

The third challenge in selecting a measure is the potential impact on the psychometric properties of a subscale that may occur when it is removed from the full scale or original measurement tool. Only one measure reviewed below is a stand-alone measure of pain-related physical function – the Pain Disability Index [6]. Another measure – the Brief Pain Inventory [7] – includes an assessment of pain in a previous section before the patient reports on pain-related interference. The other two measures – the West Haven Yale Multidimensional Pain Inventory [8] and the Sickness Impact Profile [9] – have pain-related physical function scales embedded in other scales. Some investigators hypothesize that the items surrounding an item impact on ratings of the item, thereby contributing to high cross-loadings in factor analyses [10]. The context of any single question, including both the subject's perceptions of the orientation of the questioner as well as adjacent questions, can influence subjects' responses as much as scaling and question format [11].

Behavioral and Psychopharmacologic Pain Management, ed. Michael H. Ebert and Robert D. Kerns. Published by Cambridge University Press. © Cambridge University Press 2011.

Table 5.1 Summary of key dimensions for four scales of interest

Scale	Number of items	Time (mins)	Scoring procedure	Comments
BPI	7	<5	Sum of items	
PDI	7	<5	Sum of items	
SIP				
Physical function	136	15	Weighted sum of items	Embedded in other scales
WHYMPI/MPI				
Interference	11	<5	Average of items	Embedded in other scales
General activity	18	<5	Average of items	

BPI: Brief Pain Inventory; PDI: Pain Disability Index; SIP; Sickness Impact Profile; WHYMPI: The West Haven-Yale Multidimensional Pain Inventory.

Table 5.2 Summary of instruments for assessing physical disability in specific pain populations

Target pain population	Instrument	Review article reference number
Arthritis	Arthritis Impact Measurement Scales (AIMS-2) [115] Health Assessment Questionnaire (HAQ) [116]	[123]
Back Pain	Oswestry Disability Questionnaire [117] Roland-Morris Disability Questionnaire [118]	[124]
Osteoarthritis/knee pain	Western Ontario and McMaster (WOMAC) Osteoarthritis Index [119]	[125]
Fibromyalgia	Fibromyalgia Impact Questionnaire (FIQ) [120] Fibromyalgia Health Assessment Questionnaire (FHAQ) [121]	[121]
Migraine	Migraine Disability Assessment (MIDAS) Questionnaire [122]	[122]

Overview

Measures that are widely or predominantly used within a specific pain population (e.g., low back pain) and measures that combine pain intensity and a dimension of physical function, such as the Graded Chronic Pain Scale or the SF-36 Bodily Pain scale, were excluded from this discussion. Studies using physician ratings of disability or scales designed specifically for the study also will not be included in this review.

Four measures that include five scales assessing pain-related physical function are reviewed in detail below, followed by a discussion of measures of physical performance. Each measure is reviewed separately by providing some background on the development of the scale and the extent to which it is currently used, discussing the scale itself and its psychometric properties, reviewing briefly validity data on the scale, and finally, presenting available literature addressing the responsivity of the scale to treatment effects, both from observational studies and randomized trials when available.

Each of the selected scales shows adequate psychometric properties, although some have been more extensively studied than others. Table 5.1 summarizes some of the characteristics of each scale reviewed. Following this review of scales assessing broad pain-related physical function, we include a section discussing the measurement of sleep, where the scaling is quite heterogeneous. The final section suggests some future directions for research in the area of pain-related physical function.

Table 5.2 presents a summary of measures designed for specific pain conditions, as well as relevant review articles for further reading on a specific measure.

Brief Pain Inventory – interference scale

Background

The Brief Pain Inventory (BPI [12]) was originally developed by the Pain Research Group of the WHO

Collaborating Center for Symptom Evaluation in Cancer Care [13] to measure pain severity and pain-related interference in patients with cancer. This scale is widely used in the assessment of cancer pain [12], but recently its use has been extended to non-cancer pain assessment, as discussed in the following sections.

Scales

The BPI includes two primary dimensions: pain intensity and pain interference [13]. The most widely used version of the pain interference scale uses 11-point numeric rating scales (0 – no interference to 10 – interferes completely) to assess pain-related interference in seven areas: general activity, mood, walking ability, normal work including outside the home and housework, relations with other people, enjoyment of life, and sleep [13]. Some investigators have added additional domains: self-care, recreational activities, and social activities, or changed walking to general mobility for disabled individuals [3]; for the purposes of this review, this scale will be referred to as the modified BPI Interference scale. The time frame for assessment can vary from "the past week" [13] to "the past 24 hours" [12].

Factor analyses of the pain intensity and pain interference scales support a two-factor structure that is robust across cultures [13]. Using data from the four country BPI database [1], multidimensional scaling analyses designed to control for response biases inherent to self-report questionnaires demonstrated two dimensions to the BPI Interference scale after controlling for worst pain intensity: *affect* (relations with others, mood, enjoyment of life) and *activity* (walking, work, general activity, sleep) [14].

Psychometrics

The psychometric properties of the BPI Interference scale have been examined in a wide variety of pain populations. Analyses of the BPI Interference scale used in four different countries – USA, France, China, and the Philippines – yielded excellent internal stability coefficients, ranging from 0.86 to 0.91 [1]. These authors demonstrated remarkable internal consistency of the BPI Interference scale across different levels of pain – mild, moderate, and severe (ranging from 0.80 to 0.91 across the four countries and levels of pain).

Validity: General

A large literature has germinated from the wide use of the BPI with cancer pain, helping to establish the scale's

validity. Work on the BPI has demonstrated strong correlations between pain intensity ratings and pain interference ratings across different diseases [15]. Detailed analyses indicate that the relationship between pain intensity and pain-related interference is non-linear, providing additional support for separating these two dimensions [1]. Analyses using the BPI Interference scale have used both the total score and individual items. Multivariate analyses indicate independent contributions of pain severity and mood in predicting total BPI Interference scores [15]. The German version of the BPI Interference scale correlates significantly with deteriorated performance scores and relevant SF-36 scales, including bodily pain, physical function, vitality, and general health [16].

The BPI may be particularly suited to the assessment of episodic or fluctuating pain states, such as can occur with pain due to cancer. In this regard, patients with neoplastic disease who report no pain at the time of a medical visit but pain during the past week report higher levels of interference in every domain measured by the BPI Interference scale as compared to patients who reported no pain at either the visit or during the past week [17].

Validation of the BPI Interference scale also comes from other populations, including patients with HIV/AIDS. Patients with HIV/AIDS reporting moderate to severe pain for the past 2 weeks and symptoms of post-traumatic stress disorder (PTSD) not only report higher levels of distress and lower quality of life, but also report higher BPI Interference scores as compared to individuals who do not report significant PTSD symptoms [18]. This effect was observed on the two dimensions of BPI Interference – affect and activity – and remained significant across a 6-month period [18].

Responsivity: Pre-post changes

The BPI Interference scale has been used to track responses to a variety of pain management interventions. In a small descriptive investigation of sodium valproate in reducing pain and interference due to cancer-related neuropathic pain, pain-related interference scores decreased to a similar extent as pain intensity scores, except in the area of sleep [19]. Patients with chronic cancer pain reported significantly reduced pain interference, coupled with decreased pain severity, after having their medical regimen changed from standard opioid therapy to once-daily oral extended-release hydromorphone [20]. Furthermore, patients with post–herpetic neuralgia, painful diabetic neuropathy, and low back pain reported significant combined improvements in general activity, normal work, walking ability, relationships, sleep, and enjoyment of life, parallel with decreased pain intensity, after a lidocaine 5% patch was added to a current analgesic drug regimen that already included gabapentin [21].

Randomized clinical trials

Randomized clinical trials (RCTs) evaluating cancer pain treatments have not been widely conducted, although a few trials are available which include use of the BPI Interference scale. In this regard, a randomized, prospective trial of a cancer pain treatment algorithm – including a comprehensive assessment and evidence-based analgesic guidelines – did not demonstrate a significant reduction in pain intensity, pain relief, or pain-related interference compared to a standard pain management program, although patient satisfaction scores were higher in the intervention group. The intervention yielded higher adherence to "best practice" guidelines, although there was no significant difference between groups in total 24-hour opioid dosing. Across both groups, however, opioid dosing was significantly correlated with reductions in pain interference [22].

The BPI Interference scale has been used to measure outcomes in RCTs involving non-cancerous painful conditions. Patients with Fabry disease reported a significant reduction in pain and pain-related interference in response to enzyme replacement therapy as compared to placebo treatment [23]. Three 12-week, double-blind studies revealed significantly reduced pain interference for patients with diabetic peripheral neuropathic pain receiving duloxetine 60 mg once per day or 60 mg twice per day compared to patients receiving placebo [24]. Furthermore, patients with fibromyalgia receiving unilateral repetitive transcranial magnetic stimulation of the motor cortex reported significant decreases in pain interference in the general activity, sleep, and walking domains for 30 days, as well as decreased pain severity for up to 2 weeks, in comparison to patients receiving sham stimulation [25]. In a study examining the effects of morphine discontinuation, patients with chronic non-cancer pain indicated significantly increased difficulty with general activity, walking, normal work, sleep, and enjoyment of life, as well increased pain intensity, during a placebo phase compared to a period of morphine administration [26].

In a randomized trial comparing cognitive-behavioral therapy (CBT) for HIV-related neuropathic pain to supportive psychotherapy, both groups showed reductions in pain and pain-related interference over the course of the trial [27]. Older adults with non-cancer pain receiving a pain self-management training group intervention, as compared with an education-only control condition, reported no significant reductions in pain-related interference or pain intensity [28]. Furthermore, women with fibromyalgia using either 024 essential oil or sham oil reported comparable, non-significant reductions in pain interference and pain intensity following a 12-week exercise program [29].

Pain Disability Index

Background

The Pain Disability Index (PDI) was specifically developed to be a brief measure of the degree to which chronic pain interferes with normal role functioning and consistent with the Institute of Medicine's Committee on Pain, Disability and Illness Behavior's definition of disability [6, 30]. While most data come from patients with heterogeneous pain conditions [31, 32], the PDI has been used to measure function/disability in a number of specific painful conditions, including low back pain [33], post-herpetic neuralgia [34], diabetic neuropathy [35], and spinal cord injury [36].

Scales

The PDI includes seven items assessing perceived disability in each of seven areas of normal role functioning: family/home responsibilities, recreation, social activity, occupation, sexual behavior, self-care (e.g., taking a shower, driving, getting dressed), and life-support activity (e.g., eating, sleeping, breathing). Each item is rated on an 11-point scale (0 – no disability to 10 – total disability) and the responses are summed. Recent analyses of a large group of patients ($n = 1361$) with heterogeneous pain conditions presenting for care at a hospital-based pain clinic support a single factor that accounts for 49% of the variance in items [30].

Psychometrics

The PDI shows excellent internal consistency (alpha = 0.85–86; [6, 31] and test-retest stability [6, 37].

Validity

As is seen with other measures of physical function, PDI scores correlate significantly with pain intensity [32, 38], but the moderate level of these correlations indicates only partial overlap [37]. In addition to correlating with other self-report scales such as the Oswestry [37], PDI scores have showed expected correlations with physical tests of function [33]. Total PDI and factor 1 scores (discretionary activities) showed stronger correlations with the Oswestry (r of 0.83 and 0.84, respectively) than with factor 2 scores (obligatory activities; $r = 0.41$; [37]). As seen with other measures of physical function, response biases may influence responses to the PDI. Social desirability, or the tendency to present oneself in a positive light, correlates with PDI scores only after controlling for depressive symptoms, a factor that often inflates disability ratings [4]. Other correlates of PDI ratings include depressive symptoms, work-related factors, medication use [32], and litigation status [30].

Responsivity: Pre-post changes

The responsivity of the PDI to the beneficial effects of spinal cord stimulation (SCS) for treating postherpetic neuralgia were recently documented in a consecutive case series; 23 long-term responders to SCS (long-term pain relief with a median rating of 1/10) reported concurrent reductions in pain-related disability [34]. Additionally, patients receiving standard occlusal splint therapy for chronic orofacial pain reported decreased pain-related physical disability on the PDI, as well as decreased pain severity [39].

Randomized control trials

In a study examining the efficacy of static magnetic field therapy for chronic pelvic pain, patients receiving active magnets revealed significantly lower disability levels, but not significantly decreased pain intensity, compared with patients receiving placebo [40]. In a placebo-controlled trial, patients with neuropathic pain receiving sativex revealed significant decreases in pain-related disability, as well as pain intensity [41]. Patients with central neuropathic pain administered 75 mg S(+)-ketamine reported improved physical functioning in comparison to a placebo group, despite the absence of decreased pain severity [42]. Following 7 days of treatment with controlled-release codeine in a placebo-controlled crossover clinical trial, a heterogeneous group of patients with painful conditions

reported a significant reduction in pain intensity that was associated with a significant reduction in PDI score [31], with analyses of individual items indicating significant improvements in total PDI and in each area of role functioning, with the exception of life-support activities.

The PDI was also used in a RCT evaluating lamotrigine in reducing pain due to diabetic neuropathy. While significant reductions in pain intensity occurred following treatment with lamotrigine relative to placebo, no significant effects were observed on the PDI [35], although a preliminary report of the same trial suggested a trend for PDI scores to decline in response to lamotrigine [43]. In a small group of patients with pain following a spinal cord injury, topiramate reduced pain ratings after the highest dose (800 mg) was accomplished for 3 weeks, but no concomitant change in PDI score was observed [36]. A study examining the effects of pregabalin on patients with central neuropathic pain found no significant differences in disability scores between the pregabalin group and the placebo group [44], although patients receiving pregabalin reported decreased pain intensity. Low-back pain patients receiving flexion-distraction chiropractic manipulation and trigger point therapy reported similar improvement on the PDI compared to a control group receiving sham manipulation and effleurage [45].

Sickness Impact Profile

Background

The Sickness Impact Profile (SIP) was originally developed as a behaviorally based outcome measure of overall health status and refined with randomly selected samples of patients with different types of disease, using different assessment methods and interviewers [46]. After extensive refinement, the final version includes 136 items in 12 categories of function, yielding three summary scores – psychosocial, physical, and other impairment [9]. The SIP has been used in an extremely broad number of painful conditions, as discussed in the following sections.

Scales

The SIP includes a list of 136 statements (e.g., "I do not do any of the shopping that I would usually do" or "I do not walk at all"). Respondents mark only those statements that describe the respondent "today" and are related to health, and its instructions are typically changed from "your state of health" to "your pain." Each statement is weighted and percentage scores for three areas are computed as weighted sums: Physical Function (personal care, mobility, and walking), Psychosocial Function (emotions, cognitive function, social interactions, and communication), and Other Function (sleep/rest, household, work, recreation, and eating). A total score is calculated as a weighted sum of these three subscales.

Psychometrics

The SIP was originally developed and refined on randomly selected group practice enrollees through a series of field trials; enrollees were selected to represent a range of characteristics and sampling was weighted towards inclusion of the sick and disabled [46]. The internal consistency of the overall score is excellent (alphas in the range of 0.81 to 0.94) and test-retest stability is also good (r values in the range of 0.87 to 0.97; [9]).

Validity: General

As is the case with other measures of physical function, the SIP Physical Function scale correlates with pain intensity ratings [47]. Early work with the SIP validated the Physical Function scale against daily activity logs, demonstrating a significant inverse correlation between uptime and SIP physical function score [48]. The SIP Physical Function scale was further validated in a sample of women with rheumatoid arthritis (RA) and found to correlate significantly with a variety of measures of disease activity, joint involvement, and joint function [49]. Consistent with a behavioral/operant model of pain expression, directly observed attentive responses from spouses to patients' non-verbal expressions of pain are associated with lower physical function in those patients who also report high levels of depressive symptoms [50]. Finally, overall SIP scores predict the transition from acute to chronic pain [51].

Responsivity: Pre-post changes

The SIP has been used widely to evaluate function in a variety of different pain conditions and with a range of different types of treatment. The Physical Functioning scale in particular has evidenced responsivity to change across treatments and painful conditions. Early work with a small group of patients participating in a multidisciplinary rehabilitation program demonstrated significant changes in SIP Physical Function following treatment [48], and its responsivity to

change with multidisciplinary rehabilitation has been shown repeatedly [52]. Changes in SIP Physical Function scores correlated with changes in pain severity, joint involvement and joint function in a group of women with RA followed over a 1-year period [49]. A recent and systematic evaluation of a group of patients undergoing SCS demonstrated significant improvements in SIP Physical Function 1 year following implantation [53].

Randomized control trials

Many RCTs of various pain treatments have focused on specific SIP subscales, notably the SIP Physical Function scale. In this regard, SIP Physical Function scores improved in a group of low back pain patients randomized to receive exercises for lumbar extensor muscles as compared to a waiting list control group [54]. Patients with chronic limb ischemia receiving SCS in addition to medical treatment experienced significantly improved mobility, as measured by the SIP mobility subscore, compared to patients receiving medical treatment alone, while treatment groups did not differ in pain levels or quality of life [55]. Older adults participating in an 8-week exercise program involving strength training and lifestyle advice reported significantly decreased disability, as measured by the SIP Physical subscale, as well as pain severity, compared to a control group at 3-month follow-up [56].

In a randomized, crossover placebo-controlled study of opioids, the SIP Physical Function scale did not show any improvements, despite significant pain reduction [57]. Similarly, significant changes in SIP Physical Function scores did not coincide with short-term benefits of amitriptyline and cyclobenzaprine in the treatment of fibromyalgia [58] or the pain reducing effects of nortriptyline in low back pain [59]. In the context of no apparent reductions in pain, SIP Physical Function scores also did not improve following biofeedback or fitness training for fibromyalgia patients [60].

West Haven-Yale Multidimensional Pain Inventory

Background

The West Haven-Yale Multidimensional Pain Inventory (WHYMPI [8]) and the slightly expanded version referred to as the Multidimensional Pain Inventory (MPI [61]) have provided an important tool for measuring the experience of pain. Use of this scale has contributed to the extensive knowledge base that has developed over the past two decades of pain research, particularly in understanding the psychosocial aspects of the pain experience. It has most widely been used to study non-cancerous, chronically painful conditions.

Scales

The perceived Interference scale is embedded in the first section of the instrument, which includes items assessing pain severity, support, life control and affective distress. The perceived Interference subscale includes items rated on Likert-type scales (0 – no to 6 – extreme) of interference (I), change (C), or change in satisfaction (CS). Items assess day-to-day activities (I), work (C;CS), social/recreational activities (C), marriage/family activities (C; CS), household chores (C), friendships (C) and sleep (I [8]). A second scale from the WHYMPI/MPI that deserves consideration as a potential measure of pain-related function is the General Activity subscale. This scale is in its own section of the instrument and is a compilation of four activity scales (social activities, activities away from home, household chores, and outdoor work). Similar to the perceived Interference subscale, each of 18 items is rated on a Likert-type scale (0 – never to 6 – very often).

Factor structure

Analyses of the factor structure of the WHYMPI/MPI generally confirm the original subscales [62], even when translated into Dutch [10]. A high correlation between pain severity and perceived Interference [63] is often seen with the WHYMPI/MPI, possibly due in part to the inclusion of pain-related suffering in the pain severity score, inclusion of a general interference item (In general, how much does your pain interfere with your day-to-day activities?), or item ordering effects [10]. A smaller, but still significant correlation is typically seen with General Activities [63]. A more general factor comprising multiple scales of physical function correlate with a pain severity factor also comprised of multiple scales [2], again suggesting a fundamental association between these two constructs. A recent factor analysis of all items from the WHYMPI/MPI found three factors, one of which was titled "suffering" and included items assessing pain severity, perceived interference, and punishing responses from a significant other, but confirmed the General Activity factor previously identified [64].

Psychometrics

The psychometric properties of this instrument have been examined in a large variety of settings and pain conditions. The psychometric properties of the perceived Interference and General Activity subscales demonstrate good internal consistency (alphas ranging from 0.86–0.90 for Interference and 0.74–0.78 for General Activity) and 2-week stability (test-retest coefficients for 2 weeks ranging from 0.85 to 0.87 for Interference and 0.80 to 0.87 for General Activity [8, 10, 65].

Validity: General

Validation of these two subscales is provided by an extensive literature from multiple countries and many different types of pain conditions documenting expected relationships with other measures of interference, activity level, disability, and function. An important *construct* validation study used experience sampling methods and daily diaries to examine the relationship between WHYMPI/MPI subscales and daily ratings of pain-related interference and daily activities [66]. Eight ratings made each of 6 days on diary ratings of interference due to pain were highly correlated ($r = 0.60$, $p < 0.001$) with WHYMPI/MPI perceived interference scores. Although diary ratings of household chores correlated with the relevant WHYMPI/MPI subscale ($r = 0.40$, $p < 0.01$), diary recordings of overall activity level did not correlate with the similar WHYMPI/MPI subscale ($r = 0.16$, $p > 0.05$; [66]). Similar results were reported in an earlier German study comparing diary data to WHYMPI/MPI reports (see Flor *et al.* 1990 reported in [66]). Bicycle ergometer performance correlates with WHYMPI/MPI General Activity [10]. Confirmatory factor analysis of a sample of individuals with post-amputation pain or pain with paraplegia demonstrated a physical functioning factor – WHYMPI/MPI Interference and General Activity scores and SF-36 physical and role functioning scores – that was highly correlated with physical performance outcomes during lifting and wheel turning, as well as pain severity and emotional functioning [2].

Another important *predictive* validation study demonstrated that WHYMPI/MPI Interference scores reported during a medical consultation for neck pain following a motor vehicle accident were significantly higher in the group of individuals who continued to experience residual pain from the accident 1 year later [67]. The General Activity scores were not significantly different for these individuals, and multivariate analyses indicated that the Interference score was the single effective measure in identifying individuals who report continued pain 1 year following the initial accident [67].

Responsivity: Pre-post changes

Further validation of the WHYMPI/MPI Interference and General Activity subscales comes from studies that demonstrate change on these measures following treatment for pain. Patients with fibromyalgia experienced decreased life interference, improved general activity level, and reduced pain severity following multidisciplinary pain rehabilitation involving CBT and concurrent withdrawal from analgesic medications [68]. In a similar study evaluating gender differences in fibromyalgia patients participating in multidisciplinary pain rehabilitation, women reported significantly greater pre- to post-treatment improvement in life interference, but not in general activity level or pain severity, compared to men [69]. In a similar vein, WHYMPI/MPI Interference scores declined following interdisciplinary outpatient treatment for fibromyalgia [70]. Importantly, the Oswestry scale did not show significant improvement when the WHYMPI/MPI Interference scale did [70]. However, following effective cognitive-behavioral treatment of fibromyalgia that reduced pain behavior, worry, and perceived control, Interference ratings were not reduced and General Activity scores were not increased [71].

Randomized control trials

The WHYMPI Interference and General Activity subscales have been used to evaluate the efficacy of psychological and rehabilitative treatments in a number of chronic pain populations, including temporomandibular disorders [72], musculoskeletal pain [73], and chronic back pain [74, 75]. One RCT used the WHYMPI/MPI Interference and General Activity subscales to evaluate opioids and tricyclic antidepressants in the treatment of post-herpetic neuralgia [76], and a crossover trial evaluated the effects of mexilitine on neuropathic pain with allodynia [77]. While some of these interventions reduced perceived Interference [74, 75], others did not demonstrate expected reductions in Interference scores with active treatment relative to an appropriate control [72, 76]. No study demonstrated a treatment effect on the WHYMPI/MPI General Activity subscale [73, 76]. The mexilitine trial was largely negative and results for Interference

and General Activity were not reported [77]. Finally, fibromyalgia patients receiving true acupuncture did not evidence reduced Interference or increased General Activity scores compared to patients receiving simulated acupuncture, although the true acupuncture group did report significantly decreased pain severity 1 month following treatment compared to the control group [78].

Performance outcomes

Validity

Acceptable validity and reliability have been established for several objective clinical measures of physical performance, including 5-minute walk distance, 1-minute stair climb, 1-minute standing up and sitting down from a chair, and arm endurance [79]. Furthermore, the PDI and the Oswestry Disability Questionnaire were significantly related to physical performance measures (repetitive sit-up, arch-up, and squatting) in patients with chronic low-back pain [33]. In a study of older adults participating in inpatient geriatric rehabilitation, the Timed Up & Go test and the 2-minute walk test correlated with the Functional Independence Measure (FIM) at both admission and discharge; functional reach was not significantly correlated with the FIM [80]. In another comparison of self-report and performance-based measures of physical functioning in knee osteoarthritis patients, the WOMAC (Western Ontario and McMaster Universities) osteoarthritis index and SF-36 correlated robustly with pain, whereas physical performance measures were strongly related to self-efficacy [81].

Responsivity: Pre-post changes

Relatively few studies evaluate the responsivity of performance measures following specific chronic pain interventions. One of the few such studies revealed that patients with chronic low back pain evidenced significantly increased 5-minute walk distance both immediately and 9 months following an outpatient multidisciplinary pain management program [82].

Randomized control trails

Tests of physical performance have been utilized in a substantial number of RCTs. Compared to an outpatient program, patients participating in an inpatient cognitive-behavioral pain management program displayed greater improvement in meters walked in 10 minutes, seconds of arm endurance, number of stairs climbed in 2 minutes, and stand-ups in 2 minutes at 1-month follow-up, while both groups improved significantly on performance measures over a control group [83]. Inpatient and outpatient groups did not differ on ratings of pain intensity and pain distress at 1-month follow-up. Osteoarthritis patients performing baduanjin, a traditional Chinese exercise, displayed significant improvements on the 6-minute walk test and the peak torque of the isokinetic strength of the knee extensors, as well as pain reduction, compared with a control group [84]. Patients with chronic low back pain who were informed that performing a simple leg-flexion task would slightly increase their pain evidenced poorer performance outcomes as measured by the number of flexion movements, mean range of motion, and mean work ratio compared to control patients who were told the leg-flexion task would not exacerbate their pain [85]. Older adults with chronic low back pain receiving percutaneous electrical nerve stimulation (PENS) and physical therapy demonstrated improved performance on tasks of dynamic lifting and chair rise, as well as decreased pain intensity, compared to participants receiving sham PENS, while both groups evidenced improved gait speed [86]. Improvements in 6-minute walk distance, as well as decreased pain, were observed in subjects with osteoarthritis of the knee given either glucosamine sulfate or Aquamin, a seaweed-based multi-mineral supplement, but not in a placebo or combined treatment group [87]. Finally, older adults with osteoarthritis of the hip demonstrated improvements on the timed Up & Go test, but not on three other performance tasks at 3 months after following an 8-week exercise program involving strength training and lifestyle advice, despite improved pain ratings made by observers [56].

In a study examining the effects of essential oil in women with fibromyalgia, however, no significant differences were found in performance measures – second chair stands, 6-minute walk distance, multidimensional balance scores – or pain severity between women using 024 essential oil and women given sham oil, with both groups also using an exercise regimen [29]. Patients with chronic radicular pain receiving bupivacaine and methylprednisolone did not evidence significantly greater improvement in claudication walking distance than patients receiving bupivacaine alone [90]. Physical training combined with operant-behavioral graded activity with problem solving training did not produce significant improvements in walking, fast walking, sit to stand task, loaded forward reach, number of stairs climbed, and lifting compared to either intervention alone [91].

Measures of sleep

Pain-related sleep difficulties are an important facet of the physical disability observed in chronic pain populations, as high rates of sleep disturbance are noted among samples of patients with chronically painful conditions [92]. Standardized measures of sleep used in the sleep literature, such as the Pittsburgh Sleep Quality Index (PSQI [93, 94]) and sleep diaries [92], are not frequently used in the assessment of sleep disturbance in chronic pain, particularly the treatment outcome literature. These widely used sleep measures quantify the overall quality, nature, and duration of sleep. In the pain literature, sleep is most frequently measured in terms of how much pain interferes with sleep [95], either in diary form or as part of the overall assessment of physical function using the scales described above (e.g., the WHYMPI/MPI Interference scale, the BPI, and the PDI all include items that assess pain interference with sleep). Single item sleep disturbance ratings vary from using a 10-cm visual analog scale [96, 97] to an 11-point numerical rating [98, 99].

Responsivity

Measures of pain-related sleep interference are generally responsive to a variety of pain treatments. For example, pain-related sleep interference diaries indicated improved sleep following administration of pregabalin for neuropathic pain [100], although this effect has not been consistent across pharmacological treatments [101]. Summary ratings of pain-related sleep interference, such as that included in the BPI, also may be responsive to pharmacological intervention [102]. Recent studies also have documented reductions in pain-related sleep disturbances using the Chronic Pain Sleep Inventory, which is comprised of five 100-mm visual analog scales assessing the impact of pain on sleep onset, the need for sleep medications, awakening due to pain both at night and in the morning, and overall sleep quality [103], to evaluate the efficacy of tramadol [104] and oxymorphone extended release [105] in treating osteoarthritis.

Other studies have evaluated global sleep quality in chronic pain populations. In this regard, a single rating of overall quality of sleep found no differential impact of two tricyclic antidepressants (amitriptyline and nortriptyline) in patients with post-herpetic neuralgia [97]. Moreover, a more extensive assessment of sleep quality in patients with diabetic neuropathy, including ratings of quantity of sleep, sleep adequacy, sleep disturbance, and somnolence, did not change in response to tramadol, despite reductions in pain and improvement in some areas of quality of life [106]. In a more recent study, overall sleep quality, as measured by the 12-item MOS-Sleep Scale and a daily 11-point rating scale, was improved following 14 weeks of pregabalin administration in fibromyalgia patients [107]. Furthermore, CBT of insomnia secondary to chronic pain improved an array of sleep measures, including diary measures of sleep onset latency, sleep efficiency, and minutes awake after sleep onset as well as overall sleep quality ratings [108].

Summary and recommendations

As demonstrated by this review, physical function is an important domain of measurement in the comprehensive assessment of individuals with chronic pain. Consistent with the prominence of this domain, clinical trials in the pain literature are increasingly including physical function as outcomes following the recommendations of expert groups such as OMERACT [109] and IMMPACT [110]. Recent years have witnessed an improvement in the quality of RCTs of chronic pain treatment and interventions, with an expansion in the outcome measurement to include measures of physical function. We recommend that investigators consider including multiple measures of pain-related physical function so that comparisons of these various measures can be made across populations, treatment modalities (e.g., pharmacological and behavioral), and patient groups. Of note, the Patient-Reported Outcomes Measurement Information System (PROMIS) network is developing measures of physical function to be ultimately administered using computerized adaptive testing. Evaluation of a preliminary physical function item bank supported the expected advantages of PROMIS [111]. Availability of this innovative approach will require testing and validation by outcome researchers in the pain literature. Whether this approach yields a responsive measure of physical function for pain clinical trials will need to be carefully investigated.

The reliance on self-report remains a major challenge for the assessment of pain-related physical function. Studies examining responsivity of performance-based measures to pharmacological and behavioral treatments have produced inconsistent results. The lack of uniform impact on physical performance across different painful conditions and treatment modalities limits the utility of any one measure of physical performance (e.g., walking speed) across conditions. There is a need for additional studies establishing the validity of performance measures in detecting treatment outcomes in chronic pain populations. While many studies discussed in this review utilized both performance-based and subjective measures, not all studies reported associations between these measures to establish construct validity. We recommend that future studies continue to use performance measures in tandem with self-report measures of physical function, and include correlations between these measures in order to provide solid and comprehensive evidence for specific interventions for chronic pain. Additional intervention studies examining the responsivity of performance measures are also warranted.

The measurement of sleep as a specific domain of physical function deserves greater attention in the pain literature, given the known reciprocal relationships observed between sleep disturbance and clinical pain outcomes [112]. We recommend the measurement of both daily sleep using a diary assessing sleep latency, time awake after the onset of sleep, total sleep time, and length of time in bed, as well as summary scales such as the Pittsburgh Sleep Quality Inventory [113]. Pain-specific measures of sleep interference, such as visual analogue scales or numerical rating scales, can be expected to detect changes in pain-related sleep disturbance following treatment in chronic pain populations. The sleep-improving benefits of pharmacological treatments have been documented [104, 107]. However, more interesting is the recent investigation of cognitive-behavioral treatment of insomnia secondary to chronic pain that demonstrated promising improvements in sleep quality [114]. We recommend that investigators consider carefully the use of both pain-related sleep interference and overall sleep quality indices, since the latter may have broader implications for both short- and long-term outcomes in chronic pain.

Acknowledgments

We would like to thank Ms. Amy Kwan for her extensive and thorough work in collating materials, identifying references, and doing many support tasks needed to compile the literature reviewed, and Dr. Robert Edwards for his helpful comments on an earlier draft of this chapter.

References

1. Serlin RC, Mendoza TR, Nakamura Y, *et al.* When is cancer pain mild, moderate or severe? Grading pain severity by its interference with function. *Pain* 1995; **61**: 277–84.

2. Rudy TE, Lieber SJ, Boston JR, *et al.* Psychosocial predictors of physical performance in disabled individuals with chronic pain. *Clin J Pain* 2003; **19**: 18–30.

3. Tyler EJ, Jensen MP, Engel JM, *et al.* The reliability and validity of pain interference measures in persons with cerebral palsy. *Arch Phys Med Rehabil* 2002; **83**: 236–9.

4. Deshields TL, Tait RC, Gfeller JD, *et al.* Relationship between social desirability and self-report in chronic pain patients. *Clin J Pain* 1995; **11**: 189–93.

5. de Bock GH, Hermans J, van Marwijk HW, *et al.* Health-related quality of life assessments in osteoarthritis during NSAID treatment. *Pharm World Sci* 1996; **18**: 130–6.

6. Tait RC, Pollard CA, Margolis RB, *et al.* The Pain Disability Index: Psychometric and validity data. *Arch Phys Med Rehabil* 1987; **68**: 438–41.

7. Daut RL, Cleeland CS, Flanery RC. Development of the Wisconsin Brief Pain Questionnaire to assess pain in cancer and other diseases. *Pain* 1983; **17**: 197–210.

8. Kerns R, Turk D, Rudy T. The West Haven-Yale Multidimensional Pain Inventory (WHYMPI). *Pain* 1985; **23**: 345–56.

9. Bergner M, Bobbitt RA, Carter WB, *et al.* The sickness impact profile: Development and final revision of a health status measure. *Med Care* 1981; **19**: 787–805.

10. Lousberg R, Van Breukelen GJ, Groenman NH, *et al.* Psychometric properties of the Multidimensional Pain Inventory, Dutch language version (MPI-DLV). *Behav Res Ther* 1999; **37**: 167–82.

11. Schwarz N. Self-reports: How the questions shape the answers. *Am Psychol* 2003; **54**: 93–105.

12. Anderson KO, Syrjala KL, Cleeland CS. How to assess cancer pain. In *Handbook of Pain Assessment*. 2nd edn, eds. DC Turk DC and R Melzack. (New York: Guilford Press, 2001), pp. 579–600.

13. Cleeland CS, Ryan KM. Pain assessment: Global use of the Brief Pain Inventory. *Ann Acad Med Singapore* 1994; **23**: 129–38.

14. Cleeland CS, Nakamura Y, Mendoza TR, *et al.* Dimensions of the impact of cancer pain in a four country sample: new information from multidimensional scaling. *Pain* 1996; **67**: 267–73.

15. Portenoy RK, Miransky J, Thaler HT, *et al.* Pain in ambulatory patients with lung or colon cancer. Prevalence, characteristics, and effect. *Cancer* 1992; **70**: 1616–24.

16. Radbruch L, Loick G, Kiencke P, *et al.* Validation of the German version of the Brief Pain Inventory. *J Pain Symptom Manage* 1999; **18**: 180–7.

17. Owen JE, Klapow JC, Casebeer L. Evaluating the relationship between pain presentation and health-related quality of life in outpatients with metastatic or recurrent neoplastic disease. *Qual Life Res* 2000; **9**: 855–63.

18. Smith MY, Egert J, Winkel G, *et al.* The impact of PTSD on pain experience in persons with HIV/AIDS. *Pain* 2002; **98**: 9–17.

19. Hardy JR, Rees EA, Gwilliam B, *et al.* A phase II study to establish the efficacy and toxicity of sodium valproate in patients with cancer-related neuropathic pain. *J Pain Symptom Manage* 2001; **21**: 204–9.

20. Wallace M, Rauck RL, Moulin D, *et al.* Conversion from standard opioid therapy to once-daily oral extended-release hydromorphone in patients with chronic cancer pain. *J Int Med Res* 2008; **36**: 343–52.

21. White WT, Patel N, Drass M, *et al.* Lidocaine patch 5% with systemic analgesics such as gabapentin: A rational polypharmacy approach for the treatment of chronic pain. *Pain Med* 2003; **4**: 321–30.

22. Du Pen SL, Du Pen AR, Polissar N, *et al.* Implementing guidelines for cancer pain management: Results of a randomized controlled clinical trial. *J Clin Oncol* 1999; **17**: 361–70.

23. Schiffmann R, Kopp JB, Austin HA, III, *et al.* Enzyme replacement therapy in Fabry disease: A randomized controlled trial. *JAMA* 2001; **285**: 2743–9.

24. Armstrong DG, Chappell AS, Le TK, *et al.* Duloxetine for the management of diabetic peripheral neuropathic pain: Evaluation of functional outcomes. *Pain Med* 2007; **8**: 410–8.

25. Passard A, Attal N, Benadhira R, *et al.* Effects of unilateral repetitive transcranial magnetic stimulation of the motor cortex on chronic widespread pain in fibromyalgia. *Brain* 2007; **130**: 2661–70.

26. Cowan DT, Wilson-Barnett DJ, Griffiths P, *et al.* A randomized, double-blind, placebo-controlled, cross-over pilot study to assess the effects of long-term opioid drug consumption and subsequent abstinence in chronic noncancer pain patients receiving controlled-release morphine. *Pain Med* 2005; **6**: 113–21.

27. Evans S, Fishman B, Spielman L, *et al.* Randomized trial of cognitive behavior therapy versus supportive psychotherapy for HIV-related peripheral neuropathic pain. *Psychosomatics* 2003; **44**: 44–50.

28. Ersek M, Turner JA, Cain KC, *et al.* Results of a randomized controlled trial to examine the efficacy of

a chronic pain self-management group for older adults [ISRCTN11899548]. *Pain* 2008; **138**: 29–40.

29. Rutledge DN, Jones CJ. Effects of topical essential oil on exercise volume after a 12-week exercise program for women with fibromyalgia: A pilot study. *J Altern Complement Med* 2007; **13**: 1099–106.

30. Chibnall JT, Tait RC. The Pain Disability Index: Factor structure and normative data. *Arch Phys Med Rehabil* 1994; **75**: 1082–6.

31. Arkinstall W, Sandler W, Goughnour B, *et al*. Efficacy of controlled-release codeine in chronic non-malignant pain: A randomized, placebo-controlled clinical trial. *Pain* 1995; **62**: 169–78.

32. Jerome A, Gross RT. Pain disability index: Construct and discriminant validity. *Arch Phys Med Rehabil* 1991; **72**: 920–2.

33. Gronblad MMD, Jarvinen EMS, Hurri HMD, *et al*. Relationship of the Pain Disability Index (PDI) and the Oswestry Disability Questionnaire (ODQ) with three dynamic physical tests in a group of patients with chronic low-back and leg pain. *Clin J Pain* 1994; **10**: 197–203.

34. Harke H, Gretenkort P, Ladleif HU, *et al*. Spinal cord stimulation in postherpetic neuralgia and in acute herpes zoster pain. *Anesth Analg* 2002; **94**: 694–700.

35. Eisenberg E, Lurie Y, Braker C, *et al*. Lamotrigine reduces painful diabetic neuropathy: A randomized, controlled study. *Neurology* 2001; **57**: 505–9.

36. Harden RN, Brenman E, Saltz S, *et al*. Topiramate in the management of spinal cord injury pain: A double-blind, randomized, placeb-controlled pilot study. In *Spinal Cord Injury: Assessment, mechanisms, management*. 23rd edn, eds. RP Yezierski and KJ Burchiel. (Seattle: IASP Press, 2002), pp. 393–407.

37. Gronblad M, Hupli M, Wennerstrand P, *et al*. Intercorrelation and test-retest reliability of the Pain Disability Index (PDI) and the Oswestry Disability Questionnaire (ODQ) and their correlation with pain intensity in low back pain patients. *Clin J Pain* 1993; **9**: 189–95.

38. Gronblad M, Jarvinen E, Airaksinen O, *et al*. Relationship of subjective disability with pain intensity, pain duration, pain location, and work-related factors in nonoperated patients with chronic low back pain. *Clin J Pain* 1996; **12**: 194–200.

39. Rochmon DL, Ray SA, Kullch RJ, *et al*. Validity and utility of the Canadian occupational performance measure as an outcome measure in a craniofacial pain center. *OTJR: Occupation, Participation and Health* 2008; **28**: 4–11.

40. Brown CS, Ling FW, Wan JY, *et al*. Efficacy of static magnetic field therapy in chronic pelvic pain: A double-blind pilot study. *Am J Obstet Gynecol* 2002; **187**: 1581–7.

41. Nurmikko TJ, Serpell MG, Hoggart B, *et al*. Sativex successfully treats neuropathic pain characterised by allodynia: A randomised, double-blind, placebo-controlled clinical trial. *Pain* 2007; **133**: 210–20.

42. Vranken JH, Dijkgraaf MGW, Kruis MR, *et al*. Iontophoretic administration of S(+)-ketamine in patients with intractable central pain: A placebo-controlled trial. *Pain* 2005; **118**: 224–31.

43. Lurie Y, Brecker C, Daoud D, *et al*. Lamotrigine in the treatment of painful diabetic neuropathy: A randomized, placebo-controlled study. In *Proceedings of the 9th World Congress on Pain*. 16th edn, eds M. Devor, MC Rowbotham and Z. Wiesenfeld-Hallin. (Seattle: IASP Press, 2000), pp. 857–61.

44. Vranken JH, Dijkgraaf MGW, Kruis MR, *et al*. Pregabalin in patients with central neuropathic pain: A randomized, double-blind, placebo-controlled trial of a flexible-dose regimen. *Pain* 2008; **136**: 150–7.

45. Hawk C, Long CR, Rowell RM, *et al*. A randomized trial investigating a chiropractic manual placebo: A novel design using standardized forces in the delivery of active and control treatments. *J Altern Complement Med* 2005; **11**: 109–17.

46. Bergner M, Bobbitt RA, Kressel S, *et al*. The sickness impact profile: Conceptual formulation and methodology for the development of a health status measure. *Int J Health Serv* 1976; **6**: 393–415.

47. Jensen MP, Turner JA, Romano JM, *et al*. Relationship of pain specific beliefs to chronic pain adjustment. *Pain* 1994; **57**: 301–9.

48. Follick MJ, Smith TJ, Ahern DK. The sickness impact profile: A global measure of disability in chronic low bakc pain. *Pain* 1985; **21**: 67–76.

49. Sullivan M, Ahlmen M, Bjelle A. Health status assessment in rheumatoid arthritis. I. Further work on the validity of the sickness impact profile. *J Rheumatol* 1990; **17**: 439–47.

50. Romano JM, Turner JA, Jensen MP, *et al*. Chronic pain patient-spouse behavioral interactions predict patient disability. *Pain* 1995; **63**: 353–60.

51. Epping-Jordan JE, Wahlgren DR, Williams RA, *et al*. Transition to chronic pain in men with low back pain: Predictive relationships among pain intensity, disability, and depressive symptoms. *Health Psychol* 1998; **17**: 421–7.

52. Jensen MP, Turner MA, Romano JM. Correlates of improvement in multidisciplinary treatment of chronic pain. *J Consult Clin Psychol* 1994; **62**: 172–9.

53. Burchiel KJ, Anderson VC, Brown FD, *et al*. Prospective, multicenter study of spinal cord

stimulation for relief of chronic back and extremity pain. *Spine* 1996; **21**: 2786–94.

54. Risch SV, Norvell NK, Pollock ML, *et al.* Lumbar strengthening in chronic low back pain patients. Physiologic and psychological benefits. *Spine* 1993; **18**: 232–8.

55. Spincemaille GH, Klomp HM, Steyerberg EW, *et al.* Pain and quality of life in patients with critical limb ischaemia: Results of a randomized controlled multicentre study on the effect of spinal cord stimulation. *Eur J Pain* 2000; **4**: 173–84.

56. Tak E, Staats P, Van HA, *et al.* The effects of an exercise program for older adults with osteoarthritis of the hip. *J Rheumatol* 2005; **32**: 1106–13.

57. Moulin DE, Iezzi A, Amireh R, *et al.* Randomized trial of oral morphine for chronic non-cancer pain. *Lancet* 1996; **347**: 143–7.

58. Carette S, Bell MJ, Reynolds WJ, *et al.* Comparison of amitriptyline, cyclobenzaprine, and placebo in the treatment of fibromyalgia. A randomized, double-blind clinical trial [see comments]. *Arthritis Rheum* 1994; **37**: 32–40.

59. Atkinson JH, Slater MA, Williams RA, *et al.* A placebo-controlled randomized clinical trial of nortriptyline for chronic low back pain. *Pain* 1998; **76**: 287–96.

60. van Santen M, Bolwijn P, Verstappen F, *et al.* A randomized clinical trial comparing fitness and biofeedback training versus basic treatment in patients with fibromyalgia. *J Rheumatol* 2002; **29**: 575–81.

61. Rudy TE. *Multiaxial assessment of pain Multidimensional pain inventory Computer program user's manual Version 2.1.* (Pittsburgh: University of Pittsburgh School of Medicine, 1989), 1–72.

62. Riley JL, III, Zawacki TM, Robinson ME, *et al.* Empirical test of the factor structure of the West Haven-Yale Multidimensional Pain Inventory. *Clin J Pain* 1999; **15**: 24–30.

63. Strong J, Westbury K, Smith G, *et al.* Treatment outcome in individuals with chronic pain: Is the Pain Stages of Change Questionnaire (PSOCQ) a useful tool? *Pain* 2002; **97**: 65–73.

64. Deisinger JA, Cassisi JE, Lofland KR, *et al.* An examination of the psychometric structure of the Multidimensional Pain Inventory. *J Clin Psychol* 2001; **57**: 765–83.

65. Bergstrom G, Jensen IB, Bodin L, *et al.* Reliability and factor structure of the Multidimensional Pain Inventory – Swedish Language Version (MPI-S). *Pain* 1998; **75**: 101–10.

66. Lousberg R, Schmidt AJ, Groenman NH, *et al.* Validating the MPI-DLV using experience sampling data. *J Behav Med* 1997; **20**: 195–206.

67. Olsson I, Bunketorp O, Carlsson SG, *et al.* Prediction of outcome in whiplash-associated disorders using West Haven-Yale Multidimensional Pain Inventory. *Clin J Pain* 2002; **18**: 238–44.

68. Hooten WM, Townsend CO, Sletten CD, *et al.* Treatment outcomes after multidisciplinary pain rehabilitation with analgesic medication withdrawal for patients with fibromyalgia. *Pain Med* 2007; **8**: 8–16.

69. Hooten WM, Townsend CO, Decker PA. Gender differences among patients with fibromyalgia undergoing multidisciplinary pain rehabilitation. *Pain Med* 2007; **8**: 624–32.

70. Turk DC, Okifuji A, Sinclair JD, *et al.* Interdisciplinary treatment for fibromyalgia syndrome: Clinical and statistical significance. *Arthritis Care Res* 1998; **11**: 186–95.

71. Nielson WR, Walker C, McCain GA. Cognitive behavioral treatment of fibromyalgia syndrome: Preliminary findings. *J Rheumatol* 1992; **19**: 98–103.

72. Turk DC, Rudy TE, Kubinski JA, *et al.* Dysfunctional patients with temporomandibular disorders: Evaluating the efficacy of a tailored treatment protocol. *J Consult Clin Psychol* 1996; **64**: 139–46.

73. Spence SH, Sharpe L, Newton-John T, *et al.* Effect of EMG biofeedback compared to applied relaxation training with chronic, upper extremity cumulative trauma disorders. *Pain* 1995; **63**: 199–206.

74. Flor H, Birbaumer N. Comparison of the efficacy of electromyographic biofeedback, cognitive-behavioral therapy, and conservative medical interventions in the treatment of chronic musculoskeletal pain. *J Consult Clin Psychol* 1993; **61**: 653–8.

75. Kjellby-Wendt G, Styf J, Carlsson SG. Early active rehabilitation after surgery for lumbar disc herniation: A prospective, randomized study of psychometric assessment in 50 patients. *Acta Orthop Scand* 2001; **72**: 518–24.

76. Raja SN, Haythornthwaite JA, Pappagallo M, *et al.* Opioids versus antidepressants in postherpetic neuralgia: A randomized, placebo-controlled trial. *Neurology* 2002; **59**: 1015–21.

77. Wallace MS, Magnuson S, Ridgeway B. Efficacy of oral mexiletine for neuropathic pain with allodynia: A double-blind, placebo-controlled, crossover study. *Reg Anesth Pain Med* 2000; **25**: 459–67.

78. Martin DP, Sleyren CD, Williams BA, *et al.* Improvement in fibromyalgia symptoms with

acupuncture: Results of a randomized controlled trial. *Mayo Clin Proc* 2006; **81**: 749–57.

79. Harding VR, de CW, Richardson PH, *et al*. The development of a battery of measures for assessing physical functioning of chronic pain patients. *Pain* 1994; **58**: 367–75.

80. Brooks D, Davis AM, Naglie G. Validity of 3 physical performance measures in inpatient geriatric rehabilitation. *Arch Phys Med Rehabil* 2006; **87**: 105–10.

81. Maly MR, Costigan PA, Olney SJ. Determinants of self-report outcome measures in people with knee osteoarthritis. *Arch Phys Med Rehabil* 2006; **87**: 96–104.

82. Walsh DA, Kelly SJ, Johnson PS, *et al*. Performance problems of patients with chronic low-back pain and the measurement of patient-centered outcome. *Spine* 2004; **29**: 87–93.

83. Williams AC, Richardson PH, Nicholas MK, *et al*. Inpatient vs. outpatient pain management: Results of a randomised controlled trial. *Pain* 1996; **66**: 13–22.

84. An B, Dai K, Zhu Z, *et al*. Baduanjin alleviates the symptoms of knee osteoarthritis. *J Altern Complement Med* 2008; **14**: 167–74.

85. Pfingsten M, Leibing E, Harter W, *et al*. Fear-avoidance behavior and anticipation of pain in patients with chronic low back pain: A randomized controlled study. *Pain Med* 2001; **2**: 259–66.

86. Weiner DK, Rudy TE, Glick RM, *et al*. Efficacy of percutaneous electrical nerve stimulation for the treatment of chronic low back pain in older adults. *J Am Geriatr Soc* 2003; **51**: 599–608.

87. Frestedt J, Walsh M, Kuskowski M, *et al*. A natural mineral supplement provides relief from knee osteoarthritis symptoms: A randomized controlled pilot trial. *Nutr J* 2008; **7**: 9.

90. Ng L, Chaudhary N, Sell P. The efficacy of corticosteroids in periradicular infiltration for chronic radicular pain: A randomized, double-blind, controlled trial. *Spine* 2005; **30**: 857–62.

91. Smeets RJEM, Vlaeyen JWS, Hidding A, *et al*. Chronic low back pain: Physical training, graded activity with problem solving training, or both. The one-year post-treatment results of a randomized controlled trial. *Pain* 2008; **134**: 263–76.

92. Haythornthwaite JA, Hegel MT, Kerns RD. Development of a sleep diary for chronic pain patients. *J Pain Symptom Manage* 1991; **6**: 65–72.

93. Menefee LA, Frank ED, Doghramji K, *et al*. Self-reported sleep quality and quality of life for individuals with chronic pain conditions. *Clin J Pain* 2000; **16**: 290–7.

94. Smith MT, Perlis ML, Smith MS, *et al*. Sleep quality and presleep arousal in chronic pain. *J Behav Med* 2000; **23**: 1–13.

95. Rowbotham M, Harden N, Stacey B, *et al*. Gabapentin for the treatment of postherpetic neuralgia: A randomized controlled trial. *JAMA* 1998; **280**: 1837–42.

96. Ahn SH, Park HW, Lee BS, *et al*. Gabapentin effect on neuropathic pain compared among patients with spinal cord injury and different durations of symptoms. *Spine* 2003; **28**: 341–6.

97. Watson CP, Vernich L, Chipman M, *et al*. Nortriptyline versus amitriptyline in postherpetic neuralgia: A randomized trial. *Neurology* 1998; **51**: 1166–71.

98. Bone M, Critchley P, Buggy DJ. Gabapentin in postamputation phantom limb pain: A randomized, double-blind, placebo-controlled, cross-over study. *Reg Anesth Pain Med* 2002; **27**: 481–6.

99. Finnerup NB, Sindrup SH, Bach FW, *et al*. Lamotrigine in spinal cord injury pain: A randomized controlled trial. *Pain* 2002; **96**: 375–83.

100. Tolle T, Freynhagen R, Versavel M, *et al*. Pregabalin for relief of neuropathic pain associated with diabetic neuropathy: A randomized, double-blind study. *Eur J Pain* 2008; **12**: 203–13.

101. Bone M, Critchley P, Buggy DJ. Gabapentin in postamputation phantom limb pain: A randomized, double-blind, placebo-controlled, cross-over study. *Reg Anesth Pain Med* 2002; **27**: 481–6.

102. Fishbain DA, Hall J, Meyers AL, *et al*. Does pain mediate the pain interference with sleep problem in chronic pain? Findings from studies for management of diabetic peripheral neuropathic pain with duloxetine. *J Pain Symptom Manage* 2008; **36**: 639–47.

103. Kosinski M, Janagap CC, Gajria K, Schein J Psychometric testing and validation of the Chronic Pain Sleep Inventory. *Clin Ther* 2007; **29** (Suppl 1): 2562–77.

104. Florete OG, Xiang J, Vorsanger GJ. Effects of extended-release tramadol on pain-related sleep parameters in patients with osteoarthritis. *Expert Opin Pharmacother* 2008; **9**: 1817–27.

105. Kivitz A, Ma C, Ahdieh H, *et al*. A 2-week, multicenter, randomized, double-blind, placebo-controlled, dose-ranging, phase III trial comparing the efficacy of oxymorphone extended release and placebo in adults with pain associated with osteoarthritis of the hip or knee. *Clin Ther* 2006; **28**: 352–64.

106. Harati Y, Gooch C, Swenson M, *et al*. Double-blind randomized trial of tramadol for the treatment of the pain of diabetic neuropathy. *Neurology* 1998; **50**: 1842–6.

107. Arnold LM, Russell IJ, Diri EW, *et al.* A 14-week, randomized, double-blinded, placebo-controlled monotherapy trial of pregabalin in patients with fibromyalgia. *J Pain* 2008; **9**: 792–805.

108. Currie SR, Wilson KG, Pontefract AJ, *et al.* Cognitive-behavioral treatment of insomnia secondary to chronic pain. *J Consult Clin Psychol* 2000; **68**: 407–16.

109. Tugwell P, Boers M, Brooks P, *et al.* OMERACT: An international initiative to improve outcome measurement in rheumatology. *Trials* 2007; **8**: 38.

110. Dworkin RH, Turk DC, Wyrwich KW, *et al.* Interpreting the clinical importance of treatment outcomes in chronic pain clinical trials: IMMPACT Recommendations. *J Pain* 2008; **9**: 105–21.

111. Rose M, Bjorner JB, Becker J, *et al.* Evaluation of a preliminary physical function item bank supported the expected advantages of the Patient-Reported Outcomes Measurement Information System (PROMIS). *J Clin Epidemiol* 2008; **61**: 17–33.

112. Smith MT, Haythornthwaite JA. How do sleep disturbance and chronic pain inter-relate? Insights from the longitudinal and cognitive-behavioral clinical trials literature. *Sleep Med Rev* 2004; **8**: 119–32.

113. Buysse DJ, Reynolds CF, III, Monk TH, *et al.* The Pittsburgh Sleep Quality Index: A new instrument for psychiatric practice and research. *Psychiatry Res* 1989; **28**: 193–213.

114. Edinger JD, Wohlgemuth WK, Krystal AD, *et al.* Behavioral insomnia therapy for fibromyalgia patients: A randomized clinical trial. *Arch Intern Med* 2005; **165**: 2527–35.

6

Assessment of pain and psychiatric comorbidities

Jon Streltzer

Overview

A condition that fits perfectly within the biopsychosocial model is pain. This applies to all clinical pain states: acute, cancer, and non-cancer chronic pain. Psychosocial and sociocultural factors are part and parcel of pain states, with personal, situational, and cultural factors all influencing the pain experience. The type of medical condition causing the pain state, and its meaning to the individual can also profoundly influence the pain experience and the associated degree of suffering. That being understood, however, pain states are also often comorbid with defined psychiatric disorders. In the case of chronic pain conditions, comorbid psychiatric disorders are particularly important to recognize and incorporate into treatment plans. Patients with cancer pain and terminal pain may also be prone to certain mental disorders, such as depression and delirium. In general, however, psychiatric comorbidity with cancer pain has more to do with the meaning of cancer than with pain.

Current understanding of the etiology and knowledge about effective treatments are strongest for acute pain disorders, but it is chronic pain populations that are of particular interest to psychiatrists, for it is this population that is likely to be the most troublesome to assess and treat. Several mental disorders are found to be more common in chronic pain populations, and the prevalence of mental disorders overall is substantially higher.

Mental disorders are common in pain populations. With regard to acute pain, most mental disorders are probably present in similar proportions to the general population. Certain mental disorders, including substance dependence disorders, and disorders involving impulsivity may actually be overrepresented in acute populations because they render the individual prone to accidents and other trauma. Available data are indirect, however.

Psychiatric comorbidity can be conceptualized in four categories: (1) psychiatric disorders that happen to be present in addition to a pain state without any etiological connection between the two; (2) psychiatric disorders that are, at least in part, presumed to be caused by the pain state; (3) psychiatric disorders that contribute to the experience of pain; and (4) psychiatric disorders that are part and parcel of the pain state, usually a somatoform pain disorder. Each of these four categories will be discussed in turn.

Psychiatric disorders that happen to be present in addition to a pain state include any psychiatric diagnosis. There may or may not be significant influence on the pain state. The psychiatric condition may influence communication style, which can affect the reporting of pain, making it more difficult to assess. This is particularly apparent in schizophrenia, or delirium, as examples. The mental disorder can also alter the perception of pain and influence the affective response to pain. A flat affect and loose or illogical associations of thought make evaluation of the subjective pain experience quite difficult, particularly if the schizophrenic disorder is not recognized.

> Case example: Schizophrenia: An acutely paranoid woman beginning hemodialysis for end-stage renal disease complained of pain and discomfort when needles were inserted to begin dialysis. She concluded that the dialysis machine was the devil, and the nursing staff were the devil's assistants. After treatment with antipsychotic medication, this delusion disappeared and she accepted thrice weekly dialysis treatment.

Perhaps of even greater importance, comorbid psychiatric conditions can complicate the doctor–patient relationship and affect compliance with and response to treatment. The patient with comorbid substance abuse may continually seek narcotic analgesics, feigning or exaggerating pain, making the actual pain state very difficult to assess. From a clinical perspective, many consider substance abuse or

Behavioral and Psychopharmacologic Pain Management, ed. Michael H. Ebert and Robert D. Kerns. Published by Cambridge University Press. © Cambridge University Press 2011.

"addiction" to be the major comorbid condition of concern.

Psychiatric disorders that are, at least in part, presumed to be caused by the pain state can include depressive, anxiety, and adjustment disorders. Pain itself is accompanied by emotional reactions. These reactions are determined by the context of the pain state, the meaning of the pain, and the patient's constitutional tendency to worry, be fearful, be discouraged, be resilient, and so forth. When chronic pain is poorly responsive to treatment, or associated with substantial disability, a mood or anxiety disorder is often present. Because chronic pain states are typically difficult to evaluate, some clinicians automatically accept the pain complaints at face value and view most psychiatric issues as responses to the pain state. The induction of a psychiatric condition in response to the pain state has been termed the "diathesis-stress model." [1]. This model posits that there is a pre-existing vulnerability that precipitates a psychiatric disorder under the stress of a painful condition.

Psychiatric disorders that contribute to the experience of pain are most often thought to be anxiety or depression. An anxious person, say, one who has experienced severe life stresses, might react with increased pain from a painful physical condition. A patient in the midst of a depression also might dwell on his or her pain excessively. In terms of personality factors, there is a great deal of interest in the so-called "catastrophizing" cognitive style, which makes the pain state more disabling and less responsive to treatment [2].

Psychiatric disorders in which the pain state is part of the disorder include the somatoform disorders, primarily pain disorder associated with psychological factors with or without a general medical condition, and somatization disorder, using DSM-IV terminology. In these conditions the pain cannot be adequately explained on medical grounds and is presumed to have primarily psychological determinants. Diagnostic criteria for these conditions are less precisely defined than other mental disorders, and these disorders are considered rare in some settings and common in others. Even clinics specializing in pain management will vary from diagnosing somatoform disorder rarely if at all, to diagnosing such in a majority of the patient population.

Case example: Somatoform pain disorder: A 42-year-old married woman immigrated to the USA, and was only able to obtain employment as a laundry worker. One day she bumped her head unloading a large washing machine. She initially complained of headaches, and over a period of a few weeks she complained of neck pain, back pain, shoulder pain, and dizziness. She was unable to work. Medical evaluations and imaging tests were unrevealing of significant pathology to explain the various pains. Physical therapy caused increased pain complaints.

This woman had multiple sites of pain following a trivial injury. Her condition was intractable to all treatment attempts. She was focused on verifying her disability rather than seeking ways to get better. Her family took over all her responsibilities at home, and she sought medical disability from work. Because her pains were not explainable by a medical condition and psychological factors were likely involved, her chronic pains were due to a somatoform pain disorder.

Comorbidity of psychopathology in general

A national comorbidity study, sampling over 9000 subjects in 2001/2, found that 19% reported a 1-year prevalence of chronic spinal (i.e., neck or back) pain. Of these, 35% had a comorbid mental disorder, mostly depression and anxiety disorders. In addition, almost 69% had another chronic pain condition, suggesting a high percentage of somatoform pain disorder [3]. The authors concluded that comorbidity contributes greatly to societal burdens of chronic spinal pain. This study used questionnaires and trained lay interviewers. The only mental disorders evaluated were depressive, anxiety, and substance dependence disorders. The prevalence of substance use disorders was quite low in contrast to depression and anxiety, yet no data was obtained regarding opioid or benzodiazepine use. Given the likelihood that many of the chronic pain subjects had multisomatoform pain, it is probable that a significant number of these had somatoform disorders not diagnosable by the study methodology.

Using data from the same survey, comorbidities of arthritis pain were examined: 27.3% of subjects reported a clinical condition of arthritis, and of these, 24.3% had a comorbid DSM-IV mood, anxiety, or substance use mental disorder. Alcohol and substance use disorders were uncommon, less than 4%. Anxiety disorders were the most common. Again, the most common comorbidity was another pain condition, reported by 45.6%, most of which was spine (back-neck) pain [4].

Most population studies have similar findings, and similar limitations, that is, demonstrating a high prevalence of anxiety and depressive disorders, but not evaluating for somatoform disorders, and not evaluating whether prescribed drugs are part of a substance use disorder. Personality disorders are not often assessed, but when they are the prevalence is usually high.

While most population studies are cross-sectional, a prospective study, surveying over 6600 respondents in 1998 and again in 2001 looked not at the association of mental disorders with pain, but at the association of mental disorders with the initiation of opioid treatment for pain. The prospective design revealed that the presence of a mental disorder (major depression, dysthymia, generalized anxiety disorder or panic disorder) greatly increased the likelihood of initiation into regular use of prescribed opioids for chronic pain. This was also true to a lesser extent for the presence of substance abuse in 1998, but not alcohol abuse. This period of time in the USA is associated with the encouragement and rapid rise of opioid prescribing for chronic pain. The authors of the study suggested that practitioners might have been attempting to treat relatively poorly differentiated states of mental and physical pain [5].

A problem with most studies is that opioid therapy can be a confounder. Opioids produce their own mental effects. In addition, patients may worry about their ability to function, which may be compromised by chronic opioids. There is substantial evidence that this can be the case, although some authors assert that unmanaged pain would be more disabling.

In a study of veterans receiving opioids for chronic back pain compared to those only receiving non-steroidal anti-inflammatory drugs (NSAIDs), but with identical pain ratings, depression, personality disorders, and history of substance abuse were more common in the veterans receiving opioids. Comparing the opioid-treated group to the non-opioid treated group, depression was found in 65% vs. 20%, substance use disorder was present in 43% vs. 13%, and a personality disorder was found in 14% vs. 1%, all significant at $p < 0.001$. There was no difference in the two groups in anxiety disorders or psychosis. In this sample, the average daily morphine equivalent dose was only 46 mg, a low dose in today's clinical population [6]. It is possible that the comorbidity in opioid-using chronic pain patients would be even greater in a population using larger doses.

In a study of patients presenting to the emergency room seeking refills of opioid prescriptions for pain, more than 80% were deemed to have a propensity for prescription drug abuse. A substantial portion had a comorbid psychiatric condition, with personality disorders, post-traumatic stress disorder (PTSD), and trait anxiety accounting for 38% of the variance in propensity for prescription drug abuse [7].

In conclusion, a great deal of psychiatric comorbidity is present in chronic pain states, and particularly so in those being prescribed opioids. Whether opioid prescription causes psychiatric disorders or is a response to them cannot be determined by these mostly cross-sectional studies.

Substance use disorders

Substance abuse is associated with pain states and chronic pain is associated with substance abuse. Acute pain is common because substance abusers are particularly prone to accidents and physical trauma while under the influence. This is recognized in the emergency room where drug screens are routinely done for patients with acute trauma, and a high percentage are positive for drug abuse.

Of particular concern, however, is the relationship of opioid dependence to chronic pain. A great deal of evidence supports the proposition that opioid dependence is not only associated with chronic pain, but that it actually enhances sensitivity to pain. A study by Rosenblum et al. [8] of patients receiving methadone maintenance treatment for narcotic addiction found that the subjects reported remarkably high levels of physical pain, both in intensity and frequency. It is well known that if an opioid-dependent patient suffers from acute trauma or has surgery requiring post-operative pain medication, he or she will need larger doses, not smaller, of opioid analgesics to control the acute pain. For example, a patient in a methadone maintenance treatment program for opioid addiction might be taking 100 mg of methadone daily. That dose would cause respiratory depression and likely death in an opioid-naïve individual. Methadone is a powerful analgesic, but this patient will not be protected from acute pain. To the contrary, pain will be very difficult to control.

Methadone maintenance patients have also been shown to have less tolerance for experimentally induced pain [9]. Neurophysiologic mechanisms explaining this phenomenon, called opioid-induced hyperalgesia [10], have recently been found. Chronic stimulation of the mu opioid receptor by ongoing opioid intake results in a cascade of cellular responses with multiple overlapping mechanisms, which can result in enhanced pain sensitivity. Cellular responses to chronic opioid-intake that contribute to this "drug-opposite" [11] effect include an increase in the production and activity of neuropeptides such as dynorphin [12], cholecystokinin [13], and substance P [14], all of which have been demonstrated to enhance pain sensitivity. Activation of glial cells producing inflammatory cytokines also results in amplified pain [15].

Despite the above, studies of opioid dependence in chronic pain patients have reported contradictory conclusions. Some consider opioid dependence to be part of the normal sequelae of daily opioid therapy, but one that is of relatively minimal consequence unless "addictive" behaviors" are present. "Addictive behaviors" include lying, seeking additional prescriptions from other doctors, using street drugs, and escalating doses beyond prescribed levels, seeking early refills, and related behaviors that are antisocial and manipulative for the purpose of obtaining more narcotic prescriptions. The compliant patient, even the one who convinces the doctor that dose escalations are necessary despite lack of a new acute problem, is not considered an "addict." Patients can be quite resourceful at minimizing past histories of addictive behaviors, and they can be quite convincing to physicians who assume the patient is trustworthy [16]. Essentially, if the opioid-dependent pain patient is likeable and adopts the patient role satisfactorily, he or she is unlikely to be considered an "addict." Thus, in some series, there are reports of extremely low rates of a substance disorder, even lower than the base rate in the general population. Underlying this interpretation is the assumption that opioids remain efficacious for pain even when taken daily in high doses. Increasingly, as described above, however, evidence shows the opposite!

Others have found high rates of opioid dependence in chronic pain populations. In one Veteran's Administration multidisciplinary pain clinic, 136 patients being maintained on opioids for chronic pain were followed for a year. Thirty-eight had flagrant addictive behaviors during that time period, resulting in being discharged from the clinic [17]. In another academic pain clinic, of 196 patients prescribed opioids for chronic pain, the 1-year incidence of opioid misuse was 32%. A history of drug or alcohol abuse was a strong predictor of opioid misuse [18].

Studies that show benefit and lack of substance use problems with opioid therapy have methodological deficiencies. These include low mean doses of opioids, inadequate followup, and deficient evaluation methods. Short-term clinical studies of opioids for pain tend to report benefits, whether they involve putting patients on opioids or taking patients off [19]. Long-term clinical studies are essentially absent. A meta-analysis of the effectiveness of opioids for chronic back pain found evidence, at best, of short-term benefit only, and found a high rate of past and current substance abuse disorders [20].

It has been proposed that significant opioid use in chronic pain conditions can lead to a downhill spiral of increasing pain, disability, and dependence on the opioids [21]. A study that attempted to test this hypothesis compared opioid users vs. non-users who were seen at a pain treatment center [22]. Aspects of the downhill spiral hypothesis were confirmed in the group of opioid users, but this result was confounded by benzodiazepine use within the opioid user group. This study had a significant limitation in addition in that the opioid user group had a very small median dose of opioids.

A Danish epidemiological community study demonstrated a large increase in disability and pain in the opioid-using group of chronic pain patients vs. the non-opioid using group [23]. This study specifically controlled for benzodiazepines, and this time the results were not influenced. Thus, this large, population-based study supports the downhill spiral hypothesis.

A large population study of veterans prescribed opioids for chronic pain found that mental health disorders were the strongest predictor of an opioid abuse/dependence diagnosis, with non-opioid substance abuse also a predictor. Only 2.8% of patients receiving opioids more than 211 days in 2002 received a clinically recognized diagnosis of opioid abuse/dependence in 2003–5, however. The authors suggested that the true rate might be higher [24]. This is probable for several reasons, including the likelihood that prescribers of maintenance opioids for chronic pain would consider the prescriptions necessary and appropriate rather than diagnose iatrogenic opioid dependence. Furthermore, it is possible that many of these veterans could be considered to be receiving office-based opioid maintenance therapy for opioid dependence, rather than an efficacious treatment for chronic pain.

Case report: Opioid dependence: Mr. M, a 56-year-old married man, was referred to a psychiatric pain specialist for evaluation. He complained of low back pain that had been quite severe for the past 10 years. The pain was present at all times, worsening when his medication would wear off. Every day he performed back exercises that he had learned in physical therapy, and he walked slowly for 30 minutes on days that he felt up to it. He was able to work in a limited fashion in a home business. Because he had run out of medication and experienced withdrawal symptoms in the past, his wife had taken control of his pain medications, dispensing them at specified times. Otherwise, he would take extra medication when his back pain was particularly troublesome, and this pattern would continue even after several substantial dose increases.

The first time he had difficulty with back pain was 16 years previously following heavy lifting at work. Five years after that he slipped and fell, and the back pain became excruciating from that time on. Treatments since then included multiple courses of physical therapy, chiropractic manipulation, epidural injections and nerve ablations. He underwent placement of a spinal cord stimulator, which was later removed. Analgesic doses gradually increased over several years until he was taking more than 1000 mg of extended release oxycodone daily. Despite these treatments, his back pain evidenced only occasional temporary improvements, and, over the years, it gradually worsened.

When his prescribing physician moved away, he had difficulty finding another physician who would prescribe sufficient oxycodone. He then experienced painful withdrawal symptoms. Finally, he found a physician who agreed to treat him with his desired narcotics as long as he gradually decreased the dose of oxycodone. This was done at a rate of 20 mg every month or two. After a couple years, the dose was 160 mg daily, but Mr. M found it impossible to reduce the dose further. In addition, for several years he was taking zolpidem, 20 mg, at night-time for sleep. Despite this, he awoke at approximately 2–3 a.m. every night and could not go back to sleep until his 6 a.m. dose of oxycodone was taken.

The pain specialist found Mr. M to be a pleasant man, eager for help, but fearful of any change in his medication regimen despite the immense burden that his painful condition was causing. On exam he had no neurological abnormalities. Pressure placed on the top of his head elicited complaints of his typical low back pain. This was a positive Waddell sign, a non-physiological finding [25]. This was thought to be consistent with psychological factors being important in the maintenance of the pain state. The psychological factors were thought to include the patient's fearfulness about his pain, and his opioid dependence. Treatment involved explaining to the patient how long-term high-dose opioids can enhance pain sensitivity, not allowing his condition to improve. With his wife's encouragement, he was willing to try a new approach, despite his fears. Oxycodone was discontinued and he was initiated on buprenorphine/naloxone. In addition zolpidem was discontinued and he was placed on a tapering dose of chlordiazepoxide. He soon found that he was able to sleep through the night for the first time in years. He gradually expanded his exercise regimen to include active, strenuous exercises, and walking briskly more than an hour daily. His concentration improved and he was able to devote more time to his home business, resulting in an increase in income. He felt most comfortable taking 16 mg of buprenorphine daily. After 1 year, he wanted to maintain this dose, but indicated that his goal was to eventually reduce and eliminate it.

During the time that he was on over 1000 mg of oxycodone daily, if asked, both he and his physician would have reported that he was stable on a dose that had not changed for over a year, and allowed him to cope with his pain. In fact, however, the patient was functioning well below his abilities, and it was a constant struggle to control the dose, necessitating giving his wife the task to dispense his medications on a strict schedule. In retrospect, he and his wife described that he had been quite moody with frequent episodes of mild intoxication, or mild withdrawal. He did not evidence "addictive behaviors" such as seeking prescriptions from other doctors, lying about his intake, claiming to have lost prescriptions, or taking medications to get high. He maintained good relations with all his physicians. Nevertheless, the diagnosis of opioid dependence seems clear, contributing immensely to the burden caused by his pain state.

Depression

Most studies confirm a high comorbidity between pain and depression, but being cross-sectional do not reveal whether depression leads to pain or pain leads to depression. Prospective studies seem to indicate that both directions occur. This is in conformity with clinical experience. Whichever the direction, it seems clear that comorbidity is associated with more functional disability, poorer response to treatment, worse quality of life, and more healthcare utilization. Numerous studies have found a high incidence of depression in pain states.

In a review of such studies, Bair et al. [26] found most clinical settings reported an incidence of major depression of more than 20%, with a range of 1.5–100%. Their review found that chronic pain patients with and without depression were not different in the frequency in which antidepressants were prescribed. Chronic pain patients who were depressed often were not treated for depression and those that were did not respond well to treatment. Depression was associated with an array of poor pain outcomes and worse prognosis. Patients with pain and comorbid depression experienced more pain complaints, more intense pain, more amplification of pain symptoms, and longer duration of pain. Depressed pain patients were more likely to have persistent pain and non-recovery than non-depressed pain patients.

In population surveys from 17 countries around the globe, people who reported suffering from a single pain site were almost twice as likely to have a comorbid major depressive disorder or dysthymia than those without pain. If multiple sites of pain were present, comorbid depression was almost four times as likely. There was remarkably little difference in the findings from the various countries, implying that comorbidity of depression and pain appears to be universal with relatively minimal cultural influence. Essentially the same results were found for comorbid anxiety disorders.

Abdominal pain is usually present in irritable bowel syndrome, a functional condition with altered gastrointestinal function, but in the absence of structural abnormalities. Perhaps half of those with irritable bowel symptoms do not seek treatment, but of those who do, diagnosable psychopathology, primarily anxiety and depressive disorders, are present in 50–90% [27].

A study of 148 geriatric patients admitted to an inpatient psychiatry unit with a depressive disorder found that 62% of those patients reported chronic pain. Those patients were more likely to report suicidal ideation and to be diagnosed with a personality disorder. The authors suggested that adequate treatment of the chronic pain could perhaps improve the depression. Adequate treatment is not defined but in the current cultural environment, some clinicians would take this as an invitation to try opioids, despite the likelihood that opioids may be neither safe nor effective in this population [28].

Studies of comorbidity of pain and depression rarely take into account chronic opioid use. Daily opioid intake, especially in high doses, is accompanied by more severe pain, more disability, and, most likely, depressive symptoms, if not initially, then eventually [23]. A reasonable assumption is that chronic pain plus daily opioids leads to a high incidence of depression. It is unlikely that daily opioid treatment of pain relieves primary depression. When depressive symptoms occur in association with opioid dependence and periodic withdrawal states, then opioid prescriptions may appear to alleviate depression, at least temporarily.

Case example: Depression and opioid dependence: A 41-year-old divorced woman suffered chronic low back, mid-back, and neck pain for 8 years, subsequent to a slip and fall injury at work. A few months after the injury, she had a laminectomy and diskectomy at L5–S1. Post-operatively, pain increased and she was maintained on opioids. She never returned to work. Prior to her injury, she was unhappy with her marriage, and she was also unhappy with her work supervisor. Over the years, her opioid dose gradually increased. She became more despondent, had difficulty with simple chores, slept erratically, and entertained suicidal fantasies. Eventually, after 2 years of resisting, she agreed to buprenorphine treatment for her opioid dependence. Although pain complaints continued essentially unchanged, family and friends reported that her old personality had returned, and her activities markedly increased.

Buprenorphine maintenance essentially eliminated the subtle states of withdrawal and intoxication present with her opioid analgesic regimen. She stopped having mood fluctuations, slept better, and had more energy and better concentration. She was reluctant to acknowledge the changes, perhaps because she was receiving disability compensation, but others clearly saw the improvements.

Anxiety

Case example: Generalized anxiety disorder: Mr. B, 24-years-old, complained of a painful aching throughout his body, associated with chronic fatigue. He was an anxious man, preoccupied with his symptoms. He always had numerous questions for his physicians. In addition to constant worries about his health, he worried about his appearance, his finances, and his relationships. He was diagnosed with generalized anxiety disorder with hypochondriacal tendencies. He was prescribed various medications, but he was always too anxious about side effects to take them more than once or twice. He entered psychotherapy, and his anxieties diminished. He learned to be less preoccupied with his physical symptoms. Fatigue and pain stopped bothering him and he was able to obtain employment.

This was a man with chronic somatoform pain and an anxiety disorder. In this case, the anxiety disorder seemed primary, and with successful treatment for the anxiety, the pain also diminished. In this case attempting to treat the pain and the physical symptoms with medications only continued or increased his anxiety tendencies.

The literature suggests that anxiety is as common and possibly even more common than depression in terms of comorbidity with chronic pain, and anxiety disorders rival depression in the risk for developing chronic pain and in predicting a poorer outcome of the pain state [29].

In the multinational comorbidity study cited above in the depression section, anxiety disorders (including generalized anxiety disorder, panic disorder, social anxiety disorder and PTSD) were found to be as commonly comorbid as depression, with a similar increase in the likelihood of a comorbid anxiety disorder with multiple pain sites [30].

A population study surveyed a nationally representative sample that included 588 individuals that reported arthritis pain, 614 with back pain, and 340 with migraine headaches. Three types of psychopathology were diagnosed. Compared to the surveyed individuals without pain, panic attacks and generalized anxiety disorder were more than two times as likely to be present in the back pain and arthritis subjects, and almost four times as likely in those reporting migraine headaches. Depression was 1.5–2 times more common in all pain groups [21].

Panic disorder and atypical chest pain are common comorbid conditions [33]. A patient suffering a panic attack typically finds it hard to breathe, feels chest pain, has light-headedness and dizziness, and will rush to the emergency room fearful of a heart attack. Cardiac workup is negative, and psychiatric evaluation confirms the presence of an anxiety disorder, often panic disorder, but panic attacks can be present in other anxiety disorders, also. Twenty-five percent of chest pain patients seen in emergency rooms have been reported to have panic disorder. Most commonly, the patients are young, anxious females [32]. Headache pain is also common among panic disorder patients [33].

Post-traumatic stress disorder, an anxiety disorder, engenders emotional pain and suffering, and it also has been associated with chronic somatic pain in several studies, particularly of military veterans. Up to 80% of combat veterans with PTSD report chronic pain. Patients whose pain developed after a work injury or motor vehicle accident commonly experience PTSD-like symptoms in chronic pain [34].

Case example: Cancer pain, PTSD, and substance abuse: Mr. W. was a 49-year-old single man when he was diagnosed with squamous cell carcinoma of the tonsil with lymphatic spread. He was a Vietnam combat veteran who had not adjusted well after the war. He had abused drugs and alcohol. He was employed sporadically and was occasionally homeless. Nightmares of combat experiences had diminished over the years, but he remained reluctant to talk about his experiences. Treatment of his cancer included radical neck surgery and radiation. Prognosis was for a survival of about 1 year. Post-operatively, he complained of great neck pain and was treated with high-dose opioids. As an outpatient, he was extremely demanding insisting on high-dose opioids for pain and a very high dose of alprazolam for sleep. At times, he came to clinic intoxicated on his medications, and he was so demanding of getting immediate prescriptions for more that two security guards had to be called to escort him off the premises.

He was referred to the specialty pain clinic. He was then switched to methadone to replace his several short-acting opioid analgesics that he had been demanding. He was no longer given alprazolam, but was prescribed a long-acting benzodiazepine that was systematically reduced in dose until it was eliminated. The patient complained about these changes, but he soon accepted this structure and his improved mental status. The methadone dose was then slowly decreased although periodically it had to be increased again due to infections or further surgery. After 3 years he began revealing some of his combat experiences, and also his persistent anxieties. After 5 years, the cancer did not recur. By that time he was managed with non-opioid analgesics only.

Animal models associate PTSD behavior with increased sensitivity to pain. When rats are subjected to electric shocks, or are terrified by exposure to cats, they behave in ways that appear to be models of PTSD. A number of physiological responses become altered, including an increased sensitivity to pain [35]. In humans, the association between PTSD and pain has been repeatedly demonstrated. Victims of accidents or rape who develop PTSD have an increased rate of pain disorders; in a similar manner, rates of PTSD are increased in chronic pain populations. In addition, PTSD is associated with increased severity of pain. In contrast to common lore, however, a history of childhood abuse has not been shown to be strongly related to chronic pain syndromes [36].

Case example: PTSD: Miss D, a 22-year-old woman from China had been recruited for what she thought was an employment opportunity in another country. Instead, it turned out that she was sold into sexual slavery. After her 1½ years of sexual abuse, she was rescued, but she did not adapt well to freedom. She was frightened to leave her apartment. She had nightmares every night. She complained of severe pelvic pain. She was diagnosed with post-traumatic stress disorder accompanied by severe depression. She would not talk about her experiences. She focused on her pelvic pain. Numerous medications were prescribed, but none of them helped, and she complained of side effects. Antidepressants did not relieve her depression. After 2 years, she still refused to talk about her experiences, but she became more functional, and was able to leave her apartment. She stopped focusing on her pelvic pain, although if asked, she indicated that it was unchanged.

Somatoform disorders

Case example: Mr. A was 33-years-old when he injured his back. He was a delivery truck driver who stumbled getting out of his truck one day. As he described it, from "Day one" he experienced severe low back pain that never went away, day or night. The pain continued for the next 15 years. For the first few years, he was resistant to treatment with opioid medications, disliking the way they made him feel. He had several courses of physical therapy, massage therapy, acupuncture, and biofeedback. Nothing helped, and he remained unable to return to his job. Multiple consultations failed to explain the cause of his ongoing pain. Because of the lack of neurological findings and the benign imaging studies, several surgeons found nothing on which to operate.

After several years, he agreed to a series of epidural injections. The injected solution included an opioid. The patient grew to like the injections, and sought them frequently. He claimed they gave him temporary relief, but the pain returned in less than 24 hours. He soon accepted a trial of opioid medication, which he began taking daily. Over the next couple years, the dose gradually increased and he became preoccupied with receiving his prescriptions even to the point of threatening his physician at one time. His pain did not improve with opioid medication, but his activities at home diminished, his relationship with his wife deteriorated leading to divorce, and he gave up the volunteer work that he had been doing.

This patient suffered back pain that disabled him from work and many other activities. Over the years, the pain spread, intermittently involving other areas of his body, including his upper back, shoulders, and legs. He developed frequent headaches in addition. He clearly had a somatoform pain disorder. Although he had no past history of drug or cigarette use, and only minimal alcohol use, he eventually became dependent on prescription opioids. This led to a worsening of his behaviors, and for the first time symptoms of depression.

Throughout history, cases have been well described in which prominent pain complaints appeared to have psychological origins. In more recent times, many celebrities have been treated for prescription drug dependence in which chronic pain complaints were blamed for ongoing opioid addiction. Some of Freud's seminal cases when he began practice as a neurologist involved chronic pain complaints labeled as "hysteria" because of the lack of structural abnormalities and the psychological presentation of the complaints, which differed from better understood pain syndromes. In some of these cases, painful symptoms were ameliorated as their origins were successfully analyzed.

Kirmayer and Sartorius outline seven distinct "loops" or processes in which a somatoform disorder can be reinforced so that the resulting pain symptoms are sustained by psychosocial factors [37]. Among these processes are an attention to sensations that increases the salience of the sensations and their intensity, which in turn leads to more focused attention. At another level sensations that are attributed to pathology lead to the conviction that one is ill, and this increases the tendency to further attribute sensations to pathology. At another level the reactions of others to the somatic distress can reinforce that experience and increase the likelihood of expressions of distress. If disability benefits are available, either materially or socially, this sanctions the avoidance of unpleasant circumstances and thus reinforces disability status. Thus, the psychology behind somatoform disorders can be complex and self-reinforcing.

All editions of the American Psychiatric Association's Diagnostic and Statistical Manual have included categories for psychologically based pain. Despite its prominent place in history, some clinicians

and investigators are reluctant to grant credence to the category of somatoform pain disorders [38]. Furthermore, neurophysiologic theories have arisen to explain medically unexplained pain. These theories typically involve "central sensitization", a phenomenon demonstrable in animal models of acute pain. Chronic pain sensitivity is most clearly understood as a consequence of ongoing opioid stimulation of the mu opioid receptor, however, as described above.

There have been relatively few studies of somatoform pain disorder, some even preferring terms such as "medically unexplained symptoms" rather than accepting an actual diagnostic category. Most large epidemiological studies of psychiatric conditions have not included somatoform pain disorder, probably because of the difficulty in making the diagnosis by questionnaires or for non-medically trained interviewers. Somatoform pain disorders may be most commonly seen in specialty pain clinics. In a clinic designed to consult on cases difficult to manage, 69% of 101 consecutive patients had multiple pain sites, and 88% met DSM-IV criteria for a somatoform pain disorder [39].

A community study that employed clinical interviewers who were psychologists or psychiatrists utilizing a standardized diagnostic module did diagnose DSM-IV Pain Disorder. It found a prevalence of 8.1% in a random population sample of over 4000. More than two-thirds were female, and most had multiple pain symptoms. Somatoform pain disorder was present in a quarter of all those with clinically significant pain in the past year. Mental disorders were more likely in those with clinically relevant pain compared to those without, and much more likely in those with somatoform pain disorder. Of those with a somatoform pain disorder, 53% had comorbid mood or anxiety disorders. Somatoform pain disorder was particularly associated with generalized anxiety disorder (7.1%; odds ratio = 7.3) and dysthymia (16.7%; odds ratio = 5.6). There was a substantial increase in disability days and healthcare utilization, even when controlling for comorbid mental disorders. The number of pain sites correlated with the number of disability days, doctor visits, and hospital days [40].

This study, using strict criteria, found a significant portion of a random population to have DSM-IV Pain Disorder. These results imply that somatoform pain disorders are often unrecognized or ignored, which in turn suggests treatment needs are unmet. It is likely that some of these somatoform patients are subject to invasive procedures, or are prescribed dependency-producing drugs, explaining some of the excess healthcare burden that these patients have.

In a review of the few studies of the comorbidity of somatoform pain disorders, comorbidity with anxiety disorders seemed to be the rule, and there was a high comorbidity with depressive disorders, also. Pain disorder appears to precede depressive disorders the majority of the time. Anxiety disorders precede or follow somatoform pain disorders about equally [41].

In a quasi-experimental study of somatoform pain disorder (DSMIIIR), 90 subjects evaluated a mean of 2½ years after a physical injury were divided into two groups: a somatoform group that had pain grossly disproportionate to the injury and any objective medical findings, and a control group whose pain was associated with clearly objective findings. In the somatoform group, injuries were trivial such as a minor fall or bump on the head with no actual bruises on initial exam. Over time this group had far more imaging and electrodiagnostic studies than the other group. The non-somatoform group had serious injuries, such as fractures and amputations. The somatoform group experienced statistically significantly more treatment episodes of physical therapy, massage therapy, and alternative modalities, without documented benefit. Antidepressant treatment was common in both groups, and helped depression, but not pain. The number of pain sites averaged more than five in the somatoform group, almost always spreading beyond the original site of pain, which did not occur in the control group. Daily opioid use was present in 50% of the somatoform pain disorder group compared to 9% of the control group. Daily benzodiazepine use was present in 34% of the somatoform pain disorder group compared to 5% of the controls [42]. This study provides evidence that somatoform pain disorder results in more healthcare utilization. Opioid dependence is a substantial risk when the pain is intractable and medically unexplained.

Personality disorders

Personality disorders are difficult to investigate because of the unreliability of diagnosis [43]. They appear to be common in chronic pain patients, however, with a prevalence of over 30% being reported [44], especially in somatoform pain disorder patients [42, 45].

A recent study from Germany investigated temperament as well as personality disorders in 207 chronic pain patients compared to controls [45].

Forty-one percent of chronic pain patients fulfilled criteria for having at least one personality disorder compared to 7% of controls. Paranoid and borderline types were most common. Fully 60% had somatoform disorders. Harm avoidance, a trait with strong genetic origins, was much more common in the chronic pain patients. This is consistent with the fear-avoidance model that postulates that fear of pain and avoidance of feared pain producing activities may be more disabling than the pain itself, and may maintain pain [46].

Patients with borderline personality disorder are notorious for self-mutilation, often cutting themselves or swallowing objects, for example. Thus, it has been thought that borderlines may be unusually insensitive to pain. When subjected to experimental pain, this indeed proved to be the case [47]. This may seem in contrast to the findings of the German study cited above [45], but the explanation may lie in the differences between acute and chronic pain, being subject to different psychological influences.

Psychotic disorders

Impaired processing of perceptual stimuli can make it difficult for a physician to obtain a correct or complete history of symptoms in a medically ill psychotic patient. Psychotic patients may not be able to describe their symptoms in ways that are comprehensible, and the complaints may be delusional or sound bizarre [48].

> Case example: A 50-year-old woman was the resident of a long-term psychiatric facility because of schizophrenia. While on a pass to take a vacation trip with her husband, they were involved in a motor vehicle accident, both suffering widespread burns. They were hospitalized for several weeks for treatment of these burns. The husband initially suffered excruciating pain. The woman had similar injuries, but never complained of pain, nor did she demonstrate any pain behaviors. This was so unusual that the staff sought to bring in a psychiatric consultant.

For more than a century, it has been observed that schizophrenics can be insensitive to acute pain [49]. The question arises, is this pain insensitivity part of the state of schizophrenia, or is it associated with the susceptibility to schizophrenia, a trait marker that is present prior to the onset of the disorder? In a study comparing pain thresholds in subjects with a family history of schizophrenia to controls, these subjects, indeed, had relative pain insensitivity [50]. It seems reasonable that in a disorder involving perceptual disturbance, such as hallucinations, and a thought disorder with defective reasoning, the lack of recognition of painful stimuli is quite consistent.

Dementia affects the person's ability to communicate pain states – it is unclear how it affects perception of pain. Experimentally, facial expression has been shown to match pain intensity when no verbal information is available [51]. If a demented patient has a painful medical condition, it would seem appropriate for the clinician to judge the presence of pain by not only facial expression, but also activity levels, appetite, and sometimes sleep.

Summary

Comorbid mental disorders are common in pain populations, particularly in those with chronic pain. Mental disorders can influence, be caused by, or just coexist with pain states. Comorbid conditions are associated with more disability and worse outcomes. This is true to an even greater extent in opioid-using patients that have comorbid disorders. Anxiety disorders are at least as common and may be even more common than depressive disorders. Substance use disorders are not that common in some population surveys, but they are frequently reported in populations of opioid using chronic pain patients. Prescription drug dependence is probably underdiagnosed. Substance abusers are subject to accidents and injuries, and thus are at higher risk for acute pain from trauma. Somatoform disorders are not often looked for, but when they are assessed, they represent a major portion of chronic pain populations. Personality disorders are rarely assessed, but appear to be common when somatoform disorders and opioid dependence are present with the pain state. Psychosis primarily affects communication about pain, and, at least in schizophrenia, may cause an insensitivity to pain. Particularly with regard to chronic pain, treatment should involve not just treating the comorbid conditions separately, but understanding how the comorbid condition interacts with the pain.

References

1. Dersh J, Gatchel RJ, Polatin P. Chronic spinal disorders and psychopathology. Research findings and theoretical considerations. *Spine J* 2001; **1**: 88–94.

2. Wolff B, Burns JW, Quartana PJ, *et al*. Pain catastrophizing, physiological indexes, and chronic pain severity: Tests of mediation and moderation models *J Behav Med* 2007; **31**: 105–14.

3. Von Korff M, Crane P, Lane M, *et al*. Chronic spinal pain and physical-mental comorbidity in the United States: Results from the national comorbidity survey replication. *Pain* 2005; **113**: 331–9.

4. Stang PE, Brandenburg NA, Lane MC, *et al*. Mental and physical comorbid conditions and days in role among persons with arthritis. *Psychosom Med* 2006; **68**: 152–8.

5. Sullivan M, Edlund MJ, Zhang L, Unutzer J, Wells KB. Association between mental health disorders, problem drug use, and regular prescription opioid use. *Arch Inter Med* 2006; **166**: 2087–93.

6. Breckenridge J, Clark JD. Patient characteristics associated with opioid versus nonsteroidal anti-inflammatory drug management of chronic low back pain. *J Pain* 2003; **4**: 344–50.

7. Wilsey BL, Fishman SM, Tsodikov A, *et al*. Psychological comorbidities predicting prescription opioid abuse among patients in chronic pain presenting to the emergency department. *Pain Med* 2008; **9**: 1107–17.

8. Rosenblum A, Joseph H, Fong C, *et al*. Prevalence and characteristics of chronic pain among chemically dependent patients in methadone maintenance and residential treatment facilities. *JAMA* 2003; **289**: 2370–78.

9. Doverty M, White JM, Somogyi AA, *et al*. Hyperalgesic responses in methadone maintenance patients. *Pain* 2001; **90**: 91–6.

10. Chang G, Chen L, Mao J. Opioid tolerance and hyperalgesia. *Med Clin North Amer* 2007; **91**: 199–211.

11. White JM. Pleasure into pain: The consequences of long-term opioid use. *Addict Behav* 2004; **29**, 1311–24.

12. Vanderah TW, Suenaga NM, Ossipov MH, *et al*. Tonic descending facilitation from the rostral ventromedial medulla mediates opioid-induced abnormal pain and antinociceptive tolerance. *J Neurosc* 2001; **21**: 279–86.

13. Xie JY, Herman DS, Stiller CO, *et al*. Cholecystokinin in the rostral ventromedial medulla mediates opioid-induced hyperalgesia and antinociceptive tolerance. *J Neurosci* 2005; **25**: 409–16.

14. King T, Gardell LR, Wang R, *et al*. Role of NK-1 transmission in opioid-induced hyperalgesia. *Pain* 2005; **116**: 276–88.

15. Watkins LR, Hutchinson MR, Ledeboer A, *et al*. Norman Cousins Lecture Glia as the "bad guys": implications for improving clinical pain control and the clinical utility of opioids. *Brain Behav Immun* 2007; **21**: 131–46.

16. Streltzer J, Johansen L. Prescription drug dependence and evolving beliefs about pain management. *Am J Psychiatry* 2006; **163**: 594–8.

17. Wu S M, Compton P, Bolus R, *et al*. The addiction behaviors checklist: Validation of a new clinician-based measure of inappropriate opioid use in chronic pain. *J Pain Symptom Manage* 2006; **32**: 342–51.

18. Ives TJ, Chelminski PR, Hammett-Stabler CA, *et al.* Predictors of opioid misuse in patients with chronic pain: A prospective cohort study. *BMC Health Services Research* 2006; **6**: 46.

19. Miller NS, Swiney T, Barkin RL. Effects of opioid prescription medication dependence and detoxification on pain perceptions and self-reports. *Am J Ther* 2006; **13**: 436–44.

20. Martell BA, O'Connor PG, Kerns RD, *et al.* Systematic review: Opioid treatment for chronic back pain: prevalence, efficacy, and association with addiction. *Ann Intern Med* 2007; **146**: 116–27.

21. McWilliams LA, Goodwin RD, Cox BJ. Depression and anxiety associated with three pain conditions: Results from a nationally representative sample. *Pain* 2004; **111**: 77–83.

22. Ciccone DS, Just N, Bandilla EB, *et al.* Psychological correlates of opioid use in patients with chronic nonmalignant pain: A preliminary test of the downhill spiral hypothesis. *J Pain Symptom Manage* 2000; **20**: 180–92.

23. Eriksen J, Sjøgren P, Bruera E, Ekholm O, Rasmussen NK. Critical issues on opioids in chronic non-cancer pain: An epidemiological study. *Pain* 2006; **125**: 172–9.

24. Edlund MJ, Steffick D, Hudson T, Harris KM, Sullivan M. Risk factors for clinically recognized opioid abuse and dependence among veterans using opioids for chronic non-cancer pain. *Pain* 2007; **129**: 355–62.

25. Waddell G, McCulloch JA, Kummel E, Venner RM. Nonorganic physical signs in low back pain. *Spine* 1980; **5**: 117–25.

26. Bair MJ, Robinson RL, Katon W, Kroenke K. Depression and pain comorbidity: A literature review. *Arch Inter Med* 2003; **163**: 2433–45.

27. Lydiard RB. Irritable bowel syndrome, anxiety, and depression: What are the links? *J Clin Psychiatry* 2001; **62** Suppl 8: 38–45.

28. Meeks TW, Dunn LB, Kim DS, *et al.* Chronic pain and depression among geriatric psychiatry inpatients. *Am J Ther* 2007; **23**: 637–42.

29. Roy-Byrne PP, Davidson KW, Kessler RC, *et al.* Anxiety disorders and comorbid medical illness. *Gen Hosp Psychiatry* 2008; **30**: 208–25.

30. Gureje O, Von Korff M, Kola L, *et al.* The relation between multiple pains and mental disorders: Results from the World Mental Health Surveys. *Pain* 2008 **135**: 82–91.

31. Katerndahl D. Panic plaques: Panic disorder coronary artery disease in patients with chest pain. *J Am Board Fam Pract* 2004; **17**: 114–26.

32. Huffman JC, Pollack MH. Predicting panic disorder among patients with chest pain: An analysis of the literature. *Psychosomatics* 2003; **44**: 222–36.

33. Schmidt NB, Santiago HT, Trakowski JH, Kendren JM. Pain in patients with panic disorder: Relation to symptoms, cognitive characteristics and treatment outcome. *Pain Res Manage* 2002; **7**: 134–41.

34. Asmundson GJ, Coons MJ, Taylor S, Katz J. PTSD and the experience of pain: Research and clinical implications of shared vulnerability and mutual maintenance models. *Can J Psychiatry* 2002; **47**: 930–7.

35. Stam R. PTSD and stress sensitisation: A tale of brain and body Part 2: Animal models. *Neurosci Biobehav Rev* 2007; **31**: 558–84.

36. Stam R. PTSD and stress sensitisation: A tale of brain and body Part I: Human studies. *Neurosci Biobehav Rev* 2007; **31**: 530–57.

37. Kirmayer LJ, Sartorius N. Cultural models and somatic syndromes. *Psychosom Med* 2007; **69**: 832–40.

38. Fishbain D. Where have two DSM revisions taken us for the diagnosis of pain disorder in chronic pain patients? *Amer J Psychiatry* 1996; **153**: 137–8.

39. Anooshian J, Streltzer J, Goebert D. Effectiveness of a psychiatric pain clinic. *Psychosomatics* 1999; **40**: 226–32.

40. Fröhlich C, Jacobi F, Wittchen H. DSM-IV pain disorder in the general population. *Eur Arch Psychiatry Clin Neurosci* 2006; **256**: 187–96.

41. Lieb R, Meinlschmidt G, Araya R. Epidemiology of the association between somatoform disorders and anxiety and depressive disorders: An update. *Psychosom Med* 2007; **69**: 860–3.

42. Streltzer J, Eliashof BA, Kline AE Goebert D. Chronic pain disorder following physical injury. *Psychosomatics* 2000; **41**: 227–34.

43. Zimmerman M. Diagnosing personality disorders. *Arch Gen Psychiatry* 1994; **51**: 225–45.

44. Reich J, Tupin JP, Abramowitz SL. Psychiatric diagnosis of chronic pain patients. *Am J Psychiatry* 1983; **140**: 1495–98.

45. Conrad R, Schilling G, Bausch C, *et al.* Temperament and character personality profiles and personality disorders in chronic pain patients. *Pain* 2007; **133**: 197–209.

46. Waddell G, Newton M, Henderson I, Sommerville D, Main C. A Fear-avoidance Beliefs Questionnaire (FABQ) and the role of fear-avoidance beliefs in chronic low back pain and disability. *Pain* 1993: **52**: 157–68.

47. Schmahl C, Greffrath W, Baumgärtner U, *et al.* Differential nociceptive deficits in patients with borderline personality disorder and self-injurious behavior: laser-evoked potentials, spatial discrimination of noxious stimuli, and pain ratings. *Pain* 2004; **110**: 470–9.

48. Reeves RR, Torres RA. Exacerbation of psychosis by misinterpretation of physical symptoms. *South Med J* 2003; **96**: 702–4.

49. Singh MK, Giles LL, Nasrallah HA. Pain insensitivity in schizophrenia: Trait or state marker? *J Psychiatr Pract* 2006; **12**: 90–102.

50. Hooley JM, Delgado ML. Pain insensitivity in the relatives of schizophrenia patients. *Schizophr Res* 2001; **47**: 265–73.

51. Kunz M, Scharmann S, Hemmeter U, Schepelmann K, Lautenbacher S. The facial expression of pain in patients with dementia. *Pain* 2007; **133**: 221–8.

Assessment of emotional functioning in persons with pain

Robert D. Kerns and Renata Okonkwo

The measurement of emotional functioning as an important dimension of the experience of chronic pain has not yet been generally adopted in the field. This observation is puzzling given the large and ever expanding empirical literature on the relationship between the experience of pain and negative mood, symptoms of affective distress, and frank psychiatric disorder. For example, Turk [1], despite noting the high prevalence of psychiatric disorder, particularly depression, among patients referred to multidisciplinary pain clinics, failed to list the assessment of mood or symptoms of affective distress as one of the commonly cited criteria for evaluating outcomes from these programs. In a more recent review, Turk [2] also failed to identify emotional distress as a key index of clinical effectiveness of chronic pain treatment. A casual review of the published research in the past several years fails to identify the inclusion of measures of emotional distress in most studies of pain treatment outcome, other than those designed to evaluate the efficacy of psychological interventions.

The primary goal of this chapter is to encourage the routine inclusion of specific measures of emotional functioning in the conduct of comprehensive pain assessments in both clinical and research settings, and to provide specific recommendations for the selection of appropriate measures of emotional functioning. This chapter will begin with the presentation of a rationale for the importance of assessing emotional functioning in this context. Specific dimensions of the broader experience of affective distress will be highlighted, particularly the experiences of depression, anxiety, and anger. The importance of discriminating mood states, from mood symptom clusters, and from psychiatric disorders will be discussed. This discussion will be followed by a comprehensive review of the key measures of these constructs and the data related to their reliability, validity, and utility. Recommendations will be offered

for the selection of specific measures of emotional functioning. The chapter will conclude with a few specific suggestions for future research in this area.

Why include assessment of emotional functioning in a comprehensive pain assessment?

Kerns [153] argued that psychosocial variables, including measures of emotional functioning, should be considered to be of primary importance, rather than continuing to be viewed as secondary to measures of pain relief, per se. Furthermore, Kerns and colleagues contended that the dominant contemporary models of pain emphasize the multidimensional nature of the experience of pain [3] and that the sole reliance on pain reports is inadequate for capturing the breadth and complexity of the experience of pain. He also cited the high prevalence and enormous costs associated with the experience of emotional distress and disorder among persons with persistent pain [e.g., 4, 5]. Finally, support comes from empirical demonstrations of the relative independence of pain and emotional distress [6] and from studies that have identified subgroups of persons with chronic pain on the basis of their high level of reported interpersonal and emotional distress [7, 8].

Dimensions of emotional functioning

An extensive empirical literature from both laboratory and clinical settings highlights the important relationship between mood states and symptoms of emotional distress and the experience of pain [9, 10]. The three most commonly studied dimensions of negative emotion are anxiety, depression, and anger [10]. Studies generally have focused on developing estimates of the prevalence of mood disorders among persons with chronic

Behavioral and Psychopharmacologic Pain Management, ed. Michael H. Ebert and Robert D. Kerns. Published by Cambridge University Press. © Cambridge University Press 2011.

pain, the development and refinement of models that describe and explain the impact of negative emotions on pain and pain-related disability and vice versa, and strategies for reliable assessment of these constructs.

The experience of anxiety and fear in association with the experience of pain is almost ubiquitous. An anxious mood state has long been recognized as having a dramatic and reliable effect on pain perception in the laboratory setting [11, 12]. Rates of anxiety disorders have been consistently found to be high among persons with chronic pain [4, 13]. There is also evidence that specific anxiety disorders may be particularly common among persons with certain painful medical conditions. For example, Beitman and colleagues [14] have reported that between 34% and 59% of persons with chest pain of unknown etiology may meet diagnostic criteria for panic disorder. Beckham and colleagues [15] have reported that up to 80% of Vietnam veterans with post-traumatic stress disorder (PTSD), another specific anxiety disorder, report chronic pain, and other studies have documented rates of PTSD to be as high as 50–100% among persons receiving treatment at pain treatment centers [16].

Of growing interest are observations of the specifically important role of pain-relevant anxiety, and in particular, a specific phobia, that is fear of pain [17]. Patterns of pain-related fear and behavioral avoidance related to pain have been observed to affect reports of pain and pain-related disability as well as physical performance measures [18, 19].

A particularly high rate of the coprevalence of pain and depression is well documented [5, 20], as is evidence that depression among persons with chronic pain may be associated with increased healthcare system utilization and increased disability. Romano and Turner [20] noted that reported prevalence rates of depression range from as low as 10% to as high as 100%, and Banks and Kerns [5] have suggested that, on average, rates of depression among persons presenting for multidisciplinary pain treatment are approximately 50%. The latter authors have suggested that the rates of depressive disorder are higher among persons with chronic pain than among persons with any other acute or chronic illness. There is also evidence that the presence of depression may negatively influence response to treatment [21]. These observations have led to an extensive body of research designed to examine putative neurobiological and psychosocial mediators of the relationship between pain and depression.

Anger among persons with pain has also been widely observed [10, 17], and has been found to be a particularly strong correlate of pain intensity, even relative to other negative emotional states [22, 23], and has also been demonstrated to interfere with treatment [24]. The style of expressing intense negative emotion, particularly anger, has been hypothesized to play a role in the development and perpetuation of persistent pain, pain-related disability, and depression [25–27]. Perhaps due to the relative lack of attention to anger in psychiatric nomenclature, research on the prevalence of problems with anger among people with chronic pain, and empirical research designed to investigate the relationship between anger and pain remains in their relative infancy.

Conceptual and empirical challenges in the assessment of anxiety, depression, and anger

Emotions are subjectively experienced private events that vary in intensity and are generally experienced as positive, or pleasant, or negative or unpleasant. Fernandez [17] listed several specific emotions as being of particular clinical interest: joy, anger, fear, sadness, shame, guilt, and envy. Among these, anxiety, depression, and anger have drawn the greatest attention among clinicians and researchers in the field of pain.

Fernandez [10, 17] also emphasizes the differences between emotions as a discrete episode, and mood as a relatively continuous process. These phenomena are further distinguished from temperament and personality, that is the tendency to experience certain emotions at a relatively high frequency, or certain moods for extended periods of time. The term "trait" is often used to describe this tendency, whereas "state" commonly refers to the momentary feelings. Among measures of anxiety, the most commonly used measure, the State-Trait Anxiety Inventory [28], is one that includes both a "state" form and a "trait" form that attempt to discriminate between transient experiences of anxiety and a more general tendency to be anxious. As will be discussed in more detail below, it is important to distinguish the experience of negative mood from a pathological state or disorder of emotion or mood. An affective disorder, for example, is characterized by an intensity and/or frequency that leads to an experience of dysfunction or concern on the part of the person experiencing the disorder or significant others.

The nature of the relationship between pain and emotion has been the target of considerable attention. Fernandez [10, 17] provides an overview of the several hypothesized models that can be articulated to describe, if not explain, the nature of the relationship. Each model generally attempts to ascribe a temporal relationship between pain and affect, and some incorporate a notion of causal direction. Perhaps the model with the greatest support is the simplest or most parsimonious one, as well. This model suggests simply that pain and emotion are correlates. Five other dynamic models of the relationship between pain and affect hypothesize that (1) affect is a predisposing factor in the experience of pain, (2) affect is a precipitating factor in pain, (3) affect is an exacerbating factor in pain, (4) affect is a consequence of pain, and (5) affect as a perpetuating factor in pain.

The importance of discriminating among the transient experience of a negative mood state, the experience of a cluster of symptoms commonly associated with emotional distress, and the diagnosis of a psychiatric disorder is critical in a discussion of the assessment of emotional functioning among persons with pain in the context of a comprehensive pain assessment. The construct of "depression", its operationalization, and its measurement represent the most common example of this challenge. The experience of sadness or even frank depression may be reliably and validly measured by a self-report questionnaire that asks persons to endorse a set of adjectives commonly accepted as representing this mood state, e.g., the Profile of Mood States [29]. In contrast, the two most commonly employed self-report measures of the broader construct of depressive symptom severity are the Beck Depression Inventory (BDI) [30] and the Center for Epidemiological Studies – Depression scale (CES-D) [31] that are comprised of numerous items reflecting not only the state of depressed mood, but commonly associated symptoms such as sleep difficulties, loss of interest in pleasurable activities, and loss of appetite and weight.

The diagnosis of Major Depressive Disorder (MDD), a particularly common psychiatric diagnosis among persons with chronic pain, requires the use of a clinical interview to ensure that several specific criteria for the diagnosis are met. Structured psychiatric interviews and diagnostic decision trees have been developed for facilitating reliable and valid diagnosis. As described below, the sensitivity and specificity of symptom severity measures such as the BDI and CES-D in making a diagnosis of MDD have also been described.

Sullivan [32] has argued that diagnosis of psychiatric disorders should not be considered only after a "medical disorder" has been "ruled out" as the cause

for persistent pain. He suggests that such a process leads to unnecessary and costly medical diagnostic procedures, iatrogenic injury, and poor clinical management. As an alternative, Sullivan suggests that psychiatric disorder should be considered any time a pain disorder becomes chronic. In support of this argument, Sullivan and others cite an extensive epidemiological literature that documents a high prevalence of primary psychiatric disorder among persons with chronic pain. Most commonly cited are depressive disorders, anxiety disorders, particularly panic disorders and PTSD, substance abuse and dependence disorders, somatization disorder, and personality disorders. An extensive body of research has attempted to address the question of whether pain most commonly leads to the development of subsequent psychiatric disorder [33] vs. whether psychiatric disorder serves as a vulnerability or predisposing factor for the development of persistent pain conditions [34]. Ultimately, Von Korff and Simon [35] have proposed that pain and psychiatric disorder should be viewed as reciprocal processes of illness expression and social adaptation.

Another important question that has led to extensive discussion and some empirical research is whether a model of depressive disorder that is inclusive of "physical symptoms" that may be attributable to the experience of pain (e.g., insomnia, fatigue) vs. a diagnostic conceptualization that excludes these symptoms is more appropriate and valid [36, 37]. The question has been raised in the context of reviews of epidemiological studies of the prevalence of MDD where some have suggested that rates of psychiatric disorder have been inflated and by others who suggest that treatment for the psychiatric disorder may be inappropriate and ineffective unless or until the pain condition is addressed. Koenig et al. [38] have argued that the evidence supports the reliability and sensitivity or "inclusive" models of MDD, in particular, and provide a compelling review suggesting that somatic symptoms of this disorder are not a direct function of the experience of pain.

Measures of emotional distress

The following review of measures of emotional distress begins with a consideration of primarily self-report measures of anxiety, particularly measures of pain-related fear, depressive symptom severity, and anger that may have relevance in the comprehensive assessment of persons with chronic pain as well as the evaluation of interventions for pain. Not reviewed are single item measures of emotional functioning (e.g., visual analog and numeric rating scale measures) as these strategies for the assessment of emotional distress, although appearing with some frequency in the pain literature, have largely been displaced by other multi-item standardized measures that have substantial evidence of reliability and validity. Also not considered are measures of other domains of emotional distress, including emotions other than anxiety, depression, and anger, since these have not generally been the target of particular interest and investigation in the pain field. Notable in their absence, however, are measures of marital and family distress that represent an increasingly important and interesting area of investigation in the pain literature. The decision not to review these measures is because relational distress has not become a primary target of intervention in the pain field, and when this dimension of distress has been investigated, it has largely not been affected by pain treatment. The review of measures of anxiety, depression, and anger is followed by a review of several multidimensional measures of emotional functioning and distress. The section concludes with a brief review of two semistructured psychiatric diagnostic interviews that serve as the primary methods for reliable diagnosis of disorders of emotional functioning.

Unfortunately, with the exception of measures of pain-related anxiety and fear that have recently been developed, virtually none of the other measures were developed for use in the assessment of emotional distress among persons with clinical pain conditions. Furthermore, most were developed with the intent of characterizing or quantifying the presence and severity of emotional distress or for use in screening for the presence of psychiatric disorder. Nevertheless, in several cases, these measures have subsequently been evaluated for their roles and utility as measures of emotional distress among persons with pain, and their value as measures of change in levels of emotional distress has been investigated in the context of studies of the efficacy of pain interventions.

Measurement of anxiety

The measurement of anxiety in the field of pain and pain management is increasingly dominated by measures of the construct of fear of pain. Recent data suggest that pain-related fear may be a key component in the development and maintenance of pain-related physical disability [39]. Pain-related fear (also referred to as kinesiophobia) may be defined as the constellation of fearful feelings and avoidance behaviors in anticipation of a re-experiencing of painful sensations or of a re-injury [40]. Research has demonstrated that for some individuals with chronic pain pain-related fear may mediate treatment-related improvement [41]. A brief consideration of more general measures of anxiety will be considered, followed by more detailed reviews of three measures of fear of pain, namely the Pain Anxiety Symptoms Scale [42] the Tampa Scale of Kinesiophobia [40], and the Fear-Avoidance Beliefs Questionnaire [43]. A fourth measure, the Fear of Pain Questionnaire – III (FPQ-III) [44], is not reviewed because of its recent development and the relative absence of empirical research that addresses its reliability and validity. Although none of these measures have been employed in an evaluation of pain treatment, they are briefly reviewed here because of their potential importance as pain-specific alternatives to the Spielberger measure of more general anxiety.

Spielberger State-Trait Anxiety Inventory

By far the most commonly used measure of anxiety in the pain literature has been the Spielberger State-Trait Anxiety Inventory (STAI) [28]. The measure was specifically designed to aid in the discrimination of situational (state) anxiety and dispositional (trait) anxiety. The STAI consists of two 20-item self-report inventories of each of these constructs. Respondents rate the degree of agreement with brief statements (e.g., "I feel calm") on four-point scales ranging from "not at all" to "very much so" in terms of either their present state or their frequency over time (trait version). There is a high concordance between pain and anxiety as measured by the STAI [45], and it has been widely used as a pain outcomes measure. It has acceptable psychometric properties [46], and it is sensitive to change [47].

Pain Anxiety Symptom Scale

The Pain Anxiety Symptom Scale (PASS) [42] was designed to assess the cognitive, physiological, and behavioral domains of pain-related fear. It includes 53 items distributed across four subscales measuring Fear of Pain, Cognitive Anxiety, Somatic Anxiety, and Escape and Avoidance. Respondents use 0 (never) to 6 (always) scales to endorse the frequency of each of the symptoms. The PASS has been demonstrated to have adequate internal consistency [42] with indices of internal consistency ranging from 0.81 to 0.89 for each of the four scales, and 0.94 for the total scale. Good predictive validity [48], and acceptable validity [49] have also been demonstrated. The PASS has been criticized for its poor prediction of disability relative to other pain-related fear measures [50] and its factor structure has also been challenged [51].

The Tampa Scale of Kinesiophobia

The Tampa Scale of Kinesiophobia (TSK) [40] is a 17-item instrument with items assessing pain-related fear of movement or of pain sensations due to concerns about injury or reinjury. Recent data suggest that the TSK may be a better predictor of a range of pain symptoms and behaviors than the other pain-related anxiety scales [40], and it has been found to be a better predictor of disability than pain intensity, biomedical signs and symptoms, or negative emotionality measures [50, 52].

Fear-Avoidance Beliefs Questionnaire

The Fear-Avoidance Beliefs Questionnaire [FABQ] [43] is a 21-item self-report measure based on fear theory and avoidance behavior and was specifically designed to assess patients' beliefs about the effects of activity and work on the experience of pain. Five statements are included about the relationship between pain and physical activity and respondents use a 0 (completely disagree) to 6 (completely agree) scale to rate their endorsement of the statement. Eleven additional items reflect beliefs about the relationship between pain and work. Instructions require respondents to use a similar seven-point scale. The authors of the measure demonstrated two subscale scores related to these two domains, although other investigators have reported three distinct factors [53, 54]. Results of each of these groups, as well as others [50, 55, 56], generally support the validity of the measure as a predictor of behavioral performance and treatment outcome. Buer and Linton [55] recently suggested that accumulating evidence suggests that fear-avoidance beliefs may be an appropriate target for intervention. To date, the measure has not been used to evaluate outcome following pain treatment.

Measures of depressive symptom severity

The two most commonly employed measures of depressive symptom severity are the Beck Depression Inventory [30, 57] and the Center for Epidemiological Studies – Depression scale [31]. Both measures have strong evidence of reliability, stability, and validity for use among the general population and among persons with known psychiatric disorder, and both have been employed extensively in the pain literature, including

use in studies of pain treatment outcome. Numerous additional measures of depressed mood and depressive symptom severity have also been developed, and several of these have been employed to a limited extent in the pain literature.

Beck Depression Inventory

The BDI was developed to measure the behavioral manifestations of depression in adolescents and adults and to standardize the assessment of depressive symptom severity in order to monitor change over time [30]. In its original form, the BDI consisted of 21 groups of four to five statements describing symptoms in each cluster from low to high. In 1978 the full scale was revised to eliminate redundancy among some of the items and the time frame for assessment was altered to "during the last week, including today". Only four possible responses for each symptom cluster are now included, so that scores on the measure range from 0 to 63. In 1996, the BDI-II was published and included revisions to some items and the time frame for assessment to be consistent with the DSM-IV. Although the BDI-II has advantages in terms of the content of the items and consistency with current diagnostic nomenclature, concerns have been raised about the sensitivity to change during brief periods of time as a function of the lengthened time frame for assessment [58].

The reliability and several dimensions of validity of the measure have been extensively reported. In a review of 25 years of research with the BDI, Beck and colleagues reported on 25 studies that evaluated the internal consistency of the measure [59]. Across psychiatric, healthy, and medically ill samples, indices of internal consistency (alphas) ranged from 0.73 to 0.95. Stability estimates (i.e., test-retest correlations) have consistently been high as well, typically varying in the 0.80 to 0.90 range depending on the assessment interval and sample. Validity estimates for psychiatric patients have been assessed by examining the correlation between BDI scores and clinical ratings of depression (e.g., using the Hamilton Rating Scale for Depression) average about 0.72. For non-psychiatric patients, the average validity estimate is 0.60.

Correlations with other common self-report measures of depressive symptom severity are reported to be 0.76 for the Symptom Checklist-90 and 0.60 with the Depression scale of the Minnesota Multiphasic Personality Inventory (MMPI) [58, 60]. In a review of eight studies of sensitivity to change, Moran and

Lambert [61] found that the BDI was sensitive to change as a function of psychotherapy and pharmacotherapy outcome studies.

The BDI has been used extensively in studies designed to evaluate the efficacy of pharmacologic and non-pharmacologic treatments for chronic pain [62–67], and there is ample evidence of its sensitivity to change. Results of most studies provide compelling support for the use of the BDI in assessing improvements in depressive symptom severity as a function of pain treatment.

Center for Epidemiologic Studies – Depression Scale

The CES-D was developed to screen for the presence of depressive illness and to measure levels of symptoms of depression in community samples [31]. Items were selected from existing scales (e.g., BDI, MMPI Depression scale, Zung Self-Rating Depression Scale) to represent the major components of depression on the basis of clinical and empirical studies. The measure includes 20 items that measure depressed mood, feelings of worthlessness, feelings of helplessness, loss of appetite, poor concentration, and sleep disturbance. Respondents are asked to rate the frequency of each symptom on a 0 (rarely or none of the time) to 3 (most or all of the time) scale with reference to the past week. Four items are worded in the positive direction to partially control for response bias. Scores on the measure range from 0 to 60. The CES-D takes about 5 minutes to complete [68].

Indices of internal consistency (Cronbach's alpha) have been reported to be 0.85 for community samples and 0.90 in psychiatric samples. Split-half reliabilities are also high, ranging from 0.77 to 0.92. Test-retest correlations over a 6–8 week period range from 0.51 to 0.67 [68]. Roberts [69] reported that studies of African-American and Mexican-American respondents revealed similar reliability estimates. The reliability and validity of the measure have also been examined in Asian-American, French, Greek, Hispanic, Japanese, and Yugoslavian populations [70], and it has been translated into several other languages, as well [68]. Overall, high levels of internal consistency have been reported across numerous samples from the general population and patient samples, irrespective of age, gender, race, and geographic location. In a sample of chronic pain patients, the level of internal consistency was found to be 0.90 [71]. Indices of criterion-related validity have generally been reported to be moderate to high. For example, correlations between the CES-D and the Depression scale of the SCL-90 for samples of

psychiatric patients have been reported to range from 0.73 to 0.90.

In a study of the CES-D in a primary care sample, the investigators provided evidence of the ability of the measure to discriminate between mild and severe, but not mild and moderate, or between moderate and severe, depression [72]. Sensitivity to change as a function of treatment for depression has been demonstrated [73]. Investigators in the pain field have called for modifications of the measure in terms of item content [33, 74] or scale cut-offs for the diagnosis of depression [75,76]. Ultimately, it is fair to say that the measure lacks the sensitivity and specificity for supporting its use in clinical diagnosis without concurrent use of a psychiatric interview. The CES-D has increasingly been used for the assessment of outcome following pain interventions, and in numerous cases, the measure has been demonstrated to be sensitive to change [77, 78].

Hamilton Rating Scale for Depression

The Hamilton Rating Scale for Depression (HAM-D) [79] represents a potentially valuable alternative to self-report questionnaires for the assessment of depressive symptom severity. Using this method, trained interviewers or clinicians make ratings of the presence and severity of specific symptoms of depression to derive a total score reflecting symptom severity. The HAM-D is almost certainly the most frequently employed observer-rated measure of depressive symptom severity.

Although the original version of the measure had 21 items, a 17-item version is the most commonly employed measure at the present time. Items are formatted as a checklist of symptoms with ratings of severity for each item ranging from either 0 to 4 or 0 to 2. Presumably, the decision to use only a 0–2 range was based on an assumption of the difficulty of making further discriminations in terms of severity for some symptoms. The range for each interviewer for the 17 items ranges from 0 to 50. A version of the scale with a manual for training interviewers was developed as part of the Early Clinical Drug Evaluation Program, and it is this version that is most commonly used [80], although several others have published guidelines designed to enhance its reliability [81–83]. Computerized versions have also been published [84], and the measure has been translated into numerous languages. Relatively recently, a self-report measure based on the HAM-D has been developed, termed the Hamilton Depression Inventory (HDI) [83]. The HAM-D usually takes between 15 and 20 minutes to administer.

Indices of internal consistency appear to vary considerably depending on the population and context. An international study yielded indices of only 0.48 before treatment, but 0.85 after treatment [85]. Other published reports generally have yielded indices of greater than 0.80 when structured interview methods are employed [82]. Indices of interrater agreement have also tended to be adequate, ranging from 0.65 [86] to 0.90 [79, 87].

Indices of criterion-related validity have also tended to be very good. Correlations with global measures of depressive symptom severity have been reported to be in the 0.65 to 0.90 range, and correlations with other clinician ratings have typically been in the 0.80 to 0.90 range [58].

Like other measures of depressive symptom severity that include a high number of somatic items, concerns have been raised that the HAM-D may yield inflated rates of depressive disorder when employed in medical populations or the elderly in which a high prevalence of medical conditions is known to be present. Another concern that has been raised is the ability of the HAM-D to reliably discriminate depression from anxiety symptoms [86]. The HAM-D has not been updated since prior to the publication of the DSM-III, and this fact may limit its current sensitivity and specificity as a method for screening for the presence of depressive disorder or for reliable monitoring of symptoms included in the current psychiatric nomenclature. Although the HAM-D has been encouraged because of its reliance on clinician interview and ratings rather than solely relying on respondent self-reports, data strongly suggest that its reliability can be improved with the use of a manual and adequate training of interviewers. Finally, the HAM-D has not been used extensively in the pain and pain management literatures and its sensitivity to change as a function of pain treatment has not been established.

Zung Self-Rating Depression Scale

The Zung Self-Rating Depression Scale (Zung SDS) [88] is another self-report measure of depressive symptom severity. The scale was developed to be short and simple to administer while at the same time including items reflecting the affective, cognitive, behavioral, and physiological components of depression. Items were specifically selected on the basis of diagnostic criteria at the time of its development and available factor analytic studies. The scale does not include several somatic symptoms acknowledged to be present in atypical depression including appetite and weight gain and hypersomnia. The original version of the Zung SDS included 20 items, with 10 items keyed in the positive direction and 10 in the negative direction to control for response bias. Respondents report frequency of occurrence of each symptom on four-point scales. A revised version altered the original wording of two items, but the measure has largely remained the same since its original development and publication. The scale takes between 5 and 30 minutes to complete, depending on the level of functioning of the respondent. The measure has been extensively translated, and data supporting its strong psychometric properties are available for many of these versions [58].

In one study of healthy volunteers, the index of internal consistency (Cronbach's alpha) was reported to be 0.79 and the split-half reliability coefficient was found to be 0.73. The criterion-related validity of the Zung SDS has been reported in several published studies, including correlations with other self-report (MMPI-Depression scale) and clinical interview measures (e.g., HAM-D) of depression ranging from 0.45 to 0.76 [89]. Although there have been several reports of the measure's sensitivity to change as a function of treatment for depression, a review of drug treatment studies found that the Zung SDS was specifically not sensitive to change relative to other depressive symptom severity measures [61]. There have also been significant challenges to its ability to yield reliable diagnoses of depression relative to other diagnostic categories [90]. There are few reports of its use with chronic pain patients, and psychometric data to support its reliability and validity in this population are lacking.

Geriatric Depression Scale

The Geriatric Depression Scale (GDS) [91] was specifically developed to assess depressive symptom severity among elderly persons. The development of the instrument was encouraged by observations of the fact that all of the other self-report measures of the construct were developed and validated with medically healthy younger adults. These measures suffer from the criticism that they include numerous somatic symptoms that are common among non-depressed elderly persons and that their format for responding may be difficult for some elderly persons.

The GDS consists of 30 "yes" vs. "no" questions; 10 are negatively keyed and 20 are positively keyed. Questions are ordered with more "acceptable" items presented first. A shorter version of the measure has also been published that consists of 15 items [92]. The total score for this version has been found to be highly correlated with the original version. An interview-based version has also been published that also is highly correlated with the original version and with the HAM-D [93]. Finally, a telephone version has been demonstrated to have good agreement with the original version [94].

In the original publication, indices of internal consistency (0.94) and split-half reliability (0.94) were extremely high. These indices were significantly higher than those for the Zung SDS in the same sample. Correlations with the Zung SDS (0.84) and HAM-D (0.83) were also reported to be high, and the GDS was successful in discriminating mild from severe depressed groups in this same study. In this study, depressed elderly persons with arthritis were discriminated from non-depressed persons with arthritis. Brink *et al.* [95] reported a high degree of sensitivity and specificity in discriminating depressed from non-depressed persons in a separate sample. This measure seems to have substantial advantages for the assessment of depressive symptom severity among elderly persons. However, additional research with chronic pain samples will be necessary before its use in pain treatment outcome research can be supported.

Hospital Anxiety and Depression Scale

The Hospital Anxiety and Depression Scale (HADS) [96] was specifically designed to screen for the presence of emotional distress among medically ill patients. In partial response to concerns raised about other measures of depression, in particular, the authors of this measure included only items that focus on the subjective experience of emotional distress, rather than physical signs. In addition, to further discriminate the experience of mood disturbance among medically, as opposed to psychiatrically, ill individuals, the depression subscale focuses on the experience of anhedonia, rather than on sadness.

The HADS is a self-report measure that includes only 14 items rated on four-point Likert-type scales. There are two subscales: depression and anxiety. Each subscale is comprised of seven items. A test manual has been published [97]. The HADS has been translated into numerous languages.

Indices of internal consistency of the depression subscale have been reported to generally be above 0.90 [96, 98]. Evidence of the criterion-related and discriminate validity of the HADS depression scale has

also been reported. Advantages of the measure for the assessment of depressive symptom severity are its brevity and its development and standardization for medically ill, as opposed to psychiatric, populations.

West Haven-Yale Multidimensional Pain Inventory – Affective Distress scale (MPI-AD)

The West Haven-Yale Multidimensional Pain Inventory Affective Distress scale (MPI-AD) [99] has become one of the most commonly employed measures of psychosocial functioning in the field of pain. Among its several subscales is a three-item Affective Distress scale. Indices of internal consistency and factorial validity have repeatedly been found to be adequate. Although data on the utility of the Affective Distress subscale as a valid measure of depressive symptom severity are limited, the fact that the measure was developed specifically for the assessment of distress among persons with pain, the extensive experience with the measure in the pain field, and its brevity encouraged attention as a potentially useful measure of emotional distress among persons with pain. The fact that the MPI has been used extensively to evaluate outcome from pain interventions also encourages its use in pain intervention research. Several studies have reported on the sensitivity of the Affective Distress scale to change as a function of treatment, in particular [67, 100].

Measures of anger

This section will provide only a cursory review of the available measures for the assessment of anger and the related construct of hostility, largely because of the absence of data supporting the relevance and utility of the measurement of anger in the context of pain treatment studies. As implied earlier, the failure to consider anger in the context of pain treatment is clearly not because of the rarity of anger or anger control problems among persons with chronic pain. On the contrary, as already noted, attention to the prevalence of anger among persons with chronic pain, and its potential role in the perpetuation, if not the development, of chronic pain and disability, is rapidly increasing in the literature on the psychosocial aspects of pain. More likely, the failure to include anger as a target of pain treatment or to include measurement of anger as an important outcome of treatment rests with the dominance of historical attention on anxiety and depression, the absence of specific "anger" disorders in the psychiatric nomenclature, and the relative absence of efficacious treatments for excessive anger and anger control problems.

Fernandez [17] provides a brief review of several different measures of anger, hostility, and anger expression that might have potential utility in the assessment of these variables among persons with clinical pain disorders. These include the following:

Buss Durkee Hostility Inventory [101]
Overcontrolled Hostility Scale [102]
Hostility and Direction of Hostility Questionnaire [103]
Cook-Medley Hostility Scale [104]
Anger Self-Report [105]
Reaction Inventory [106]
Anger Inventory [107]
Multidimensional Anger Inventory [108]
Targets and Reasons for Anger in Pain Sufferers [109]
State-Trait Anger Expression Inventory [110, 111]

Multidimensional measures of emotional (psychological) functioning

Minnesota Multiphasic Personality Inventory

The Minnesota Multiphasic Personality Inventory (MMPI) [112] is by far the most commonly used objective measure of personality, and it is similarly the most commonly employed measure for the evaluation of psychological functioning of persons with pain. A recently revised version, known as the MMPI-2, is comprised of 567 true–false items that are used to derive scores on ten clinical scales, three validity scales, and fifteen new content scales [113]. The ten clinical scales are the most commonly examined scales in clinical settings. These scales are named: Hypochondriasis, Depression, Hysteria, Psychopathic Deviate, Masculinity–Femininity, Paranoid, Psychasthenia, Schizophrenia, Mania, and Social Isolation. Respondent scores on these scales are converted into standard T-scores so that they may be compared to normative data. The revised version of the measure is thought to be more culturally sensitive and advantageous relative to the original version because the validation samples were more representative of the population of the USA.

Nevertheless, significant concerns have been raised about the appropriateness of either the MMPI or the MMPI-2 for use in the assessment of persons with chronic pain [114]. Observed differences on the clinical scales between pain and non-pain samples have been demonstrated to more likely reflect disease status rather than psychological functioning [115]. An extensive research effort has focused on the identification of

reliable subgroups of patients with chronic pain based on their MMPI profiles. The sum of this literature suggests that, although reliable subgroups can be identified, and despite evidence that the subgroups differ in terms of behavioral correlates of the experience of pain, it has yet to be demonstrated in a compelling fashion that the MMPI has value in characterizing patterns of coping with chronic pain over and above data derived from pain-specific measures [114].

In addition, inconsistent results from several studies challenge support for the value of the MMPI profiles as reliable predictors of pain treatment responsiveness [116–118]. Two recent studies stand in contrast to these relatively disappointing findings. In one study, Clark [119] reported that the Negative Treatment Indicators content scale from the MMPI-2 reliably predicted male patients' improvements in depressive symptom severity and physical capacity evaluations after multidisciplinary treatment. A study by Vendrig and colleagues demonstrated that scores on several MMPI-2 scales reliably predicted post-treatment changes on measures of pain intensity and disability [120]. Interestingly, in contrast to the Clark study findings, MMPI-2 scores did not predict post-treatment change on a similar measure of physical capacity. Similarly, results of studies designed to examine the sensitivity of the measure to change as a function of pain treatment have not been consistent or compelling.

Symptom Checklist-90 Revised

The Symptom Checklist-90 Revised (SCL-90R) [121] requires respondents to rate the extent to which they have been bothered by each of 90 physical or mental health symptoms in the past week. Responses are used to derive nine specific standardized indices of psychological disturbance labeled as Somatization, Obsessive-Compulsive, Interpersonal Sensitivity, Depression, Anxiety, Hostility, Phobic Anxiety, Paranoid Ideation, and Psychoticism. A Global Severity Index may also be derived. The reliability and validity of the SCL-90R for the evaluation of psychiatric patients have been extensively reported in a manual for the instrument [121] and by others [122].

Like the MMPI-2, the appropriateness of this measure for use in the assessment of persons with chronic pain has numerous critics. Jamison et al. [123] identified three reliable subgroups of patients with chronic pain using the SCL-90R. These investigators demonstrated that patients with elevations on the subscales of the measure, relative to those with a profile consistent with normative data, reported significantly higher levels of disability, sleep disturbance, and emotional distress. Unfortunately, no data have been published in support of the ability of these subgroups or the individual scales to predict pain treatment response [114]. A 53-item version of the measure, the Brief Symptom Inventory (BSI) [124] has also been published, but its psychometric strengths have been the focus of little research in the chronic pain field. Finally, the sensitivity of the SCL-90R or the BSI to change as a function of treatment has not been adequately demonstrated.

Millon Behavioral Health Inventory

The Millon Behavioral Health Inventory (MBHI) [125] is a 150-item true–false measure specifically developed to evaluate the psychological functioning of persons with physical health problems. Numerous scales measure styles of patients' interactions with healthcare providers (e.g., Cooperative), major psychological stressors (e.g., Social Alienation), and response to treatments (e.g., Pain Treatment Responsivity) and illness (e.g., Gastrointestinal Susceptibility). Adequate indices of reliability and validity have been reported, and the measure has clear advantages over either the MMPI or the SCL-90R since it was specifically designed and evaluated for use with physical health and illness populations. Despite these apparent advantages, results of studies designed to evaluate its predictive validity relative to treatment outcome evaluations have been discouraging [126, 127]. Again, although the MBHI may have some utility in the characterization of persons with chronic pain, its utility as an outcome measure in pain treatment studies is not clear and demonstration of its sensitivity to change as a function of treatment have not been forthcoming.

Illness Behavior Questionnaire

The Illness Behavior Questionnaire (IBQ) [128, 129] is a 62-item true–false questionnaire designed to identify patterns of abnormal illness behavior. Seven scales are labeled: General Hypochondriasis, Disease Conviction, Psychological vs. Somatic Focus of Disease, Affective Inhibition, Affective Disturbance, Denial of Life Problems Unrelated to Pain, and Irritability. Serious challenges to the reliability, factor structure, and validity of the IBQ have been raised, including concerns that it may be largely confounded by the respondent's level of anxiety or neurotic features [114]. Dworkin and his colleagues [130], in a recent published report, suggested that elevated scores on the IBQ may reflect an appropriate, rather than an abnormal, response to chronic pain.

On the other hand, several investigators have reported data that appear to support the validity of at least some aspects of the IBQ as a measure of chronic illness (pain) behavior among chronic pain patients [131, 132]. Ultimately, concerns about the validity of this measure seem to outweigh its apparent strengths.

The Medical Outcomes Study 36-Item Short-Form Health Survey

The Short-Form Health Survey (SF-36) was developed as a general measure of perceived health status [133]. The measure is generally self-administered, although it has been used extensively in telephone administrations or in other interview settings. The measure contains 36 items that are combined to form eight scales: Physical Functioning, Physical Role Functioning, Bodily Pain, General Health, Vitality, Social Functioning, Emotional Role Functioning, and Mental Health. Respondents use yes–no or five- or six-point scales to endorse the presence of degree of specific symptoms, problems, and concerns. The standard version of the measure employs a four-week recall period, but a more recent version uses a one-week timeframe. Scores on the scales range from 0–100 with higher scores indicating better health status and functioning. The measure takes about 10–15 minutes to complete.

The SF-36 has been extensive validated with large samples from the general population and across several demographic subgroups, including samples of healthy persons over 65 [134, 135]. A manual provides normative data for several medically ill groups [136]. Estimates of internal consistency (alphas) for most samples range from 0.62 to 0.94 for the subscales, with most estimates ranging over 0.80. Test–retest coefficients ranged from 0.43 to 0.81 for a 6-month period, and from 0.60 to 0.81 for a 2-week period [137]. Factor analytic studies have supported the presence of two distinct factors labeled Physical Health and Mental Health Functioning that account for 82% of the measure's variance [134].

The SF-36 has only recently begun to be studied in chronic pain populations, including use as an outcome measure in pain intervention trials [138, 139]. Rogers and his colleagues [140] reported that the SF-36 lacked reliability for the assessment of outcomes following multidisciplinary pain treatment and also questioned aspects of the measure's validity in discriminating dimensions of functional limitations. Similar concerns about the sensitivity of the SF-36 to change have also been raised [141].

Continued examination of the sensitivity of the SF-36 Mental Health Functioning component to change as a function of pain interventions is indicated.

Profile of Mood States

The Profile of Mood States (POMS) [29] is a self-report instrument designed to assess six dimensions of mood: Tension-Anxiety (i.e., heightened musculoskeletal tension including reports of somatic tension and observable psychomotor manifestations of anxiety), Depression-Dejection (i.e., depression accompanied by a sense of personal inadequacy), Anger-Hostility (i.e., anger and antipathy toward others), Vigor-Activity (i.e., vigorousness, ebullience, and high energy), Fatigue-Inertia (i.e., weariness, inertia, and low energy level), and Confusion-Bewilderment (i.e., bewilderment, muddle-headedness appearing to be an organized-disorganized dimension of emotion). It is comprised of a list of 65 mood-related adjectives that requires respondents to report the degree to which each feeling or mood state has applied to them "for the past week, including today" using 0 (not at all) to 4 (extremely) Likert-type scales.

Reliability and validity of the measure were initially derived from a sample of persons presenting for healthcare at an academic medical center ($n = 1000$). Persons who were illiterate, alcoholic, actively psychotic, and non-English speaking were excluded from the sample, and the age range was limited to those 60 years of age and under. Indices of internal consistency (alphas) for the six mood scales ranged from 0.84 for Confusion-Bewilderment to 0.95 for Depression-Dejection. Stability estimates (test-retest reliability correlations) ranged from 0.65 for Vigor-Activity to 0.74 for Depression-Dejection. Concurrent validity was examined via correlations with MMPI-2 scales. Correlations between scales of the POMS and analogous scales from the MMPI-2 were largely in the expected direction and significant, with coefficients ranging from -0.58 to 0.69. The POMS requires only about 3–5 minutes to administer.

The POMS has been used extensively in the pain treatment literature, and has been shown to be sensitive to change as a function of pain treatment [138, 142]. Interestingly, however, its use has been largely limited to pharmaceutical trials, and it has yet to be employed in a large, randomized controlled trial of any psychological intervention.

Advantages of the POMS include its ease of administration, its brevity, its development on non-psychiatric populations, and its design to capture both negative and positive dimensions of emotional functioning. In particular, since the POMS has scales for anxiety, depression, and anger, three of the most important dimensions of emotional distress among persons with pain, the scale has an explicit advantage over any alternative scale. The inclusion of an Anger-Hostility scale is particularly novel and potentially an advantage of the POMS relative to any other comparable instrument. The Vigor-Activity scale represents a relatively unique opportunity to assess improvements in this key dimension of emotional functioning rather than relying on a reduction in negative mood and symptoms of emotional distress. The Fatigue-Inertia scale provides an opportunity to measure this common concomitant of the experience of chronic pain, especially when assessing pain treatment among persons with clinical pain conditions in which fatigue is particularly prevalent (e.g., pain in multiple sclerosis). The opportunity to attempt to discriminate effects of a pain intervention on fatigue and anergia, on the one hand, and other symptoms of emotional distress, on the other, may have particular utility in certain cases. Finally, given concerns about the effects of certain pain medications on cognitive functioning, the Bewilderment-Confusion scale may also have some benefit.

Psychiatric diagnostic interviews

The use of structured psychiatric interviews is viewed as the "state of the art" for reliable determination of the presence of psychiatric disorder. Having said this, unstructured clinical interviewing remains a more commonly used method for determining psychiatric diagnosis in the clinical setting [32], and even in most published clinical trials, the presence of a psychiatric diagnosis is generally not reported to be based on one of the more reliable methods for making this determination.

The two most commonly employed and widely researched psychiatric interviews are the Diagnostic Interview Schedule (DIS) [143, 144] and the Structured Clinical Interview for DSM (SCID) [145]. Neither the DIS nor the SCID has been used to examine psychiatric diagnosis among samples of persons with chronic pain. Even more important in the current context, neither measure has been used to examine effects of pain treatment on remission from psychiatric disorder, or even for examination of moderating effects of psychiatric disorder on pain treatment outcome. Nevertheless, these measures are briefly reviewed here because of their potential utility in characterizing pain treatment study samples, to control for psychiatric diagnosis in pain outcome studies, and for their potential utility, as yet unrealized, as reliable and valid measures of the efficacy of pain treatments as a contributor to remission from psychiatric disorder.

Diagnostic Interview Schedule

The Diagnostic Interview Schedule (DIS), originally developed to provide reliable and valid diagnosis based on earlier versions of the Diagnostic and Statistical Manual of Mental Disorders (DSM), has been updated to correspond to the most recent edition (DSM-IV) [146]. Use of the DIS requires specialized training available at Washington University, home of its authors. Studies of the original version of the DIS revealed adequate test-retest stability estimates, with kappa coefficients ranging from 0.37 to 0.59 for lifetime psychiatric diagnosis over 1-year periods [147, 148]. Kappa coefficients for diagnoses made by psychiatrists and lay interviewers ranged from 0.47 to 1.00 [144]. Eaton and colleagues [149] have provided evidence that the DIS may lead to underestimations of psychiatric diagnosis among the elderly, males, and those who have a relatively low level of impairment.

Structured Clinical Interview for DSM

The SCID has also been recently updated to correspond to the DSM-IV [150]. Detailed materials are available to facilitate training in the use of this method. A computerized version of the measure has also been published [151]. Published rates of interrater agreement for primary psychiatric diagnosis hover around 0.70 [152].

Recommendations for the measurement of emotional distress in a comprehensive pain assessment

The introductory sections of this chapter provided a brief review of a broad array of issues that should be taken into account in making decisions about the selection of measures for assessing emotional functioning in the context of a comprehensive assessment of chronic pain. In addition, an outline of the most salient issues for assessing the efficacy or effectiveness of pain interventions was provided. These issues include: the efficacy or effectiveness of pain interventions; how to reliably and validly assess emotional distress given its private, subjective, and complex nature;

the importance of discriminating "levels" of analysis of emotional distress (i.e., mood, symptom clusters, disorders of emotional regulation) and dimensions of emotional distress (e.g., anxiety, depression, anger); and disagreements among clinicians and researchers alike about the nature of the relationship between pain and emotional distress. Perhaps as a function of both the theoretical and empirical complexity of these issues and the lack of a consensus about any of them, it is not surprising that routine measurement of emotional distress has not been generally accepted as being of central importance in the comprehensive assessment of persons with chronic pain nor outcome of pain interventions. On the other hand, the sheer prevalence of emotional distress among persons with clinical pain conditions, the pervasive negative effects of emotional distress on the experiences of pain and pain-related disability, the high costs associated with emotional distress among persons with pain, and the influence of emotional distress on pain treatment participation and outcomes all contribute to a view that emotional distress among persons with pain should be addressed in the context of any pain-relevant intervention, and should be assessed as an important, if not necessary, outcome of pain treatment.

Having reviewed these issues and agreed upon the importance of including reliable and valid measure(s) of emotional distress in both comprehensive assessments of persons with chronic pain and in pain treatment outcome research, it is equally clear that there is no current consensus on the appropriate targets for assessment of emotional distress, let alone their measurement. Particularly problematic is the fact that none of the most likely candidates for the assessment of emotional distress in pain treatment and intervention research were specifically developed for use in the assessment of persons with painful conditions. The few exceptions to this observation include measures that lack strong intuitive appeal as primary outcome measures of emotional distress due to their simplicity (e.g., MPI-Affective Distress scale), because they were not specifically designed to be used as outcome measures and likely lack sensitivity to change (e.g., Fear-Avoidance Beliefs Questionnaire), or have only recently been proposed and lack sufficient reliability and validity data.

One final problem in the existing pain outcome literature that deserves serious attention is the apparent discrepancy between the pharmacological and non-pharmacological pain intervention literature in terms of the selection of measures of emotional distress. The

POMS [24] is identified as the most commonly used measure of emotional distress in pharmacological treatment trials. This may be due to the simplicity of the measure and its low response burden, and perhaps most importantly, to the more general lack of specific attention to issues of coprevalent psychiatric disorder, particularly depression. On the other hand, the inclusion of a measure of depressive symptom severity (e.g., the BDI or CES-D), and often a measure of level of anxiety (e.g., STAI), appears to represent the state of the art for the assessment of outcomes from psychological pain treatments. Evaluations of the efficacy or effectiveness of multidisciplinary pain treatment programs have more often included measures of depressive and/or anxiety symptom severity.

Ultimately, the inclusion of a multidimensional measure of emotional functioning, such as the POMS, as well as a measure of depressive symptom severity, such as the BDI or CES-D, is recommended for all comprehensive pain assessments and intervention studies. The inclusion of a combination of these measures has distinct advantages over the selection of either one or the other of these measures alone. Support for this recommendation will highlight the known advantages of each of these measures, and will contrast their selection with alternative multidimensional and symptom-specific measures.

Among multidimensional measures of emotional functioning, the POMS appears to be the strongest candidate for inclusion in comprehensive pain assessments and pain intervention research. The POMS has the distinct advantage of having been developed for the assessment of mood among non-psychiatric populations, and numerous psychometric studies have provided evidence to support its use in healthy and medically ill samples, including samples of persons with clinical pain conditions. It is simple to administer and has a particularly low response burden, requiring only 3–5 minutes for most persons to complete. As already emphasized, the POMS includes dimensions of emotional functioning that may provide the most comprehensive characterization of persons with chronic pain. The inclusion of positive, in addition to negative, dimensions of emotional functioning may prove to have advantages for pain treatment programs that are explicitly designed to promote wellness and adaptation, in addition to reduction in pain and disability, per se. Results of numerous studies provide evidence of very good to excellent indices of reliability and stability of the measure. Published

validity indices have largely been strong, and in particular, are based on the some of the best, and most contemporary, alternative measures of emotional functioning (e.g., the MMPI-2). The increasing use of the measure in pain outcome research, and demonstrations of sensitivity to change as a function of pain interventions, is a particularly compelling reason for this recommendation.

Limitations of the POMS are primarily two-fold. First, like all other multidimensional measures of emotional functioning, are concerns about the intercorrelation of its subscales designed to measure discrete mood states. For most purposes, the use of a single composite score is indicated, and analyses focusing on change in the individual mood scales should be viewed with caution. Secondly, the measure is designed to serve as a measure of mood state, rather than as a more comprehensive measure of mood-related symptoms or disorder. For this reason, the importance of including a measure representative of a broader cluster of symptoms of emotional distress is strongly recommended when conducting pain outcome research.

As already described, the three most prevalent dimensions of emotional distress among persons with clinical pain disorders are anxiety, depression, and anger. Perhaps not surprisingly, assessment of anger and associated problems has not been a routine target in pain treatment nor in pain intervention research. Future research may help to identify the utility of targeting anger and its measurement in pain treatment, but to date, there is not strong support for a recommendation to include its measurement as a routine component of clinical pain interventions or pain outcome studies.

Anxiety, on the other hand, has an extensive history of dedicated attention in the pain field, including efforts to reduce this aspect of emotional distress in the context of pain treatment. For this reason, the pain research literature continues to focus on examination of the relationship between pain and anxiety, to refine pain treatments to further reduce pain-related anxiety, and to assess changes in anxiety as a function of treatment. The most commonly used measure of anxiety in the pain intervention literature is by far the Spielberger State-Trait Anxiety Inventory. The STAI was initially developed for use with psychiatric populations, but fails to incorporate dimensions of anxiety disorders in its content. The correlation of its scores with other dimensions of emotional distress is known to be particularly high. It is particularly noteworthy that the last decade has seen the emergence of a theory of pain-related fear and fear-avoidance and the proliferation of several alternative measures of pain-specific anxiety. None of these measures have been employed as part of a comprehensive assessment of individuals with chronic pain nor as indices of outcomes following pain treatment. It is likely that future research will incorporate such tests and may lead to recommendations for use of any one of these new measures as an important target for intervention and evaluation of its efficacy.

In contrast to these substantive concerns about inclusion of a measure of anxiety in pain treatment and research, there is compelling evidence to support the selection of a measure of depressive symptom severity. The apparently high prevalence of discrete symptoms of depression (i.e., depressed or irritable mood, loss of interest in normally pleasurable activities, sleep dysfunction, anergia and fatigue, pervasive negative thinking, suicidal ideation), and of major depressive disorder and dysthymic disorder argue strongly for routine inclusion of a measure of depressive symptoms, as opposed to the sole reliance on a measure of depressed or dysphoric mood, in the comprehensive assessment of individuals with chronic pain. Additional support comes from evidence of the analgesic potential of medications developed for the treatment of depressive disorder, observations that alleviation of depressed mood and other symptoms of depression may mediate the effectiveness of certain pain interventions, and evidence that depression may disrupt or interfere with successful pain treatment.

Among the several measures of depressive symptom severity, two have drawn the most attention from pain researchers and represent the state-of-the-art for assessment of this construct. Based on a comprehensive review of the issues salient to making a recommendation for the adoption of a single measure of depressive symptom severity, if not an exhaustive review of the published literature, the BDI and CES-D clearly have the strongest support. Ultimately, the preponderance of the evidence led to the recommendation to employ the BDI.

A particularly important distinction between the BDI and the CES-D was the stated intent of the authors of these measures. Beck and colleagues specifically designed the BDI to be a reliable measure of depressive symptom severity *and* to assess change over time as a function of treatment. Indeed, the measure has a long and impressive history in this regard, and there is ample evidence to support its sensitivity to change as

a function of both psychological and pharmacological treatments. As for the CES-D, it was designed to assess the level of depressive symptoms and to screen for the presence of depressive disorder in epidemiological studies of community, as opposed to clinical, samples. Although it has been employed extensively as a measure of change as a function of treatment, and it has ample evidence to support its sensitivity to change, this use has not been without its critics.

Both measures are simple to use and have a low response burden, although the BDI may take slightly longer to complete than the CES-D. Comparison of the evidence supporting the reliability and validity of each of these measures reveals few differences that can be upheld in support of one measure over the other. Both have evidence supporting their psychometric strengths across the broadest possible array of populations, including racial and ethnic minorities, women, and the elderly. Each measure has been challenged in terms of its inclusion of somatic symptoms that may inflate estimates of the prevalence of depressive disorder, although the preponderance of the evidence suggests that this is largely unfounded. There is over 25 years of research supporting the reliability and validity of the BDI and it is clearly the most extensively studied measure of emotional distress in the field of pain and pain management. The sheer volume of research on this instrument is the most compelling reason for its selection in this context.

Implications for future research

This review does not represent an exhaustive consideration of the available measures of pain-related emotional distress. The conduct of a rigorous meta-analysis that could be employed to substantiate or dispute the recommendations of this chapter would be welcomed. Research designed to directly compare the reliability and sensitivity to change of the primary measures of emotional distress reviewed in this paper is also indicated. Similar studies have proved beneficial in evaluating the value of measures of pain-related disability and interference. Continued development and examination of measures of pain-related fear and fear-avoidance holds promise in advancing our understanding of the importance of these constructs, their potential for influencing refinements in pain interventions, and the measurement of this potentially important construct, particularly as a pain-specific alternative to more general measures of anxiety. Similarly, research on the construct of anger and its measurement is strongly encouraged. Finally, although it is likely that the routine inclusion of the POMS and BDI in comprehensive assessments of individuals with chronic pain and pain intervention research will contribute substantially to our ability to sharpen our focus on the effects of pain interventions on emotional distress, continued development of pain-specific measures of emotional distress, including depressive symptom severity, is encouraged.

References

1. Turk DC. Efficacy of multidisciplinary pain centers in the treatment of chronic pain. In *Pain Treatment Centers at a Crossroads: A practical and conceptual reappraisal*, eds. MJM Mitchell and JN Campbell. (Seattle, WA: IASP Press, 1996).

2. Turk DC. Clinical effectiveness and cost-effectiveness of treatments for patients with chronic pain. *Clin J Pain* 2002; **18**: 355–65.

3. Flor H, Birbaumer N, Turk DC. The psychobiology of chronic pain. *Adv Behav Res Ther* 1990; **12**: 47–84.

4. Atkinson JH, Slater MA, Patterson TL, Grant I, Garfin SR Prevalence, onset, and risk of psychiatric disorders in chronic pain patients: A controlled study. *Pain* 1991; **45**: 111–21.

5. Banks SM, Kerns RD. Explaining high rates of depression in chronic pain: A diathesis-stress framework. *Psychol Bull* 1996; **119**: 95–110.

6. Holroyd KA, Malinoski P, Davis, MK, Lipchik JL. The three dimensions of headache impact: Pain, disability, and affective distress. *Pain* 1999; **83**: 571–8.

7. Jamison RN, Rudy TE, Penzein DB, Mosley TH. Cognitive-behavioral classifications of chronic pain: Replication and extension of empirically derived patient profiles. *Pain* 1994; **57**: 277–92.

8. Klapow JC, Slater MA, Patterson TL, Atkinson JH, Weickgenant AL, Grant I, Garfin SR. Psychosocial factors discriminate multidimensional clinical groups of chronic low back pain patients. *Pain* 1995; **62**; 349–55.

9. Robinson ME, Riley III, JL. The role of emotion in pain. In *Psychosocial Factors in Pain: Critical perspectives*, eds RJ Gatchell and DC Turk. (New York: Guilford Press, 1999).

10. Fernandez E, Kerns RD. Anxiety, Depression, and Anger: Core components of negative affect in medical populations. In *The SAGE Handbook of Personality Theory and Assessment: Personality Theories and Models (Vol 1)*, eds. GJ Boyle, G Matthews and DH Saklofske. (Trowbridge: Cromwell Press Ltd, 2008).

11. Chaves J, Barber TX. Hypnotism and surgical pain. In *Behavior Control and Modification of Psychological Activity*, ed. DI Mostovsky. (Englewood Cliffs: Prentice Hall, 1976).

12. Mersky, H. Pain and personality. In *The Psychology of Pain*, ed. R. Sternbach. (New York: Raven Press, 1978).

13. Asmundson GJ, Jacobson SJ, Allerdings MD, Norton GR. Social phobia in disabled workers with chronic musculoskeletal pain. *Behav Res Ther* 1996; **34**: 939–43.

14. Beitman BD, Mukerji V, Kushner M, *et al*. Validating studies for panic disorder in patients with angiographically normal coronary arteries. *Med Clin North Amer* 1991; **75**: 1143–55.

15. Beckham JC, Crawford AL, Feldman ME, *et al*. Chronic posttraumatic stress disorder and chronic pain in Vietnam combat veterans. *J Psychosom Res* 1997; **43**: 379–89.

16. Kulich RJ, Mencher P, Bertrand C, Maciewicz R. Comorbidity of post-traumatic stress disorder and pain: Implications for clinical and forensic assessment. *Curr Rev Pain* 2000; **4**: 36–48.

17. Fernandez, E. *Anxiety, Depression, and Anger in Pain*. (Dallas, TX: Advanced Psychological Resources, Inc, 2002).

18. Asmundson GJ, Jacobson SJ, Allerdings, MD. Fear and avoidance in dysfunctional chronic back pain patients. *Pain* 1997; **69**, 231–6.

19. Lethem J, Slade, PO, Troup, JPG, Bentley G. Outline of a fear-avoidance model of exaggerated pain perception. *Behav Res Ther* 1983; **21**: 401–8.

20. Romano JM, Turner JA. Chronic pain and depression: Does the evidence support a relationship? *Psychol Bull* 1985; **97**: 18–34.

21. Haythornthwaite JA, Sieber WJ, Kerns RD. Depression and the chronic pain experience. *Pain* 1991; **46**: 177–84.

22. Summers JD, Rapoff, MA, Varghese G, Porter K, Palmer RE. Psychosocial factors in chronic spinal cord injury pain. *Pain* 1991; **47**: 183–9.

23. Feeney SL. The relationship between pain and negative affect in older adults: Anxiety as a predictor of pain. *J Anx Disord* 2004; **18**: 733–44.

24. Fernandez E, Turk DC. The scope and significance of anger in the experience of chronic pain. *Pain* 1995; **61**: 165–75.

25. Beutler LE, Engle D, Oro-Beutler, ME, Daldrup R. Inability to express intense negative affect: A common link between depression and pain? *J Consult Clin Psychol* 1986; **54**: 752–9.

26. Catchlove RFH, Braha RED. A test to measure the awareness and expression of anger. *Psychother Psychosom* 1985; **43**: 113–9.

27. Kerns RD, Rosenberg R, Jacob, MC. Anger expression and chronic pain. *J Behav Med* 1994; **17**: 57–67.

28. Spielberger CD, Gorsuch RL, Lushene R. *Manual for the State-Trait Anxiety Inventory* (Palo Alto, CA: Consulting Psychologists Press, 1970).

29. McNair DM, Lorr M, Doppleman LF. *Profile of Mood States*. (San Diego, CA: Educational and Industrial Testing Service, 1971).

30. Beck AT, Ward CH, Mendelsohn M, Mock J, Erbaugh J. An inventory for measuring depression. *Arch Gen Psychiatry* 1961; **4**: 561–71.

31. Radloff LS. The CES-D Scale: A self-report depression scale for research in the general population. *Appl Psychol Meas* 1977; **1**: 385–401.

32. Sullivan MD. Assessment of psychiatric disorders. In *Handbook of Pain Assessment, 2nd edn.*, eds. DC Turk and R Melzack. (New York: Guilford Press, 2001).

33. Brown GK. A causal analysis of chronic pain and depression. *J Abnorm Psychol 1990*; **99**: 127–37.

34. Katon W, Egan K, Miller D. Chronic pain: Lifetime psychiatric diagnosis and family history. *Am J Psychiatry* 1985; **142**: 1156–60.

35. Von Korff M, Simon G. The relationship between pain and depression. *Br J Psych* 1996; **168**(Supplement 30): 101–8.

36. Geisser ME, Roth RS, Robinson ME. Assessing depression among persons with chronic pain using the Center for Epidemiological Studies – Depression Scale and the Beck Depression Inventory: A comparative analysis. *Clin J Pain* 1997; **13**: 163–70.

37. Rodin G, Voshart K. Depression in the medically ill: An overview. *Am J Psychiatry* 1986; **143**: 696–705.

38. Koenig HG, George LK, Peterson, BL, Pieper CF. Depression in medically ill hospitalized older adults: Prevalence, characteristics, and course of symptoms according to six diagnostic schemes. *Am J Psychiatry* 1997; **164**: 1376–83.

39. McCracken, LM, Faber SD, Janeck AS. Pain-related anxiety predicts nonspecific physical complaints in persons with chronic pain. *Behav Res Ther* 1998; **34**: 927–33.

40. Kori SH, Miller RP, Todd DD. Kinesiophobia: A new view of chronic pain behavior. *Pain Manage*, January/February, 35–43.

41. Vlaeyen JW, de Jong J, Geilen M, Heuts PH, van Breukelen G. Graded exposure in vivi in the treatment of pain-related fear: A replicated single-case experimental design in four patients with chronic low back pain. *Behav Res Ther* 2001; **39**: 151–66.

42. McCracken LM, Zayfert C, Gross RT. The Pain Anxiety Symptoms Scale: Development and validation of a scale to measure fear of pain. *Pain* 1992; **50**: 67–73.

43. Waddell G, Newton M, Henderson I, Somerville D, Main C. A Fear-Avoidance Beliefs Questionnaire (FABQ) and the role of fear-avoidance beliefs in chronic low back pain and disability. *Pain* 1993; **52**: 157–68.

44. McNeil DW, Rainwater III AJ. Development of the Fear of Pain Questionnaire – III. *J Behav Med* 1998; **21**: 389–410.

45. Polatin PB, Kinney RK, Gatchel RJ, Lillo E, Mayer TG. Psychiatric illness and chronic low-back pain. The mind and the spine – which goes first? *Spine* 1993; **18**: 66–71.

46. Spielberger CD, Gorsuch RL, Lushene R, Vagg PR, Jacobs GA. *Manual for the State-Trait Anxiety Inventory (Form Y)* (Palo Alto: Consulting Psychologists Press, 1983).

47. Mongini F, Defilippi N, Negro C. Chronic daily headache. A clinical and psychological profile before and after treatment. *Headache* 1997; **37**: 83–7.

48. McCracken LM, Faber SD, Janeck AS. Pain-related anxiety predicts nonspecific physical complaints in persons with chronic pain. *Behav Res Ther* 1998; **36**: 621–30.

49. McCracken LM, Gross RT, Aikens J, Carnrike CLM. The assessment of anxiety and fear in persons with chronic pain: A comparison of instruments. *Behav Res Ther* 1996; **34**: 927–33.

50. Crombez G, Vlaeyen JWS, Heuts PHTG, Lysens R. Pain-related fear is more disabling than pain itself: Evidence on the role of pain-related fear in chronic back pain disability. *Pain* 1999; **80**: 329–39.

51. Larsen DK, Taylor S, Asmundson GJG. Exploratory factor analysis of the Pain Anxiety Symptoms Scale in patients with chronic pain complaints. *Pain* 1997; **69**: 27–34.

52. Vlaeyen JW, Seelen HA, Peters M, *et al.* Fear of movement/(re)injury and muscular reactivity in chronic low back pain patients: An experimental investigation. *Pain* 1999; **82**: 297–304.

53. Pfingsten M, Kroner-Herwig B, Leibing E, Kronshage U, Hildebrandt J. Validation of a German version of the Fear Avoidance Beliefs Questionnaire (FABQ). *Eur J Pain* 2000; **4**: 259–66.

54. Pfingsten M, Leibing E, Harter W, *et al.* Fear-avoidance behavior and anticipation of pain in patients with chronic low back pain: A randomized controlled study. *Pain Med* 2001; **2**: 259–66.

55. Buer N, Linton SJ. Fear-avoidance beliefs and catastrophizing: Occurrence and risk factor in back

pain and ADL in the general population. *Pain* 2002; **99**: 485–91.

56. Klenerman L, Slade PD, Stanley IM. The prediction of chronicity in patients with an acute attack of low back pain in a general medical practice. *Spine* 1995; **20**: 478–84.

57. Beck AT, Steer RA. *Beck Depression Inventory* (San Antonio, TX: Psychological Corporation, 1983).

58. Yonkers, KA, Samson J. Mood disorders measures. In *American Psychiatric Association: Handbook of Psychiatric Measures*. (Washington, DC: American Psychiatric Association, 2000).

59. Beck AT, Steer RA, Garbin MG. Psychometric properties of the Beck Depression Inventory: Twenty-five years of evaluation. *Clin Psychol Rev* 1988; **8**: 77–100.

60. Beck AT, Steer RA, Brown GK. *Beck Depression Inventory-Second Edition Manual* (San Antonio, TX: Psychological Corporation, Harcourt Brace, 1986).

61. Moran PW, Lambert MJ. A review of current assessment tools for monitoring changes in depression. In *The Assessment of Psychotherapy and Outcomes*, eds. MD Lamber, ER Christiensen and SS Dejolie. (New York: Wiley, 1983).

62. Applebaum KA, Blanchard EB, Hickling EJ, Alfonso M, *et al.* Cognitive-behavioral treatment of a veteran population with moderate to severe rheumatoid arthritis. *Behav Ther* 1988; **19**: 489–502.

63. Burns JW, Johnson BJ, Mahoney N, Devine J, Pawl R. Cognitive and physical capacity process variables predict long-term outcome after treatment for chronic pain. *J Consult Clin Psychol* 1998; **66**: 434–9.

64. Kerns RD, Turk DC, Holzman AD, Rudy TE. Comparison of cognitive-behavioral and behavioral approaches to the outpatient treatment of chronic pain. *Clin J Pain* 1986; **1**: 195–203.

65. Khatami M, Rush AJ. A one-year follow-up of the multimodal treatment for chronic pain. *Pain* 1982 **14**: 45–52.

66. Kleinke CL. How chronic pain patients cope with pain: Relation to treatment outcome in a multidisciplinary pain clinic. *Cognit Ther Res* 1992; **16**: 669–85.

67. Marhold C, Linton SJ, Melin L. A cognitive-behavioral return-to-work program: Effects on pain patients with a history of long-term versus short-term sick leave. *Pain* 2001; **91**: 155–63.

68. Radloff LS, Locke BZ. Center for Epidemiologic Studies Depression Scale (CES-D). In *Handbook of Psychiatric Measures*. (Washington, DC: American Psychiatric Association, 2000).

69. Roberts RE. Reliability of the CES-D in different ethnic contexts. *Psychiatry Res* 1980; **2**: 125–34.

70. Naughton MJ, Wiklund I. A critical review of dimension-specific measures of health-related quality of life in cross-cultural research. *Qual Life Res* 1993; **2**: 397–432.

71. Arnstein P, Caudill M, Mandle CL, Norris A, Beasley R. Self efficacy as a mediator of the relationship between pain intensity, disability, and depression in chronic pain patients. *Pain* 1999; **80**: 483–91.

72. Fechner-Bates S, Coyne JC, Schwenk TL. The relationship of self-reported distress to depressive disorders and other psychopathology. *J Consul Clin Psychol* 1994; **62**: 550–9.

73. Weissman MM, Sholomskas D, Portenger M, *et al.* Assessing depressive symptoms in five psychiatric populations: A validation study. *Am J Epidemiol* 1977; **106**: 203–14.

74. Blalock, SJ, DeVellis RF, Brown GK, Wallston KA. Validity of the Center for Epidemiological Studies Depression Scale in arthritis populations. *Arthritis Rheum* 1989; **32**: 991–7.

75. Magni G, Caldieron C, Rigatti-Luchini S, Merskey H. Chronic musculoskeletal pain and depressive symptoms in the general population: An analysis of the 1st National Health and Nutrition Examination Survey data. *Pain* 1990; **43**: 299–307.

76. Turk DC, Okifuji A. Detecting depression in chronic pain patients: Adequacy of self-reports. *Behav Res Ther* 1994; **32**: 9–16.

77. Nielsen WR, Walker C, McCain GA. Cognitive-behavioral treatment of fibromyalgia: Preliminary findings. *J Rheumatol* 1992; **19**: 98–103.

78. Turner JA, Clancy S, McQuade KJ, Cardenas DD. Effectiveness of behavioral therapy for chronic low back pain: A component analysis. *J Consult Clin Psychol* 1990; **58**: 573–9.

79. Hamilton M. A rating scale for depression. *J Neurol Neurosurg Psychiatry* 1960; **23**: 56–62.

80. Zitman FG, Mennen MFG, Griez E, *et al.* The different versions of the Hamilton Depression Rating Scale. In *The Hamilton Scales (Psychopharmacology Series 9)*, eds. P Bech and A Coppen. (Berlin: Springer-Verlag, 1990).

81. Carroll BJ, Feinburg M, Smouse PE, *et al.* The Carroll Rating Scale for Depression: Development, reliability, and validation. *Br J Psychiatry* 1981; **138**: 194–200.

82. Potts MK, Daniels M, Burnam A, *et al.* A structured interview version of the Hamilton Depression Rating Scale: Evidence of reliability and versatility of administration. *J Psychiatr Res* 1990; **24**: 335–50.

83. Reynolds WM., Kobak KA. Reliability and validity of the Hamilton Depression Inventory: A paper and

pencil version of the Hamilton Rating Scale Clinical Interview. *Psychol Assess* 1990; **7**: 472–83.

84. Kobak KA, Reynolds WM, Rosenfeld R, *et al.* Development and validation of a computer-administered version of the Hamilton Depression Rating Scale. *Psychol Assess* 1990; **2**: 56–63.

85. Gastpar, M, Gilsdorf, U. The Hamilton Depression Rating Scale in a WHO collaborative program. In *The Hamilton Scales (Psychopharmacology Series 9)*, eds. P Bech and A Coppen (Berlin: Springer-Verlag, 1990).

86. Maier W, Phillip M, Heuser I, *et al.* Improving depression severity assessment, I: Content, concurrent, and external validity of three observer scales. *J Psychiatr Res* 1988; **22**: 3–12.

87. Rehm L, O' Hara M. Item characteristics of the Hamilton Rating Scale for Depression. *J Psychiatr Res* 1985; **19**: 31–41.

88. Zung WWK. A self-rating depression scale. *Arch Gen Psychiatry* 1965; **12**: 63–5.

89. Biggs JT, Wylie LT, Ziegler VE. Validity of the Zung Self-Rating Depression Scale. *Br J Psychiatry* 1978; **132**: 381–5.

90. Guy W. *ECDEU Assessment Manual of Psychopharmacology-Revised (DHEW Publ No ADM 76–338)*. Rockville, MD: US Department of Health, Education, and Welfare, Public Health Service, Alcohol, Drug Abuse, and Mental Health Administration, NIMH Psychopharmacology Research Branch, Division of Extramural Research Programs. (1976).

91. Yesavage JA, Brink TL. Development and validation of a geriatric depression screening scale: A preliminary report. *J Psychiatr Res* 1983; **17**: 37–49.

92. Sheikh JI, Yesavage JA. Geriatric Depression Scale (GDS): Recent evidence and development of a shorter version. *Clin Gerontol* 1986; **5**: 165–73.

93. Jamison C, Scogin F. Development of an interview based geriatric depression rating scale. *Int J Aging Hum Dev* 1992; **35**: 193–204.

94. Burke WJ, Roccaforte WH, Wengel SP, *et al.* The reliability and validity of the Geriatric Depression Rating Scale administered by telephone. *J AmGeriatr Soc* 1995; **43**: 674–9.

95. Brink TA, Yesavage JA, Lum O, *et al.* Screening tests for geriatric depression. *Clin Gerontol* 1982; **1**: 37–43.

96. Zigmond AS, Snaith RP. The Hospital Anxiety and Depression Scale. *Acta Psychiatr Scand* 1983; **67**: 361–70.

97. Snaith RP, Zigmond AS. *The Hospital Anxiety and Depression Scale Manual* (Windsor: Nfer-Nelson, 1994)

98. Moorey S, Greer S, Watson M, *et al.* The factor structure and factor stability of the Hospital Anxiety and Depression Scale in patients with cancer. *Br J Psychiatry* 1991; **158**: 255–9.

99. Kerns RD, Turk DC, Rudy TE. The West Haven-Yale Multidimensional Pain Inventory (WHYMPI). *Pain* 1985; **23**: 345–56.

100. McCarberg B, Wolf J. Chronic pain management in a health maintenance organization. *Clin J Pain* 1999; **15**: 50–7.

101. Buss AH, Durkee A. An inventory for assessing different kinds of hostility. *J Consult Psychol* 1957; **21**: 343–9.

102. Megargee EI, Cook PE, Mendelsohn GA. Development and validation of an MMPI scale of assaultiveness in overcontrolled individuals. *J Abnorm Psychol* 1967; **72**: 519–28.

103. Caine TM, Foulds GA, Hope K. *Manual of the Hostility and Direction of Hostility Questionnaire* (London: University of London, 1967).

104. Cook W, Medley D. Proposed hostility and pharisaic-virtue scales for the MMPI. *J Appl Psychol* 1954; **38**: 414–18.

105. Zelin ML, Adler G, Myerson PG. Anger self-report: An objective questionnaire for the measurement of aggression. *J Consult Clin Psychol* 1972; **39**: 340.

106. Evans DR, Strangeland M. Development of the Reaction Inventory to measure anger. *Psychol Rep* 1971; **29**: 412–14.

107. Novaco RW. *The effect of disposition of anger and degree of provocation on self-report and physiological measures of anger in various modes of provocation.* Unpublished manuscript, Indiana University, Bloomington, IN. (1974)

108. Siegel JM. The Multidimensional Anger Inventory. *J Pers Soc Psychol* 1986; **51**: 191–200.

109. Fernandez E. *The Targets and Reasons for Anger in Pain Sufferers: A structured interview.* Unpublished manuscript, Southern Methodist University. (1996).

110. Spielberger CD. *State-Trait Anger Expression Inventory Professional Manual* (Odessa, FL: Psychological Assessment, 1988).

111. Spielberger CD. *The State-Trait Anger Expression Inventory-2 Professional Manual* (Odessa, FL: Psychological Assessment, 1999).

112. Hathaway SR, McKinley J. *The Minnesota Multiphasic Personality Inventory* (Minneapolis: University of Minnesota Press, 1943).

113. Hathaway SR, McKinley JC, Butcher JN, *et al. Minnesota Multiphasic Personality Inventory-2: Manual*

for administration (Minneapolis: University of Minnesota Press, 1989).

114. Bradley LA, McKendree-Smith NL. Assessment of psychological status using interviews and self-report instruments. In *Handbook of Pain Assessment*, 2nd edn., eds. DC Turk and R Melzack. (New York: Guilford Press, 2001).

115. Pincus T, Callahan LF, Bradley LA, Vaughn WK, Wolfe F. Elevated MMPI scores for hypochondriasis, depression, and hysteria in patients with rheumatoid arthritis reflect disease rather than psychological status. *Arthritis Rheum* 1986; **29**: 1456–66.

116. Guck TP, Meilman PW, Skultety M, Poloni ID. Pain-patient Minnesota Multiphasic Personality Inventory subgroups: Evaluation of long-term treatment outcome. *J Behav Med* 1988; **11**: 159–69.

117. McCreary C. Empirically derived MMPI profile clusters and characteristics of low back pain patients. *J Consult Clin Psychol* 1985; **53**: 558–60.

118. Moore JE, Armentrout DP, Parker JC, Kivlahan DR. Empirically-derived pain-patient MMPI subgroups: Prediction of treatment outcome. *J Behav Med* 1986; **9**: 51–63.

119. Clark ME. MMPI-2 Negative Treatment Indicators Content and Content Component Scales: Clinical correlates and outcome prediction for men with chronic pain. *Psychol Assess* 1996; **8**: 32–8.

120. Vendrig AA, Derksen JL, deMey HR. Utility of selected MMPI-2 scales in the outcome prediction for patients with chronic back pain. *Psychol Assess* 1999; **11**: 381–5.

121. Derogatis L. *The SCL-90R Manual – II: Administration, scoring and procedures* (Towson, MD: Clinical Psychometric Research, 1983).

122. Preveler RC, Fairburn CG. Measurement of neurotic symptoms by self-report questionnaire: Validity of the SCL-90-R. *Psychol Med* 1990; **20**: 873–9.

123. Jamison RN, Rock DL, Parris WCV. Empirically derived Symptom Checklist 90 subgroups of chronic pain patients: A cluster analysis. *J Behav Med* 1988; **11**: 147–58.

124. Derogatis L, Spencer P. *BSI Manual I: Administration and procedures* (Baltimore, MD: Johns Hopkins University, Clinical Psychometric Unit, 1983).

125. Millon T, Green C, Meagher R. *Millon Behavioral Health Inventory manual 3rd edn.* (Minneapolis, MN: National Computer Systems, 1983).

126. Gatchell RJ, Mayer TG, Capra P, Barnett J, Daimond P. Millon Behavioral Health Inventory: Its utility in predicting physical function in patients with low back pain. *Arch Phys Med Rehabil* 1986; **67**: 878–82.

127. Sweet JJ, Breuer SR, Hazlewood LA, Toye R, Pawl RP. The Millon Behavioral Health Inventory: Concurrent

and predictive validity in a pain treatment center. *J Behav Med* 1985; **8**: 215–26.

128. Pilowsky I, Spence ND. Patterns of illness behavior in patients with intractable pain. *J Psychosom Res* 1975; **19**: 279–87.

129. Pilowsky I, Spence ND. *Manual for the Illness Behavior Questionnaire* (IBQ). Unpublished manual (available from the authors) (1994).

130. Dworkin RH, Cooper EM, Siegfried RN. Chronic pain and disease conviction. *Clin J Pain* 1996; **12**: 111–7.

131. Keefe FJ, Crisson JE, Maltbie A, Bradley LA, Gil KM. Illness behavior as a predictor of pain and overt behavior patterns in chronic low back pain patients. *J Psychosom Res* 1986; **30**: 543–51.

132. Waddell G, Pilowsky I, Bond MR. Clinical assessment and interpretation of abnormal illness behavior in low back pain. *Pain* 1989; **39**: 41–53.

133. Ware JE, Sherbourne CD. The MOS 36-item Short-Form Health Survey (SF-36), I: Conceptual framework and item selection. *Med Care* 1992; **30**: 473–83.

134. Kazis LE, Skinner K, Rogers W, *et al.* Health status and outcomes of veterans: physical and mental component summary scores (sf-36v). 1998 national survey of ambulatory care patients. Mid-year executive report. Office of Performance and Quality, Health Assessment Project, Center for Health Quality Outcomes and Economic Research, HSRD Service, Veterans Administration, Washington, D.C. and Bedford (MA), (1998).

135. Ware JE, Bayliss MS, Rogers WH, Kosinski M, Tarlov AR. Differences in 4-year health outcomes for elderly and poor, chronically ill patients treated in HMO and fee-for-service systems. *JAMA* 1996; **276**: 1039–47.

136. Ware JE, Kosinski M, Keller SD. *SF-36 Physical and Mental Health Summary Scales: A users manual* (Boston, MA: Health Assessment Lab, New England Medical Center, 1994).

137. McHorney CA, Ware JE, Lu JFR, *et al.* The MOS 36-item Short-Form Health Survey (SF-36), III: Tests of data quality, scaling assumptions, and reliability across diverse patient groups. *Med Care* 1994; **32**, 40–66.

138. Backonja M, Beydoun A, Edwards KR, *et al.* for the Gabapentin Diabetic Neuropathy Study Group. Gabapentin for the symptomatic treatment of painful neuropathy in patients with diabetes mellitus. *JAMA* 1998; **280**: 1831–6.

139. Katz JN, Harris TM, Larson MG, *et al.* Predictors of functional outcomes after arthroscopic partial meniscectomy. *J Rheumatol* 1992; **19**, 1938–42.

140. Rogers WH, Wittink H, Wagner A, Cynn D, Carr DB. Assessing individual outcomes during outpatient

multidisciplinary chronic pain treatment by means of an augmented SF-36. *Pain Med* 2000; **1**: 44–54.

141. McHorney C, Tarlov A. Individual-patient monitoring in clinical practice: Are available health status surveys adequate. *Qual Life Res* 1995; **4**: 293–307.

142. Rowbotham M, Harden N, Stacey B, Bernstein P, Magnus-Miller L. for the Gabapentin Postherpetic Neuralgia Study Group. Gabapentin for the Treatment of Postherpetic Neuralgia A Randomized Controlled Trial. *JAMA* 1998; **280**: 1837–42.

143. Helzer JE, Robins LN. The Diagnostic Interview Schedule: Its development, evaluation and use. *Soc Psychiatry Psychiatr Epidemiol* 1988; **23**: 6–16.

144. Robins LN, Helzer JE, Croughan J, Ratcliff KS. National Institute of Mental Health Diagnostic Interview Schedule. *Arch Gen Psychiatry* 1981; **38**, 381–9.

145. Spitzer RL, Williams JBW, Gibbon M, First MB. *Structured Clinical Interview for DSM-III-R* (Washington, DC: American Psychiatric Press, 1990).

146. American Psychiatric Association. *Diagnostic and Statistical Manual of Mental Disorders.* 4th edn. (Washington, DC: American Psychiatric Association, 1994).

147. Helzer JE, Spitznagel EL, McEvoy L. The predictive validity of lay Diagnostic Interview Schedule diagnoses in the general population: A comparison with physician examiners. *Arch Gen Psychiatry* 1987; **44**: 1069–77.

148. Vandiver T, Sher KJ. Temporal stability of the Diagnostic Interview Schedule. *Psychol Assess* 1991; **3**: 277–81.

149. Eaton WW, Neufeld K, Chen LS, Cai G. A comparison of self-report and clinical diagnostic interviews for depression: Diagnostic Interview Schedule and Schedules for Clinical Assessment in Neuropsychiatry in the Baltimore Epidemiologic Catchment Area follow-up. *Arch Gen Psychiatry* 2000; **57**: 217–22.

150. First MB, Spitzer RL, Williams JBW, Gibbon M. *User's Guide for the Structured Clinical Interview for the DSM-IV Axis I Disorders: SCID –I clinician version* (Washington, DC: American Psychiatric Press, 1997).

151. First MB, Gibbon M, Williams JBW, Spitzer RL. *SCID Screen Patient Questionnaire Computer Program* (North Tonawanda, NY: Multi-Health Systems, 2000).

152. Williams JB, Gibbon M, First MB, *et al.* The Structured Clinical Interview for DSM-III-R (SCID) II: Multisite test-retest reliability. *Arch Gen Psychiatry* 1992; **49**: 630–6.

153. Kerns, R.D. Psychosocial factors: Primary or secondary outcomes? In *Pain Treatment Centers at a Crossroads: A Practical Conceptual Reappraisal,* eds. JN Campbell and MJ Mitchell. (Seattle: IASP Press, 1996).

Psychopharmacologic, behavioral, and psychotherapeutic approaches

Interdisciplinary pain rehabilitation programs

Cynthia O. Townsend, Jeffrey D. Rome, Barbara K. Bruce and W. Michael Hooten

"For so long I had been searching for a cure for my pain. Injections, pain medications, surgeries, massage, chiropractors, herbals… I tried everything. Nothing worked. My family, my doctor and I were frustrated and demoralized. I had never heard of an interdisciplinary pain rehabilitation program. My pain is still there but now I feel like I have my life back. I'm using all of the tools I've learned in the program to manage my pain. I feel like I have control over my life again. Now I'm making plans for the future rather than barely surviving through the day." A 45-year-old woman after completing a 3-week interdisciplinary pain rehabilitation program

Interdisciplinary pain rehabilitation programs (IPRPs) are the embodiment of the biopsychosocial model of care for patients with chronic pain. The biopsychosocial perspective suggests pain results from one's perception of the pain based on sensory phenomena, as well as beliefs and appraisals that interact with emotional factors, social influences, environmental reinforces and behavioral responses. All too frequently, the interaction of these factors contributes to significant distress and debilitation in the context of persistent pain. Treatment that is based on a biopsychosocial model addresses the biological basis of pain symptoms and teaches the patient techniques to gain a sense of control over the effects of pain by modifying the affective, behavioral, cognitive and sensory facets of the experience [1]. There appears to be no other treatment that more effectively addresses these important components of chronic pain than IPRPs.

It has long been recognized that the complexities of chronic pain require the collaborative expertise from multiple disciplines. A single clinician, working in isolation, cannot evaluate and manage all aspects of chronic pain. Although the professional staff of IPRPs may vary from one practice setting to another, the treatment team commonly includes a physician (or group of physicians) who specialize in pain medicine and/or psychiatry, neurology, anesthesiology or

physiatry, pain psychologists/therapists, nurse practitioners, registered nurses, physical therapists, occupational therapists, pharmacists, biofeedback therapists, and vocational specialists. Ancillary services are provided by social workers, dieticians, chaplains/ministers, chemical dependency counselors, and nicotine dependence counselors. Financial managers and billing staff, knowledgeable in pre-authorization and pre-certification requirements of various insurance carriers, workers' compensation system guidelines and the appeal process, have become increasingly important members of the IPRP team in the current healthcare environment.

The following are descriptions of the roles of each major discipline in an IPRP:

- *Physician* – The IPRP physician is usually the director of the treatment program and is clinically responsible for the medical management and psychiatric care of all of the patients in the program. S/he has extensive training and experience treating patients with chronic pain and co-morbid mood disorders such as depression and anxiety. Moreover, s/he is responsible for synthesizing clinical information from the various disciplines to assess patients' progress and make appropriate recommendations or referrals for further diagnostic or therapeutic services. Additionally, the physician addresses the patients' and families' questions regarding medical history, test results, diagnosis, restrictions, treatment options, and rehabilitation focus. Each patient's current medication use is assessed by the physician to determine baseline use of pain and psychotropic medications. S/he collaborates with the patient's local physicians and/or pharmacist, orders tapering of opioid and other medications, and monitors the progress of medication taper(s) and physiologic symptoms of medication use and

Behavioral and Psychopharmacologic Pain Management, ed. Michael H. Ebert and Robert D. Kerns. Published by Cambridge University Press. © Cambridge University Press 2011.

withdrawal. Regarding mood-related goals, the physician regularly assesses the patient's emotional status and initiates psychopharmacotherapy for symptom management as indicated, and coordinates discharge care.

- *Pain psychologist/mental health therapist* – Pain psychologists and mental health therapists in IPRPs have extensive training in cognitive-behavioral interventions for pain management. They play a vital role in determining patients' appropriateness for treatment by assessing patients' motivation for treatment, expectations about treatment outcomes and barriers to rehabilitation progress. Often serving as co-leader of the treatment team with the pain physician, the pain psychologist guides the treatment team's application of cognitive-behavioral interventions, conceptualizes patients' pain beliefs and coping style, and assesses psychosocial and cognitive functioning. The pain psychologists/therapists address concerns about adherence to treatment recommendations, and use cognitive-behavioral interventions to manage comorbid mood disorders and pain-complicated disorders (e.g., panic disorder, post-traumatic stress disorder, functional vomiting) prevalent in pain populations. Often trained in behavioral research, the pain psychologist uses standardized tools to assess patient's baseline and discharge functioning, improve program quality and conduct clinical research. Mental health therapists facilitate group therapy sessions which are part of the rehabilitation treatment protocol.

- *Clinical Nurse Specialists and Certified Nurse Practitioners* – Clinical Nurse Specialists (CNSs) in IPRPs are certified in psychiatry or other medical specialties, and in some states have prescriptive privileges within their practice agreement with the pain physician. Other IPRPs employ Certified Nurse Practitioners (CNPs) who are trained as generalists and have full prescriptive authority. Both types of providers collaborate with the pain physician to monitor and address medication issues, develop medication tapers, coordinate with patient's local physicians and pharmacy to discuss patients' medication use and prescription availability, and provide education in groups regarding various

medication and health issues. With the medical director, the CNS/CNP can help ensure that medications support a patient's health, overall functioning and well-being. Clinical Nurse Specialists trained in psychiatry also play a primary role in facilitating group therapy sessions with patients and family members by providing information about managing chronic pain, and exploring strategies to manage interpersonal issues facing patients with chronic pain.

- *Nurse Care Coordinator* – In many IPRP settings nurses play a major role as care coordinators for patients throughout their course of treatment. Nurses meet with patients regularly to review recommendations from the various IPRP disciplines, develop treatment plans, and assess progress toward treatment goals. They also coordinate discharge plans and communicate treatment progress and recommendations to local healthcare providers. During frequent individual meetings with the patient, nurse care coordinators support patients' efforts to individualize program concepts to meet specific treatment goals. This includes assisting with return-to-work meetings, addressing family members' concerns, and advocating for a balanced, healthy lifestyle. Throughout the course of treatment, nurse care coordinators assess changes in physical and/or mental status, vital signs and medication use.

- *Physical therapist* – The physical therapy staff meets with the patients daily throughout the course of treatment to provide personalized instruction on strengthening exercises, stretching, and aerobic conditioning. Additionally, they provide group education on proper body mechanics, lifting techniques, proper posture, benefits of aerobic exercise and discussions on pain behaviors. Most patients have received passive physical therapies focused on the site of pain before admission to the IPRP. In contrast, physical therapy in an IPRP entails a comprehensive focus to increase overall strength and stamina. Patients learn more efficient ways of moving their bodies so their daily activities can be accomplished more easily. The gradual and progressive exercises are designed to help decrease patients' fear of movement that can be more debilitating than the pain itself. Additionally, physical therapists in IPRPs reinforce the importance of continuing a home exercise program to maintain physical gains made during the program. In the case of complex regional pain syndrome (CRPS), the physical therapists may collaborate with the pain psychologist to develop a desensitization hierarchy for graded exposures to painful and feared stimuli.

- *Occupational therapist* – The IPRP occupational therapy staff provide daily instruction on techniques that will increase the control and independence patients have over activities of daily living and daily schedules. The instruction is designed to be practical and focus on creating a balance between work, self-care, and leisure activities. This includes discussion of weekend planning, observation of proper body mechanics for functional tasks including home chores and cleaning tasks, work-related tasks (e.g., computer ergonomics), as well as volunteer and recreational activities (e.g., golfing, needlework).

- *Biofeedback therapist* – Biofeedback therapists teach patients how to modulate the physiologic processes of the autonomic nervous system that are being negatively affected by chronic pain. Through electrodes placed on one's body, a computerized instrument receives information about physiological processes such as breathing rate and muscle tension. The feedback is used to increase patients' awareness of these physical processes and positive changes that can be experienced through appropriate use of relaxation training. Biofeedback therapists meet with patients on multiple occasions during the course of treatment to provide individualized instruction and treatment.

- *Pharmacist* – Upon admission to the IPRP, a pharmacist reviews the medication list for every patient to ensure accuracy and adherence to the prescribed pharmacologic regimen. Importantly, this establishes a baseline of opioid analgesic and psychotropic medication use. This review also includes over-the-counter and herbal medication use. The pharmacist is available to meet with patients on an as-needed basis to address questions and concerns regarding pharmacologic issues. Additionally, the pharmacist may teach group sessions on the use of medications in chronic pain management. The pharmacist also serves as a consultant to the staff in addressing medication selection, interactions, and side effects.

- *Vocational specialist* – The vocational specialist has expertise in counseling psychology and has extensive training in the measurement of aptitudes, values, needs and vocational interests. The vocational psychologist uses standardized tools to assess the patient in these domains, provides systematic feedback on the results, and develops a life plan that includes either return to paid employment or alternative but meaningful life roles (e.g., volunteerism, hobbies). Patients typically report reclaiming their lost sense of self and a renewed sense of direction after intervention by the vocational psychologist.

The patient is an essential member of the treatment team. In contrast to the biomedical model of care in which patients are passive recipients of numerous interventions, IPRPs encourage patients to be active agents of change in their response to pain. Patients are actively involved in establishing their treatment goals, treatment plan development, and reviewing progress toward these goals. The IPRP treatment team meets regularly with the patient to give the patient feedback on his/her progress, reinforce rehabilitation efforts, and encourage specific areas for continued growth. While the various disciplines in the IPRP may be experts in pain management, the patients are considered the experts in determining how they are going to implement the treatment into their lives.

In the ideal setting, the disciplines forming the IPRP treatment team practice at the same location to concurrently provide comprehensive patient care and lend their expertise toward the common goal of maximizing patients' functioning. In frequent face-to-face patient care team meetings, each discipline contributes to the treatment planning, implementation, progress assessment, and follow-up care for every patient throughout the course of treatment. Because of the medical and psychological complexities and large number of disciplines involved, active collaboration and interdisciplinary communication is necessary to ensure treatment success during the intensive rehabilitative process. Each discipline offers perspectives from their area of expertise; reports observations of patients' physical progress, social interactions, and pain behaviors; and collaborates to address motivational, emotional, cognitive, familial, and personality concerns [2]. The success of IPRPs is derived from the collegial attitude, clinical contribution, and cooperation of the entire pain management team. In this way, IPRPs differ from single-modality clinics that offer a specific treatment modality (i.e., pharmacotherapy, surgery, interventional procedures) without the availability and/or integration of other disciplines.

Interdisciplinary pain rehabilitation program treatment objectives

The evidence-based clinical practice guidelines for chronic non-cancer pain recommend interdisciplinary rehabilitation that is goal-directed and time-limited [3]. The emphasis of rehabilitative treatment is on educating patients in active self-management techniques that focus on maximizing function through integrated therapies involving medical, psychological/behavioral, physical therapy, occupational therapy, and disability/vocational interventions. As opposed to the treatment of acute pain, guidelines for chronic pain management de-emphasize pain relief as a specific measure of treatment success and instead focus on improved physical and psychosocial functioning. This shift in the treatment paradigm is evident in a recently published physician guide for opioid prescribing by the Federation of State Medical Board that advocates for treatment plans that incorporate functional goals rather than the relief of nociception [4].

Interdisciplinary pain rehabilitation programs' treatment goals include improvement in physical functioning (e.g., improved range of motion, standing and walking), general functional status (e.g., increased activities of daily living, social, leisure, and domestic responsibilities), increase in self-management of the chronic pain condition, improvement of vocational/disability status (e.g., return to work, job training, academic coursework), reduction/discontinuation of non-indicated medications including opiate and sedatives, reduction of healthcare utilization, and improvement in pain severity.

The IPRP treatment approach is based on a cognitive-behavioral perspective, which enhances patients' functional improvement, by teaching adaptive attitudes and behaviors to manage the pain. Discussed in detail elsewhere [5], the essential components of cognitive-behavioral therapy (CBT) for chronic pain include reconceptualizing pain as under one's control, skill acquisition to self-manage pain through self-regulation of physiological responses and stress-management, skill consolidation through practice and rehearsal, and skill generalization and maintenance through relapse prevention.

Specific cognitive-behavioral techniques include: differentiating acute from chronic pain, cognitive restructuring, relaxation training with or without biofeedback, teaching positive self-coping statements while decreasing pain catastrophizing, stress management, anger management, assertive communication, understanding and decreasing pain behaviors, adaptive problem-solving, goal setting to lead a plan-rather than pain-contingent lifestyle, activity pacing, proper body mechanics for activities of daily living, time management, healthy lifestyle behaviors such as proper sleep and nutrition, chemical health education, and maintaining gains and preventing relapses. Additionally, by engaging in daily quota-based exercise programs, patients progressively increase their physical strength and endurance while also decreasing their fear of injury, which can be a strong predictor of functional limitations [6]. In a sense, physical therapy in an IPRP adopts a cognitive-behavioral perspective rather than a physical-mechanistic approach [5]. Consistent with increasing patients' autonomy and decreasing illness behaviors, patients are taught exercise programs they can maintain independently outside of a hospital setting.

No single coping technique has been proven to be universally effective in the management of chronic pain. It is usually a combination of multiple personalized cognitive-behavioral techniques incorporated into one's lifestyle that leads to success in restoring patients' functioning and quality of life. When successful rehabilitation occurs, there is an important shift from helplessness and passivity to resourcefulness and ability to function regardless of pain [7].

Due to the potential for significant debilitation, and detrimental effects of chronic pain on one's physical functioning, health, mood, family, work, and quality of life, cognitive-behavioral pain management concepts should not be introduced as a last resort, after all other forms of treatment have failed. Instead, CBT for chronic pain management should be integrated into the treatment plan at the earliest stages of chronic pain and with every intervention. The benefits of pharmacotherapy and interventional treatments may be limited if the patient does not improve physical conditioning while learning to moderate excessive activity levels (i.e., sedentary, overexertion) that exacerbate pain. The primary care provider or pain specialist accomplishes this integration with brief educational interventions during routine assessments of patients' functioning. As the chronic pain persists, physicians' treatment plans and communication with patients should clearly reflect a biopsychosocial perspective of pain. More in-depth and cost-effective patient education groups on CBT strategies can be arranged in the primary care setting or pain specialty clinic. Additionally, individualized cognitive-behavior treatment by therapists with specialty training in pain management provides specific instruction on CBT strategies and assistance with implementation.

For some patients, particularly those with impaired mobility or advanced debilitation, severe medication overuse, and associated medical or psychiatric co-morbidity, this level of care will not be adequate for functional restoration. In such instances, comprehensive and intensive interdisciplinary treatment will be necessary to reverse the downward spiral of deconditioning and promote healing. Success with rehabilitative objectives is then strengthened when the patient's primary care providers, pain specialists and pain psychologist/therapist reinforce the applied cognitive-behavioral techniques. Ideally, the rationale and benefits of interdisciplinary care should be considered before significant depression, deconditioning, loss of job, and adverse impact on family relationships have developed. Please refer to Figure 8.1 for an illustration of the continuum of intensity of cognitive-behavioral interventions for chronic pain. This figure also illustrates the ideal bi-directional nature of this care as each provider and level of CBT intervention supports the others.

Medication management

A reduction or discontinuation of analgesic and psychotropic medications is a common IPRP treatment goal. Patients with chronic pain are vulnerable to polypharmacy. They commonly have numerous sources of medications, which include prescriptions from multiple providers, over-the-counter medications, medications borrowed from relatives, and herbal preparations. The risks of polypharmacy are a significant concern given these numerous sources, potential adverse side effects, and possible drug–drug interactions. Frequently patients admitted to an IPRP are taking medication "cocktails" to address pain, insomnia, fatigue, anxiety, and depression, while also taking medications to counter adverse side effects of these medications (e.g., sedation, difficulty concentrating, constipation, weight gain).

Medication management in IPRPs includes a review of each patient's medication regimen to evaluate dosing and duration. Medications are discontinued

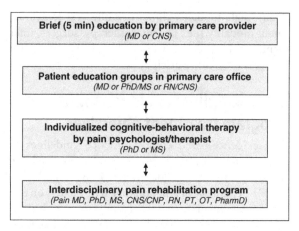

Figure 8.1 Continuum of cognitive-behavioral interventions for chronic pain.

Note. MD, primary care provider or physician pain specialist; CNS, clinical nurse specialist; CNP, certified nurse practitioner; PhD, pain psychologist; MS, master's level therapist; RN, registered nurse; PT, physical therapist; OT, occupational therapist; PharmD, pharmacist.

when therapeutic efficacy is limited, when adverse effects are clinically significant, and when it is determined that specific objectives are better addressed by non-pharmacological interventions.

Opioid withdrawal as a treatment objective

The use of opioid therapy for chronic non-cancer pain is actively debated by healthcare professionals and the public at large. At the heart of the debate is a disagreement about the primary goal of treatment: pain relief or improved functioning. In fact, both of these objectives should be considered when evaluating treatment efficacy [8, 9]. Nevertheless, patients' observed pain behaviors were found to be the best predictor of a physician's decision to prescribe opioids for chronic pain [10]. Additionally, large doses of opioids may be prescribed, often in the absence of improvement in patients' pain or level of functioning and in spite of evidence that suggests that prolonged, high-dose opioid therapy may be neither safe nor effective [11]. Problems arise when medications provide only limited symptomatic benefit and are accompanied by adverse effects (e.g., sedation, nausea, constipation), yet patients and physicians are reluctant to discontinue them, fearing symptoms may grow worse [12]. Despite the high prevalence of chronic opioid therapy in clinical practice, a recent systematic review of research on the use of opioids for chronic noncancer pain found the presence of large and persistent evidence gaps on the use of chronic opioid therapy for chronic noncancer pain [13]. Specifically, critical research gaps include lack of effectiveness studies on the long-term benefits and harm of opioids (including drug abuse, addiction, and diversion); insufficient evidence about optimal approaches to risk stratification, monitoring, or initiation and titration of opioid therapy; and lack of evidence on the utility of opioid rotation, the benefits and harms of methadone or higher dose of opioids, and treatment of patients with chronic noncancer pain who are at risk for drug abuse or misuse. Meta-analyses and several reviews of randomized, double-blind, placebo-controlled trials of opioids used for chronic non-cancer pain [3, 14–18] suggest only a minority of patients benefit from long-term opioid treatment.

Interdisciplinary pain rehabilitation programs vary in their stance of opioid withdrawal within the context of rehabilitative treatment. In some programs complete opioid withdrawal is mandatory. Other programs may support opioid maintenance therapy or elective decreases in opioid dosing. The practice of opioid therapy for chronic pain will continue to undergo scrutiny as evidence emerges suggesting opioid tolerance and opioid-induced hyperalgesia can occur within 1 month of initiating oral morphine therapy [19], withdrawal from high-dose opioids can decrease pain [20], and IPRPs that incorporate opioid withdrawal can be effective for improving functioning, mood, and pain for patients with diverse types of pain [21, 22], chronic headaches [23], and fibromyalgia [24].

The elevated levels of pain, distress, and debilitation reported by patients referred to IPRPs suggests that opioid therapy has not led to substantial improvements in these parameters. In IPRPs that incorporate analgesic withdrawal, opioid and simple analgesics are gradually reduced utilizing structured drug tapers. These take place while patients are learning and practicing cognitive-behavioral strategies to more adaptively manage pain and mood. Factors such as medication efficacy, safety, drug interactions, and practical issues such as cost are taken into consideration when making medication adjustments.

Addiction treatment within IPRPs

The diagnosis and treatment of addiction within the context of chronic pain is challenging – particularly when the chemicals to which patients are addicted are prescribed for pain and mood management. These include opioids, sedatives, stimulants, anxiolytics, muscle relaxants, and cannabinoids. The misuse of prescription drugs jumped by 94% from 1992 to 2003,

according to the National Center on Addiction and Substance Abuse at Columbia University (CASA) [25]. Opioids, in particular, raise concerns for misuse, addiction and possible diversion for non-medical use. Additionally, the presence of current substance abuse disorders (e.g., abuse of alcohol, marijuana, and methamphetamine) can detract from a patient's need for pain management treatment. Individuals who have a history of alcohol or illicit drug abuse may turn toward the use of prescription opioids for legitimate medical reasons and become addicted after years of sobriety. Chemical dependency programs are often ill-equipped to manage chronic pain and have difficulty distinguishing true addiction from pseudoaddiction, which involves aberrant drug-seeking behaviors in an effort to obtain pain relief. In a population already noted for its medical and psychological complexities, the issue of chemical dependency and addiction can add considerable confusion and frustration.

Like chronic pain, the management of substance abuse requires a multidisciplinary approach. The treatment team recognizes that drug abuse is often chronic and progressive; therefore, it requires a treatment approach aimed at enhancing social support, maximizing treatment compliance and containing harm from episodic relapse [26]. The management of chronic pain in patients with a history of addiction may require additional monitoring, documentation and consultation, or referral to an addictions expert.

Interdisciplinary pain rehabilitation programs vary in the role the treatment team plays in evaluating and providing interventions for substance abuse and addiction. They may intermix patients with chronic pain with those patients receiving chemical dependency treatment. The majority of IPRPs, however, identify addiction and substance abuse concerns within the course of the pre-candidacy evaluation or rehabilitative treatment. Spot urine toxicology screens are frequently utilized to diagnose potential abuse problems and monitor patients with a history of abuse. During the course of the 3- to 4-week intensive treatment, the treatment team empathically addresses patient's and family member's defensiveness toward seeking treatment. Appropriate referrals are made to the patient and family members for a comprehensive addiction evaluation by a certified addiction specialist, focused treatment at a formal chemical dependency program, and participation in community codependency groups. Depending on the nature of the substance abuse disorder and chronic pain, this treatment may occur

Inclusion criteria

- Patient has chronic pain of sufficient severity to bring about significant dysfunction in daily social, vocational, and interpersonal activities.
- Chronic pain duration of six months or more or clinical indication that pain of a shorter duration will likely manifest into a chronic condition.
- Patient has adequate control over his/her behavior and is not judged to be imminently dangerous to self or others.
- Patient demonstrates adequate motivation to proceed with a rehabilitation approach to learn self-management of pain, which often implies awareness or some level of acceptance that medical or surgical treatments are not a presently an option.

Exclusion criteria

- Patient demonstrates an unwillingness to discontinue use of opioid analgesic medications, other psychotropic medications, or substances of abuse, including alcohol, as recommended that would preclude meaningful participation in the program.
- Patient has insufficient motivation to address the necessary components that make up the general scope of interdisciplinary pain rehabilitation, including medication management, physical and occupational therapy, and group therapy.
- There is evidence of an acute physical condition or illness that is currently being treated in a manner that would preclude adequate participation in the program and detract from rehabilitation goals.
- There is evidence of significant cognitive deficits that would interfere with patient's ability to understand and learn treatment techniques and preclude adequate participation in the program.

Figure 8.2 Example of inclusion and exclusion criteria for treatment in interdisciplinary pain rehabilitation programs.

either before or following rehabilitative treatment but often in collaboration with the IPRP treatment plan.

Candidates for IPRPs

Interdisciplinary pain rehabilitation programs commonly utilize similar criteria in evaluating patients for admission to intensive, multidisciplinary rehabilitation. See Figure 8.2 for an example of inclusion and exclusion criteria for treatment in IPRPs.

A general inclusion criterion suggests that chronic pain has been present for more than 6 months. It is common, however, that patients have often needlessly suffered for years or even decades before being referred to an IPRP. A recent review of patients admitted to the Mayo Clinic Pain Rehabilitation Center [22], an IPRP in a large tertiary care center, found that patients had experienced chronic pain for a mean of 9.4 years (range, 3 months to 60 years). Almost two-thirds of patients (64.2%) reported pain duration of 4 years or longer; one-third (33.3%) for 10 or more years; and 14% for 20 or more years.

Patients referred to IPRPs often represent the most treatment-refractory and functionally impaired subgroup of patients with chronic pain. Before rehabilitation, they have generally undergone multiple

pharmacological trials including long-term opioid therapy, extensive physical therapy, interventional pain treatments, surgical procedures, and complementary and alternative interventions without lasting benefit or improved functioning [22]. These failed efforts are costly to the individual and the healthcare system and extract a heavy toll from patients and their families. Over three-fourths (79%) of patients admitted to the Mayo Clinic IPRP endorsed depressive symptomology suggestive of minor depression with over half (54%) meeting criteria for major depression [22]. Additionally, upon admission to an IPRP, patients exhibit significant pain catastrophizing. Pain catastrophizing has been associated with heightened disability, increased pain and illness behaviors, greater use of healthcare services, longer duration of hospital stays, use of analgesic medications, and is one of the most important psychological predictors of a person's experience of pain [27]. See Table 8.1 for the demographics and characteristics of patients admitted to an IPRP.

The most common chronic pain conditions represented in an IPRP population include chronic low back pain, fibromyalgia, and chronic headache/migraine. Smaller but still significant proportions of patients have chronic generalized non-fibromyalgia pain, abdominal

Table 8.1 Demographics and characteristics of patients admitted to the Mayo Clinic Pain Rehabilitation Center, an interdisciplinary pain rehabilitation program

IPRP patient characteristics	Total participants ($n = 373$)
Age, years, mean (SD)	45 (14)
Sex, % female	79
Ethnicity, % white	96
Marital status, % married	62
Education, years, mean (SD)	15 (3)
Completed high school, %	92
Disability assistance, %	60
Litigation, pain-related, %	17
Primary pain diagnosis, %	
Back	24
Fibromyalgia	20
Chronic headache	12
Generalized (not fibromyalgia)	9
Abdominal	7
Neck	6
Other[a]	22
Pain duration, years, mean (SD)	9 (10)
Opioids upon admission, %	57
Opioid use, years, mean (SD)	4 (4)
Opioids, morphine equivalence (mg/day), mean (SD)	99 (142)
Opioids, median dose (mg/day)	45
Depression (CES-D), mean (SD)	27 (12)
Minor depression, CES-D ≥ 16, %	79
Major depression, CES-D ≥ 27, %	54
Pain catastrophizing (PCS), mean (SD)	26 (13)
≥ 75th percentile (PCS ≥ 30), %	43
Completed rehabilitation, %	91

[a] Lower/upper extremity, face, foot, jaw, chest wall, pelvis, hip, mouth.
CES-D: Center for Epidemiological Studies-Depression scale [38]; PCS: Pain Catastrophizing Scale [39].

pain, neck, lower and upper extremity pain (including pain associated with complex regional pain syndrome, CRPS), and chronic face, foot, jaw, atypical chest wall, pelvis, hip, and mouth pain.

Most commonly in IPRPs, patients with different types of pain are treated together, rather than in groups based on site or type of pain. With the progression of any type of chronic pain disorder, individuals are more meaningfully characterized by their degree of deconditioning, disability, and demoralization than by physiological characteristics of their pain condition [28]. Some IPRPs are offering treatment for chronic conditions that do not include pain but are also associated with significant debilitation, such as chronic fatigue syndrome and postural orthostatic tachycardia syndrome. These conditions benefit from intensive interdisciplinary treatment focused on functional restoration. Furthermore, cancer survivors with chemotherapy-induced neuropathic and/or radiation-related pain, patients with recurrent or metastatic disease who are surviving longer, and patients with neuropathic pain associated with diabetes are examples of medically challenging patients who can potentially obtain improved quality of life and functioning utilizing cognitive-behavioral and rehabilitation-oriented treatment.

Exclusion criteria for IPRPs include active substance abuse/dependence, the presence of acute psychiatric illness or active suicidal ideation, significant cognitive deficits that prevent learning and meaningful participation in treatment, and the inability or unwillingness to participate fully in rehabilitative therapies. Programs may vary, however, on other exclusionary criteria such as age restrictions (e.g., adult only), workers' compensation status, pain-related litigation, mandate of family involvement in treatment, and acceptance of opioid withdrawal as a treatment goal.

It is standard practice for IPRPs to conduct a pre-candidacy evaluation prior to admission. This evaluation is conducted by various members of the rehabilitation team and includes a comprehensive assessment of the patient's general health, functional impairment, and psychological status. Medical records from the patient's healthcare providers may not address these issues in sufficient detail. This evaluation provides an important opportunity to introduce a biopsychosocial approach to chronic pain. In this discussion, patients may begin to shift their expectations from pain relief to pain management. This interaction is also an opportunity to allay patients' fears that their pain is believed to be psychological in origin, factitious, or involve malingering, and instead introduces a self-management approach to chronic pain. See Figure 8.3 for a list of questions patients, primary care providers, and pain specialists should ask when determining if a patient is ready for an IPRP treatment approach.

Is a pain rehabilitation center program right for me?
Interdisciplinary pain rehabilitation is a challenging process that requires a serious commitment. Ask yourself these questions to assess your readiness: • Is my recovery from injury or illness taking much longer than my doctors or I expected?   • Are my doctors telling me that they can do nothing further to relieve my pain?   • Is my life controlled by pain?   • Am I concerned about the long-term effects of taking pain medications?   • Is my family's well-being affected by my pain?   • Am I not able to commit to events with family or friends because of worry about controlling my pain?   Answering "yes" to any of these questions may indicate that your physician and you should consider your participation in an interdisciplinary pain rehabilitation program focused on improving your quality of life and functioning.

Figure 8.3 A list of questions patients, primary care providers and pain specialists should ask when determining a patient's appropriateness for an interdisciplinary pain rehabilitation treatment approach.

From Ref [23]. Copyright by Mayo Foundation for Medical Education and Research. Adapted with permission.

Treatment structure

Treatment intensity

There is significant heterogeneity between IPRPs in treatment structure and intensity. Traditionally, IPRP treatment has been 3–4 weeks in duration and most are now outpatient programs offering patient care 5 days per week, 8 hours per day. Some programs may offer less intensive programs of shorter duration (e.g., 2 weeks) and hours (e.g., half-day treatment) for patients who are still working and/or less deconditioned but can benefit from early CBT intervention. The most effective interdisciplinary programs generaly involve cognitive/behavioral therapies combined with supervised physical therapy offered several times a week for over 100 total hours of treatment. Since there are few IPRPs nationwide, many patients travel great distances and reside in hotels or other lodgings throughout the course of treatment. Interdisciplinary pain rehabilitation programs can be found in large, not-for-profit, tertiary-care academic medical centers and in small private group practices.

The national trend of IPRPs to provide outpatient rather than inpatient care has increased opportunities for patients to consolidate skills through practice, rehearsal, and generalization in real-world situations. In the evenings and weekends during treatment, patients are encouraged to independently utilize the rehabilitative pain management strategies to which they have been introduced in formal treatment. Patients who have typically been isolated and inactive due to pain are encouraged to participate in social and leisure activities with family members and other patients. Family members practice providing non-solicitous responses to pain behaviors in order to encourage wellness rather than illness behaviors. Before the weekend, patients develop an individualized weekend schedule that incorporates daily exercise, activity pacing, relaxation, and recreational activities. The weekend plan offers an opportunity to practice a plan-contingent rather than a pain-contingent lifestyle.

Initially, the intensive treatment in IPRPs can seem overwhelming for some patients who have become extremely deconditioned and isolated. Through structured activities, graded daily exercise, and accomplishment of daily goals throughout the 3–4 weeks, patients steadily reverse the cycle of debilitation and demoralization. As treatment progresses, patients experience increased confidence in their ability to manage their pain without analgesic medications and reliance on healthcare providers.

Group therapy

While some IPRP services are offered in individual sessions (e.g., assessment of co-morbid mood disorders, dietician, vocational counselor, biofeedback, chemical dependency assessment, and psychometric

	Monday	Tuesday	Wednesday	Thursday	Friday
8:00	PT Stretch	PT Stretch	PT Stretch	PT Stretch	PT Stretch
8:30	Community: Expectations/ concerns	Openers (daily goal setting)	Openers (daily goal setting)	Openers (daily goal setting)	Openers (daily goal setting)
9:00	Physical therapy	Physical therapy	Physical therapy	Physical therapy	Physical therapy
10:00	Biofeedback	Meet with treatment team	Biofeedback	Meet with treatment team	CBT: Group family session
11:00	CBT: Overview of stress	CBT: Fears and chronic pain	CBT: Pain catastrophizing	CBT: Activity pacing	CBT: Individual family session
12:00	Lunch	Lunch	Lunch	Lunch	Lunch
1:00	OT: Kitchen and shopping	OT: Yard work, driving	OT: Time management	OT: Computer ergonomics	OT: Weekend planning
2:00	CBT: Cycle of pain	CBT: Difficult day planning	CBT: Problem solving	CBT: Goals setting	CBT: Maintaining
3:00	Pharmacist: Pain medications	Chaplain: Spirituality	CBT: Assertive communication	CBT: Sleep hygiene	CBT: Chemical health
4:00	Advanced relaxation	Advanced relaxation	Advanced relaxation	Advanced relaxation	Advanced relaxation

Figure 8.4 Sample of cognitive-behavioral group therapy incorporated with physical therapy, occupational therapy and family sessions in an interdisciplinary pain rehabilitation program.

Note. CBT, cognitive-behavioral therapy; OT, occupational therapy; PT, physical therapy.

assessment), most therapies in IPRPs take place in group settings. Although IPRPs vary in size, groups often include 6 to 12 patients with chronic pain working together with program staff.

The groups are typically facilitated by psychologists, other mental health provider or certified nurse specialist with specialty training in pain management and behavioral medicine. Such specialty training is ideal because interventions are focused on changing long-standing behaviors and beliefs. Different psychodynamic, process-oriented group treatment, or community-based support groups, group therapy in IPRPs is structured to facilitate the learning of cognitive and behavioral pain coping skills. The groups provide opportunities for skills' rehearsal and feedback as patients are encouraged to personalize CBT concepts for generalization into their work, home, and family environments. Patients affirm one another by sharing the emotional aspects of suffering with chronic pain, but more importantly, they aid one

another in problem-solving barriers to maintaining rehabilitation progress. Group therapy has several advantages including: (1) the opportunity for chronic pain patients to be exposed to individuals with similar problems; (2) patients gain a better understanding of pain and the role of their own behaviors, thoughts, and feelings on their pain experience; (3) structured groups allow teaching, demonstration, and problem-solving of specific coping skills; and (4) greater cost-effectiveness than individual sessions [29]. See Figure 8.4 for an example of one week of treatment at an IPRP that incorporates daily cognitive-behavioral group therapy sessions, physical therapy, and occupational therapy.

Often overwhelmed with pain and intense negative emotions, patients with chronic pain spend more time in isolation and away from family, work, community, religious, and volunteer networks. Within the group therapy setting, patients begin taking steps necessary to make positive changes toward a new life. In group therapy sessions, patients are encouraged to talk about how daily life has been affected by health concerns, avoid talking about symptoms and other pain behaviors, focus on present issues rather than prior difficulties, identify specific problems and issues to resolve, be open to new ideas and alternatives, identify constructive ways to respond to pain and healthier ways to manage the cycle of pain, and incorporate new skills into one's life.

Most IPRPs have an open "rolling admission" group format in which each participant may start and complete treatment at different times. This format is suited to IPRPs because patients may have varying lengths of stay, modules can be introduced at any point during treatment, and veteran participants can help allay any concerns new patients may have about medication changes and treatment expectations. Veteran participants play a vital role in the groups by frankly discussing their own initial skepticism and reservations, and modeling effective use of cognitive-behavioral approaches to pain management.

Family therapy

Interdisciplinary pain rehabilitation programs vary in their expectations and structure for the involvement of family members in treatment. All IPRPs, however, recognize the importance that family has in initiating and maintaining illness and wellness behaviors. From a biopsychosocial perspective of the family system, the debilitating effects of chronic pain extend beyond nociception. These effects create shifts in family roles, loss of income, increased family, and marital distress, which, in turn, have increased negative effects on pain and disability. As chronic pain conditions persist, spouses, parents, siblings, and even children become vigilant about assessing the patient's pain severity, need for medication and assistance. Children in the family may inappropriately assume the role of caregiver.

To address the often unintended reinforcement of disability and pain behaviors, the family members participate in time-limited and goal-oriented sessions about the cognitive-behavioral management of pain. Using the cognitive-behavioral model of family therapy for patients with chronic pain [30], the family's resources are increased through education and skills training. Through this training, they are better able to understand the adaptive management of chronic pain, decrease the negative impact of stress on the family, improve the family functioning and support the

patient's ability to maintain rehabilitation progress. Family members learn that they can play a significant role in the extinction of pain behaviors (e.g., inactivity, somatic focus) by positively reinforcing well behaviors (e.g., continued productive activity, exercise, and socializing).

It is difficult, if not impossible, to change long-standing family dynamics and maladaptive communication styles during 3–4 weeks of IPRP treatment. In cases when more intensive, individualized family therapy is warranted, patients and their family members are encouraged to find a marital or family therapist who is familiar with improving family functioning within the context of a chronic health condition.

Maintaining rehabilitation progress

The IPRP treatment team's communication of the patient's disposition and discharge plan to the primary care provider and medical specialists who may be involved is merely the beginning of efforts necessary to maintain progress following discharge. The patient's healthcare providers play a key role in reinforcing rehabilitation concepts and aiding the patient in distinguishing between pain associated with acute illness and a flare of the chronic pain condition. The home provider's awareness of specific cognitive-behavioral pain coping strategies is imperative to guide patients to utilize these techniques. This may help avoid a return to opioid therapy, the initiation of unnecessary and costly diagnostic testing, or reinforcement of a pain-contingent lifestyle. The knowledge and confidence the primary provider has in these pain management strategies enhances his/her ability to adhere to a biopsychosocial model of care and empirically supported treatment for chronic pain. Physicians and other healthcare providers are regularly encouraged to visit and form professional relationships with the IPRP treatment team.

Throughout the IPRP treatment, as patients improve their mental and physical functioning, they also grow in their independence for managing their chronic pain and decrease their reliance on medical providers. Patients are commonly assisted in identifying a cognitive-behavioral psychologist or therapist for time-limited and goal-directed assistance following discharge. Some IPRPs offer formal aftercare or "booster" programs for IPRP graduates to review rehabilitation concepts, gain additional support for making lifestyle changes, and address barriers to achieving rehabilitation goals.

Treatment efficacy of IPRPs

At a time when much attention is devoted to new pharmacological, interventional, and surgical procedures for "pain relief," IPRPs have stood the test of time. There is abundant evidence to suggest that they are an effective treatment for managing chronic pain and improving patients' functioning and quality of life. It has been suggested that IPRP treatment is more effective than any other form of treatment for chronic pain [31].

In a recent review of the literature on chronic pain, the American Pain Society's Comprehensive Pain Rehabilitation report concluded IPRPs that focus on functional restoration and include a cognitive-behavioral treatment component are associated with substantive long-term improvements in functioning and positive outcomes for various chronic pain conditions (e.g., back pain, upper extremity disorders, fibromyalgia, headache, musculoskeletal disorders, temporomandibular joint disorder) [32]. Additionally, compared to other treatment modalities for chronic pain, IPRP is the only therapeutic approach that has demonstrated treatment efficacy and cost-effectiveness for major outcome variables such as improved functioning, physical activity, and working ability, decreased pain, decreased healthcare utilization, decreased medication use, decreased disability claims, and decreased healthcare costs and insurance claims. Similarly, in a review of cost effectiveness of IPRPs, rehabilitation was more cost effective than implantation of spinal cord stimulators, intraspinal implantable drug delivery systems, or surgery. The IPRP treatment approach resulted in significantly greater reduction in medication use and healthcare utilization and in significantly greater increases in functional activities, return to work, closure of disability claims, as well as substantially fewer iatrogenic consequences and adverse events [33]. McCracken *et al.* [34] found that interdisciplinary treatment offered in IPRPs demonstrated effectiveness for even highly disabled chronic pain sufferers with limited mobility and need of assistance with self-care – a group of patients whose pain has been refractory to conventional and unimodal treatments. Based on a systematic review of the literature, recently published evidence-based clinical practice guidelines from the American Pain Society [13] gave a "strong recommendation" based on "high-quality" evidence that patients with nonradicular low back pain who do not respond to usual, noninterdisciplinary intervention should be considered for intensive interdisciplinary rehabilitation with cognitive/behaviral emphasis.

Research in the field of chronic pain is ongoing and exciting. Quality research demonstrating the efficacy of rehabilitative treatment is needed to combat the ever-present biomedical model approach to chronic pain management. Equally important is the dissemination of such research to front-line medical care providers who oversee the healthcare of patients from the onset of acute pain through the development of a chronic pain condition.

Challenges for the future of IPRPs

The durability of the IPRP treatment approach for over three decades is a testament that the biopsychosocial model of care is the optimum care for this complex patient population. However, like any treatment modality, there are many challenges to overcome in order to ensure progress in an ever-changing healthcare environment. These challenges include declining reimbursement rates for IPRPs, lack of quality training opportunities in interdisciplinary pain management, and minimal funding available for pain research.

Declining reimbursement patterns and the subsequent closing of numerous IPRPs across the nation jeopardizes the futures of IPRPs and millions of patients suffering from chronic pain. The steady decrease in IPRPs across the nation is concurrent with the rise in utilization of analgesic medications and interventional pain treatments. These approaches to pain management differ from IPRPs, which focus on optimizing functioning rather than solely addressing pain relief. Although ample evidence documents the treatment efficacy of interdisciplinary pain rehabilitation programs, third-party payers continue to erect barriers to IPRPs. They incorrectly use terms such as "investigational" or "not medically necessary" when denying requests for IPRP treatment. Paradoxically, insurers have increasingly reimbursed interventional and surgical procedures for which there is minimal scientific evidence and few functional gains. Declining reimbursement patterns and the denial of treatment is the number one problem for the survival of IPRPs, which are inaccurately characterized as costly and inefficient [35, 36]. Unfortunately, hospital administrators, who are focused on cost-containment, are also responding to the decline in reimbursement and decreased profit generation by terminating IPRPs. The survival of IPRPs largely depends on the administrative team's ability to carefully monitor changes in reimbursement trends, be proactively involved in all financial aspects of the program, have flexibility to make programmatic changes necessary to meet financial demands, and willingness to partner with insurers.

Consistent with reimbursement trends, training opportunities in pain more often focus on training interventionists rather than pain rehabilitation specialists. There is a great need for behaviorally trained pain specialists who are well-versed in fundamental theories of operant conditioning and its relevance to reinforcing wellness behaviors, as well as cognitive-behavioral treatment of pain. Interdisciplinary pain rehabilitation programs trying to remain financially viable typically have limited resources to allocate to training or to compete for grant funding to hire pain residents and fellows. The programs that are able to offer training positions often compete amongst themselves for the few candidates who are interested in pursuing subspecialty training in pain management. Recently, legislatures and state boards of medical practice have begun to require or encourage participation in continuing medical education courses on pain management and palliative care. Even greater efforts will be needed, however, to educate providers regarding empirically based treatment plans which describe when to initiate (and cease) pharmacotherapy (particularly opioids), surgical and interventional pain treatments, and cognitive-behavioral pain management.

Funding for pain research is dismal and unproportional to the millions of people suffering from pain. In 2003, only 1% of funding from the National Institutes of Health was dedicated to primary pain grants [37]. Until increased pain research funding is available, IPRPs face the challenge of developing clinical research projects and demonstrating treatment efficacy within the existing program. There is often a separation between the research being conducted by scientists in largely academic laboratory settings and behavioral pain specialists providing mostly direct clinical care. Interdisciplinary pain rehabilitation programs that continue to focus solely on providing clinical care do a disservice by not contributing to the empirical data needed to secure their future existence. In the absence of research funding and faced with demanding clinical schedules, collaboration with academic pain researchers who have minimal patient access but greater research resources may be an ideal but often underutilized option to maximize research efforts for IPRPs.

Conclusion

The superiority of the biopsychosocial model of care for chronic pain is most evident within the IPRP treatment approach. Orchestrating the expertise of multiple disciplines concurrently focused on restoring patients' functioning and quality of life is a worthwhile challenge. The rewards are great for the patients, families, healthcare providers, pain specialists, IPRP treatment team, and society as a whole. The availability of IPRPs nationwide will be an ongoing struggle as insurers are educated on the long-term efficacy and cost-effectiveness of interdisciplinary rehabilitation-oriented treatment. Patients' inability to access IPRP treatment due to healthcare providers' lack of knowledge, however, is avoidable with continued education and training opportunities within IPRPs. Comprehensive treatment planning for patients with chronic pain is essential and referrals to IPRPs should be (but are often not) a part of standardized practice. The recommendation for treatment in an IPRP should be considered earlier in the course of patient care and before patients have endured years of suffering and disability.

Acknowledgments

We express profound appreciation for the numerous care providers and staff at the Mayo Comprehensive Pain Rehabilitation Center whose commitment to excellent patient care is inspiring.

References

1. Turk DC, Monarch ES. Biopsychosocial perspective on chronic pain. In *Psychological Approaches to Pain Management: A practitioner's handbook,* 2nd edn., eds. DC Turk RJ Gatchel. (New York: Guilford Press, 2002), pp. 3–29.

2. Townsend CO, Bruce BK, Hooten WM, Rome JD. The role of mental health professionals in multidisciplinary pain rehabilitation programs. *J Clin Psychol* 2006; **62**: 1433–43.

3. Sanders SH, Harden RN, Vicente PJ. Evidence-based clinical practice guidelines for interdisciplinary rehabilitation of chronic nonmalignant pain syndrome patients. *Pain Pract* 2005; **5**: 303–15.

4. Fishman SM. *Responsible Opioid Prescribing: A Physician's Guide* (Federation of the State Medical Board, 2008).

5. Turk DC. A cognitive-behavioral perspective on treatment of chronic pain patients. In *Psychological*

Approaches to Pain Management: A practitioner's handbook, 2nd edn., eds. DC Turk RJ Gatchel (New York: Guilford Press, 2002). pp. 138–58.

6. Crombez G, Vlaeyen JW, Heuts PH. Pain-related fear is more disabling than pain itself: Evidence on the role of pain-related fear in chronic pain disability. *Pain* 1999; **80**: 329–39.

7. Boothby JL, Thorn BE, Stroud M, Jensen MP. Coping with pain. In *Psychosocial Factors in Pain*, eds. RJ Gatchel and DC Turk. (New York: Guilford Press, 1999), pp. 343–59.

8. Turk DC. Clinicans' attitudes about prolonged use of opioids and the issue of patient heterogeneity. *J Pain Symptom Manag* 1996; **11**: 218–30.

9. Nishimori M, Kulich, RJ, Carwood CM, *et al.* Successful and unsuccessful outcomes with long-term opioid therapy: A survey of physicians' opinions. *J Palliat Med* 2006; **9**: 50–5.

10. Turk DC, Okifuji A. What factors affect physicians' decisions to prescribe opioids from chronic noncancer pain patients? *Clin J Pain* 1997; **13**: 330–6.

11. Ballantyne JC, Mao J. Opioid therapy for chronic pain. *N Engl J Med* 2003; **349**: 1943–53.

12. Loder E, Herbert P, McAlary P. Chronic pain rehabilitation. In *The Massachusetts General Hospital Handbook of Pain Management,* 2nd edn., eds. J Ballantyne, SM Fishman and S Abdi. (Philadelphia, PA: Lippincott, Williams Wilkins, 2002), pp. 262–71.

13. Chou R, Ballantyne JC, Fanciullo GJ, Fine PG. Research gaps on use of opioids for chronic noncancer pain: findings from a review of the evidence for an American Pain Society and American Academy of Pain Medicine Clinical Practice Guideline. *J Pain* 2009; **10**: 147–59.

14. Kalso E, Edwards JE, Moore RA, McQuay HJ. Opioids in chronic non-cancer pan: A systemic review of efficacy and safety. *Pain* 2004; **112**: 372–80.

15. Moore RA, McQuay HJ. Prevalence of opioid adverse events in chronic non-malignant pain: Systematic review of randomized trials of oral opioids. *Arthritis Res Ther* 2005; **7**: 46–51.

16. Martell BA, O'Connor PG, Kerns RD, *et al.* Systematic review: Opioid treatment for chronic back pain: prevalence, efficacy and associated with addiction. *Ann Intern Med* 2007; **146**: 116–27.

17. Furlan AD, Sandoval JA, Mailis-Gagnon A, Tunks E. Opioids for chronic noncancer pain: A meta-analysis of effectiveness and side effects. *CMAJ* 2006; **174**: 1589–94.

18. Chou R, Clark E, Helfand M. Comparative efficacy and safety of long-acting oral opioids for chronic non-cancer pain: A systematic review. *J Pain Symptom Manage* 2003; **26**: 1026–48.

19. Chu LF, Clark DJ, Angst MS. Opioid tolerance and hyperalgesia in chronic pain patients after one month of oral morphine therapy: A preliminary prospective study. *J Pain.* 2006; 7: 43–8.

20. Baron MJ, McDonald PW. Significant pain reduction in chronic pain patients after detoxification from high-dose opioids. *J Opioid Manag* 2006; **2**: 277–82.

21. Rome JD, Towsnend CO, Bruce BK, *et al.* Chronic noncancer pain rehabilitation with opioid withdrawal: Comparison of treatment outcomes based on opioid use status at admission. *Mayo Clin Proc* 2004; **79**: 759–68.

22. Townsend CO, Hooten WM, Bruce, BK, *et al.* Pain rehabilitation with opioid withdrawal: Longitudinal study of treatment outcomes for chronic noncancer pain. *J Pain* 2007; **8**: S41.

23. Bruce BK Hooten WM. *Mayo Clinic Guide to Pain Relief: How to Manage, Reduce and Control Chronic Pain* (Rochester, MN: Mayo Clinic Health Solutions), 2008.

24. Hooten WM, Townsend CO, Sletten CD, Bruce BK, Rome JD. Treatment outcomes after multidisciplinary pain rehabilitation with analgesic medication withdrawal for patients with fibromyalgia. *Pain Med* 2007; **8**: 8–16.

25. National Center on Addiction and Substance Abuse (CASA). *Under the Counter: The Diversion and Abuse of Controlled Prescription Drugs in the US* (New York, NY: Columbia University, 2005).

26. Passik SD, Kirsh KL. Identifying and treating patients with drug abuse problems. In *Psycholocial Aspects of Pain: A Handbook for Health Care Providers, Progress in Pain Research and Management,* Vol. 27, eds. R.H. Dworkin W.S. Breitbart (Seattle, WA: IASP Press, 2004) pp. 465–78.

27. Sullivan MJ, Thorn B, Haythornthwaite JA, *et al.* Theoretical perspectives on the relation between catastrophizing and pain. *Clin J Pain* 2001; 17: 52–64.

28. Bruce BK, Townsend CO, Hooten WM, Rome JD, Moon JS, Swanson JW. Chronic pain rehabilitation in chronic headache disorders. *Current Neurol Neurosci Rep* 2008; **8**: 94–9.

29. Keefe FJ, Beaupre PM, Gil KM, Rumble ME, Aspnes AK. Group therapy for patients with chronic pain. In *Psychological Approaches to Pain Management: A practitioner's handbook,* 2nd edn., eds. DC Turk, RJ Gatchel (New York: Guilford Press, 2002) pp. 234–55.

30. Kerns RD, Otis JD, Wise EA. Treating families of chronic pain patients: Application of a cognitive-behavioral transactional model. In *Psychological Approaches to Pain Management: A practitioner's handbook,* 2nd edn., eds. DC Turk RJ Gatchel (New York: Guilford Press, 2002) pp. 256–75.

31. Loeser JD. Multidisciplinary pain management. In *The Paths of Pain 1975–2005*, eds. H Merskey, JD Loeser, R. Dubner, (Seattle, WA: IASP Press, 2005), pp. 503–11.

32. Gatchel, RJ, Okifuji, A. Evidence-based scientific data documenting the treatment and cost-effectiveness of comprehensive pain programs for chronic nonmalignant pain. *J Pain*, 2006; 7: 779–93.

33. Turk DC. Clinical effectiveness and cost-effectiveness of treatments for patients with chronic pain. *Clin J Pain* 2002; 18: 355–65.

34. McCracken LM, MacKichan F, Eccleston C. Contextual cognitive-behavioral therapy for severely disabled chronic pain sufferers: Effectiveness and clinically significant change. *Eur J Pain*, 2007; 11: 314–22.

35. Gatchel RJ. Clinical essentials of pain management. In *Reimbursement Issues in Pain Management* (Washington, DC: American Psychological Association, 2005), pp. 241–54.

36. Thomsen AB, Sorensen J, Sjogren P, Ericksen J. Economic evaluation of multidisciplinary pain management in chronic pain patients: A qualitative systematic review. *J Pain Symptom Manag* 2001; 22: 688–98.

37. Bradshaw DH, Nakamura Y, Chapman CR. National Institutes of Health grant awards for pain nausea, and dyspnea research: An assessment of funding patterns in 2003. *J Pain* 2005; 6: 277–93.

38. Radloff L. The CES-D scale: A self-report depression scale for research in the general population. *Appl Psychol Meas* 1977; 1: 385–401.

39. Sullivan MJ, Bishop S, Pivik J. The Pain Catastrophizing Scale: Development and validation. *Psychol Assess* 1995; 7: 524–32.

Pharmacologic approaches to pain management

Robin M. Gallagher

Pain management in the continuum from injury to disease

Successful pharmacologic treatment of pain in a population of patients usually rests on the success of the provider–patient relationship. However, in modern medicine this relationship is already challenged by a distancing technology and the constraints on time and trust imposed by the intrusions of other social systems, such as managed systems of care, shrinking insurance reimbursement fees, and forensic/regulatory concerns. To these burdens, chronic pain or "maldynia" (bad pain, or pain as a disease) adds its unique strains. Whether the condition causing pain is considered "benign," such as often the case in low back pain or arthritis, or considered "malignant," such as in cancer or complex regional pain syndrome (CRPS), chronic pain is almost always difficult for a patient to endure. Pain makes people unhappy and irritable, clinically depressed, suicidal, and even violent [1–4]. Doctors must endure and manage these secondary co-morbidities and their behavioral manifestations in abnormal illness behavior. They also must endure the strain of treating pain with opioid analgesics under state and federal regulation [5], managing the hassles of prescribing defensively in a fear-inspiring social context of variable state and federal regulations and variable, at times perniciously erratic, enforcement and even criminal prosecution [6, 7]. It's no wonder primary physicians pull the pain consult trigger so readily – although often unsuccessfully as pain specialists become inundated with these tasks and responsibilities. The conflict between caring about patients' suffering and fear of being "duped" is very real. Physicians expressing their natural empathy to ease suffering – a high calling of their profession – are being asked to identify potential criminal behavior! [7–9]. No other medical condition so consistently demands that in every encounter a prescribing clinician plays dual roles as healer and regulator/sheriff. The longitudinal strain on both doctor and patient and their relationship is enormous. This cost is the ultimate rationale for risk management strategies, such as treatment agreements [10], and structured programs, such as the opioid renewal clinic [11], that reduce these risks and by clarifying patient and provider roles and responsibilities in opioid analgesia, also reduce the strain on the provider–patient relationship.

How does the system prepare clinicians for this struggle? A provider's ability to care for patients with chronic pain can be conceptualized as depending on a hierarchy of at least three factors: first, whether their inherent capacity for empathy is enhanced or diminished by their rigorous premedical and medical education and by their prolonged and difficult skill-based training caring for sick patients [12, 13]; second, whether this process trains them to understand the concept of biopsychosocial, multifactorial causal models of chronic disease and trains them in the general methods of chronic disease management [14, 15]; and third, whether their training exposes them to chronic pain in a manner that is both intellectually stimulating and provides them with role models that skillfully practice and teach chronic pain assessment and management. The hierarchy implied by these factors' order of presentation suggests that certain personality types might be more naturally predisposed to choose this path and better endure the required training. For the public health, standardized training reduces the variability of clinical performance when caring for an illness somewhat independently of personality factors. Some doctors will never master the manual skills of a surgeon, and others will

Behavioral and Psychopharmacologic Pain Management, ed. Michael H. Ebert and Robert D. Kerns. Published by Cambridge University Press. © Cambridge University Press 2011.

never master the patience and patient-centeredness of family medicine or psychiatry. But within the broad groups of doctors, variability will be reduced by rigorous standardized training. For example, every family doctor and internist learns to manage problems such as hypertension, diabetes, depression, and pneumonia; thus patients (and the public generally – even actuarial types!) can assume core skills based upon a standardized national system of monitoring medical student education and residency training programs through the Assocation of American Medical Colleges and the US Accreditation Council for Medical Education, respectively. Unfortunately for the public, this is not the case for chronic pain [15–17]. Despite the fact that pain is the most common reason patients see doctors, unfortunately pain management is the stepchild of many training programs, and a focus of none. Anesthesia, which presently runs most hospital pain programs, focuses its training on surgical anesthesia, with lesser attention to acute pain management in the hospital and to regional anesthesia. In most of this training there is little exposure to the outpatient settings in which chronic pain is generally encountered and managed, and little training in the core concepts and skills of chronic disease management, such as biopsychosocial formulation, managing co-morbidities, and managing the doctor–patient relationship. Neurology focuses on finding the neurological causes of pain symptoms, but traditionally has been little interested in the biopsychosocial model of chronic disease and in pain procedures. Psychiatry focuses on the neurosciences and mental health consequences or co-morbidities of chronic pain, the doctor–patient relationship, and on theories of psychogenic causation, but with little training in assessment or management of peripheral pain generators. Pain management in rehabilitation traditionally focuses on the musculoskeletal system and its rehabilitation without an examination of the neurobehavioral contributions to pain and, until recently, little attention to neural blockade and neuromodulation. Thus, most specialty clinicians are ill-prepared by their education and training to manage effectively the challenges of caring for chronic pain disorders and diseases and must learn from practice experience supplemented with continuing medical education.

Providers seeking the immediate gratification of dramatically treating life threatening conditions or sleuthing a medical conundrum, may lack the capacity for the sustained empathic response required to support a suffering patient through the clinical trials of what is often a tedious pathway to satisfactory pain control and improved quality of life. Good training in some instances may unlock their latent capacity. Conversely, those with an abundance of unrestrained empathy may be consumed by the long and arduous process of uncertainty, repeated disappointments, and lack of cure associated with chronic pain management. Either way, without education and training that is specific to chronic pain assessment and treatment, pain management becomes a burden rather than the intellectually stimulating and rewarding specialty it really can be. This book aims to redress this knowledge deficit and outline the intellectual and training challenges for the field. This chapter specifically reviews the core knowledge and skills required to prescribe medications effectively for chronic pain disorders and diseases, with the caveat that medications alone are rarely as effective as a comprehensive management plan that integrates various modalities of treatment. These modalities are covered in other chapters.

The science and the art of pain management using medications

The science of pain medicine is rapidly evolving, spurred by our advances in epidemiology and neuroscience. We now appreciate many of the neurobiological mechanisms underlying the progression from acute injury or disease onset to the pathophysiology of what we now consider as chronic pain diseases. We know much more about the corresponding mechanisms of action of the medications used to treat pain [18–20]. In addition to understanding the peripheral systems involving inflammation and mechanical nociception in pain perception and modulation, the field is also learning how complex neural networks in the brain and spinal cord, subserved by a variety of neurotransmitter systems, process environmental sensory stimuli such as nociception [21, 22]. Genetic phenotypes interact with life's experiences with pain and with psychosocial and environmental factors to shape these neural systems. Appreciation of this science forms the substrate for an informed and rational approach to the pharmacotherapy of pain. Peripheral mechanical, inflammatory, and neural systems governing the activation of pain, and the central neural systems governing the pain experience, both can be modified by medications; additionally,

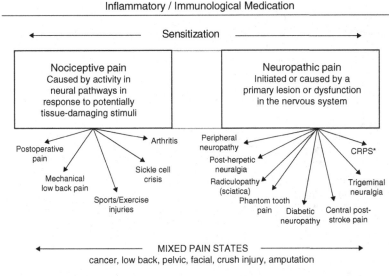

Inflammatory / Immunological Medication

Sensitization

Nociceptive pain
Caused by activity in neural pathways in response to potentially tissue-damaging stimuli

Neuropathic pain
Initiated or caused by a primary lesion or dysfunction in the nervous system

Postoperative pain

Arthritis

Mechanical low back pain

Sickle cell crisis

Sports/Exercise injuries

Peripheral neuropathy

Post-herpetic neuralgia

Radiculopathy (sciatica)

Phantom tooth pain

Diabetic neuropathy

CRPS*

Trigeminal neuralgia

Central post-stroke pain

MIXED PAIN STATES
cancer, low back, pelvic, facial, crush injury, amputation

*Complex regional pain syndrome.

Figure 9.1 Conditions causing chronic pain, differentiated by mechanism.

Adapted from from: Gallagher RM, Verma S. *Semin Clin Neurosurgery. 2004.* This information concerns uses that have not been approved by the US FDA.

the effectiveness of medications can be modified by neural systems influenced by past pain experience, cognitive processes and emotions. Finally, discrete psychiatric, neurological, and other medical co-morbidities can importantly influence patients' responses to the pharmacotherapy of pain and must be managed if the clinician is to maximize treatment response [1, 19, 20].

In addition to maintaining a current understanding of pain mechanisms and the clinical efficacy of available pharmacotherapies, physicians must cultivate the ability to assess pain in a comprehensive manner. While *intensity* is the dimension of pain most often assessed in clinical trials, the assessment of pain *quality* (e.g., burning, sharp, stabbling) and other dimensions such as *impact on mood, sleep and physical, psychosocial,* and *vocational functioning* are also important to evaluate the success of pharmacotherapy, especially in light of the fact that pain perception and pain behavior are modulated by a variety of neurophysiologic systems. A number of new tools for the assessment of multiple pain dimensions have been developed which, if put into use, may aid the physician in the development of individual treatment plans for patients. However, in the busy clinic, simple questions would include: How much does it hurt, how bad is it – 0 (no pain) to 10 (pain as bad as it can be) scale [23]? What does it prevent you from doing – work, household activities, exercise, sex, hobbies, and activities of daily living? How does pain affect your

sleep? Your mood? Your relationships? How is treatment moderating these effects? Physicians should be aware of the strengths and weaknesses of the available assessment tools so that they may be used most effectively. These tools are reviewed in Section 2 of this volume.

Chronic pain conditions are conveniently identified as either neuropathic or nociceptive because the evidence-based treatment algorithm for managing pain with medication usually involves this differentiation, as outlined in Figure 9.1.

These conditions are rarely cured but rather should be considered, like diabetes or heart disease, as chronic diseases that may or may not progress depending on factors related to the disease itself and to the effectiveness of its management along the causal pathway to chronicity. Various pathophysiologic processes underlie the progression of acute pain to chronic pain as a disease of the central nervous system (CNS) with bodily, CNS and psychosocial manifestations, as suggested by Figure 9.2. Pharmacotherapy aims to interrupt or attenuate this process by medications' specific effects on the pathophysiology of each stage of the process.

Pharmacotherapy of chronic pain

Analgesic medications act both peripherally and centrally by a variety of mechanisms to modulate nociception, pain perception, and, ultimately, pain

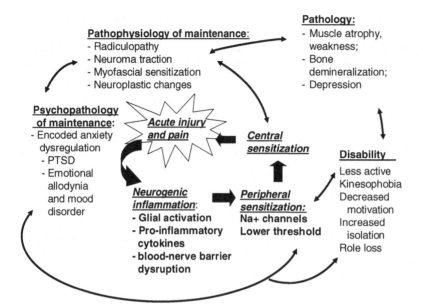

Figure 9.2 Acute to chronic pain pathophysiologic cycle.

behavior [21, 22]. Medications are provided through several routes: oral, topical patches and gels, intramuscular and intrafascial, intravenous, transdermal, subcutaneous, transmucosal (nasal, buccal, rectal), and intrathecal (epidural space). Non-steroidal anti-inflammatory drugs (NSAIDs), given by oral, parenteral, and transdermal routes, act primarily in the periphery to reduce nociception through the inhibition of prostaglandin. Anticonvulsants, usually acting on sodium and/or calcium channels, and tricyclic antidepressants, acting on sodium channels, stabilize neuronal membranes to reduce ectopic nerve impulse generation and neuropathic pain. Topical lidocaine, administered by transdermal patches or gels and injections, also acts on sodium channels to inhibit pain transmission and to inhibit both peripheral and central sensitization. The mechanism of the efficacy of serotonin-norepinephrine re-uptake inhibitors (SNRIs) and tricyclic antidepressants (TCAs) in neuropathic pain is due, purportedly, to their inhibition of reuptake of norepinephrine and serotonin, thereby enhancing descending pain modulating systems from the midbrain to the spinal cord dorsal horn. Tricyclic antidepressants in gel form have been shown to be effective topically, presumably by sodium channel activity. Opioids, which can be provided in local, oral, rectal, transmucosal, intramuscular, intravenous, and intrathecal forms, act on opioid receptors distributed widely in the peripheral tissues and the CNS. Topical opioids can be applied directly to wounds to beneficial effect.

Adequate analgesia by itself, when effective, can modify maladaptive emotional and behavioral responses. Some analgesic drugs powerfully influence emotions and behavior. Opioids, besides their strong analgesic effects, calm agitated patients. Antidepressants such as the tricyclics, selective serotonin reuptake inhibitors (SSRIs), and SNRIs (e.g., duloxetine and venlafaxine) effectively treat depression or anxiety and may modify maladaptive emotional and behavioral responses to pain [1]. Emotional states such as anger and anxiety activate the noradrenergic system, which heightens attention to pain, and in turn activates the descending sympathetic system, which increases the firing of damaged pain neurons in neuropathic pain conditions [24]. By alleviating secondary depression or anxiety, antidepressants (and psychotherapies discussed in other chapters) may moderate these pathophysiologic responses and enhance patients' ability to comply with pain management instructions such as regimens in exercise, pacing, relaxation, and medication. These improvements also may enable patients to cope more effectively with the negative consequences of pain such as job stress or loss, relationship stress, and workers' compensation stress.

In designing a treatment plan, the physician should consider not only how the intervention will affect the pathophysiologic processes causing chronic pain (Figures 9.1, and 9.2) but also each intervention's potential for adverse side effects and drug interactions. For example, *physical therapy* may aggravate

Table 9.1 Functions of record keeping

1. A major problem for pharmacologic pain treatment is the clinicians' and patients' lack of clear objective tests of response to treatments, such as a blood pressure in hypertension or hemoglobin A1C in diabetes. Patients can learn a 0–10 scaling system that has intra-rater reliability.

2. Patients deliver an accurate record of changes in pain within a reasonable time frame of the change. Pain patterns are notorious for being poorly remembered, and in fact are inaccurate in retrospect [44]. By keeping a diary, patients can establish a baseline for daily pain levels that will enable the reliable monitoring of treatment effects.

3. By recording circumstances of the changes in pain, including factors associated with flares and remissions, patients may learn about the multiple other biopsychosocial factors that may precipitate and perpetuate their pain.

4. Record-keeping is therapeutic. The patient finally can do something that helps their treatment, an activity that improves, often immediately, their sense of control and self-efficacy. Rather than "catastrophizing" (see Chapter 3), they can begin taking control.

5. By providing a numerical scale to communicate pain levels, record-keeping serves to extinguish maladaptive pain behavior (grimacing, stooping, complaining) that serve as their only means of communicating pain levels and distress, but do not help the provider make effective treatment decisions.

nerve injury and/or muscle damage. *Interventional procedures* are associated with complications and if repeated regularly high cost and potential complications: for example, steroids used repeatedly may not be effective longitudinally and are potentially toxic to damaged neurons and cause osteopenia [25]. Thus interventional procedures, including neuromodulation, should be undertaken within the context of selectively comprehensive treatment that addresses the most salient factors contributing to pain and functional impairment [26] Otherwise, even if they temporarily relieve pain, they often fail to improve longitudinal outcomes.

The pain diary for evaluation and management of pain

At initial presentation, patients may be taking a variety of medications. Barring an immediate medical reason to change medications, clinicians should consider asking the patient to keep a pain diary for 1–2 weeks to assess baseline pain and functional status on existing medications (reviewed in Chapter 20). Functions of record-keeping are summarized in Table 9.1. Having this baseline will help the clinician evaluate and monitor the response to various treatments. Diaries can provide important information about factors that alleviate or worsen pain, about patient behavior and coping, and about the effects of treatment. The diary should be reviewed subsequently at each visit until a stable medication regimen is obtained. This procedure also encourages adherence to treatment plans and gives the patient some responsibility for outcome.

Principles of prescribing medications for chronic pain

The author recommends ten general principles when prescribing medication for patients with chronic non-cancer or cancer pain, as in Table 9.2.

Detailed information about pharmacological doses and regimens in specific clinical situations is beyond the scope of this chapter. Importantly, clinicians should consider risks and burdens associated with different medication classes. Over-use of some drugs, such as NSAIDs or acetaminophen, is associated with serious risks such as gastrointestinal bleeding or liver disease, respectively. Benzodiazepines must be used cautiously, especially in the elderly or those operating machinery, because they increase the risk for falls and accidents, they can cause dependency, they increase the risk of respiratory depression when combined with opioids, and they inhibit new learning, which may be problematic in pain treatment requiring that patients learn new coping skills (see below). Opioids, with organ system toxicity limited to constipation and hypogonadism in some cases, and with less drug or disease interactions than most other medications used for pain, can be safe and effective, especially when used within a comprehensive pain program or structured setting [27–31]. However, animal literature and clinical experience suggests that some patients develop tolerance and even hyperalgesia after long-term exposure to opioids for pain [32–35] through the activation of N-methyl-D-aspartate receptors and protein kinase C as well as the regulation of glutamate transporters. As yet, we cannot predict which patients will develop tolerance or hyperalgesia

Table 9.2 Principles for prescribing medication in patients for chronic pain

Principle	Examples
1. Prioritize safety in non-malignant chronic pain	Older patients are at greater risks for falls if given tricyclic anti-depressants or anti-convulsants. Low dose opioids, supervised appropriately, may be safer. Patients with COPD are at greater risk for clinically significant respiratory depression when titrating opioids when combined with benzodiazepines. Patients with substance abuse histories are more likely to develop aberrant behaviors and relapse to active addiction if exposed to opioid analgesics without adequate structure and support.
2. Prioritize effectiveness in terminally ill patients with pain	Titrating opioid analgesia to sedation may be the only way to assure the relief of suffering in a dying cancer patient.
3. Consider potential interactions with existing medical conditions and other medications	Gabapentin titration must be slow and at lower doses in older patients and those with renal disease. Methadone must be titrated cautiously in patients taking anti-depressants and anti-convulsants for depression, pain or seizures because of individual differences in their effects on the CYP450 isoenzymes in the liver.
4. Selectively choose drugs for pain disorders and co-morbid psychiatric disorder	Consider efficacy for individual pain diseases – for example, tricyclics, which have proven efficacy in diabetic neuropathy, have not demonstrated efficacy in clinical trials for HIV neuropathy.
5. Balance side-effect profile and toxicity risk against efficacy	TCAs are effective in neuropathic pain in lower doses than needed for depression, thus avoiding much of the side effect burden, particularly in younger patients. SSRIs and SNRIs (antidepressants) are much more likely to cause sexual side effects than buproprion when treating depression in patients with chronic pain. Regular long-term use of NSAIDs is associated with higher organ system risk (e.g., renal, gastrointestinal) than opioids.
6. Consider cognitive and behavioral effects	Tricyclics are more likely than SSRIs to cause cognitive impairment in older persons. Benzodiazepines may inhibit learning new coping skills in patients with chronic pain.
7. Select combinations of medications from difference classes based on complementary mechanisms of action.	For neuropathic pain, SNRIs enhance descending modulating systems, TCAs combine SNRI and Na channel blocking effects, gabapentin and pregabalin act at voltage gated calcium channels, and opioids act at opioid receptor sites.
8. Monitor pain and activity levels and response measures during therapeutic trials	Use pain and activity diaries to establish effectiveness of treatment.
9. Avoid irrational poly-pharmacy and optimize methods of medication delivery	Look for potential drug interactions, such as SSRIs and tegretol affecting methadone metabolism through effects on cytochrome P-450 enzymes in the liver.
10. Integrate medications with behavioral and physical therapies	Not all pain must be treated with medications. Neuromodulation with simple techniques such as icing, stretching, TENS, and acupuncture and behavioral techniques such as pacing, relaxation, and hypnosis should be used by the patient to minimize unnecessary reliance on medications.

COPD: Chronic obstructive pulmonary disease; TCAs: tricyclic antidepressants; SSRIs: selective serotonin re-uptake inhibitors; SNRIs: serotonin-norepinephrine reuptake inhibitors; NSAIDs: non-steroidal anti-inflammatory drugs; TENS: trans-cutaneous electrical nerve stimulation.

Algorithm for medication selection in chronic pain with and without co-morbid depression

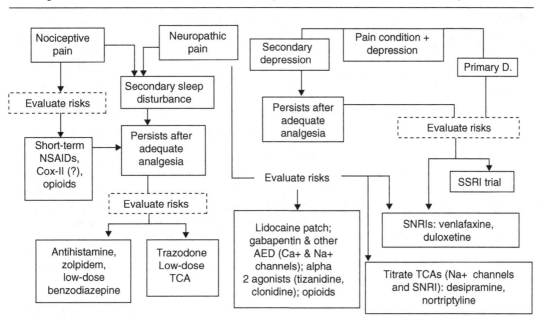

Figure 9.3 Evidence-based algorithm for pain pharmacotherapy.
Adapted from Gallagher RM, Verma S. *Semin Clin Neurosurgery* 2004. This information concerns uses that have not been approved by the US FDA.

[36], although clinical experience indicates that psychiatric co-morbidity, particularly sensitized states such as post-traumatic stress disorder, appears to be associated with such tolerance. Preliminary evidence suggests several promising methods for preventing opioid tolerance such as the co-administration of the N-methyl-D-aspartate (NMDA) antagonist ketamine [36]. To reduce the risks of misuse and diversion, all patients prescribed regular opioids for pain should be asked basic substance abuse questions to identify the potential for activating pre-morbid addiction or worsening existing addiction disorder [37]; when risks or aberrant behavior become apparent, structured risk management programs should be applied [11, 38, 39].

In terminally ill patients, pain management's highest priority is to maintain quality of life. Treatment aims to not only reduce pain and suffering, but importantly to improve function, such as enabling quality time with family and friends, and time to organize business and personal affairs. In these cases, it is important to continuously reassess the risk-to-benefit ratio of medications, in an attempt to control pain while minimizing undesirable physiological, cognitive, emotional, and behavioral effects.

In persistent, non-terminal pain, the safety of medications when two or more are used together, or

when there is co-morbid illness (e.g., diabetes, heart disease, cancer, rheumatoid arthritis) should be evaluated, especially in older patients. A key example in this area of risk assessment is cardiac toxicity, such as heart block, orthostatic hypotension leading to falls, and urinary retention associated with TCAs. In addition, the pharmacokinetics and metabolism of many drugs are altered in the elderly and those taking certain anti-depressants and anti-convulsants, leading to toxicity or altered effectiveness. For example, 5–10% of Caucasians are poor metabolizers via the cytochrome P450 enzyme 2D6 system, which is inhibited by SSRIs such as paroxetine and fluoxetine, lowering the rate of methadone metabolism and inadvertent overdose [41, 42].

Figure 9.3 presents a general evidence-based algorithm for considering medications appropriate for nociceptive and neuropathic pain with and without sleep disturbance and depression, which are commonly co-morbid with chronic pain – with the caveat that medical therapy should be but one component of a comprehensive, multidimensional treatment approach. Optimally, pain treatment should be embedded in a trusting doctor–patient relationship that involves the patient in reporting outcomes such as pain relief, mood, sleep, and physical, social, and occupational functioning

Table 9.3 Prioritized goal-oriented management plan: case no. 1

Problem list	Goal	Plan
A. Immediate problems		
1) Poor pain control	Obtain pain control to enable him to stay at work for the immediate future	1. Trial of tramadol 50 mg three times per day and 100 mg at bedtime as tolerated 2. Back up by Percocet 1–2 tabs as needed (up to 4 daily) 3. Naprosyn 500 mg three times per day on regular basis for 10 days, then twice per day 4. Call in one week, and return to clinic in 2 weeks
	Establish pain pattern	Pain diary
2) Sleep disturbance	Provide sleep relief	1. Improve pain control. 2. Evaluate effects of analgesics and gabapentin (see below) 3. Evaluate effects of tizanedine (see below)
3) Fear and job insecurity	Control symptoms	1. Improve pain control 2. Improve sleep 3. Advise about helpful websites and provide informative literature
	Establish work parameters – ergonomics	1. Explore realistically his vacation, sick leave, and disability options
B. Pivotal problems		
1) Neuropathic pain	1) Establish neuropathic pain medication program	1. Titrate gabapentin (starting at 300 mg at bedtime and increasing to 600 mg three times per daily as tolerated to start) or pregabalin (starting at 50 mg twice per day and increasing to 150 mg twice per day as tolerated to start) 2. Consider starting with duloxetine or venlafaxine, particularly if mood symptoms prominent
2) Myofascial pain and muscle spasms.	1) Reduce muscle spasm	1. Tizanedine 2 mg at bedtime for 5 days, then 4 mg at bedtime. Evaluate for sleep effect.
	2) Improve flexibility	1. Train in ice and stretch routine 2. Consider trigger point therapy followed by physical therapy
3) Mood disorder and poor coping	1) Improve mood and coping	1. Consider anti-depressants if persists after good pain control. 2. Pain coping skills training, in group.
4) Nociceptive, facet arthritis	1) Reduce biomechanical strain	1. Learn ergonomics at home and work 2. Weight loss
C. Background problems		
1) Weight management	Establish weight control program	1. Diet 2. Light exercise program
2) Marital stress	Inform and involve wife	1. Meeting with patient and wife to obtain her input and participation in management plan
3) Deconditioning, poor ergonomics, and poor pacing	Improve muscle strength, flexibility Learn ergonomics and pacing at work	1. Exercise program and PT if necessary 2. Pacing skills – rest flat on back at lunch, rise and stretch every 30 minutes 3. Review desk chair

Table 9.4 Indications for polypharmacy

1. To minimize treatment intolerance to a medication by utilizing a second drug which enables a lower dose of the first agent (this may increase adherence).
2. To create analgesic efficacy for different parts of the day by giving immediate-release medications combined with long-acting agents (e.g., to control breakthrough pain in a patient on long-acting opioids when certain unavoidable tasks, which predictably activate nociception, must be completed at work; or when a stumble or fall activates nociception). Rather than relying on a short-acting opioid for every contingency, clinicians should help patients also use NSAIDs, acetomenophen and physical measures such as icing and stretching can be useful taken periodically for flare-up due to minor re-injury. This strategy, as well as avoidance of predictable risks, will reduce the tendency to develop tolerance to opioid analgesia and possible hyperalgesia when a patient regularly adds short-acting opioids to long-acting opioids.
3. To utilize a lower dose of a drug by utilizing a second medication for purposes other than reduction of side effects (e.g., opioid-sparing, as in using an NSAID for osteoarthritic low back pain)
4. To utilize a second drug in order to facilitate synergy (the combination of the two medications given together has greater efficacy than the mathematically combined efficacy of the two agents given individually) (e.g., when treating spinal stenosis with NSAIDs, adding gabapentin for the neuropathic component)
5. To address non-response or partial response to monotherapy by utilizing a second drug to increase the efficacy of treatment either by administering two medications for the same indication but with different mechanisms of action (e.g, a tricyclic [sodium channel blocker and SNRI] at bedtime to help structure sleep and treat neuropathic pain from radiculopathy, while also using gabapentin or pregabalin for the neuropathic pain of radiculopathy) or by utilizing an augmentation strategy (e.g., addition of a pharmacological agent not considered to have analgesic properties but which may boost or enhance the effect of analgesic or, as another example, to add an NMDA receptor antagonist to an opioid to boost efficacy or decrease tolerance)

NSAIDs: non-steroidal anti-inflammatory drugs; SNRI: serotonin-norepinephrine reuptake inhibitor; NMDA: N-methyl-D-aspartate.

and in which the physician is available to treat flare-ups and respond to medication problems. This relationship is best achieved when a goal-oriented management plan is negotiated between doctor and patient (see case example 1, Table 9.3). Together, the doctor and patient should establish that pain control is a shared value. The physician can help control negative emotions and maladaptive illness behaviors with cognitive reframing, treatment agreements, and medications. When seeing a patient for the first time, factors to be evaluated include the patient's symptom patterns, coping skills, and psychosocial context. Then, precipitating factors are noted (including biological, such as an injury; psychological, such as hurried behavior at work; or social/cultural, such as an increased work load). Predisposing background factors (such as diseases, disorders, and coping styles), and current factors that may be perpetuating the pain (such as untreated depression, joblessness, or neurological sensitization) are also important to recognize. Effective pain treatment requires not only a comprehensive understanding of available therapies, pain mechanisms, and the complex neuropsychology of co-morbidities, but the ability to generate a unique treatment plan for each patient, because each patient is very different from the next. In this context, to help manage

the regulatory requirements of opioid prescribing, an opioid treatment agreement should always be created in patients taking regular, daily opioids for more than 90 days [5, 10, 37]. A model treatment agreement can be found on the website of the American Academy of Pain Medicine (www.painmed.org). As part of this agreement, to establish and protect the integrity of the provider–patient relationship and to avoid the appearance of biased treatment of patients by "profiling" since stereotypes rather than data often drive opioid prescribing [43], all patients should undergo periodic urine testing for controlled substances.

Case example 1: A 45-year-old man presents with low back pain with radiation into the buttocks and down his right leg to the outside of his foot, which started when he was downhill skiing 6 months ago. He was started on ibuprofen by his doctor and told to rest for 3–4 days, which helped and he returned to his office job at a bank. However, sitting more than 2 hours caused pain to flare, such that often he couldn't concentrate well, and he had trouble sitting through meetings. He was sent for a series of three epidural injections, which helped his leg pain for about 2 weeks each, and the pain returned. Oxycodone 5 mg with acetomenophen 325 mg has been prescribed and he now takes two tablets twice daily – mid-afternoon and bedtime – to get through the day at work and to get to sleep. He has suffered no bowel or bladder symptoms, no fever or persistent pain when lying down, no muscle weakness

Table 9.5 Clinical strategies and tactics in the pharmacotherapy of chronic pain

1. *Identify pain pattern and pain diagnosis and formulate mechanisms.* A database should include a complete medical and pain history, selective physical, mental status and laboratory examinations, response to other treatment trials, and a baseline record of pain levels (using a daily pain diary for at least one week).

2. *Inquire about patient's and significant others' knowledge, beliefs and attitudes about medication.* Family, social and cultural values may strongly influence a patient's adherence to medication trials and response to side effects. When necessary and appropriate, meet with significant others to establish rapport and common goals.

3. *Develop a goal-oriented management plan for each problem.* Specify time-limited target outcome measures such as pain relief, improved sleep, less social irritability, and improved function at home and work.

4. *Select medication carefully.* Choose medication according to diagnosis, efficacy, tolerability, ease of use, and cost (if this applies). Consider the mechanism of pain (e.g., nociceptive, neuropathic), mechanisms perpetuating pain (e.g., deconditioning, sleep disturbance, depressive illness, poor compliance with treatment), medical problems (co-morbid illness or psychiatric disturbance) and psychosocial factors that might influence treatment.

5. *Plan medication trials carefully with patient.* Establish outcome measures with patient. Be sure adequate trials are achieved. If patient consistently achieves at least a 2 point or greater reduction in pain intensity on a 0–10 (eleven point) scale, remain on the lowest dose that achieves that effect and is also tolerable; then add another medication that addresses a different mechanism (add a sodium channel blocker to a calcium channel blocker; add an SNRI or tricyclic to an anti-convulsant; add an opioid to any; add an NSAID for PRN flares).

6. *When titrating medication, closely follow patients at least every 2 weeks until stable, occasionally with contact several times weekly, to establish optimal dosing and to maximize adherence.* This behavioral approach facilitates the completion of an adequate medication trial, much like a protocol in a clinical trial study of a drug. Patient's concerns – such as about side effects, inadequate response, and stigma – can be managed more effectively.

7. *Consider alternate management strategies for pain fluctuations.* Often, physical therapy interventions (e.g., icing, TENS, stretching, exercise), behavioral techniques (e.g., avoidance of nociceptive activity, relaxation training, pacing, cognitive restructuring, stress management) and trigger point therapies (e.g., spray and stretch with ethyl chloride or injections) can control pain without the need for additional medications. For psychological symptoms, reassurance, brief support and cognitive-behavioral techniques may be sufficient to restore a patient's sense of control and comfort, without the need for a full therapeutic trial of psychotropic medication.

8. *If a drug trial fails to help, or if the physician or patient is uncertain if it is helping, gradually reduce the dose (while keeping other medications stable) and closely monitor the response, before initiating a trial with another medication.* If a patient stops a medication suddenly, this may precipitate a withdrawal syndrome, including seizures in the case of anti-convulsants or short-acting benzodiazepines, and worsening of pain through activation of the sympathetic system. The physician should counsel the patient to discuss concerns and ideas about medication before making a change.

or loss, and no other sensory symptoms. He has stopped playing tennis (hurts to serve) and taking regular walks and has gained 20 pounds. He started smoking again after abstaining for 5 years. His sleep is interrupted by pain after about 4–5 hours, and he has difficulty returning to sleep. His mood is depressed almost every day although he has no suicidal ideation. His sex drive is diminished. He has tried taking days off from work, and often leaves work early – but in an economic downturn, he is getting behind and is worried about his job. On examination he has positive sciatic signs on the right side with sitting leg extension and straight leg raising, but no loss of sensation, motor strength or reflexes. His range of motion is limited by pain in his low back and his low back paraspinal muscles are tight. MRI completed prior to epidural injections showed a partially herniated disk at L5-S1 on the right without foraminal encroachment.

The efficacy and side effects of a particular drug should be evaluated in the context of every clinical encounter with the individual patient. For example, an overweight patient with radicular low back pain or diabetic neuropathy should not be prescribed amitriptyline. Although amitriptylene is effective in some neuropathic pain diseases, it often causes weight gain; thus in the case of low back pain causing further biomechanical strain on spinal structures and in the case of diabetes, complicating management. Gabapentin, pregabalin, and other anticonvulsants (topiramate, oxycarbazine, lamotrigene, etc.) and SNRI antidepressants (e.g., duloxetine and venlafaxine) may be preferred, as well as lidocaine patches which have no systemic effects. Neuropsychologic functions such as learning, memory, and psychomotor performance, which are critical to improving functional outcomes in rehabilitation, can be interfered with by benzodiazepines, which also disinhibit anger, a frequent co-morbidity of disabled workers for example. An outline of the rationale for polypharmacy is presented in Table 9.4 [20].

When combining analgesics, it is reasonable to combine medications with pharmacological activity at different receptor sites in the pain pathway (e.g., combined use of a centrally acting opioid, a TCA or SNRI, an anti-convulsant, and a peripherally acting NSAID) [19, 34]. If treatment with a specific medication fails, it is often useful to consider a trial with an alternate drug in the same therapeutic class but with a different purported mechanism of action (e.g., when using an anti-convulsant, switch from a calcium channel blocker (gabapentin, pregabalin) to a sodium channel blocker (e.g., topiramate); or when using an anti-depressant switch from a selective serotonin reuptake inhibitor (SSRI – paroxetine, fluoxetine, sertraline, citalopram) to a serotonin norepinephrine reuptake inhibitor (SNRI – duloxetine or venlafaxine) or dopamine-norepinephrine reuptake inhibitor (bupropion). Common reasons for pharmacotherapy failure are underdosing (e.g., a drug trial that is too short or at a dose that is too low), non-adherence, or inadequate use of rational polypharmacy. When patients report that pain is unrelieved or increased, do not reflexively increase the dose before considering other factors potentially contributing to inadequate response, such as drug interactions, side effects, toxicity, behavioral effects, increased activity level, disease progression, or non-disease factors (e.g., a change in activity or stress). Often patients improve enough to resume activities that activate damaged tissues exacerbating either or both neuropathic and musculoskeletal pain. Some useful clinical strategies to optimize pharmacotherapy incorporate the biopsychosocial approach to treatment and are detailed in Table 9.5.

Conclusion

Pain management must be timely and aggressive to prevent the inevitably negative consequences of poorly managed pain on physical, psychosocial and occupational functioning. Rational use of mechanism-based pharmacology will rely on a focused evaluation of peripheral pain generators, of peripheral and central perpetuating factors, and of co-morbidities that may affect outcomes. Rapid and effective therapy can stop the downward spiral to central nervous system pathophysiology (maldynia) and impairments in functioning and physical and psychosocial losses that require a

much larger expenditure of clinical and social resources to remediate effectively. Pain management, the easing of suffering, can be skillfully and effectively applied in all settings. The rewards of every life restored are truly wonderful for the patient and hugely satisfying for the provider who skillfully commits to this task in every patient encounter.

If I can stop one heart from breaking
I shall not live in vain;
If I can ease one life the aching
And cool one pain
And help one fainting robin
Unto its nest again,
I shall not live in vain.

Emily Dickinson

References

1. Gallagher RM, Verma S. Mood and anxiety disorders in chronic pain. In *Psychosocial and Psychiatric Aspects of Pain: A Handbook for Health Care Providers*, eds. R Dworkin and W Brieghtbart. Progress in Pain Research and Management, Vol. 27. (Seattle: IASP Press, 2004).

2. Dohrenwend B, Marbach J, Raphael K, Gallagher RM. Why is depression co-morbid with chronic facial pain? A family study test of alternative hypotheses. *Pain* 1999; **83**: 183–92.

3. Fishbain D, Bruns D, Disorbio M, Lewis J. Risk for five forms of suicidality in acute pain patients and chronic pain patients vs. pain-free community controls. *Pain Med* 2009; **10**: 1095–105.

4. Fishbain D, Bruns D, Disorbio M, Lewis J. Correlates of self-reported violent ideation against physicians in acute- and chronic-pain patients. *Pain Med* 2009; **10**: 573–85.

5. Gallagher R. Opioids in chronic pain management: Navigating the clinical and regulatory challenges. *J Fam Prac* 2004; **53**: S23–32.

6. Goldenbaum DM, Christopher M, Gallagher RM, *et al*. Physicians charged with opioid analgesic-prescribing offenses. *Pain Med* 2008; **9**: 737–47.

7. Fishman SM, Papazian JS, Gonzalez S, Riches PS, Gilson A. Regulating opioid prescribing through prescription monitoring programs: Balancing drug diversion and treatment of pain. *Pain Med* 2004; **5**: 309–24.

8. Fishman SM. Opioid-based multimodal care of patients with chronic pain: Improving effectiveness and mitigating risks. *Pain Med* 2009; **10**: S49–52.

9. Wilsey BL, Fishman SM, Casamalhuapa C, Gupta A. Documenting and improving opioid treatment: The

prescription opioid documentation and surveillance (PODS) System. *Pain Med* 2009; **10**: 866–77.

10. Fishman SM, Mahajan G, Jung SW, Wilsey BL. The trilateral opioid contract. Bridging the pain clinic and the primary care physician through the opioid contract. *J Pain Symptom Manage* 2002; **24**: 335–44.

11. Wiedemer N, Harden P, Arndt R, Gallagher R. Effects of a structured opioid therapy program, using treatment agreements, urine drug screens, and consultation, on primary care practice. *Pain Med* 2007; **8**: 573–84.

12. Banja J. Empathy in the physician's pain practice: benefits, barriers and recommendations. *Pain Med* 2006; **7**: 265–75.

13. Gallagher RM. Empathy: A timeless skill for the pain medicine toolbox. *Pain Med* **7**: 213–14.

14. Gallagher RM. Pain medicine and primary care: A community solution to pain as a public health problem. *Med Clin North Amer* 1999; **83**: 555–85.

15. Fishman S, Gallagher RM, Carr D, Sullivan L. The case for pain medicine as a medical specialty. *Pain Med* 2004; **5**: 281–6.

16. Gallagher RM, Fishman S. Pain medicine: history, emergence as a medical specialty, and evolution of the multidisciplinary approach. In *Cousins and Bridenbaugh's Neural Blockade*, 4th edn, eds. MJ Cousins, PO Bridenbaugh, D Carr and T Horlocker. (Baltimore: Lippincott, Williams and Wilkins, 2008).

17. Follett K, Dubois MY. Program requirements for GME in pain medicine released for the first time. *Pain Med* 2008; **9**: 471–2.

18. Backonja MM, Irving G, Argoff C. Rational multidrug therapy in the treatment of neuropathic pain. *Curr Pain Headache Rep* 2006; **10**: 34–8.

19. Gallagher RM. Management of neuropathic pain: Translating mechanistic advances and evidence-based research into clinical practice. *Clin J Pain* 2006; **22**(S1): S2–S8.

20. Gallagher RM. Rational integration of pharmacologic, behavioral, and rehabilitation strategies in the treatment of chronic pain. *Am J Phys Med Rehabil* 2005;**84 (S3)**: S64–76.

21. Costigan M, Woolf CJ. Pain: Molecular mechanisms. *J Pain* 2000; **1**(3 Suppl): 35–44.

22. Woolf CJ. Dissecting out mechanisms responsible for peripheral neuropathic pain: Implications for diagnosis and therapy. *Life Sci* 2004; **74:** 2605–10.

23. Farrar JT, Young JP Jr, LaMoreaux L, Werth JL, Poole RM. Clinical importance of changes in chronic pain intensity measured on an 11-point numerical pain rating scale. *Pain* 2001; **94**: 149–58.

24. Tirado CF, Gallagher RM. The diagnosis and treatment of anxiety disorders in chronic spinal pain. In *Interventional Spine: An algorithmic approach,* eds. CW Slipman, R Derby, FA Simeone, TG Mayer. (Philadelphia: Saunders, 2007), pp. 171–183.

25. Armon C, Argoff CE, Samuels J, Backonja M. Assessment: Use of epidural steroid injections to treat radicular lumbosacral pain. *Neurology* 2007; **68**: 723–9.

26. Krames E. Interventional pain medicine. *Med Clin North Amer* 1999; **83**: 555–85.

27. Gallagher RM, Rosenthal L. Chronic pain and opiates: Balancing pain control and risks in long-term opioid treatment. *Arch Phys Med Rehabil* 2008; **89**(3 Suppl 1): S77–82.

28. Bloodworth D. Issues in opioid management. *Am J Phys Med Rehabil* 2005; **84**(3 Suppl): S42–55.

29. Eisenberg E, McNicol ED, Carr DB. Efficacy and safety of opioid agonists in the treatment of neuropathic pain of nonmalignant origin: Systematic review and meta-analysis of randomized controlled trials. *JAMA* 2005; **293**: 3043–52.

30. Martell BA, O ' Connor PG, Kerns RD, *et al.* Systematic review: Opioid treatment for chronic back pain: prevalence, efficacy, and association with addiction. *Ann Intern Med* 2007; **146**: 116–27.

31. Chou R, Fanciullo GJ, Fine PG, *et al.* Clinical guidelines for the use of chronic opioid therapy in chronic noncancer pain. *J Pain* 2009: **10**: 113–30.

32. Ballantyne JC, Mao J. Opioid therapy for chronic pain. *New Eng J Med* 2003; **349**: 1943–53.

33. Mao J. Opioid-induced abnormal pain sensitivity: Implications in clinical opioid therapy. *Pain* 2002; **100**: 213–17.

34. Simonnet G. Opioids: From analgesia to anti-hyperalgesia? *Pain* 2005; **118**: 8–9.

35. Vanderah TW, Ossipov MH, Lai J, Malan Jr TP, Porreca, F Mechanisms of opioid-induced pain and antinociceptive tolerance: Descending facilitation and spinal dynorphin. *Pain* 2001; **92**: 5–9

36. Celerier E, Rivat C, Jun Y, *et al.* Long-lasting hyperalgesia induced by fentanyl in rats: Preventative effect of ketamine. *Anesthesiology* 2000; **92**: 465–72.

37. Gourlay DL, Heit HA, Almahrezi A. Universal precautions in pain medicine: A rational approach to the treatment of chronic pain. *Pain Med* 2005; **6**: 107.

38. Passik SD, Kirsch KL, Casper D. Addiction-related assessment tools and pain management: Instruments for screening, treatment planning, and monitoring compliance. *Pain Med* 2008; **9**(S2): S145–S166.

39. Meghani S, Wiedemer N, Becker W, Gracely E, Gallagher RM. Predictors of resolution of aberrant drug behavior in chronic pain patients treated in a structured opioid risk management program. *Pain Med* 2009; **10**: 858–65.

40. Fishbain D. Polypharmacy treatment approaches to the psychiatric and somatic comorbidities found in patients with chronic pain. *Am J Phys Med Rehabil* 2005; **84**(3 Suppl): S56–63.

41. Ener J, Meglathery SB, Van Decker WA, Gallagher RM. Complications of serotonergic medications. *Pain Med* 2003; **4**: 63–74.

42. Fishman SM, Wilsey B, Mahajan G, Molina P. Methadone reincarnated: Novel clinical applications with related concerns. *Pain Med* 2002; **3**: 339–48.

43. Wilsey M, Fishman SM, Ogden C, Tsodikov A, Bertakis KD. Chronic pain management in the emergency department: A survey of attitudes and beliefs. *Pain Med* 2008; **9**: 1073–180.

44. Raphael KG, Marbach JJ. When did your pain start? Reliability of self-reported age of onset of facial pain. *Clin J Pain*; 1997; **13**: 352–9.

Chronic opioid therapy in pain management

Howard S. Smith and Charles E. Argoff

Introduction

Opioids are versatile and potent broad-spectrum analgesics, which continue to have a key place among pharmacologic agents available for the treatment of chronic pain.

Throughout many, many years of opioid use, the pendulum of the medical profession, society, and regulatory agencies has been swinging between opiophilia and opiophobia camps. Based on data from the US Drug Enforcement Agency (DEA) Automation of Reports and Consolidated Order System (ARCOS), which monitors opioid production and delivery to retail pharmacies, between 1997 and 2004 the amount of oxycodone, hydrocodone, and methadone delivered increased by 640%, 275%, and 903%, respectively [1].

There has been renewed interest in opioid prescribing in the USA, perhaps in part due to a growing number of tools/instruments to help clinicians with "screening"/decisions/documentation related to opioid therapy. The Opioid Management Society (OMS), which is dedicated to the proper and adequate use of opioids for the control of all types of pain, was started during the past decade as well as their Opioid Education Program and the *Journal of Opioid Management*. Through research, education, and dissemination of leading edge information, OMS hopes to enhance the medical profession's knowledge on how to better utilize this important class of drugs. Just in 2007/2008, at least eight mini-books or major texts were published, with new editions being devoted in large part to opioids/opioid related issues [2–9].

Appropriate use of these drugs requires skills in opioid prescribing, knowledge of the principles of addiction medicine, and a commitment to performing and documenting a comprehensive assessment repeatedly over time. Inadequate assessment can lead to undertreatment, compromise the effectiveness of therapy when implemented, and prevent an appropriate response when problematic drug-related behaviors occur [10–12].

Practicing in the "middle of the road" by employing the appropriate use of opioids in the context of good medical practice, as well as focusing appropriate attention on the risk assessment and management of opioid abuse (being cognizant of potential abuse, addiction, and diversion), has become known as "balance" [13–15].

It is essential that opioids not be just "thrown at" pain problems as sole therapy but rather be utilized in an appropriate and thoughtful manner. After completing a patient's history and physical examination, the clinician should diligently pursue a discrete etiology for the pain and attempt to target a specific treatment to "match" the pathophysiologic mechanisms [16].

Mechanisms of opioid analgesia

Exogenous opioids act by activating the body's endogenous opioid receptors in the pain-modulating systems, which may dampen nociceptive input.

Opioids largely work by binding to one of three major opioid receptors (mu, kappa, delta). Almost all clinically useful opioid analgesics are mu opioid receptor (MOR) agonists. Opioid agonists produce effects by binding to membrane-bound opioid receptors and initiating activation of G protein-coupled receptors (GPCRs) [16].

Opioids may provide analgesia via peripheral, spinal, and/or supraspinal mechanisms. Furthermore, opioids targeted to or administered in the periphery [17], subarachnoid space [18], or supraspinal areas may produce analgesia.

Behavioral and Psychopharmacologic Pain Management, ed. Michael H. Ebert and Robert D. Kerns. Published by Cambridge University Press. © Cambridge University Press 2011.

Terminology related to opioid therapy

Narcotic

A term historically used to describe opium and its derivatives. The word derives from a Greek word meaning "benumbing." In modern society, the word *narcotic* has become a legal term that includes a wide range of sedating and potentially abused substances; it is no longer limited to opioid analgesics.

This term maintains an extremely negative connotation and should be avoided by clinicians in discussing opioid therapy with patients and other clinicians.

Opiate

A term used to describe substances derived from opium. The term *opiate* is often incorrectly used interchangeably with *opioid*.

Opioid

An opium-like substance. In the past, *opioid* was used to describe endogenous opium-like substances, and the term *opiate* described drugs derived from opium. Today *opioid* is the preferred term in both clinical and scientific dialogue for describing this class of analgesic medications.

Aberrant drug-related behaviors

Any behaviors that suggest the presence of substance abuse or addiction [19].

Pseudoaddiction

Behaviors resulting from inadequate analgesia that are erroneously thought to be due to inappropriate drug-seeking behavior [20].

Pseudotolerance

A situation in which opioid dose escalation occurs and appears consistent with pharmacological tolerance but, after a thoughtful evaluation, is better explained by a variety of other variables [21]. These may include increased analgesic requirements due to progressive disease, presence of new pathology, or increased or excessive physical activity. Patients may also become non-compliant, have drug interactions, or even divert medications in a manner that incorrectly produces the appearance of tolerance.

In 1999, the American Society of Addiction Medicine (ASAM), the American Academy of Pain Medicine (AAPM), and the American Pain Society (APS) formed the Liaison Committee on Pain and Addiction (LCPA), which developed a set of definitions for common addiction-related terms [22]. A symposium panel of experts [23] used those definitions, and also relevant published studies and their own findings, to define terms commonly used in addiction research (See Table 10.1).

Opioids in the pharmacologic treatment of pain

An "analgesic ladder" approach to the selection of analgesic drugs for cancer pain has been popularized by the World Health Organization and is now widely accepted as a broad guideline and educational tool [24]. No such universally accepted and validated simplistic guideline or stepwise algorithm exists for persistent non-cancer pain; however, similar principles of therapy exist, including initiating treatment conservatively with progressive titration of doses and the addition of more aggressive strategies in the face of a lack of responsiveness.

According to the analgesic ladder, selection of an analgesic should be guided by the usual severity of pain: patients with mild to moderate pain usually are first treated with acetaminophen or a non-steroidal anti-inflammatory drug (NSAID) with or without one or more adjuvant drugs. These adjuvants include drugs selected to treat a side effect of the analgesic (e.g., laxatives) and drugs with analgesic effects (the so-called adjuvant analgesics) [25].

Patients with moderate to severe pain (including those with insufficient relief after a trial of acetaminophen or an NSAID), are treated with an opioid conventionally used for moderate pain (See Table 10.2). This opioid usually is combined with or without acetaminophen or an NSAID and with or without an adjuvant drug [25].

Patients with severe pain (including those who fail to achieve adequate relief after appropriate administration of drugs on the second rung of the analgesic ladder) receive an opioid conventionally selected for severe pain (See Table 10.3). This treatment may also be combined with acetaminophen, an NSAID, or an adjuvant drug.

There is no opioid ceiling dose during this process of dose finding. The absolute dose is immaterial as long as side effects do not supervene. Occasionally patients require opioid doses equivalent to many grams of morphine per day.

Table 10.1 Definitions of the medical terms associated with opioid use

Term	Definition
Misuse	Use of a medication (for a medical purpose) other than as directed or as indicated, whether harm results or not
Abuse	Any use of an illegal drug The intentional self-administration of a medication for a non-medical purpose such as altering one's state of consciousness, e.g., getting high *Note that licit substances, e.g., alcohol, can also be abused*
Physical dependence[a]	The state of adaptation that is manifested by a drug class specific withdrawal syndrome that can be produced by abrupt cessation, rapid dose reduction, decreasing blood level of the drug, and administration of an antagonist
Tolerance[a]	The state of adaptation in which exposure to a given dose of a drug induces biologic changes that result in diminution of one or more of the drug's effects over time. Alternatively, escalating doses of a drug are required over time to maintain a given level of effect
Addiction[a]	A primary, chronic, neurobiologic disease, with genetic, psychosocial, and environmental factors influencing its development and manifestations Behavioral characteristics include one or more of the following: - Impaired control over drug use - Compulsive use - Continued use despite harm - Craving
Iatrogenic[b]	Denoting response to medical or surgical treatment induced by treatment itself; usually used for unfavorable responses
Pseudoaddiction	Syndrome of abnormal behavior resulting from undertreatment of pain that is misidentified by the clinician as inappropriate drug-seeking behavior Behavior ceases when adequate pain relief is provided Not a diagnosis; rather, a description of a clinical interaction
Diversion	The intentional removal of medication from legitimate distribution and dispensing

[a] AAPM, APS, ASAM, 2001; [b] Stedman's Medical Dictionary.
Source. Ref. [23].

Table 10.2 Pharmacokinetic data – WHO Step 2 analgesic agents

Oral agents	Bioavailability	Half-life (h)	Onset (min)	Peak effect (min)	Duration (h)
Codeine	40% (12% to 84%)	2.5 to 3.5	30 to 60	45 to 60	4 to 6
Dihydrocodeine	20%	3 to 4	30	45 to 60	3 to 4
Tramadol	75%	6	30 to 80	4 to 6	
Hydrocodone	39%	3.8 (2 to 4.5)	20 to 30	1.3 (1 to 2)	3 to 6

Source. Ref. [25].

In most cases, opioid titration identifies a dose that yields a favorable balance between analgesia and side effects, and the opioid requirement remains stable for a prolonged period; however, on occasion, analgesic tolerance is experienced.

When pain increases during long-term therapy, the development of tolerance should not be assumed. Rather, recurrent pain should signal the need to re-evaluate the nature of the pain. Dose titration should start again and should continue until the favorable balance between analgesia and side effects is regained or the therapy is determined to be ineffective because of treatment limiting toxicity [26].

Table 10.3 Pharmacokinetic data – WHO Step 3 opioids

Oral agents	Bioavailability	Half-life (h)	Onset (min)	Peak effect (min)	Duration (h)
Morphine sulfate IR	25% to 35% (15% to 64%)	2 to 3	20 to 30	60 to 90	3 to 6
Oxycodone IR	75% (60 to 87%)	2 to 3.5	20 to 30	60 to 120	3 to 6
Hydromorphone IR	37% to 62%	2.5 (2 to 3)	30	1 to 2	3 to 6
Oxymorphone IR	10%	7.3 to 9.4	15 to 23	45 to 60	4 to 6
Methadone	80%	12 to 150	30 to 90	2 to 4	Analgesia: 6 to 8; for suppressing opioid withdrawal: 24 to 48
Levorphanol	Uncertain	11 to 16 chronic dosing (up to 30)	20 to 60	1 to 2	6 to 8

SS: steady state; IR: immediate release/short-acting.
Source. Ref. [25].

Opioid-induced adverse effects

Common opioid side effects may include constipation, nausea and vomiting, sedation, and pruritus. Other adverse effects may include cognitive disturbances, perceptual distortions, delirium, myoclonus, urinary retention, headache and/or dizziness, fatigue, anorexia, dry mouth, sweating, decreased sexual desire (libido), abdominal discomfort/cramping/bloating, and infrequent respiratory depression. Opioid toxicity will be different between individuals. Individuals do not develop every potential adverse effect/toxicity and differ greatly as to the magnitude of various effects and how much distress is experienced. In general, tolerance develops to most side effects. There remains a dearth of high-quality evidence for the treatment of opioid side effects in populations both with and without cancer pain [27].

Opioid rotation

With gradual escalation of the opioid dose in most patients, a favorable balance between analgesia and side effects can be achieved. However, some patients experience intolerable side effects before adequate analgesia is reached or, more rarely, do not benefit at all. Although multiple strategies can be employed in this situation one direct approach is to change to another opioid in an attempt to allow titration to adequate pain control while limiting side effects.

The practice of changing from one opioid to another, referred to as *opioid rotation*, is most commonly undertaken when adequate analgesia is limited by the occurrence of problematic side effects. The principle of rotation is based on the observation that a patient's response can vary from opioid to opioid, both for analgesia and adverse effects. Importantly, an inadequate response or the occurrence of intolerable side effects with one opioid does not necessarily predict a similar response to another.

Mercandante and Bruera found that opioid rotation results in clinical improvement in at least 50% of patients with chronic pain presenting with a poor response to a particular opioid [28], but a Cochrane review revealed that there are no randomized controls for opioid rotation [29]. The evidence to support the practice is largely anecdotal or based on uncontrolled studies, but switching appears to be a useful maneuver.

The most common aims of opioid rotation are to improve pain control, reduce toxicity, or both. Other indications for opioid rotation include patient convenience, convenience of route, wish for a reduction in invasiveness, and cost [30].

Dose conversion

Conversion doses should be based on an equianalgesic table that provides values for the relative potencies

Table 10.4 Opioid equianalgesic conversions

Name	Equianalgesic dose		Comments	Precautions and contraindications
	Oral	Parenteral		
Morphine	30 mg	10 mg	Standard of comparison for opioid analgesics	Clearance of parent drug and active metabolite is prolonged in patients with renal failure
Hydromorphone	4 to 6 mg	≈1.5mg	Exact dose equivalence unclear	
Hydrocodone	20 mg	N/A	1.5:2 hydrocodone:morphine dose equivalence	Available in USA combined with acetaminophen; maximum daily dose of acetaminophen is 4 g
Oxycodone	20 mg	≈5 to 10 mg[a]	1.5:2 oxycodone:morphine dose equivalence	Clearance is prolonged in patients with hepatic failure
Methadone[b]	10 to 20 mg (single dose) (may vary widely)	N/A	Long plasma half-life (24 to 36 hours), unique characteristics, considerable interindividual difference in pharmacokinetics, can not be titrated in the same manner as other opioids	Accumulates with repeated dosing, unpredictable pharmacology in individual patients; use with caution
Buprenorphine			Available in 3- and 7-day transdermal formulations[c] (see manufacturer's recommendations for morphine dose equivalence range)	
Oxymorphone[d]	10 mg	1 to 1.5 mg[a]	ER matrix slowly releases oxymorphone over 12 h	
Fentanyl	N/A	200 μg	Available in transdermal preparation (see manufacturer's recommendations for morphine dose equivalence range)	Considered reasonably safe in patients with renal impairment

ER: Extended release.

[a] Parenteral not available in USA.

[b] It is extremely important to monitor all patients closely when converting from methadone to other opioid agonists. The ratio between methadone and other opioid agonists may vary widely as a function of previous dose exposure. Methadone has a long half-life and tends to accumulate in the plasma.

[c] Transdermal not available in USA.

[d] The approximate equivalent doses in this conversion table are only to be used for the conversion from current opioid therapy to oxymorphone extended release (Opana ER). Sum the total daily dose for the opioid and use the approximate equivalent doses to calculate the oxymorphone total equianalgesic daily dose. For patients on a regimen of mixed opioids, calculate the approximate oral oxymorphone dose for each opioid and sum the totals to estimate the total daily equianalgesic oxymorphone dose. The dose of Opana ER can be gradually adjusted, preferably at increments of 10 mg every 12 hours every 3 to 7 days, until adequate pain relief and acceptable side effects have been achieved.

Source. Ref. [34].

among different opioids (See Table 10.4). However, several limitations of equianalgesic tables must be acknowledged. Most conversion tables are based on studies in which opioid-naïve individuals were given single low-dose opioids, without attention to side effects, organ failure, polypharmacy, complications, or the reason for rotation. These studies also failed to take into account the interindividual variations that play a prominent role in determining the real conversion for each individual. The variation in published conversion ratios is also a problem. Oxycodone, fentanyl, and methadone show the largest differences among the available conversion tables [31]. Small variations in conversion ratios can lead to large differences in calculated equianalgesic doses, especially at higher doses. For example, reported morphine to oxycodone ratios have ranged from 1:1 to 2:1.

Methadone deserves special consideration in dose conversion. It has many advantages, including low cost, good oral and rectal absorption, no active metabolites, low tolerance development, and long duration of effect. At the same time, however, its half-life is long and unpredictable, with large interindividual variations. This can result in delayed toxicity. Moreover, methadone has been linked to prolongation of the QTc [32]. The conversion dose varies depending on the dose of the original opioid used. At morphine equivalence of less than 90 mg, a conversion of 5:1 (morphine:methadone) is recommended. At morphine equivalence of 90 to 300 mg, a conversion of 6:1 is suggested. For doses of morphine over 300 mg, a rotation of 8:1 is recommended [33]. In some individuals, steady-state blood levels are not achieved for 4 days; therefore dose adjustments should be made every 4–5 days. Despite the many advantages of methadone, the variable conversion ratios and its unpredictable half-life make this a difficult medication to use unless the provider is experienced with it.

Key points for opioid rotation

- Utilize an opioid equianalgesic table that is appropriate/relevant for your practice, and use it consistently.
- In deciding on an alternative opioid, consider all patient factors (e.g., What is the best route of drug delivery in this patient? Which drug is most convenient for the patient/treating team? Is cost going to be an issue? Is the new drug available in the community?).
- In rotating opioids, consider all medical factors that may be relevant (e.g., renal function, liver function, age, co-morbidities), and adjust equianalgesic dose based on these factors.
- In rotating to an opioid other than methadone or fentanyl, decrease the equianalgesic dose by 25% to 50%.
- In rotating to methadone, reduce the dose by 75% to 90%.

- In rotating to transdermal fentanyl, maintain the equianalgesic dose.
- In rotating because of uncontrolled pain, consider a lesser dose reduction than usual.
- Ensure that appropriate rescue/breakthrough doses are available. Use 5–15% of the total daily opioid dose as a guide, and reassess and retitrate the new opioid.

Although the above recommendations encourage the utilization of an opioid equianalgesic conversion table, healthcare providers must keep in mind that there is significant variability among opioids and significant differences among patients. Clinicians need to "practice medicine" and "actively decide" the most appropriate opioid dose to start with, tailoring their decisions to specific individual patients, rather than simply "robotically" calculating an opioid dose and prescribing this amount without deciding whether any adjustments are needed. Subsequent close patient follow-up and careful opioid titration should ensue in attempts to achieve optimal analgesia with minimal adverse effects [34].

Opioid routes of administration

Transdermal route

The transdermal route offering a 48- to 72-hour dosing interval may be very useful for patients who are unable to swallow or absorb an orally administered opioid, as well as for those who perceive non-oral administration as a convenience.

Patients who are unable to swallow or absorb opioid drugs and who do not experience intolerable side effects from systemic administration may be ideal candidates for transdermal opioid administration.

Spinal opioids

Intraspinal drug infusions via implantable intrathecal drug delivery systems are the most commonly used option for long-term spinal administration of opioids for chronic pain. They may be used for the treatment of intractable, persistent pain that is unresponsive to less invasive approaches. Efforts to review the current literature, revise the algorithm for drug selection developed in 2000, and develop current guidelines (among other goals) led to the organization of the 2003 Polyanalgesic Consensus Conference, and later the 2007 Polyanalgesic Consensus Conference [35]. Opioids have been and continue to be a mainstay agent for intraspinal therapy. The guidelines developed at the Polyanalgesic Consensus Conference suggest that the first-line intraspinal agent should be an opioid alone (e.g., preservative-free, sterile morphine sulfate), switching from one agent to another (e.g., hydromorphone) or adding agents if the suggested "maximum" dose is reached (e.g., 15 mg/day of morphine) or if side effects occur or to use ziconotide [35].

With further evidence of favorable outcomes in the oncology population, the use of intraspinal infusion in the management of cancer pain is likely to increase. Smith *et al.* [36] conducted a controlled trial comparing neuraxial infusion and comprehensive medical management, and they found that the spinal opioid treatment improved pain, side effects, quality of life, and even survival. The long-term spinal administration of combinations of analgesic agents (e.g., opioid, local anesthetic, and clonidine) may be utilized "off label" for a wide variety of populations but has not been rigorously studied. Ziconotide, an N-type calcium channel blocker, has been shown to be effective for cancer pain in controlled trials [37], and has been added to the guidelines as a potential first-line agent [35].

Clinical opioid use for analgesia

Kalso and colleagues [38] reviewed data from 1145 patients initially randomized in 15 placebo-controlled trials of potent opioids used in the treatment of severe pain; these opioids were analyzed for efficacy and safety in chronic non-cancer pain. Four studies tested intravenous opioids in neuropathic pain in a crossover design, with 115 of 120 patients completing the protocols. Using either pain intensity difference or pain relief as the endpoint, all four studies reported average pain relief of 30–60% with opioids. Eleven studies (1025 patients) compared oral opioids with placebo for 4 days to 8 weeks. Six of the 15 trials that were included had an open-label follow-up of 6–24 months. The mean decrease in pain intensity in most studies was at least 30% with opioids and was comparable in neuropathic and musculoskeletal pain. Roughly 80% of patients noted at least one adverse effect. The most common adverse effects were constipation (41%), nausea (32%), and somnolence (29%). Only 44% of 388 patients on open-label treatments were still on opioids after therapy for between 7 and 24 months. Adverse effects and lack of efficacy were two common reasons for discontinuation.

Eisenberg and colleagues [39] examined 22 studies that met inclusion criteria and were classified as short term (less than 24 hours; $n = 14$) or intermediate term (median + 28 days; range 8–56 days; $n = 8$) trials. They reported contradictory results in the short-term trials. However, all eight intermediate-term trials demonstrated opioid efficacy for spontaneous neuropathic pain. A fixed-effects model meta-analysis of six intermediate-term trials showed mean post-treatment scores of pain intensity (on a visual analog scale) after opioids to be 14 units lower on a scale from 0 to 100 than after placebo (95% confidence interval [CI] −18 to −10; $p < 0.001$). As the mean initial pain intensity recorded from four of the intermediate-term trials ranged from 46 to 69, this 14-point difference was considered to correspond to a 20–30% greater reduction with opioids than with placebo.

When the number needed to harm (NNH) is considered, the most common adverse event was nausea (NNH, 3.6; 95% CI 2.9 to 4.8), followed by constipation (NNH, 4.6; 95% CI 3.4 to 7.1), drowsiness (NNH, 5.3; 95% CI 3.7 to 8.3), vomiting (NNH, 6.2; 95% CI 4.6 to 11), and dizziness (NNH, 6.7; 95% CI 4.8 to 10.0) [39]. Eisenberg and colleagues concluded that although short-term studies provide only equivocal evidence regarding the efficacy of opioids in reducing the intensity of neuropathic pain, intermediate-term studies demonstrate significant efficacy of opioids over placebo [39]. They also concluded that further randomized, controlled trials are needed in order to establish the long-term efficacy of opioids for neuropathic pain, the safety of long-term opioids (including addiction potential), and the effects of opioids on quality of life. Rowbotham *et al.* demonstrated a dose-dependent analgesic effect in patients with mixed neuropathies and reported that high-dose levorphanol yielded significantly more pain relief than did lower doses of this agent [40].

At the end of 2007, Dworkin *et al.* [41] updated their last published recommendations of the Neuropathic Pain Special Interest Group from 2003 [42].

In the 2003 recommendations opioids and tramadol were listed as first-line medications for the treatment of neuropathic pain; however, in the 2007 recommendations they have been "cut from the starting team," and relegated to second-line therapy (except in "select clinical circumstances"). Four such circumstances which the authors list include:

1. during titration of a first-line medication to an efficacious dosage for prompt pain relief;
2. episodic exacerbations of severe pain;
3. acute neuropathic pain; and

4. neuropathic cancer pain [41].

Dworkin and colleagues add that such "first-line" use of opioids should be reserved for circumstances in which "suitable alternatives cannot be identified and should be on a short-term basis to the extent possible" [42].

One special clinical scenario where opioids may be best reserved as a second or third line treatment option is multiple sclerosis associated central pain [43]. Some of the reasons given by Dworkin and colleagues for "axing opioids from the starting line-up of analgesics for neuropathic pain" include:

1. more frequent adverse effects than some first-line agents [44–46] (some of which may persist throughout long-term treatment) [47];
2. the long-term safety of opioid therapy has not been systematically studied [39, 48], and preliminary evidence that long-term opioid therapy may be associated with immunologic changes and hypogonadism [49–51];
3. experimental data which suggest that opioid treatment may be associated with opioid-induced hyperalgesia [52–55]; and
4. the potential for opioid analgesic misuse or addiction [41].

Chronic opioid therapy

When making the decision to prescribe opioids for this type of pain, the following factors concerning long-term opioid therapy (LTOT) should be kept in mind:

- LTOT may not be optimal for all patients.
- LTOT does not provide good or excellent analgesia in all patients.
- LTOT is not devoid of side effects.
- LTOT should be monitored in an effort to assess efficacy, side effects, and aberrant drug behavior.
- Initially, when first starting opioid therapy, it should be explained that this is a trial. After patient reassessment depending on the individual case, the clinician may decide on opioid titration, fine tuning of opioid dose perhaps with long-acting and/or short-acting agents, opioid rotation, consideration of other non-opioid analgesic strategies, or may choose an exit strategy to discontinue opioid therapy.
- LTOT can be successfully withdrawn in selected patients who may do better without opioids and

thus discussion of an "exit strategy" from opioid therapy is important, ideally prior to initiating opioid therapy.
- The prescription of LTOT for persistent non-cancer pain is an art that may be used alone or in conjunction with other therapeutic options. It is not typically used as a first-line agent for patients who have not tried previous treatments [56].

The pre-opioid prescribing period

The pre-opioid prescribing period is the period during which the physician determines whether opioids should be prescribed and, if the decision to prescribe such an agent is made, which necessary controls are put in place prior to initiating therapy [57]. Activities that surround the initiation phase (and in some cases the maintenance phase) include discussions with the patient and other relevant parties (e.g., the patient's family or other healthcare providers), assessments, and documentation.

The following are other specific activities which may be associated with this period:

- obtaining and documenting informed consent
- executing opioid "contracts"/treatment agreements
- executing goal-directed therapy agreements
- evaluating the potential for substance abuse with one or more of many available screening tools
- performing a urine drug test
- performing a psychological assessment (this may be an informal assessment by the provider)
- developing a sense of the doctor–patient relationship.

Goal-directed therapy agreements

Perhaps one of the most important principles in initiating and maintaining LTOT for persistent non-cancer pain is to "know where you are and where you are going." Goal-directed therapy agreements (GDTA) may be helpful in initiating LTOT for persistent non-cancer pain [58]. Clinicians are sometimes faced with patients for whom opioid therapy was initiated without clearly defined endpoints in efforts to achieve analgesia. This may cause a patient to continue experiencing severe pain despite taking relatively high doses of opioids. In efforts to clarify patient and clinician expectations and to make expected treatment outcomes more finite and concrete, the use of some form of GDTA may be useful.

As with opioid treatment agreements, a GDTA is not necessarily advocated for all patients or all practices; it is merely suggested in situations where the clinician deems such a measure appropriate.

Such agreements should be tailored to each individual patient, should be clear and concise, should set goals that can reasonably be attained by the patient over a finite period, and optimally should be agreed upon by both patient and clinician. Examples may include increasing daily ambulation by a defined amount, increasing social/recreational activities by a defined amount, and so on. By utilizing GDTAs before instituting opioid therapy, clinicians can establish defined criteria to be met in order for opioid therapy to continue. In this manner, patients may be expected to reach certain reasonably attainable functional goals (which may have to be documented by a physical and/or behavioral therapist) in order to continue opioid therapy. The specific defined "goals" should be clearly stated in the GDTA. It would seem optimal to institute the GDTA prior to instituting opioid therapy. The GDTA is essentially felt to be a "contractually" agreed upon, realistic target of translational analgesia [58] that should be realized in order maintain opioid treatment.

It is hoped that with the use of GDTAs in certain patients or circumstances, a closer match between the expectations of both patient and clinician can be established [58].

Opioid-therapy documentation

When opioids are used for long-term therapy, the clinician must be skilled in opioid prescribing, know the principles of addiction medicine, and be committed to performing and documenting a comprehensive assessment repeatedly over time. Inadequate assessment can lead to undertreatment, compromise the effectiveness of therapy, and prevent an appropriate response when problematic drug-related behaviors occur.

There are several domains of interest in patient assessment during LTOT for those engaged in frontline practice. These include pain relief (i.e., are the medications or treatments leading to pain reduction?), functional outcomes (i.e., is the patient more engaged in life as a result of treatment?), side effects (i.e., how have the medications adversely affected the patient?), and drug-related behaviors (i.e., is the patient acting out in unusual or disturbing ways?).

Ongoing assessment of these main domains not only improves pain outcomes for the patient but protects your practice for those patients on an opioid regimen. Passik and Weinreb [59] have described a useful mnemonic for following the relevant domains of outcome in pain management. The so-called "four A's" (analgesia, activities of daily living, adverse events, and aberrant drug-taking behaviors) are the clinical domains that reflect progress toward the larger goal of a full and rewarding life.

Analgesia

Although listed as the first "A," analgesia should not necessarily be considered the most important outcome of pain management. An alternate measure is how much relief it takes for patients to feel that their lives are meaningfully changed, enabling them to work toward the attainment of their own goals.

Activities of daily living

The second "A" refers to quality-of-life issues and functionality. It is necessary for patients to understand that they must comply with all of their treatment recommendations in order to be able to return to work, leisure, and social activities in the minimum amount of time.

Adverse events

Patients must also be made aware of the adverse side effects inherent in the use of opioids and other medications to treat pain. Side effects must be aggressively managed so that sedation and other side effects do not overshadow the potential benefits of drug therapy. The most common side effects of opioid analgesics are constipation, sedation, nausea and vomiting, dry mouth, respiratory depression, confusion, urinary retention, and itching.

Aberrant drug-taking behaviors

Finally, patients must be educated about the parameters of acceptable drug taking. Even an overall good outcome in every other domain might not constitute satisfactory treatment if the patient is exhibiting worrisome drug-related behaviors. Dispensing pain medicine in a highly structured fashion may become necessary for some patients who are in violation, or constantly on the fringes, of appropriate drug taking.

A consistent method of documentation can help busy clinicians to remember which of the domains should be assessed on any given visit. Moreover, oversight by regulatory agencies, state medical boards, and various peer-review groups includes examination of appropriate medical care as well as proper documentation.

As the old axiom states, "If it isn't written, it didn't happen." In cases of LTOT for chronic pain, issues beyond typical office-visit charting deserve attention and documentation. Although no explicit requirements are spelled out as to the documentation of issues related to opioid therapy, the use of specific tools and instruments in the chart on some or all visits may boost both adherence to documentation expectations and the consistency of such documentation.

Unidimensional tools such as the numerical rating scale (i.e., "On a scale of 0 to 10, how would you rate your pain?") described in Chapter 3 are useful for ongoing assessment of a patient's pain. However, analgesia is only one of the four domains of outcome for pain management, and clinicians must continually assess all four domains. It has been proposed that the use of various tools may provide adjunctive information and help clinicians to create a more complete picture regarding longitudinal trends of overall progress and functioning for their patients with chronic pain [60]. Assessing individual outcomes during outpatient multidisciplinary chronic pain treatment is often an extremely challenging task, but, fortunately, a number of tools are now available to facilitate the ongoing assessment of patients on LTOT.

The pain assessment and documentation tool

The pain assessment and documentation tool (PADT) is a simple charting device based on the four A's concept; it is designed to help clinicians focus on key outcomes and consistently document progress in pain management therapy over time [61, 62]. The PADT has several advantages in practice:

- It is a brief, two-sided chart note that can be readily included in the patient's medical record.
- It is intuitive, pragmatic, and adaptable to clinical situations.
- It takes between 5 and 10 minutes to complete in its revised version.
- It helps clinicians meet their obligations for ongoing assessment and documentation.
- Although not intended to replace a progress note, it can complement existing documentation with a

focused evaluation of outcomes that are clinically relevant, and it addresses the need for evidence of appropriate monitoring.

Numerical opioid side effect assessment tool

The numerical opioid side effect (NOSE) assessment tool was designed specifically for the quantification of adverse effects [63]. It is not uncommon for patients on LTOT to ask to discontinue therapy because of adverse effects, even if they have attained reasonable analgesia.

Therefore, it is useful to assess opioid adverse effects in such a manner as to be able to follow trends as well as compare the patient's perceived intensity of the adverse effects vs. the intensity of pain and/or other symptoms. The NOSE was designed in an effort to provide a tool that facilitates this goal. There are several benefits to the NOSE, including the following:

- It is self-administered and can be completed by the patient in minutes while waiting for an appointment.
- It is easy to interpret and provides clinicians with important information that could potentially affect therapeutic decisions.
- It can be entered into electronic databases or inserted into a hard-copy chart on each patient visit.
- It allows for legible, clear, and concise documentation of such information in outpatient records.

The translational analgesic score

The translational analgesic score (TAS) is a patient-generated tool that attempts to quantify the degree of translational analgesia [64], or improvements in physical, social, or emotional function realized by the patient as a result of improved analgesia [64]. Improvements may be subtle and can include a range of daily-function activities or other signs (e.g., going out more with friends, doing laundry, showing improved mood, enjoying more rewarding relationships with family members). The TAS is simple, rapid, user-friendly, and suitable for use in busy pain clinics. The patient can complete the tool at each visit while in the waiting room, and the responses are averaged for an overall score, which is recorded in the chart. Patients should be encouraged to write down specific examples

Table 10.5 The SAFE Evaluation Tool

Sample SAFE Form					
Criterion	**Rating**				
Social	**1**	**2**	**3**	**4**	**5**
Marital, family, friends, leisure, recreational	Supportive, harmonious, socializing, engaged				Conflictual, discordant, isolated, bored
Analgesia	1	2	3	4	5
Intensity, frequency, duration	Comfortable, effective, controlled				Intolerable, ineffective, uncontrolled
Function	1	2	3	4	5
Work, ADLs, home management, school, training, physical activity	Independent, active, productive, energetic				Dependent, unmotivated, passive
Emotional	1	2	3	4	5
Cognitive, stress, attitude, mood, behavior, neuro-vegetative signs	Clear, relaxed, optimistic, upbeat, composed				Confused, tense, pessimistic, depressed, distressed
Total score					

The patient's status in each of the four domains is rated as follows: 1 = excellent, 2 = good, 3 = fair, 4 = borderline, 5 = poor.
Source. Smith HS, Kirsh KL. Potential documentation tools in long-term opioid therapy. *In Opioid Therapy in the 21st Century*, ed. HS Smith. (New York: Oxford University Press, 2008), pp. 109–114.

of things that they can now do or do frequently that they could not do or did rarely when their pain was less controlled.

Alternatively, the patient's responses can be entered into a computerized record (with graphs of trends) if the pain clinic's medical records are electronic. At least one or two specific examples of translational analgesia should be documented on the bottom or reverse side of the TAS score sheet. Treatment decisions regarding escalation or tapering of opioids, changing agents, adding agents, obtaining consultations, and instituting physical or behavioral medicine techniques depend on the medical judgment of practitioners and should be based on a careful re-evaluation of the patient, not on numbers. The concept of translational analgesia is not meant to imply that opioids should be tapered, weaned, and/ or discontinued. If a patient has a very low TAS that remains essentially unchanged over time, the clinician should re-evaluate the patient and consider a change in therapy. This could mean pursuing various therapeutic options including, perhaps, increasing the dose of opioids. The TAS may be helpful as an adjunctive documentation tool and still awaits rigorous validation.

The SAFE score

The SAFE score is a score generated by the healthcare provider that provides a multidimensional assessment of the outcome of opioid therapy [65]. The goals of the SAFE score are to demonstrate that the clinician has routinely evaluated the efficacy of the treatment from multiple perspectives; to guide the clinician toward a broader view of treatment options beyond adjusting the medication regimen; and to provide adjunctive data in efforts to document the rationale for continuation, modification, or cessation of opioid therapy. It is a simple, practical tool that may have clinical utility, but it has not yet been rigorously validated. It is not intended to replace more elaborate patient-based assessment tools, but it may be useful as an adjunct to illuminate differences between patients' perceptions of how they are doing on opioid treatment vs. the physician's view of the outcome. At each visit, the clinician numerically rates the patient's functioning and pain relief on a scale of 1 to 5 in four domains (Social functioning, Analgesia, Physical functioning, and Emotional functioning) (see Table 10.5). The ratings in each domain are combined to yield a SAFE score, which can range from 4 to 20. The *green zone* is a SAFE score of 4 to 12 and/or a decrease of 2 points in total score from baseline. With a score in the green zone, the patient is considered to be doing well, and the plan would be to continue with the current medication regimen or consider reducing the total dose of opioids.

The *yellow zone* is a SAFE score of 13 to 16 and/or a rating of 5 in any category and/or an increase of 2 or more from baseline in the total score. With a score in the yellow zone, the patient should be monitored closely and re-assessed frequently. The *red zone* is a SAFE score greater than or equal to 17. With a score in the red zone, a change in treatment would be warranted.

Assessment and documentation are cornerstones for both protecting your practice and obtaining optimal patient outcomes in opioid therapy. There are a growing number of assessment tools designed to guide clinicians in the evaluation of important outcomes during opioid therapy and to provide a simple means of documenting patient care. They all may prove helpful in clinical management and offer mechanisms for documenting the types of practice standards that those in the regulatory and law enforcement communities seek to insure.

Managing opioid risk

Opioid-specific screening tools

Several opioid-specific screening tools have been developed recently for risk assessment in patients with chronic pain. Most of these tools have been designed to help clinicians decide whether a patient is a candidate for LTOT and what level of monitoring would be best for a particular patient on opioids. These tools are useful as a complement to clinical assessment and as research tools.

Screening Instrument for Substance Abuse Potential

The Screening Instrument for Substance Abuse Potential (SISAP) is a five-item screen that assesses the risk of opioid abuse based on a patient's alcohol consumption, marijuana use, tobacco use, and age [66]. It is designed to be used when the clinician has sufficient collateral data to confirm the patient's responses (see Table 10.6).

Screener and Opioid Assessment for Patients with Pain

The screener and opioid assessment for patients with pain (SOAPP) is a survey tool used to predict opioid abuse and is available as a 5-, 14-, or 24-item questionnaire

Table 10.6 The Screening Instrument for Substance Abuse Potential (SISAP) tool

Questions

1. If you drink alcohol, how many drinks do you have on a typical day?

2. How many drinks do you have in a typical week?

3. Have you used marijuana or hashish in the past year?

4. Have you ever smoked cigarettes?

5. What is your age?

Interpretation of SISAP results

Use caution when prescribing opioids for the following patients:

1. Men who exceed 4 drinks per day or 16 drinks per week

2. Women who exceed 3 drinks per day or 12 drinks per week

3. A patient who admits to marijuana or hashish use in the past year

4. A patient under 40 who smokes

Adapted with permission from Ref. [66].

Table 10.7 The Screener and Opioid Assessment for Patients with Pain Short Form tool

Please answer the question below using the following scale:

0 = never; 1 = seldom; 2 = sometimes; 3 = often; 4 = very often

1. How often do you have mood swings?

2. How often do you smoke a cigarette within an hour after you wake up?

3. How often have you taken medication other than the way it was prescribed?

4. How often have you used illegal drugs (e.g., marijuana, cocaine) in the past 5 years?

5. How often in your life have you had legal problems or been arrested?

[67, 68]. Although the five-item questionnaire (SOAPP V LO-SF[5Q]) is less sensitive and specific than the longer version, it may suffice for use in primary care settings. The SOAPP-SF is scored by adding up the ratings of each of the five questions. The 5Q SOAPP uses a cut-off score of 4 or above (out of a possible 20); with a score above 4 indicating that the subject may be at increased risk for opioid abuse. Therefore, the patient may require additional or special precautions and/or monitoring when treated with LTOT (e.g., giving prescriptions at intervals of days or weeks with limited tablets). While the SOAPP is intended to predict which patients may

Table 10.8 The Opioid Risk Tool (ORT)

Item	Mark each box that applies	Item score if female	Item score if male
1. Family history of substance abuse	[]	1	3
Alcohol	[]	2	3
Illegal drugs	[]	4	4
Prescription drugs			
2. Personal history of substance abuse			
Alcohol	[]	3	3
Illegal drugs	[]	4	4
Prescription drugs	[]	5	5
3. Age (mark box if between 16 and 45)	[]	1	1
4. History of preadolescent sexual abuse	[]	3	0
5. Psychological disease			
Attention deficit disorder obsessive-compulsive disorder, bipolar, schizophrenia	[]	2	2
Depression	[]	1	1
Total ORT score (sum of 1–5)			
Interpretation of ORT Score			
Low risk (score of 0–3)			
Moderate risk (score of 4–7)			
High risk (score of 8 and above)			

Reproduced with permission from Ref. [70].

exhibit drug-related aberrant behaviors in the future, the Current Opioid Misuse Measure is designed to help clinicians identify current opioid patients who are exhibiting abuse behaviors [69]. Further information on the SOAPP is available at: www.painedu.org/soap-development.asp (see Table 10.7).

Opioid Risk Tool

The Opioid Risk Tool (ORT) is a five-question self-administered assessment that can be completed in under 5 minutes and may be utilized on a patient's initial visit [70]. Personal and family history of substance abuse, age, history of preadolescent sexual abuse, the presence of depression, attention deficit disorder, obsessive-compulsive disorder, bipolar disorder, and schizophrenia are assessed. In studies, the ORT accurately predicted which patients were at highest and lowest risk for exhibiting aberrant, drug-related behaviors associated with abuse or addiction [70] (see Table 10.8).

Current Opioid Misuse Measure

The Current Opioid Misuse Measure (COMM) was established for continued assessment of current opioid

use, examining various items reflecting those patient activities that are suggestive of current, ongoing aberrant drug-related behaviors [69].

Choice of assessment

Many factors will determine the choice of assessment tool, including the clinician's expertise or access to specialists and the time available.

Once an assessment or set of questions is chosen, it should be routinely applied, and patients should be monitored for their response to LTOT. The purpose behind assessing patients is not to deny high-risk patients pain treatment but to ensure that all patients receive appropriate monitoring and clinical vigilance. The goal is an environment where opioids may be safely prescribed and consumed, resulting in better clinical outcomes and less abuse.

Risk management plans

There is no single behavior that is pathognomonic of a substance use disorder, thus there is no foolproof instrument that can reliably assess the risk of opioid addiction [71]. As the prevalence of addiction in the general population is not insignificant, it seems prudent to utilize the ten steps of "universal precautions" in patients receiving LTOT [72]. These are: (1) reasonable attempts to make a diagnosis with an appropriate differential; (2) comprehensive patient assessment including risk of addictive disorders; (3) informed consent; (4) treatment agreement; (5) pre- and postintervention assessment of pain level and function; (6) appropriate trial of opioid therapy ± "adjunctive" medications; (7) reassessment of pain score and level of function; (8) regular assessment of the four A's of pain medicine; (9) periodic review of pain diagnosis and co-morbid conditions, including addictive disorders; and (10) documentation. Application of the universal precautions is intended to help the clinician identify and interpret aberrant behavior and, where they exist, diagnose underlying substance misuse disorders.

In the interest of "balance" as well as documentation, many have advocated utilizing a risk-management plan in prescribing LTOT. Currently, no specific elements are required as part of such a plan; however, popular risk-management elements include obtaining informed consent for chronic opioid therapy, using opioid contracts or agreements, performing urine drug tests, and implementing specific policies to manage aberrant behaviors.

Informed consent

The prescriber must discuss the opioid treatment plan clearly with the patient and answer any questions the patient may have. The patient must be informed of the anticipated benefits of LTOT as well as the foreseeable risks, including the issues of addiction, physical dependence, and tolerance [70]. The AAPM has a sample informed consent form titled "Consent for Chronic Opioid Therapy," available in both English and Spanish on their website at www.painmed.org/productpub/statements (see Figure 10.1).

Contracts/agreements

It may also be reasonable to use an opioid contract when prescribing LTOT for patients with persistent non-cancer pain. However, such a contract may not be necessary for all patients in all settings. Therefore the use of opioid contracts is left to the clinician's judgment and/or policies. Elements of opioid contracts may include the following:

- only one physician prescribing opioids while the patient is being treated at a pain clinic;
- use of only one pharmacy for medications;
- random drug (blood or urine) screens and/or pill counts allowed;
- refill requests must be made according to pain clinic policy and not on nights or weekends;
- selling, trading, or sharing opioids with anyone constitutes grounds for discontinuation of opioids and possible dismissal;
- forged or abused prescriptions constitute grounds for discontinuation of opioids and dismissal;
- use of any illegal controlled substances (e.g., marijuana, cocaine) constitutes grounds for discontinuation of opioids and possible dismissal;
- opioids must be safeguarded from loss or theft (lost or stolen opioids will not be replaced);
- the patient agrees to take medication exactly as prescribed; and
- all unused opioid medication must be brought to the pain clinic at every visit.

An extension of the traditional contract is the use of a trilateral opioid contract, which is seen, agreed upon, and signed by the pain specialist, patient, and patient's primary care physician [73]. The AAPM has a sample agreement form (see Figure 10.2).

Urine drug testing

The practice of urine drug testing (UDT) is more common in a non-cancer pain setting than in an oncology or primary care setting; however, it sometimes seems to be incorrectly utilized in a punitive manner to "catch" the patient with an inappropriate positive or negative test. Unfortunately, this often results in dismissal of the patient from the practice. While drug testing can be used in a variety of ways, it is most commonly used for two quite different purposes: to identify substances that should not be present in the urine (i.e., forensic testing) and to detect the presence of prescribed medications (compliance testing).

The use of UDT in efforts to monitor patients on LTOT treated in a pain clinic is reasonable. This type of testing is not mandatory for all patients on LTOT in all settings. It should be utilized based on the clinical judgment of the prescribing clinician; however, some clinicians and/or clinics test all patients on LTOT sporadically based on policy. Katz and Fanciullo have

Consent for Chronic Opioid Therapy

A consent form from the **American Academy of Pain Medicine**

Dr. _____is prescribing opioid medicine, sometimes called narcotic analgesics, to me for a diagnosis of_____.

This decision was made because my condition is serious or other treatments have not helped my pain.

I am aware that the use of such medicine has certain risks associated with it, including, but not limited to: sleepiness or drowsiness, constipation, nausea, itching, vomiting, dizziness, allergic reaction, slowing of breathing rate, slowing of reflexes or reaction time, physical dependence, tolerance to analgesia, addiction and possibility that the medicine will not provide complete pain relief.

I am aware about the possible risks and benefits of other types of treatments that do not involve the use of opioids. The other treatments discussed included:

_____
_____
_____

I will tell my doctor about all other medicines and treatments that I am receiving.

I will not be involved in any activity that may be dangerous to me or someone else if I feel drowsy or am not thinking clearly. I am aware that even if I do not notice it, my reflexes and reaction time might still be slowed. Such activities include, but are not limited to: using heavy equipment or a motor vehicle, working in unprotected heights or being responsible for another individual who is unable to care for himself or herself.

I am aware that certain other medicines such as nalbuphine (Nubain™), pentazocine (Talwin™), buprenorphine (Buprenex™), and butorphanol (Stadol™), may reverse the action of the medicine I am using for pain control. Taking any of these other medicines while I am taking my pain medicines can cause symptoms like a bad flu, called a withdrawal syndrome. I agree not to take any of these medicines and to tell any other doctors that I am taking an opioid as my pain medicine and cannot take any of the medicines listed above.

I am aware that addiction is defined as the use of a medicine even if it causes harm, having cravings for a drug, feeling the need to use a drug and a decreased quality of life. I am aware that the chance of becoming addicted to my pain medicine is very low. I am aware that the development of addiction has been reported rarely in medical journals and is much more common in a person who has a family or personal history of addiction. I agree to tell my doctor my complete and honest personal drug history and that of my family to the best of my knowledge.

I understand that physical dependence is a normal, expected result of using these medicines for a long time. I understand that physical dependence is not the same as addiction. I am aware physical dependence means that if my pain medicine use is markedly decreased, stopped or reversed by some of the agents mentioned above, I will experience a withdrawal syndrome. This means I may have any or all of the following: runny nose, yawning, large pupils, goose bumps, abdominal pain and cramping, diarrhea, irritability, aches throughout my body and a flu-like feeling. I am aware that opioid withdrawal is uncomfortable but not life threatening.

I am aware that tolerance to analgesia means that I may require more medicine to get the same amount of pain relief. I am aware that tolerance to analgesia does not seem to be a big problem for most patients with chronic pain, however, it has been seen and may occur to me. If it occurs, increasing doses may not always help and may cause unacceptable side effects. Tolerance or failure to respond well to opioids may cause my doctor to choose another form of treatment.

(**Males only**) I am aware that chronic opioid use has been associated with low testosterone levels in males. This may affect my mood, stamina, sexual desire and physical and sexual performance. I understand that my doctor may check my blood to see if my testosterone level is normal.

(**Females Only**) If I plan to become pregnant or believe that I have become pregnant while taking this pain medicine, I will immediately call my obstetric doctor and this office to inform them. I am aware that, should I carry a baby to delivery while taking these medicines, the baby will be physically dependent upon opioids. I am aware that the use of opioids is not generally associated with a risk of birth defects. However, birth defects can occur whether or not the mother is on medicines and there is always the possibility that my child will have a birth defect while I am taking an opioid.

I have read this form or have it read to me. I understand all of it. I have had a chance to have all of my questions regarding this treatment answered to my satisfaction. By signing this form voluntarily, I give my consent for the treatment of my pain with opioid pain medicines.

Patient signature_____ Date_____

Witness to above_____

Approved by the AAPM Executive Committee on January 14, 1999.

4700 W. Lake Avenue
Glenview, IL 60026‑1485
847/375-4731
Fax 877/734-8750
E-mail aapm@amctec.com
Web site www.painmed.org

© 1999 **American Academy of Pain Medicine**

Figure 10.1 Sample informed consent from for COT

proposed that although further research is needed, it may be easier and more uniform to conduct routine urine toxicology testing in patients with chronic pain treated with opioids [74]. By adopting a uniform policy of testing, stigma is reduced while ensuring that those persons dually diagnosed with pain and substance use disorders may receive optimal care. With careful explanation of the purpose of testing, any patient concerns can be easily addressed [75, 76]. Caveats to the use of UDT include the following:

1. ensuring the proper collection, handling, and documentation of the urine specimen;

**SAMPLE FOR ADAPTATION AND REPRODUCTION
ON PHYSICIAN LETTERHEAD**

PLEASE CONSULT WITH YOUR ATTORNEY

Long-term Controlled Substances Therapy
for Chronic Pain

SAMPLE AGREEMENT

A consent form from the American Academy of Pain Medicine

The purpose of this agreement is to protect your access to controlled substances and to protect our ability to prescribe for you.

The long-term use of such substances as opioids (narcotic analgesics), benzodiazepine tranquilizers, and barbiturate sedatives is controversial because of uncertainty regarding the extent to which they provide long-term benefit. There is also the risk of an addictive disorder developing or of relapse occurring in a person with a prior addiction. The extent of this risk is not certain.

Because these drugs have potential for abuse or diversion, strict accountability is necessary when use is prolonged. For this reason the following policies are agreed to by you, the patient, as consideration for, and a condition of, the willingness of the physician whose signature appears below to consider the initial and/or continued prescription of controlled substances to treat your chronic pain.

1. All controlled substances must come from the physician whose signature appears below or, during his or her absence, by the covering physician, unless specific authorization is obtained for an exception. (Multiple sources can lead to untoward drug interactions or poor coordination of treatment.)

2. All controlled substances must be obtained at the same pharmacy, where possible. Should the need arise to change pharmacies, our office must be informed. The pharmacy that you have selected is:

   _____ phone: _____.

3. You are expected to inform our office of any new medications or medical conditions, and of any adverse effects you experience from any of the medications that you take.

4. The prescribing physician has permission to discuss all diagnostic and treatment details with dispensing pharmacists or other professionals who provide your health care for purposes of maintaining accountability.

5. You may not share, sell, or otherwise permit others to have access to these medications.

6. These drugs should not be stopped abruptly, as an abstinence syndrome will likely develop.

7. Unannounced urine or serum toxicology screens may be requested, and your cooperation is required. Presence of unauthorized substances may prompt referral for assessment for addictive disorder.

8. Prescriptions and bottles of these medications may be sought by other individuals with chemical dependency and should be closely safeguarded. It is expected that you will take the highest possible degree of care with your medication and prescription. They should not be left where others might see or otherwise have access to them.

9. Original containers of medications should be brought in to each office visit.

10. Since the drugs may be hazardous or lethal to a person who is not tolerant to their effects, especially a child, you must keep them out of reach of such people.

11. Medications may not be replaced if they are lost, get wet, are destroyed, left on an airplane, etc. If your medication has been stolen and you complete a police report regarding the theft, an exception may be made.

12. Early refills will generally not be given.

13. Prescriptions may be issued early if the physician or patient will be out of town when a refill is due. These prescriptions will contain instructions to the pharmacist that they not be filled prior to the appropriate date.

14. If the responsible legal authorities have questions concerning your treatment, as might occur, for example, if you were obtaining medications at several pharmacies, all confidentiality is waived and these authorities may be given full access to our records of controlled substances administration.

15. It is understood that failure to adhere to these policies may result in cessation of therapy with controlled substance prescribing by this physician or referral for further specialty assessment.

16. Renewals are contingent on keeping scheduled appointments. Please do not phone for prescriptions after hours or on weekends.

17. It should be understood that any medical treatment is initially a trial, and that continued prescription is contingent on evidence of benefit.

18. The risks and potential benefits of these therapies are explained elsewhere [and you acknowledge that you have received such explanation].

19. You affirm that you have full right and power to sign and be bound by this agreement, and that you have read, understand, and accept all of its terms.

_____   _____
Physician Signature   Patient Signature

_____   _____
Date   Patient Name (Printed)

Approved by the AAPM Executive Committee on April 2, 2001.

AAPM
4700 W. Lake Avenue
Glenview, IL 60025-1485
847/375-4731   Fax 877/734-8750
E-mail aapm@amctec.com
Web site http://www.painmed.org

© 2001 American Academy of Pain Medicine

Figure 10.2 Sample "bilateral" opioid agreement

2. being knowledgeable regarding interpretation of UDT results;
3. knowing exactly what your patient consumed and when it was consumed prior to the urine collection; and
4. knowing what you are looking for and what you will do when various results come back.

The healthcare professional must know which drugs to test for and by what methods, as well as the expected use of the results. It is critical that the clinician be knowledgeable regarding the limitations of the tests (i.e., low sensitivity of immunoassay for semisynthetic and synthetic opioids). Confirmatory tests should be specifically requested. If the purpose of testing is to find unprescribed or illicit drug use, combination techniques such as GC/MS or HPLC are the most specific for identifying individual drugs or their metabolites [77].

Caution must be exercised in interpreting UDT results in a pain practice. True negative urine results for prescribed medication may indicate a pattern of binging rather than drug diversion. Time of last use of the drug(s) can be helpful in interpreting the results.

In certain cases, a UDT may detect traces of unexplained opioids secondary to drug metabolism. For example, a patient taking codeine may show trace quantities of hydrocodone (up to 11%) that is unrelated to hydrocodone use [78]. Detection of minor amounts of hydrocodone in urine containing a high concentration of codeine should not be interpreted as evidence of hydrocodone misuse. In the case of a patient who is prescribed hydrocodone, quantities of hydromorphone may also be detected due to hydrocodone metabolism [75]. Morphine may be metabolized to produce small amounts of hydromorphone (up to 10%) through a minor metabolic pathway [79].

If UDT is utilized, it is crucial to avoid inappropriate interpretation of results, which may adversely affect clinical decision making. Healthcare providers should not jump to conclusions of non-compliance or appropriate opioid use vs. opioid misuse based on positive or negative detection of opioid in the urine. Clinicians should use the results of the drug test in conjunction with other clinical information when deciding whether to alter the treatment plan.

Public health concerns of opioids

Untreated pain results not only in unnecessary individual suffering, but in increased utilization of healthcare resources, reduced productivity, and over-utilization of disability support systems [22, 80].

Untreated addictive disorders may result in significant economic costs to society, negative public health consequences, and increased crime [81, 82]. Regulatory definitions that acknowledge addiction as a chronic illness and clearly distinguish it from physical dependence and tolerance are critical to the development of regulatory, enforcement, and healthcare policies that effectively address addictive disorders [22].

Inappropriate use can include: selling and diverting prescription drugs, seeking additional prescriptions from multiple providers, and manipulating the formulations to use them in a manner in which they were not intended (e.g., snorting, injecting) [69]. It is also important for the successful treatment of chronic, non-cancer pain to be able to frequently monitor patients on opioid regimens and to identify those patients who exhibit ongoing abuse behaviors [83, 84].

Chronic opioid therapy for pain relief may impact public health concerns since opioids may be used in various manners other than their intended, indicated, or prescribed use. Tampering was defined by a symposium panel [23] as manipulating a pharmaceutical dosage form to change its drug delivery performance in a way not specified by the manufacturer. Tampering was distinguished from abuse in that the latter can occur without manipulation of the dosage form [23]. This concept is closely related to that of extractability, which has been defined as the extent to which extraction procedures performed on a drug formulation

yield the quantities of active ingredient desired by the abuser [23]. The ease with which the active ingredient can be extracted from a prescription opioid has been widely regarded as relevant to the abuse potential of the product [24].

In the development of a proposed extractability rating system, Katz and colleagues [85] identified four dimensions of extractability:

- Ease of extractability, which encompasses a series of progressively difficult extraction steps: simple physical manipulation, single-step chemical extraction, multistep chemical extraction, and complex laboratory extraction
- Purity of the extract
- Efficiency of the extraction process, or the percent of active drug extracted
- Potency of the extract, or the number of doses needed to induce the desired effect.

Abuse-deterrent opioids, whether based on the molecule itself or a unique formulation, offer potential benefits to pain patients by decreasing inadvertent misuse, unintended exposure, and abuse and addiction and increasing the willingness of prescribers and pharmacists to support appropriate opioid therapy, and to the community by quelling the social and legal ramifications of opioid abuse and addiction [23]. Yet, abuse-deterrent opioid formulations should be viewed in the correct context, that is, as only one aspect of a comprehensive approach to prescription opioid risk management. This comprehensive approach would necessarily include proactive education that would promote appropriate patient assessment and management, and also adequate supply chain control and prescription monitoring [23].

A consensus panel agreed that, despite their higher development and production costs, prescription opioid abuse-deterrent formulations, because of the benefits that would be accrued to the patient and to the community, should ultimately replace traditional formulations, at least in high-risk populations [23].

The Federal Drug Administration (FDA) now requires sponsors of new drug submissions to submit comprehensive risk management action plans, so-called Risk MAPs, as a way of addressing some of these issues, although this requirement of Risk MAP development has not been extended to companies producing generic versions of innovator products. It has historically been the responsibility for a generic company to submit to the FDA or other appropriate regulatory bodies evidence of bioequivalence to the innovator product in order to obtain an accelerated approval of the generic version [86].

The transdermal fentanyl system (TDS-Fentanyl) has become available as a generic product. While transdermal fentanyl systems are outwardly similar, in that they both deliver measured amounts of the active drug over time, they are quite different in terms of design. The innovator product is based on a reservoir technology containing a measured quantity of fentanyl-containing gel. The new design is based on technology in which the active drug is dispersed evenly throughout the adhesive matrix of the patch. The matrix product, however, differs in one significant way: all same-sized pieces of patch contain the same amount of fentanyl base, and never more than the unused patch itself [86]. As fentanyl base is an extremely stable molecule, it lends itself to pulmonary use by vaporization; simply cutting up a matrix patch and heating a small piece in a glass pipe will provide a simple and titratable means of delivering fentanyl vapor to the drug user [86].

In some respects, the FDA may have already indicated that simple bioequivalence is not enough when a generic manufacturer makes a submission. Recently, the FDA rejected the Noven Pharmaceutical submission of a 100 µg/h fentanyl matrix patch because it contained substantially more fentanyl base than the innovator product. Even though this patch was arguably *bioequivalent* to the innovator product, it was felt that the excess fentanyl in the patch posed a public safety risk that was unacceptable [86].

Summary

A study lists behaviors that are less indicative of addiction (e.g., hoarding medications, taking someone else's pain medication, aggressively requesting more drugs from the doctor) and behaviors that are more indicative of addiction (e.g., buying pain medication from a street dealer, stealing money to obtain drugs, selling prescription drugs) [88].

Several strategies can be adopted at the initiation of or during opioid therapy based on the perceived level of risk for the patient. These strategies include the following:

- adopting a structured, strict prescription policy with no early refills and no replacement of lost prescriptions (without a police report documenting the loss);
- requiring the patient to attend frequent visits, with small quantities of opioids being prescribed;

- requiring that the patient use only one pharmacy;
- requiring the patient to bring the pill bottle to each appointment for a pill count;
- requiring unscheduled, spontaneous calls for the patient to bring the bottle in for a pill count between regular appointments;
- performing UDT at screening and informing the patient that occasional tests will be required in the future (with proper monitoring of the collection tensure that the urine is fresh and real, not imitation or another person's urine sample);
- requiring the use of non-pharmacologic/non-opioid therapies; and
- requiring that the patient see an addiction medicine specialist.

Based on the level of the problematic behavior and a reassessment of the four A's, the clinician must make the decision as to whether LTOT should be continued, whether the patient should be referred to a pain specialist or an addiction specialist, and whether the patient should be released from the practice.

References

1. Burgess F. Pain treatment, drug diversion, and the casualties of war. *Pain Med* 2006; 7: 474–5.

2. Webster LR, Dove B. *Avoiding Opioid Abuse While Managing Pain A Guide for Practitioners* (North Branch, MI Sunrise River Press, 2007).

3. Fine P, Portenoy RK, eds. *A Clinical Guide to Opioid Analgesia.* (McGraw Hill. New York, NY, 2008).

4. Smith HS, Passik SD, eds. *Pain and Chemical Dependency* (Oxford: Oxford University Press, 2008).

5. Stannard C, Coupe M, Pickering A, eds. *Opioids in Non-Cancer Pain* (Oxford: Oxford University Press, 2008).

6. Smith HS, Fine PG, Passik SD, eds. *Opioid Risk Management: Tools and Tips* (Oxford: Oxford University Press, 2008).

7. Forbes K. (Ed.) *Opioids in Cancer Pain* (Oxford: Oxford University Press, 2007).

8. Smith HS. *Opioid Therapy in the 21st Century* (Oxford: Oxford University Press, 2008).

9. Davis MP, Glare P, Hardy J. (Eds) *Opioids in Cancer Pain* (Oxford: Oxford University Press, 2005).

10. Passik SD Issues in long-term opioid therapy: unmet needs, risks, and solutions. *Mayo Clin Proc* 2009; 84: 593–601.

11. Max MB, Payne R, Edwards WT, *et al. Principles of Analgesic Use in the Treatment of Acute Pain and Cancer*

Pain, 4th edn. (Glenview, IL: American Pain Society, 1999).

12. Katz N. The impact of pain management on quality of life. *J Pain Symptom Manage* 2002; **24**(Suppl 1): S38–S47.

13. World Health Organization. *Achieving Balance in National Opioids Control Policy: Guidelines for Assessment* (Geneva: WHO, 2000).

14. Zacny J, Bigelow G, Compton P, *et al.* College on Problems of Drug Dependence taskforce on prescription opioid non-medical use and abuse: position statement. *Drug Alcohol Depend* 2003; **69**: 215–32.

15. Joint statement from 21 health organizations and the Drug Enforcement Administration. Promoting pain relief and preventing abuse of pain medications: a critical balancing act. Biomedical Computing Group, University of Wisconsin Medical School Web site. www.medsch.wisc.edu/painpolicy/Consensus 2.pdf [Accessed April 2010].

16. Smith HS. Introduction to opioids. In *Opioid Therapy in the 21st Century,* ed. HS Smith. (New York: Oxford University Press, 2008), pp. 1–6.

17. Smith HS. Peripherally-acting opioids. *Pain Physician* 2008; **11**(2 Suppl): S121–32.

18. Smith HS, Deer TR, Staats PS, *et al.* Intrathecal drug delivery. *Pain Physician* 2008; **11**(2 Suppl): S89–S104.

19. Kirsh KL, Whitcomb LA, Donaghy D, Passik SD. Abuse and addiction issues in medically ill patients with pain: Attempts at clarification of terms and empirical study. *Clin J Pain* 2002; **18**(Suppl): S52–60.

20. Weissman DE, Haddox JD. Opioid pseudoaddiction – an iatrogenic syndrome. *Pain* 1989; **36**: 363–6.

21. Pappagallo M. The concept of pseudotolerance to opioids. *J Pharm Care Pain Symptom Control* 1998; **6**: 95–8.

22. Savage SR, Joranson DE, Covington EC, *et al.* Definitions related to the medical use of opioids: evolution towards universal agreement. *J Pain Symptom Manag* 2003; **26**: 655–67.

23. Katz NP, Adams EH, Chilcoat H, *et al.* Challenges in the development of prescription opioid abuse-deterrent formulation. *Clin J Pain* 2007; **23**: 648–60.

24. World Health Organization. *Cancer Pain Relief, with a Guide to Opioid Availability,* 2nd edn. (Geneva: World Health Organization, 1996).

25. Smith HS. Optimizing pharmacologic outcomes: Individualization of therapy. In *Opioid Therapy in the 21st Century,* ed. HS Smith. (New York: Oxford University Press, 2008), 71–6.

26. Portenoy RK. Supportive and palliative care. In *Educational Review Manual in Medical Oncology,* ed. DJ Straus. (New York: Castle Connolly Graduate Medical Publishing, 2007), pp. 361–408.

27. McNichol E, Horowicz-Mehler N, Risk R, *et al.* Management of opioid side effects in cancer related and chronic noncancer pain: A systematic review. *J Pain* 2003; **4**: 231–56.

28. Mercadante S, Bruera E. Opioid switching: A systematic and critical review. *Cancer Treat Rev* 2006; **32**: 304–15.

29. Quigley C. Opioid switching to improve pain relief and drug tolerability. *Cochrane Database Syst Rev.* 2004; **3**: CD004847. DOI: 10.1002114651858.CD004847.

30. Cherny N, Ripamonti C, Pereira J, *et al.* Expert Working Group of the European Association of Palliative Care Network: Strategies to manage the adverse effects of oral morphine: an evidence-based report. *J Clin Oncol* 2001; **19**: 2542–54.

31. Anderson R, Saiers JH, Abram S, *et al.* Accuracy in equianalgesic dosing: Conversion dilemmas. *J Pain Symptom Manage* 2001; **21**: 397–406.

32. Krantz MJ, Lowery CM, Martell BA, *et al.* Effects of methadone on QT-interval dispersion. *Pharmacotherapy.* 2005; **25**: 1523–29.

33. Bruera E, Sweeney C. Methadone use in cancer patients with pain: A review. *J Palliat Med* 2002; **5**: 127–38.

34. McCarberg BH, Smith HS. Optimizing pharmacologic outcomes: Principles of opioid rotation. *In Opioid Therapy in the 21st Century,* ed. HS Smith. (New York: Oxford University Press, 2008), pp. 59–70.

35. Deer T, Krames ES, Hassenbusch SJ, *et al.* Polyanalgesic Consensus Conference 2007: Recommendations for the management of pain by intrathecal (intraspinal) drug delivery: Report of an interdisciplinary expert panel. *Neuromodulation* 2007; **10**: 300–28.

36. Smith TJ, Staats PS, Deer T, *et al.* Implantable Drug Delivery Systems Study Group. Randomized clinical trial of an implantable drug delivery system compared with comprehensive medical management for refractory cancer pain: Impact on pain, drug-related toxicity, and survival. *J Clin Oncol* 2002; **20**: 4040–9.

37. Staats PS, Yearwood T, Charapata SG, *et al.* Intrathecal ziconotide in the treatment of refractory pain in patients with cancer or AIDS: A randomized controlled trial. *JAMA.* 2004; **291**: 63–70.

38. Kalso E, Edwards JE, Moore RA, *et al.* Opioids in chronic non-cancer pain: A systematic review of efficacy and safety. *Pain* 2004; **112**: 372–80.

39. Eisenberg E, McNicol ED, Carr DB. Efficacy and safety of opioid agonists in the treatment of neuropathic pain of nonmalignant origin: Systematic review and meta-analysis trials. *JAMA* 2005; **293**: 3043–52.

40. Rowbotham MC, Twilling L, Davies PS, *et al*. Oral opioid therapy for chronic peripheral and central neuropathic pain. *N Engl J Med* 2003; **348**: 1223–32.

41. Dworkin RH, O' Connor AB, Backonja M, *et al*. Pharmacologic management of neuropathic pain: Evidence-based recommendations. *Pain* 2007; **132**: 237–51.

42. Dworkin RH, Backjona M, Rowbotham MC, *et al*. Advances in neuropathic pain: Diagnosis, mechanisms, and treatment recommendations. *Arch Neurol* 2003; **60**: 1524–34.

43. Kalman S, Osterberg A, Sorensen J, Boivie J, Bertler A. Morphine responsiveness in a group of well-defined multiple sclerosis patients: A study with I.V. morphine. *Eur J Pain* 2002; **6**: 69–24.

44. Gilron I, Bailer JM, Tu D, *et al*. Morphine, gabapentin, or their combination for neuropathic pain. *N Engl J Med* 2005; **352**: 1324–34.

45. Khoromi S, Cui L, Nackers L, Max MB. Morphine, nortriptyline and their combination vs. placebo in patients with chronic lumbar root pain. *Pain* 2007; **130**: 65–75.

46. Raja SN, Haythornthwaite JA, Pappagallo M, *et al*. Opioids versus antidepressants in postherpetic neuralgia: A randomized, placebo-controlled trial. *Neurology* 2002; **59**: 1015–21.

47. Watson CPN, Watt-Watson JH, Chipman ML. Chronic non-cancer pain and the long term utility of opioids. *Pain Res Manage* 2004; **9**: 19–24.

48. Furlan AD, Sandoval JA, Mailis-Gagnon A, Tunks E. Opioids for chronic noncancer pain: A meta-analysis of effectiveness and side effects. *CMAJ* 2006; **174**: 1589–94.

49. Daniell HW. Hypogonadism in men consuming sustained-action oral opioids. *J Pain* 2002; **3**: 337–84.

50. Rajagopal A, Vassilopoulou-Sellin R, Palmer JL, *et al*. Symptomatic hypogonadism in male survivors of cancer with chronic exposure to morphine. *Cancer* 2004; **100**: 851–8.

51. Vallejo R, de Leon-Cassola O, Benyamin R. Opioid therapy and immunosuppresion: A review. *Am J Ther* 2004; **11**: 354–65.

52. Angst MS, Clark JD. Opioid-induced hyperalgesia: A qualitative systematic review. *Anesthesiology* 2006; **104**: 570–87.

53. Chang G, Chen L, Mao J. Opioid tolerance and hyperalgesia. *Med Clin North Am* 2007; **91**: 199–221.

54. Chu LF, Clark DJ, Angst MS. Opioid tolerance and hyperalgesia in chronic pain patients after one month of oral morphine therapy: A preliminary prospective study. *J Pain* 2006; 7: 43–8.

55. Wilder-Smith OHG, Arendt-Nielsen L. Postoperative analgesia: Its clinical importance and relevance. *Anesthesiology* 2006; **103**: 601–7.

56. McCleane G, Smith HS. Opioids for persistent noncancer pain. *Med Clin North Am* 2007; **91**: 177–97.

57. Smith HS. Pre-opioid prescribing period. In *Opioid Therapy in the 21st Century*, ed. HS Smith. (New York: Oxford University Press, 2008), pp. 97–100.

58. Smith HS. Goal-directed therapy agreements. *J Cancer Pain Symptom Palliation* 2006; **1**: 11–13.

59. Passik SD, Weinreb HI. Managing chronic nonmalignant pain: Overcoming obstacles to the use of opioids. *Adv Ther* 2000; **17**: 70–80.

60. Smith HS. Perspectives in long-term therapy for persistent noncancer pain. *J Cancer Pain Symptom Palliation* 2005; **1**: 31–2.

61. Passik SD, Kirsh KL, Whitcomb LA, *et al*. A new tool to assess and document pain outcomes in chronic pain patients receiving opioid therapy. *Clin Ther.* 2004; **26**: 552–61.

62. Passik SD, Kirsh KL, Whitcomb LA, *et al*. Monitoring outcomes during long-term opioid therapy for non-cancer pain: Results with the pain assessment and documentation tool. *J Opioid Manage.* 2005; **1**: 257–66.

63. Smith HS. The numerical opioid side effect (NOSE) assessment tool. *J Cancer Pain Symptom Palliation* 2005; **1**: 75–9.

64. Smith HS. Translational analgesia and the Translational Analgesia Score (TAS). *J Cancer Pain Symptom Palliation* 2005; **1**: 15–19.

65. Smith HS, Audette J, Witkower A. Playing it "SAFE." *J Cancer Pain Symptom Palliation* 2005; **1**: 3–10.

66. Coambs RB, Jarry JL. The SISAP: a new screening instrument for identifying potential opioid abusers in the management of chronic nonmalignant pain in general medical practice. *Pain Res Manage* 1996; **1**: 155–62.

67. Butler SF, Budman SH, Fernandez K, *et al*. Validation of a screener and opioid assessment measure for patients with chronic pain. *Pain* 2004; **112**: 65–75.

68. Akbik H, Butler SF, Budman SH, *et al*. Validation and clinical application of the Screener and Opioid Assessment for Patients with Pain (SOAPP). *J Pain Symptom Manage* 2006; **32**: 287–93.

69. Butler SF, Budman SH, Fernandez K, *et al*. Development and validation of the Current Opioid Misuse Measure. *Pain* 2007; **130**: 114–56.

70. Webster LR, Webster RM. Predicting aberrant behaviors in opioid-treated patients: Preliminary validation of the Opioid Risk Tool. *Pain Med* 2005; **6**: 432–42.

71. Gourlay D, Heit HA. Universal precautions: A matter of mutual trust and responsibility. *Pain Med* 2006; **7**: 210.

72. Gourlay DL, Heit HA. Universal precautions in pain medicine: A rational approach to the treatment of chronic pain. *Pain Med* 2005; **6**: 107.

73. Fishman SM, Mahajan G, Jung SW, *et al.* The trilateral opioid contract. Bridging the pain clinic and the primary care physician through the opioid contract. *J Pain Symptom Manage* 2002; **24**: 335–44.

74. Katz N, Fanciullo G. Role of urine toxicology testing in the management of chronic opioid therapy. *Clin J Pain* 2002; **18**: 576–82.

75. Gourlay DL, Heit HA, Caplan YH. *Urine Drug Testing in Primary Care: Dispelling the Myths Designing Strategies* (Pharmacom Group, 2002).

76. Heit HA. *Use of Urine Toxicology Tests in a Chronic Pain Practice*, 3rd edn. (Chevy Chase, MD: American Society of Addiction Medicine, 2003).

77. Vandevenne M, Vandenbussche H, Verstraete A. Detection time of drugs of abuse in urine. *Acta Clin Belg* 2000; **55**: 323–33.

78. Oyler JM, Cone EJ, Joseph RE Jr, *et al.* Identification of hydrocodone in human urine following controlled codeine administration. *J Anal Toxicol* 2000; **24**: 530–35.

79. Cone EJ, Heit HA, Caplan YH, *et al.* Evidence of morphine metabolism to hydromorphone in pain patients chronically treated with morphine. *J Anal Toxicol* 2006; **30**: 1–5.

80. Strax T, Grabois M. Evaluating pain and disability. *Physical Med Rehab Clinics North Amer* 2001; **12**: 559–70.

81. Alcohol and Health: *Tenth Special Report to the U.S. Congress* (Washington DC: U.S. Department of Health and Human Services, 1997).

82. Sinha R, Easton C. Substance abuse and criminality. *J Amer Acad Psychiatry Law* 1999; **27**: 513–26.

83. Friedman R, Li V, Mehrotra D. Treating pain patients at risk: Evaluation of a screening tool in opioid-treated pain patients with and without addiction. *Pain Med* 2003; **4**: 181–84.

84. Passik SD, Kirsh KL. The need to identify predictors of aberrant drug related behavior and addiction in patients being treated with opioids for pain. *Pain Med* 2003; **4**: 186–9.

85. Katz N, Buse DC, Budman SH, *et al.* Development and preliminary experience with an ease of extractability rating system for prescription opioids. *Drug Dev Ind Pharm* 2006; **32**: 727–46.

86. Gourlay DL, Heit HA. Risk management is everyone's business. *Pain Med* 2007; **8**: 125–27.

87. Marquardt KA, Tharratt RS. Inhalation abuse of fentanyl patch. *J Toxicol Clin Toxicol* 1994; **32**: 75–8.

88. Passik SD, Kirsh KL, Konaghy KB, *et al.* Pain and aberrant drug-related behaviors in medically ill patients with and without histories of substance abuse. *Clin J Pain* 2006; **22**: 173–81.

Psychopharmacologic, behavioral, and psychotherapeutic approaches

Behavioral therapeutic interventions in pain management

Steven H. Sanders

Introduction

The application of behaviorally based concepts and methods for the better understanding and treatment of clinical pain is now well established in clinical practice. Spearheaded by the seminal work of Fordyce [1, 2] and others such as Sternbach [3], the last 40 years have produced an abundance of research on and clinical application of behavioral/learning based methods for pain. Much of the focus has been on understanding and treating patients with chronic painful conditions. The current chapter offers a review and discussion of those important behavioral/learning concepts and treatment strategies applied to clinical pain, as well as the evidence supporting them.

The chapter is divided into five main sections. The first offers a behaviorally based definition for pain. This is followed by a review of behavioral/learning models and principles, and their relationship to clinical pain. The third section offers an empirical, integrated, and interactive behavioral/learning conceptual model for the onset and maintenance of clinical pain, and summarizes the evidence basis. The fourth section reviews the details for effective application of these interactive behavioral/learning principles to clinical pain, as well as current limitations. The final section offers a summary of current clinical and research needs regarding behavioral approaches for clinical pain.

Defining clinical pain

While there are a multitude of possible ways to define clinical pain, this section focuses on a definition highlighting the various responses which together comprise the pain experience. Such constitutes a behavioral conceptual approach. As will be obvious, this provides a basis for a more complete conceptual understanding of clinical pain and the logical application of behavioral/learning based principles. The International Association for the Study of Pain (IASP) has defined pain as: "An unpleasant sensory and emotional experience associated with actual or potential tissue damage, or described in terms of such damage" [4]. While this definition recognizes that pain is not merely a sensory phenomenon, incorporating a behavioral perspective can serve to enhance the clarity and specificity of the definition.

A behavioral definition

Pain in its entirety can be conceptualized as a cluster of responses associated with actual or potential tissue damage. Specifically, an interacting cluster of neurophysiological, overt, and covert responses produced by actual or potential tissue damage [5]. Table 11.1 outlines these response categories and specific example responses. From a review of the table, we can begin to see the obvious complexity of clinical pain. Within such a behavioral model, and as the research literature has clearly demonstrated, the gross motor and cognitive/subjective pain responses should be considered as equally important and clinically significant as the neurophysiological ones. Likewise the three pain response categories can show marked desynchrony, with multiple and intense pain responding in one category, and minimal or no responses in others [6]. In addition, as will become obvious as important later in this chapter, all of the pain responses across categories are by definition associated with the aversive, nociceptive condition of actual or potential tissue damage.

When discussing clinical pain from a behavioral perspective, it is important to also introduce the concept of "well" behaviors. Such responses are typically just the opposite and/or inhibit their pain response counterparts, and are also an important target of behavioral treatment techniques. At the neurophysiological level, well responses might include such things

Behavioral and Psychopharmacologic Pain Management, ed. Michael H. Ebert and Robert D. Kerns. Published by Cambridge University Press. © Cambridge University Press 2011.

as release of beta endorphin neuropeptides or muscle relaxation. Gross motor well responses could include verbal expressions of reduced pain level, increased standing and walking behavior, and increased smiling. Possible cognitive/subjective well responses would be thoughts that one is in control of one's pain, feelings of being relaxed, and images of walking without a cane.

Having defined clinical pain within a behavioral response model, let us now review and discuss those important fundamental learning/conditioning behavioral concepts and principles that serve as a foundation for understanding and treating pain within such a model.

Fundamental learning/conditioning behavioral models

This section summarizes three major learning/conditioning behavioral models as they interact and relate to clinical pain. These include respondent, operant, and observational learning/conditioning. While the learning/conditioning models are discussed separately for increased clarity and understanding, they do not act in isolation in the clinical setting. Rather, as outlined later in this chapter, there is an ongoing rich interaction across the models [7, 8].

Respondent learning/conditioning

Respondent (also called classical) learning/conditioning was initially introduced and developed primarily through the pioneering work of Pavlov [9]. This form of conditioning involves studying "involuntary" reflex responses (e.g., salivation, pupil dilation, blushing) and those stimulus conditions which can elicit and/or maintain these responses. The focus in this paradigm is on those controlling stimulus conditions that precede a given reflexive response. The basic paradigm consists of identifying a specific reflexive response, labeled the unconditioned response (UR), and stimulus condition, labeled the unconditioned stimulus (US), which when present elicits the UR. An example used by Pavlov involves presenting food (the US) and measuring elicitation of salivation (the UR) in dogs. The US–UR association is considered to be genetically/biologically encoded, and thus, unconditioned. The respondent conditioning paradigm would then repeatedly pair a neutral stimulus such as a bell sound, labeled the conditioned stimulus (CS), with the presentation of the US. Pavlov demonstrated that

this repeated association of the CS with the US results in the CS by itself eliciting a physiological response, labeled the conditioned response (CR), similar in nature and intensity to the UR. Thus, establishing that a neutral stimulus could be conditioned to elicit a reflexive response, which represents a type of basic learning. Pavlov also demonstrated that the repeated presentation of the CS without continued pairing with the US would lead to a gradual reduction in the ability of the CS to elicit the CR. This gradual reduction is called habituation, with ongoing repeated presentation of the CS without the US eventually resulting in a loss (extinction) of the ability of the CS to elicit the CR. It has also been demonstrated that after extinction occurs, there can be a spontaneous recovery of the ability of the CS to elicit the CR. Typically, such recovery is transient, with more permanent extinction occurring over time.

The respondent conditioning paradigm has also included the use of aversive USs like electric shock and extreme cold associated with pain from nociceptive tissue damage and irritation. Research findings have demonstrated that when the paradigm involves an aversive US, conditioning of the CS can occur quite rapidly, even after one pairing with the US–UR, and the CR is almost identical to the UR in composition and strength. Likewise, this aversive respondent conditioning paradigm is quite resistant to habituation and eventual extinction [10].

Studies have also demonstrated the phenomena of both stimulus and response generalization during respondent conditioning [11, 12]. Stimulus generalization refers to the act of responding to a stimulus similar to but distinct from the CS. For example, in addition to exhibiting a CR to the CS bell sound, the dog in Pavlov's experiments might also exhibit the CR to a tone sound. Response generalization involves eliciting a different but similar CR to the same CS. An example of response generalization can be seen in experiments with the rabbit eye blink reflex. This reflex can be classically conditioned to occur to a tone conditioned stimulus. With additional conditioning, that same tone might also elicit an eye twitch response.

Since Pavlov's original work, the respondent conditioning paradigm has been subjected to extensive research scrutiny to fully understand the nature of the relationship between the stimulus and response conditions, as well as the extent and role this type of conditioning plays in animal and human behavior. Such research has resulted in a more thorough understanding of the

Table 11.1 Multiple response conceptualization of clinical pain

Response category	Examples
Neurophysiological	
Ascending	Afferent A-delta and C nerve excitation
Supraspinal/cortical	Hypothalamic, limbic, somatosensory excitation
Descending	Efferent autonomic, pyramidal, extrapyramidal nerve excitation
Chemical	Release of substance P, glutamates, prostaglandins
Physiological	Increase in heart rate, muscle tension, respiration rate, vascular tone
Gross motor	
Verbal	Moaning, crying, yelping/yelling, pain complaints, pain ratings
Non-verbal	Grimacing, rubbing, limb withdrawal, limping, taking analgesics
Cognitive/subjective	
Thoughts	The pain is horrible, unbearable, out of control
Feelings states	Perceptions of pain, fear/anxiety, anger, sadness/depression
Images	Visualizations of being crippled, having surgery, losing a job

types of reflexive responses that can be included in the respondent conditioning paradigm. As Skinner [13], Sidman [14], and Reynolds [12] all observed, reflexive responses can include more generalized emotional behaviors such as crying, fear reaction, smiling, quivering, and yelping/yelling. In addition, contemporary research findings have lead to the expansion and revision of Pavlov's original concepts. For example, the influence of cognitive processes has been demonstrated [15, 16]. Likewise, the need for a US–CS pairing has been questioned. Donahoe and Vegas have demonstrated that learning/conditioning can occur with just the CS–UR pairing [17]. Regardless of these more recent findings, the fundamentals and clinical application of respondent conditioning remains rooted in Pavlov's basic paradigm. Included in this substantial body of research are multiple studies demonstrating that respondent conditioning can play a significant role in eliciting and/or maintaining a host of pain responses (e.g., somatosensory excitation, limb withdrawal, fear of pain, crying, muscle tension, yelping/yelling) outlined in Table 11.1. [7, 18–21].

Operant learning/conditioning

Operant (also called instrumental) learning/conditioning also has a rich history, with its initial delineation and scientific basis attributed to the paradigm changing work of Skinner [13, 22]. This learning model focuses on control of behavioral responses by the contingent application of certain consequences. Skinner

labeled this basic operant conditioning paradigm as "reinforcement". The reinforcement paradigm involves contingently following an overt behavior with the application (positive reinforcement) or removal (negative reinforcement) of a consequence, which results in the maintenance and/or increase in the occurrence of the overt behavior. Consequences in the positive reinforcement category typically are pleasurable/enjoyable, such as food, social contact, or verbal praise, with negative reinforcement consequences involving unpleasant/aversive experiences like physical pain, social stress, or intense fear. Much of Skinner's research was done with white rats and pigeons within a positive reinforcement paradigm, using a lever press (for rats) or button peck (for pigeons) as the overt behavior and contingent delivery of food as the positive reinforcing consequence. Through a number of elegant and systematic observational studies, Skinner and many others have demonstrated that the occurrence and frequency of lever-pressing and button-pecking behaviors can be systematically controlled by various contingent delivery schedules of a food reinforcer.

While the negative reinforcement paradigm of withdrawing an unpleasant/aversive experience or event contingent upon the occurrence of a targeted overt behavior was defined and studied by Skinner, much of the research on this paradigm has been done by others. Sidman conducted a great deal of this research, with the negative reinforcement paradigm more descriptively labeled escape/avoidance conditioning [14]. Noting that the overt behavior serves to escape and sometimes avoid the occurrence of the unpleasant/aversive experience. Again, much of this initial work has been done using white rats, with the unpleasant/aversive experience of electric shock to the animal's feet. Sidman demonstrated that the rat could be conditioned to systematically emit the bar press response to escape the electric shock, and, with sufficient time and overt cues (discussed below), to emit the response and effectively avoid the electric shock from occurring. Initial and subsequent operant conditioning researchers have observed that escape/avoidance conditioning responses for animals and humans can include those overt generalized emotional behaviors like crying, limb withdrawal, or grimacing also involved in respondent conditioning and associated with painful, nociceptive tissue damage or irritation. In addition, responses conditioned through the escape/avoidance paradigm are also quite resistant to change and can continue indefinitely, particularly if the response serves to actually avoid the unpleasant/aversive experience.

Unpleasant/aversive experiences within the operant learning/conditioning model are also involved in the punishment paradigm. Skinner defined this paradigm as the contingent application of an unpleasant/aversive experience or removal of a pleasurable event or experience following the occurrence of a targeted overt behavior. Such a contingent application or removal can lead to a temporary reduction in the targeted overt behavior. Depending on the severity of the consequence, the punishment paradigm can sometimes lead to a more permanent cessation of the target behavior [12].

It is important to highlight the varying influence that unpleasant/aversive experiences such as painful nociception can have on behaviors within the operant learning/conditioning model. The contingent removal of an unpleasant/aversive experience following a given behavior (negative reinforcement paradigm) can increase and/or maintain the occurrence of such escape/avoidance behavior. In contrast, the contingent application of an unpleasant/aversive experience following a given behavior (punishment paradigm) can result in decreasing the target behavior. Thus, depending upon whether the unpleasant/aversive experience or event is removed or applied, it can either increase or decrease the occurrence of the target behavior.

Another fundamental operation within the operant learning/conditioning model is that of extinction. The extinction paradigm involves the removal of the contingent relationship between an overt behavior and its positive or negative consequences. Removal of the contingent relationship with a positive or negative reinforcer typically results in a reduction in the occurrence of the targeted overt behavior. In contrast, removal of a contingent punisher typically results in an increase in the frequency/occurrence of a target behavior. As already noted, a major exception to this extinction effect is commonly seen with conditioned/learned escape/avoidance behavior. This is particularly so with avoidance behavior. Simply removing the contingent consequent relationship often does not change the occurrence of such behavior. This resistance to extinction is quite understandable within the escape/avoidance learning paradigm. Once emission of a behavior consistently avoids the occurrence of an aversive/unpleasant consequence, the opportunity to learn that the aversive consequence might not actually occur in the absence of engaging in the avoidant behavior is removed. Since maintenance of the avoidant behavior does not rely on the actual application of the aversive consequence, removing the contingent relationship typically has little effect on the behavior. Changing such behavior often requires not only removing the contingent relationship with an aversive/unpleasant consequence, but also consistently limiting or preventing the avoidant behavior from occurring [11, 14].

Skinner and many other behavioral scientists/researchers have also demonstrated that a variety of environmental stimuli can acquire discriminative or cue-like properties if repeatedly paired with the occurrence of a contingent relationship between a given behavior and its consequence. These so-called discriminative stimuli can take on the role of signaling the presence of the contingency, and that emission of the target behavior is likely to result in certain consequences. Research has clearly demonstrated that discriminative stimuli can have significant influence on the occurrence of a host of overt behaviors, and, along with stimulus generalization effects, can play a major role in the maintenance of avoidant behavior.

Operant learning/conditioning has been found to be most effective when specific target behaviors and effective positive or negative consequences for such behaviors are identified and applied consistently. While the immediate application of contingent consequences has been shown to be most effective, delayed application can also be effective as long as there is awareness of the contingent relationship between the behavior and its consequence. Likewise, learning/conditioning effects are best obtained using a shaping procedure. This involves systematically reinforcing successive approximations of a given target behavior until a complete response occurs [12]. For example, a rat may first be given food for just moving close to a bar lever. Once this movement response is consistently occurring, the rat is then contingently given food only when touching the bar with its nose or paw. Finally, food is contingently given only when actually pressing the bar. This shaping method of rewarding parts or approximations of the given behavior until the actual behavior occurs can be very important for successful learning/conditioning to occur. Like respondent learning/conditioning, the phenomena of stimulus and response generalization are also present within the operant learning/conditioning process.

Also, like with the respondent model, operant learning/conditioning has undergone extensive research for over 50 years. Multiple studies have shown that most voluntary and many generalized emotional responses, including those pain responses delineated in Table 11.1, are significantly influenced by contingent consequences and surrounding environmental cues [5, 7, 22].

Observational learning/conditioning

This learning/conditioning model focuses on influencing behavior through observing others engaging in such behavior. Bandura is credited with introducing and initially researching this model [1977] [23]. He and his colleagues have demonstrated that animals and humans are able to acquire a variety of overt behaviors by simply observing like animals or humans (models) engage in such behavior. Specifically, observational learning is demonstrated when the observer's behavior changes from viewing similar behavior of a model. Consistent with operant conditioning, the observer's behavior could either increase or decrease depending upon whether the model's behavior is reinforced or punished. Bandura found that the effectiveness of observational learning requires attention to the model, retention of response details, ability to reproduce the behavior, and motivation with opportunity to engage in the behavior. Likewise, learning is more likely when the observer and model have similar characteristics such as age, sex, occupation, race, and culture. As with operant and respondent learning, observational learning has been shown to influence a variety of socially based behaviors, including various pain responses, in animals and humans [24, 25].

Having reviewed the fundamental learning/conditioning behavioral models, the next section offers an interactive/learning based conceptualization of clinical pain, combining the effects across respondent, operant, and observational learning/conditioning. The evidence basis for such an interactive model is also summarized.

An interactive learning/conditioning behavioral model for clinical pain

Table 11.2 delineates a representative functional analysis (temporal relationship) of clinical pain responses in the acute state, with the combined potential effects of antecedent and consequent stimulus conditions across the respondent, operant, and observational learning/conditioning models. Starting with the left-hand portion of the table, at least four prevalent antecedent stimulus categories are noted that can illicit/initiate and/or maintain acute pain responses. These antecedent stimuli are divided into primary and secondary contributors. As the table examples note, tissue damage/irritation, and environmental stressors are thought to play a more primary (dominant) role in the acute state, with prior conditioned and discriminative stimuli, as well as pain response models, postulated to play a more secondary role. The middle portion of Table 11.2 indicates the primary and secondary acute state pain response categories (as reviewed in Table 11.1). During the acute state, neurophysiological and gross motor pain responses are thought to be primary, with the cognitive/subjective category responses somewhat secondary. The right-hand portion of Table 11.1 lists at least four prevalent consequent conditions which have been shown to influence the maintenance of various individual pain responses. These include reduction in pain perception, reduction in tissue damage/irritation, reduction in environmental stressors, and increase in social attention. Reduced pain perception and tissue damage/irritation are considered primary consequences in the acute state.

Table 11.3 outlines a functional analysis proposed for chronic clinical pain. A review of the antecedent stimulus conditions on the left side reveals the same four categories as during the acute state, but a change in the primary/secondary status. It is postulated that environmental stressors remain primary, and with time and learning effects, the conditioned and discriminative stimuli become primary antecedent controlling

Table 11.2 Primary and secondary pain responses, antecedent, and consequent stimuli for acute pain

Prevalent antecedent stimuli initiating/maintaining responses	Pain responses	Prevalent consequent stimuli maintaining responses
	Acute state	
TISSUE DAMAGE/IRRITATION	NEUROPHYSIOLOGICAL	↓ SUBJECTIVE PAIN
e.g., ruptured disc, extracranial vascular distension in migraine headache	GROSS MOTOR *Cognitive/subjective*	PERCEPTION ↓TISSUE DAMAGE/IRRITATION *↓ Environmental stressors*
ENVIRONMENTAL STRESSORS		*↑ Social attention*
e.g., marital conflict, economic hardship, work demands		
Prior conditioned/discriminative stimuli		
e.g., spouse, physician, worksite, questions about how one is feeling		
Pain response models		
e.g., injured co-worker, spouse, friend		

Primary (i.e., important contributor) stimuli/responses in capital letters; secondary (i.e., less important contributor) stimuli/responses in italics.

Table 11.3 Primary and secondary pain responses, antecedent, and consequent stimuli for chronic pain

Prevalent antecedent stimuli initiating/maintaining responses	Pain responses	Prevalent consequent stimuli maintaining responses
	Chronic state	
ENVIRONMENTAL STRESSORS	GROSS MOTOR	↓ or AVOID ENVIRONMENTAL
CONDITIONED/DISCRIMINATIVE	COGNITIVE/	STRESSORS
STIMULI	SUBJECTIVE	↓ or AVOID SUBJECTIVE PAIN
PAIN RESPONSE MODELS	*Neurophysiological*	PERCEPTION
Tissue damage/irritation		↓ or AVOID DRUG
e.g., from acute state, iatrogenic, chronic muscle trigger points		WITHDRAWAL ↑ SOCIAL ATTENTION ↑ ECONOMIC GAINS *↓ or Avoid tissue damage/ irritation*

Primary (i.e., important contributor) stimuli/responses in capital letters; secondary (i.e., less important contributor) stimuli/responses in italics.

conditions. While tissue damage/irritation can still be present, its dominant role in maintaining chronic pain responses is thought to diminish. Likewise, the three pain response categories are present but show some changes in primary vs. secondary status. Specifically, while the gross motor pain responses persist and remain dominant, cognitive/subjective responses are also thought to take on a greater primary role. Neurophysiologically based chronic pain responses are often present, but are thought to be more secondary with chronic pain. The right hand portion of Table 11.3

lists a larger number of prevalent consequent stimulus conditions empirically demonstrated to influence the maintenance of various chronic pain responses. Also, as with the antecedent stimuli, the primary and secondary status of consequent stimuli during the chronic state are thought to change. Not only can the chronic pain responses lead to a reduction or escape from certain aversive consequences such as subjective pain level, environmental stressors, tissue damage/irritation, and the added drug withdrawal, they can also serve to actually avoid such consequences.

This sets the occasion for an escape/avoidance learning paradigm for pain responses, which along with respondent conditioning effects, make them quite resistant to change/reduction through simple extinction [2]. Table 11.3 also notes the addition of economic gains as a primary potential reinforcing consequent chronic pain behaviors.

The interactive learning based conceptual model outlined in Tables 11.2 and 11.3 offers a very useful and practical approach to understand the initiation and perpetuation of clinical pain states. It also sets the occasion for the logical application of behaviorally based therapies with clinical pain. However, it is important to note that the current interactive model should not be considered definitive, nor has all of it been empirically tested. The next section summarizes the empirical evidence that is currently available.

Evidence basis for interactive learning/ conditioning model of clinical pain

Although research support is not yet available for the entire interactional learning/conditioning model of pain, there is substantial evidence demonstrating the effects on pain responses across all three categories by operant, respondent, and observational learning/conditioning. As multiple reviews of the scientific literature have concluded, a host of well-controlled studies have clearly demonstrated that those antecedent and consequent stimulus conditions listed in Tables 11.2 and 11.3 can significantly change those pain responses delineated in Table 11.1 [5, 7, 26]. Continued support for such effects has been reported by ongoing research in this area. For example, Jolliffe and Nicholas have demonstrated operant conditioning effects on verbal pain responses [27], with researchers also showing the effects of operant learning on other overt pain behaviors such as taking opioids, resting, and guarding [28, 29, 30]. In addition, studies have shown the effects of operant conditioning on neurophysiological responses such as evoked potential responses to aversive stimuli [31], as well as the influence on pain behavior by discriminative stimuli [32, 33]. Holzl et al. also conducted a very interesting analog study demonstrating that hypersensitivity to painful stimulation can be conditioned using operant methods without the person's awareness – in other words, a form of implicit operant conditioning for acute pain responses [34].

Respondent conditioning effects have also been demonstrated for somatosensory evoked potentials

from aversive stimuli [18], muscle tone/reactivity [19], as well as fear of pain, crying, and yelping/yelling [20, 21]. Likewise, with a series of systematic animal studies, Siegel and his colleagues have demonstrated that anticipatory hyperalgesia and drug withdrawal can be classically conditioned [35, 36]. While Taddio et al. have demonstrated respondent conditioned hyperalgesic reactions in human newborns [37]. In addition, observational learning/conditioning effects on pain responses have been repeatedly reported in the animal and human research literature [38, 39, 40].

While there is strong evidence for interactive learning/conditioning effects on pain responses, specific research regarding the relative strength and persistence of these effects over time is lacking. Also, the relative importance of various antecedent and consequent stimuli and pain responses presented in Tables 11.2 and 11.3, as well as the nature and extent of potential stimulus to stimulus and response to response interactions need a great deal more empirical scrutiny.

Evidence-based behavioral therapeutics with clinical pain

Given the interactive learning/conditioning model for pain, this section describes those empirically based behavioral methods frequently used to treat clinical pain. For clarity, methods are discussed by the predominant behavioral learning/conditioning approach (respondent, operant, and observational) upon which they were originally based. A case example is also presented illustrating the application of these various behavioral therapeutic techniques.

Before reviewing the various behavioral methods, it is important to consider why such methods should be included in treating clinical pain. For the most part, many would argue that pain is an internal subjective experience. From our previous discussion, it should be obvious that pain is not simply an internal subjective experience, but rather, a complex response system with a significant overt behavioral component. Thus, overt behavior needs to be addressed, and behavioral methods have demonstrated a clear ability to produce significant improvement in pain behavior. In addition, the presence of overt pain behaviors has been found to be a significant risk factor for chronic disability and dysfunction in low back pain patients [41, 42]. Likewise, the specific clinical goal to increase and/or maintain functional overt behavior in pain patients for maximum long-term improvement is considered fundamental in current clinical practice [43]. To date, behavioral strategies have been found to be some of the best methods to achieve such overt behavioral change.

A critical initial step for proper application of behavioral strategies involves a functional behavioral analysis (assessment) of the patient [1, 44]. The next section discusses the important fundamental components of such an assessment process.

Behavioral assessment strategies

As noted, proper application of behavioral methods depends upon a functional behavioral analysis of the patient. Such an assessment should result in identifying pain and well behaviors in need of change, as well as those antecedent and consequent stimulus conditions that consistently influence the presence or absence of such behaviors. Included in this process should be a determination of whether and to what extent identified controlling stimuli can be altered to produce a clinically significant change in relevant pain and well behaviors. When possible, this should also include consideration of altering any identified ongoing neurophysiological pain responses and tissue damage or irritation present. Such information typically leads to useful monitoring of pain behaviors and controlling stimuli, as well as identification of any behavioral treatment methods to consider for a given patient.

In addition to a detailed clinical interview, specific information to complete a useful functional behavioral analysis is commonly obtained by a combination of direct observation of the patient, behavioral assessment questionnaires, and patient self-monitoring. Table 11.4 summarizes examples of such assessment methods. All of the measures listed have demonstrated reliability and validity. The table includes example self-monitoring, direct observation, and questionnaire-based measures for various chronic pain conditions for adults and elderly patients with dementia, as well as non-verbal adult patients with acute traumatic injuries. Example behavioral measures for infants and children with acute and/or chronic painful conditions are also listed. The lower part of Table 11.4 offers examples for assessing and moni toring consequent controlling stimuli using patient's self-report questionnaires. Except for the presence of tissue damage or irritation detected from medical examination and diagnostic tests, along with the

detailed clinical interview and direct observation, specific, structured methods/measures to assess and identify controlling antecedent stimuli for pain behaviors are currently lacking.

The decision on which measurement technique to employ depends on the nature of the patient's clinical presentation and practical application of any assessment. It is recommended that direct observation of overt pain behavior be incorporated in assessment and monitoring whenever possible, as well as patient self-monitoring at least on an episodic basis. This should include self-report monitoring of the patient's subjective pain level. There are a number of reliable and valid rating scales to do this, including separate and combined word, numeric, and face expression scales (see Chapter 4 for a review of these various self-report measures of subjective pain level).

Operant-based therapeutics

The initial systematic application of operant conditioning to clinical pain can be credited to Fordyce and his colleagues [1]. Their pioneering work ushered in a major advancement in understanding and effectively treating chronic painful conditions. Much of the initial work was done with chronic low back pain patients, with more recent application including other chronic pain conditions such as fibromyalgia and tension or vascular headaches [5]. When operant learning/conditioning is used in a therapeutic context, it is typically referred to as contingency management or operant therapy. This section offers a more detailed description of empirically based operant methods with clinical pain, specifically focusing on chronic pain conditions.

Contingency management/operant therapy

This method involves applying the operant principles of contingent reinforcement and punishment, as well as antecedent discriminate stimulus control to overt pain and well behaviors. Table 11.5 delineates those fundamental indicators that operant conditioning effects are present and the basic conditions needed for effective usage of contingency management. As the table denotes, the presence of three or more indicators listed in the top portion suggests operant conditioning effects are influencing the patient's pain behaviors. Obviously, even when present, operant conditioning effects do not rule out or diminish the potential additional influence of other learning/conditioning factors or the presence of ongoing tissue damage/irritation.

Table 11.4 Example overt pain behaviors and controlling stimuli measures

Measure	Purpose	Method	Patient type
Overt pain behaviors			
Daily activity diary [1]	Monitor overt sit/walk/stand behaviors	Patient self-observe across day	Adults with various chronic pain conditions
Overt Pain Behavior Rating System [64]	Monitor 5 overt pain behaviors (e. g., rubbing, sighing, grimacing)	Time-limited direct observation of live conditions or video taped behaviors	Adults with various chronic pain
UBA Pain Behavior Scale [65]	Monitor 10 overt pain behaviors (e.g., moaning, conditions lying down, med. use)	Daily observer rating of behaviors	Adults with various chronic pain
Pain Behavior Checklist [52]	Monitor 20 overt pain behaviors (e.g., limping, cane use, posturing)	Single event observer rating of behaviors	Adults with various chronic pain conditions
Pain Behavior Observation System [66]	Monitor 5 overt pain behaviors (e.g., rubbing, sounds, facial action)	Time-limited direct observation of live behaviors	Adults with sub-acute or chronic low back pain
PAINAD [67]	Monitor 5 overt pain behaviors (e.g., pain face, breathing, sounds)	Time limited direct observation of live behaviors	Elderly with dementia with various pain conditions
PAINE [68, 69]	Monitor 22 overt pain behaviors (e.g., pain face, moaning, grimacing)	Single event observer scaled rating of behaviors	Elderly with dementia with various pain conditions
EPCA-2 [70]	Monitor 8 overt pain related behaviors (e.g., pain face, contact react)	Time limited direct observation of live behaviors	Nonverbal elderly with various pain conditions
CPOT [71]	Monitor 4 overt pain related behaviors (e.g., pain face, body posture)	Time-limited direct observation of live behaviors	Nonverbal ICU adults with various traumatic injuries (pain)
Neonatal Facial Coding System [72]	Monitor 10 facial actions (e.g., open mouth, nose wrinkle) seen with pain	Time-sampled direct observation of video taped facial expressions	Infants (0–12 months) during acute painful procedures
Child Facial Coding System [73]	Monitor 13 facial actions (e.g., eye squeeze, brow furrow) seen with pain	Time-sampled direct observation of video taped facial expressions	Children (2–5 yrs) during acute and some chronic pain conditions
Pain Expression Scale 74]	Monitor 10 overt pain behaviors (e.g., resting, pain face, complaining)	Single event parent scaled rating of behaviors	Children (8–18 yrs) with chronic rheumatic pain
Controlling stimuli			
Reinforcement Survey Schedules [75]	Identify reinforcers across activities/ experiences	60-item questionnaire completed by patient	Adult and child versions
Spouse Response Inventory [29]	Assess spouse response to patient pain & well behaviors	39-item questionnaire completed by patient	Adults with various chronic pain conditions
Multidimensional Pain Inventory-Section 2 [76]	Assess spouse response to patient pain behaviors	14-item questionnaire section completed by patient	Adults with various chronic pain conditions
Behavioral Assessment of Pain Questionnaire [77]	Assess spouse & physician response to patient pain behaviors	35-item questionnaire sections completed by patient	Adults with various chronic pain conditions

Table 11.5 Indicators of operant conditioning effects and conditions for contingency management usage

Operant conditioning effect indicators [a]

Overt pain behavior has been present for 3 months or longer

Overt pain behavior occurs as a function of the environment, time of day, or person(s) present (e.g., in the clinic, at night, with spouse present)

Overt pain behavior is acknowledged by others (e.g., the family, friends, health providers)

Overt pain behavior is sometimes followed by positive or negative consequences

Overt pain behavior is in excess of known physical findings

Patient expresses significant concern about increased pain with increased physical activity or return to work

Conditions for contingency management usage

Patient exhibiting overt pain behaviors

Salient positive and negative reinforcers can be identified

Sufficient environmental control is present to contingently applied antecedent and consequent stimulus conditions

Patient is not experiencing any major non-drug-related cognitive/learning impairment

Whenever possible, patient is willing to actively participate in treatment

[a] Operant conditioning effects are considered present given three or more indicators.

Even if no operant indicators are present, contingency management can be included in a treatment protocol when more adaptive well behaviors such as independent walking, laughing, or sustained exercising, are targeted for increase.

While there are analog studies showing the ability of operant conditioning techniques to influence acute pain behaviors (see evidence section), clinical application has for the most part involved adult chronic pain syndrome patients exhibiting low back, myofascial, and/or headache pain. Chronic pain syndrome is present when a patient exhibits any set of behaviors that involves complaints of enduring or recurring pain, pain has persisted longer than expected for a given condition, patient has responded inadequately to appropriate care, and pain is associated with significant impairment of function [43]. Chronic pain syndrome patients often may demonstrate significant mood disturbance and/or anger/hostility, but these symptoms are not considered necessary to make a diagnosis. When such patients are encountered,

contingency management/operant therapy should be considered.

Likewise, contingency management/operant therapy has been applied both in inpatient and outpatient settings. A functional behavioral analysis should provide useful information regarding which treatment setting is most appropriate. When a patient demonstrates the presence of very potent controlling conditions in the natural environment that cannot be altered or exhibits problem non-compliance, inpatient intervention is preferable. Also, those patients showing a need for close monitoring due to excessive medication usage with physical dependency and/or extreme physical deconditioning, are typically better served in an inpatient environment whenever possible. In practice, the majority of chronic pain patients suitable for such treatment receive contingency management within an outpatient treatment model.

Table 11.6 outlines basic application guidelines for effective use of contingency management/operant therapy. They should be considered generic guidelines for chronic pain syndrome patients presenting with various painful conditions. As highlighted in previous sections, the upper portion of the table focuses on behavioral assessment and the need to maintain some type of monitoring system during treatment to help guide decisions regarding revision and effectiveness. With this functional behavioral analysis information, a treatment plan can be established using the guidelines outlined in Table 11.6. This includes strategies to decrease various pain responses and increase well behaviors. As the table indicates, reduction in pain medication taking behavior should include changing the medication delivery schedule to a time contingent one, thus removing the contingent negative reinforcement effects (i.e., reduce, escape, or avoid increased nociception and/or physical withdrawal) typical with as needed pain contingent delivery. Such a change in the medication delivery strategy can be viewed as a form of response prevention in that patients are not allowed (prevented) from taking pain medication to contingently escape/avoid a specific increase in nociception and/or physical withdrawal symptoms. The guidelines also address the need to slowly reduce the frequency of reinforcers with an increase in well responses. This is based upon multiple studies showing that behavior reinforced intermittently is much more resistant to extinction or gradual reduction over time [12, 22]. Table 11.6 also recommends applying contingency management/operant therapy across as many environments and people as possible to

Table 11.6 Application guidelines for effective use of contingency management – operant therapy with chronic pain syndrome patients

Assessment and monitoring

Complete a functional behavioral analysis on patient including level of patient and family cooperation

Determine nature and extent of ongoing tissue damage/irritation as a contributing antecedent controlling stimulus. Incorporate this in setting realistic goals for pain and well behavior change

Maintain at least episodic, time sampled monitoring of relevant pain and well behaviors throughout treatment and follow-up. Use this information to make decisions about any treatment revisions and to demonstrate effectiveness

Treatment application guidelines

Focus on specific overt pain and well behaviors to change, using extinction, as well as positive and negative reinforcement strategies. Common behaviors might include pain medication usage, subjective pain ratings, standing/walking, working, limping, lying down

For escape avoidance pain responses include response prevention as part of the extinction process

To reduce medication-taking behavior, use scheduled, time contingent dose delivery, with gradual reduction in amount of medication per dose and/or day

To increase activity level, uptime, and/or physical exercise, determine baseline level and gradually increase at preset amounts, as determined by staff and patient, with frequent reinforcement

Apply the concept of shaping and gradual change for the initiation and increase in well behaviors

With consistent increase in well behaviors, slowly reduce the amount of positive and/or negative reinforcement to an intermittent varying schedule which reinforces the well behavior approximately 50% of the time

Use contingency management for overt pain and well behaviors in as many different environmental conditions and people to maximize ongoing generalization of the response and establishment of discriminate stimuli effects

Minimize/eliminate as many external controlling stimulus conditions that have been maintaining overt pain behavior in the natural environment as possible

Incorporate the cooperation of the patient and family if possible to directly apply contingency management strategies in the treatment and natural environments

Allow adequate time for contingency management to affect behavioral change, including following patients for at least 3–6 months after active treatment to promote long-term maintenance

When possible, incorporate contingency management methods within interdisciplinary treatment approaches

maximize generalization of effects, as well as to reduce the potential controlling effects of naturally occurring stimulus conditions. These two strategies are intended to strengthen maintenance of therapeutic change seen during treatment in the patient's natural environment over time. To further enhance longer-term maintenance, the guidelines also recommend following patients for 3–6 months after active treatment. Finally, the need to incorporate contingency management/operant therapy within a more comprehensive, interdisciplinary treatment model is emphasized. Given current access to and need for treatment methods across various disciplines and modalities typically seen with chronic pain syndrome patients, isolated application of contingency management/operant therapy is not only difficult and impractical, but also can be insufficient to accomplish maximum treatment effectiveness (see Chapter 3 and Chapter 8).

Biofeedback

While a more detailed description, evidence review, and application discussion is offered elsewhere in the current book (Chapter 13), the biofeedback paradigm is briefly highlighted in this section because of its original and fundamental operant basis. This involves the contingent reinforcement (with signal feedback and social praise) of certain neurophysiological pain responses such as striated muscle tension, peripheral blood flow, and somatosensory excitation. Likewise, it typically includes contingent social praise for changes in subjective pain ratings. Biofeedback has been successfully used to treat adult chronic pain patients with low back pain, headaches, phantom limb pain, and temporomandibular pain disorders [45, 46]. It has also been successfully applied to children with chronic pain conditions. Studies have shown that biofeedback techniques can produce significant improvement in subjective pain ratings, use of pain medications, and for low back pain patients, increased activity level. As with contingency management/operant therapy, research indicates that biofeedback is best applied in combination with other treatment modalities.

Respondent-based therapeutics

As the empirical research summarized in this chapter denotes, respondent learning effects can occur with those pain responses falling in the category of unconditioned reflexes (e.g., grimacing, withdrawal), escape/avoidant behavior (e.g., lying down, taking pain medications), and generalized emotional responses (e.g., crying, fear reaction to nociception). Given this, respondent-based therapeutics applied to clinical pain have shown an increase in acceptance and popularity. While the original explanation basis for Pavlovian conditioning has been expanded and modified with additional research findings [11, 16], the fundamental application remains rooted in Pavlov's respondent conditioning model, specifically, Pavlovian B conditioning involving use of the aversive unconditioned stimulus of nociceptive tissue damage or irritation. Exposure/desensitization and progressive muscle relaxation training are the two respondent-based approaches with the most empirical support. They are summarized in this section; see Chapters 12 and 13 for in-depth description, evidence review, and application recommendations. With a focus on musculoskeletal based chronic pain problems in adults, respondent methods have been shown to improve subjective pain ratings, increase activity, promote return to work, and reduce pain medication usage.

Exposure/desensitization

The fundamental paradigm involves gradually exposing patients to stimulus conditions – situations and/or behaviors which naturally elicit or have been classically conditioned to elicit pain nociception, fear of pain, and escape/avoidant pain behaviors. For example, a patient may be asked to engage in gradually increasing normal gait, exercise, and activities like stair climbing, which are time or distance based. It is important that this gradual increase in relevant well behaviors does not elicit or significantly exacerbate perceived pain nociception. Given that, repeated controlled exposure to engaging in these targeted well behaviors, while preventing the occurrence of incompatible escape/avoidant pain behaviors, leads to the extinction of respondent conditioning effects influencing pain and

well behaviors. Vlaeyen and colleagues [26,47,48] have shown that this paradigm results in a reduction in the fear of pain when present, as well as fear of increased activity level and/or movement. Such a reduction in fear is thought to "desensitize" the patient and lead to an increase in willingness to engage in more adaptive well behaviors.

While the consequences of targeted well behaviors are not really emphasized within the exposure/desensitization paradigm, the possible concurrent presence of operant conditioning here is obvious. This includes the real opportunity for positive and negative reinforcement through physical relief and/or absence of increased nociception, social praise, and self-praise. This point underscores the clear interactive nature between the various learning models.

Progressive muscle relaxation

As originally introduced, this method involves conditioning reduction in pain-related neurophysiological muscle excitation reaction in targeted striated muscles. This is accomplished by eliciting a reflex reaction in each targeted muscle by briefly tensing the muscle and then releasing it. This action is completed for all targeted muscle groups sequentially, thus pairing/associating these reflex responses across muscle groups and environmental stimuli. With repeated trials, these muscular reflex reactions are classically conditioned to occur across muscle groups with voluntary tension of just a few muscles. Given this conditioned reflex across striated muscles, patients can then trigger this response when needed to reduce pain-related muscle tension. Although research findings have called into question the actual presence of and need for a conditioned reflex response with progressive muscle relaxation [49], the utility of this method is widely acknowledged in clinical practice, including application with tension and vascular-based headaches in adults and children.

Observational based therapeutics

While there is good evidence that observational learning effects are present and influence at least overt pain responses [38], the development of empirically based observational therapeutics and the systematic application of observational learning in clinical pain are lacking. This section briefly describes those clinical strategies/situations where observational learning effects are most likely to be present, specifically, those situations where social modeling is present and may influence pain and well behaviors. Obviously, given the lack of systematic evidence, any specific guidelines or recommendations regarding the general application of observational-based therapeutics would be premature. Regardless of this and within the clinical arena, it is important to at least be aware of potential observational learning effects. The most obvious clinical situation rich with potential opportunities for observational learning to occur involves group therapy/treatment methods.

Group therapy/treatment

Within the clinical environment, it is not uncommon for pain patients to receive psychological and physical therapy using a group format. Detailed descriptions and recommendations on group therapy are given elsewhere [50, 51]. While the specific content, duration, and frequency of such groups can vary greatly, all involve pain patients observing one another participating in a structured activity. Herein lies the occasion for ongoing social modeling/observational learning. Unfortunately, the extent and appropriateness of such effects are for the most part not known or controlled. Thus, patients might receive either positive and/or negative therapeutic effects on pain behaviors from such observational learning. Negative effects might be particularly likely if there are few or no patients in the group exhibiting more appropriate and adaptive well behaviors.

Given the potential for actual negative therapeutic effects from observational learning and while no clear evidence is currently available to support it, an obvious point to consider is to include patients in both psychological and physical therapy groups that can serve as positive, appropriate social models. Obviously, this may not be possible in all cases, but can be accomplished most of the time if efforts are made to have patients at various stages of treatment and improvement participate in the group. Based upon observational learning theory, it should also be advantageous to focus on the commonalities across patients to increase perceived similarities. This should increase the probability and salience of any social modeling effects. In addition and realizing the presence of and opportunity for operant learning within groups, the potential influence of observational learning might be increased significantly by

ensuring that the social model's well behaviors are clearly and frequently reinforced during the group process.

Hopefully, the clinical and research communities will pay more attention to the potential effects and utility of observational learning with pain patients. There is certainly a great deal to gain from studying such effects, leading to the development of clinically useful observational therapeutic methods.

Case example of clinical application

The following example represents an actual case treated in an interdisciplinary outpatient pain rehabilitation program. It serves to illustrate the effective application of those behaviorally based methods just reviewed. The description will also include application of other treatment modalities such as physical therapy and certain medications, which typically occur in concert with behavioral intervention. The focus of this clinical example will be on process as opposed to outcome, with some basic outcome information included.

Patient demographics and medical presentation

The patient was a 51-year-old mildly obese, married, white male with a high school education. He was currently off work and receiving workers' compensation. He presented with a 2-year history of bilateral low back pain, with radiation into the right lower extremity, subsequent to a lifting injury sustained on the job as a truck driver. The pain was described as an aching sharp pain in the low back bilaterally, with secondary burning/shooting pain with numbness in the right lower extremity. The patient rated his subjective pain level at 8 on a 0–10 numerical scale. Initial post injury MRI showed a ruptured/herniated disk at lumbar vertebrae 4–5 (L4–5), while a more recent MRI showed some residual scar tissue at L4–5. Recent electromyography (EMG) of right lower extremity showed some residual nerve damage. All laboratory findings were within normal limits. Physical examination was within normal limits except for bilateral muscle tenderness with trigger points over the paraspinal lumbar region, as well as dermatomal sensory loss and mild muscle wasting in the right lower extremity. The patient did report suffering from hypertension, which was well-controlled with medication. Prior treatments included three lumbar epidural steroid injections with only time-limited benefit, multiple trials of passive and active physical therapy, partial diskectomy and laminectomy at L4–5 about 1 year after original injury, and medication management. Medications included ongoing opioids, anti-seizure medications for neuropathic based pain, muscle relaxants, and various sleep medications. The patient was also showing some dysphoria, poor appetite and sleep pattern, increased fatigue, reduced sex drive, and moderate anhedonia, indicating the presence of a major depression.

Functional behavioral analysis

In addition to the medical evaluation and history, behavioral/psychological information was obtained during a separate evaluation interview with the patient and his wife. This included specific questions to identify acute and chronic controlling stimuli for various pain behaviors, as well as the patient's fear of pain with activity and return to work. Direct behavioral observation was obtained during the medical and psychological/behavioral evaluations using the Pain Behavior Checklist [52], with the patient also completing the Spouse Response Inventory [29].

Table 11.7 summarizes the findings from this behaviorally based assessment. (Note: All of the information about controlling stimuli and pain responses delineated during the acute state, except the ruptured disc, were obtained from patient and spouse historical self-reports.) A review of the acute state portion of the table shows that the patient's pain responses were influenced by a number of other antecedent and consequent stimulus conditions besides just the disk herniation. These included multiple environmental stressors along with the brother's modeling effects, as well as at least four significant contingent consequent stimulus groups delivering both negative reinforcement (reduction in the aversive experience of subjective pain perception, tissue damage/irritation, and environmental stressors) and positive reinforcement (increase in social attention). These acute conditions along with those controlling stimuli which occurred as the patient's pain became more chronic, were sufficient to initiate and maintain the patient's clinical pain presentation. The bottom portion of Table 11.7 describes in more detail the observed pain responses and controlling stimuli present for the patient's chronic state as identified during the initial behavioral based assessment. A review of this portion of the table shows the presence of some additional chronic pain responses (e.g., use of brace and cane, images of being in a wheelchair), as well as a host of antecedent

and consequent stimuli influencing pain behavior. These included the development of antecedent conditioned/discriminative stimuli and residual tissue damage/irritation, and the addition of contingent escape/avoidance of drug withdrawal and positive economic gains.

Both the patient and his wife were interested in improving his pain responses, increasing his general level of function, as well as reducing his opioid medication usage. Given the level of interest and cooperation, it was determined that application of behavioral techniques on an outpatient basis would be possible. The patient was asked to monitor his subjective pain rating using the 0–10 scale on a daily basis, with The Pain Behavior Checklist completed by staff on a weekly basis. In keeping with recent recommendations regarding outcome evaluation [53], the Brief Pain Inventory [54, 55], and Beck Depression Inventory (see Chapter 13), along with these other measures, were used to assess treatment outcome. The patient's ICD-9 [57] based diagnoses included low back pain with radicular symptoms, chronic pain syndrome, and major depression.

Behavioral/interdisciplinary treatment

The patient was scheduled to participate in an outpatient pain rehabilitation program for 6 weeks, 3 days a week for 4–6 hours per day. This included individual and group therapy. The patient also received physical therapy and medication management concurrently with the behaviorally based treatments, with the wife being seen once a week to receive information to better understand the patient's pain presentation and appropriate responses to the patient's pain and well behaviors within the natural environment. Table 11.8 summarizes the behavioral treatment methods used for targeted pain and well responses. A review of the table indicates that a number of responses were targeted, with behavioral methods across the operant, respondent, and observational therapies utilized. Likewise, the basic recommendations specified in Table 11.6 regarding proper application of contingency management were followed. The specific dosing and rate reduction for opioid withdrawal followed clinical protocols and guidelines [58, 59].

Physical therapy treatment focused on active methods to gradually increase range of motion, gait, strength, and activities of daily living, with behavioral treatment concurrently applied to those relevant targeted behaviors occurring during physical therapy.

Table 11.7 Case example. Primary and secondary pain responses and controlling stimuli by acute and chronic pain states (52-year old male with 2-year history of work-related low back pain)

Controlling antecedent stimuli	Pain responses	Controlling consequent stimuli
	Acute state	
TISSUE DAMAGE/IRRITATION with ruptured disc at L4–5 ENVIRONMENTAL STRESSORS	NEUROPHYSIOLOGICAL ascending, cortical, descending, chemical excite	↓ SUBJECTIVE PAIN PERCEPTION: with opioids, lying down, guarding, limping
with workboss issues and physical strain with age, $ expenses from child injury, wife lost job *Pain Response Models* *with brother disabled from low back injury*	GROSS MOTOR moaning, pain complaints guarding, limping, taking opioids, lying down *Cognitive/Subjective* *fear of pain, pain is unbearable*	↓TISSUE DAMAGE/IRRITATION with rest, limping, guarding ↓ ENVIRONMENTAL STRESSORS with ↓ work issues-strain, delay of bill payments due to injury ↑ SOCIAL ATTENTION with friend visits, waited on by family, more wife affection
ENVIRONMENTAL STRESSORS	Chronic state GROSS MOTOR	↓ or AVOID STRESSORS
with no return to work=$ demands & boss demands to return, marital conflict, suggestions pain not real	acute state responses plus brace/cane COGNITIVE/SUBJECTIVE fear of pain, pain is unbearable, depression, images in wheelchair *Neurophysiological diminished acute state responses plus ↑ muscle tension*	with ↓ demands from wife-boss- bill collectors, justify no return to work & pain not real
CONDITIONED/DISCRIMINATIVE STIMULI with stairs, contact with wife-boss, sexual arousal, thoughts of work		↓ or AVIOD SUBJECTIVE PAIN PERCEPTION with increase in acute state behavior, use of TENS, message, sleeping
PAIN RESPONSE MODELS with more disabled brother contact		↓ or AVOID DRUG WITHDRAWAL with increase in opioid medication
Tissue damage/irritation *with L4–5 scar tissue & nerve fiber irritation*		↑ SOCIAL ATTENTION with more contact by children, brother, friends, other patients
		↑ ECONOMIC GAINS with workmans' compensation & short-term disability $ *↓ or avoid* *tissue damage/irritation with* *continued acute state behavior plus* *back brace & cane*

Primary (i.e., important contributor) stimuli/responses in capital letters; secondary (i.e., less important contributor) stimuli/responses in italics.

TENS: transcutaneous electrical nerve stimulation.

The patient also received clinically appropriate non-opioid medications. These included pregabalin for nerve fiber irritation (neuropathic) nociception, tizanidine for lumbar muscle tension (myofascial) nociception, and trazodone for improvement in sleep and mood.

Outcome and follow-up

Post-treatment assessment showed significant improvement in all targeted pain and well responses, in addition to significant positive changes in the patient's Brief Pain Inventory and Beck Depression Inventory scores. The patient had been successfully withdrawn

Table 11.8 Case example. Behavioral treatment methods by targeted pain and well responses

Target behaviors	Behavioral treatment methods	Rationale/effects
Pain responses		
Verbal pain complaints, moaning, guarding, limping, lying down	Extinction (withhold social attention to behaviors in clinic and at home) Reduce Environmental $ Stressor (wife gets job) Reduce Pain Model (limit contact with brother)	Stop contingent positive reward, reduce antecedent stressor & modeling effects
Use of back brace and cane, fear of pain	Extinction (withhold social attention & pain contingent usage) Exposure/Desensitization (initial very limited time contingent standing to walking without back brace and repeat without cane, with gradual increase in across time/distance across multiple settings)	Stop contingent positive & negative reward, gradually reduce escape/avoid fear, generalized settings
Taking opioids, fear of withdrawal & pain increase	Extinction (withhold pain contingent usage) Exposure/Desensitization (time contingent delivery, with gradual preset reduction in 24-hour dose until discontinued)	Stop contingent negative reward, gradually reduce escape/avoid fear of withdrawal/pain
Increase in lumbar muscle tension	Progressive muscle relaxation (daily practice using CD recording with restorative and preventive daily use)	Conditioned reflex muscle relaxation response to reduce muscle tension
Well responses		
Increases in activity/ standing- walking without brace/cane, exercise tolerance, smiling/ laughing, reduced pain reports/ subjective ratings	Contingency Management (ongoing contingent delivery of positive reinforcers, including social praise-massage-free time, across multiple settings using shaping technique) Social Modeling (daily exposure individually and in groups to patients engaging in reinforced well behaviors across settings)	Start contingent positive reward to increase well behaviors across multiple settings, with addition of observational learning effects
Climbing stairs, driving	Contingency Management (ongoing contingent delivery of positive reinforcers using shaping technique) Exposure/Desensitization (gradual, repetitive, exposure to stairs and sitting in car within reinforced shaping technique)	Start contingent positive reward to increase stair climbing and driving, while reducing avoidance fear

Note: Positive reinforcers were initially delivered continuously and gradually reduced to intermittent delivery approximately 50% of the time.

from opioids and was showing significant improvement in sleep, sex drive, and appetite. At six-month follow-up gains were maintained, with the patient also having been able to discontinue his trazodone medication. He reported having settled his worker's compensation case and currently being in school to acquire necessary skills for pursuing a job within his physical restrictions/limitations.

This case example describes a successful application of behaviorally based therapeutics within an interdisciplinary treatment setting. Obviously, all patients may not show the kind of positive response demonstrated here. Although, the vast majority of chronic pain syndrome patients can benefit significantly from inclusion of behavioral therapeutics in their treatment plan. There are, however, application limits with the behavioral therapeutics that should be considered.

Application limits

While behaviorally based therapeutics with chronic pain have solid empirical support, the majority of this research has been on chronic low back, headache, and musculoskeletal pain patients. Substantial evidence is lacking regarding application of behavioral methods with a number of other painful conditions such as complex regional pain syndrome, cancer pain, and some visceral pain syndromes. This is not to say that behavioral methods might not apply or work with these patient groups, but rather, to date, there is an absence of clear substantiating research. Likewise, application of behavioral therapeutics has not been adequately studied in acute pain, children (except for biofeedback with headaches), adolescents, or advanced geriatric patient groups. Given this, systematic, broad-based application of behavioral therapeutics for these painful conditions and patient groups can not yet be routinely recommended until more evidence is available. However, if any such patients demonstrate a chronic pain syndrome, the possible application of behavioral therapeutics should be explored.

Clinical and research needs

As the field of pain medicine and rehabilitation continues to evolve and expand, there are some important clinical and research issues/needs regarding behavioral therapeutics. At the clinical level, there is a growing need to reinforce and heighten awareness within the medical and insurance communities about the real potential benefits of considering and incorporating behavioral assessment and therapeutics within treatment planning for pain patients. Given the clear influence of interactional learning/conditioning effects on clinical pain, appreciating and incorporating behaviorally based assessment and treatment approaches could significantly improve the care of these patients. This is particularly true when looking at primary and secondary prevention of chronic painful conditions. As has now been demonstrated in the literature [60], early detection and intervention using behavioral and cognitive-based assessment and treatment can significantly reduce the occurrence of pain chronicity and disability, at least for back pain patients.

There are a multitude of research needs. These include such areas as more substantiation and testing of the various components and assumptions within the interactional conditioning/learning model for pain, studies to better understand the learning mechanisms involved in transition from acute to chronic states, and more detailed delineation of interactions and effects within and between pain response and stimulus categories. In addition, clinical studies are needed to better determine patient to behavioral treatment matching, comparative effectiveness to other types of psychological, physical therapy, procedural, and pharmacological methods, as well as comparative cost effectiveness

with other treatment approaches. More research determining the effectiveness and upper limits of behavioral methods with a variety of other chronic and acute painful conditions, clinical settings, and patient populations is needed. Likewise, studying and developing clinically useful methods using observational learning effects need to be done. Research on possible strategies to reduce/prevent relapse with behavioral techniques is lacking [61, 62], as well as more studies examining the potential utility of more broad-based environmental stimulus control strategies to better manage clinical pain [63].

Behaviorally based therapeutics have enjoyed a rich history of research and clinical application. However, only with continued scientific efforts focused on such concepts and treatment methods can they evolve and maintain an important role in the understanding and management of clinical pain. The alternative is a gradual decline to "extinction" of this critical body of knowledge.

References

1. Fordyce, WE. *Behavioral Methods for Chronic Pain and Illness* (St. Louis, MO, Mosby, 1976).

2. Fordyce WE, Shelton JL, Dunmore DE. The modification of avoidance learning pain behaviors. *J Behav Med* 1982; **5**: 415–14.

3. Sternbach R. *Pain: A psychophysiological analysis* (NY: Academic Press, 1968).

4. Merskey, H Bogduk, N. *Classification of Chronic Pain* (Seattle, WA: IASP Press, 1994).

5. Sanders SH. Operant therapy with pain patients: Evidence for its effectiveness. *Sem Pain Med* 2003; **1**: 90–8.

6. Evers AWM, Kraaimaat FW, van Riel PLCM, *et al*. Cognitive, behavioral, and physiological reactivity to pain as a predictor of long-term pain in rheumatoid arthritis patients. *Pain* 2001; **93**: 139–46.

7. Flor H, Hermann C. Biopsychosocial models of pain. In *Psychosocial Aspects of Pain: A handbook for health care providers*, eds. RH Dworkin, WS Breitbart. (Seattle, WA: IASP Press, 2004), pp. 47–75.

8. Staats PS, Hekmat H, Staats AW. The psychological behaviorism theory of pain: A basis for unity. *Pain Forum* 1996; **5**: 194–207.

9. Pavlov I. *Conditioned Reflexes* (London: Oxford University Press, 1927).

10. Grant, DA. Classical and operant conditioning. In *Categories of Human Learning*, ed. AW Melton. (New York: Academic Press, 1964), pp. 1–31.

11. Mowrer RR, Klein SB, eds. *Hand Book of Contemporary Learning Theory* (Mahwah, NJ: Lawrence Erlbaum Associates, 2001).

12. Reynolds GS. *A Primer of Operant Conditioning* (Glenview, Il: Scott, Foresman, Co., 1968).

13. Skinner, BF. *Science and Human Behavior* (New York: McMillan, 1953).

14. Sidman M. Operant techniques. In *Experimental Foundations Of Clinical Psychology,* ed. AJ Bachrach. New York: Basic Books, 1962), pp. 170–210.

15. Hollis KL. Contemporary research on Pavlovian conditioning: A "new" functional analysis. *Am Psychol* 1997; **52**: 956–65.

16. Mineke S, Zinburg P. A contemporary learning theory perspective on the analogy of anxiety disorders. It's not what you thought it was. *Am Psychol* 2006; **61**; 20–6.

17. Donahoe JW, Vegas R. Pavlovian conditioning: The CS–UR relation. *J ExpPsychol Anim Behav Processes* 2004; **30**: 3–16.

18. Diesch E, Flor H. Alteration in the response properties of the primary somato-sensory cortex related to differential aversive Pavlovian conditioning. *Pain* 2007; **131**: 171–80.

19. Schneider C, Palomba D, Flor H. Pavlovian conditioning of muscular responses in chronic pain patients: Central and peripheral correlates. *Pain* 2004; **112**: 239–47.

20. Klinger R, Soost S, Flor H, Worm M. Classical conditioning and expectancy in placebo hypoalgesia: A randomized controlled study in patients with atopic dermatitis and persons with healthy skin. *Pain* 2007; **128**: 31–9.

21. Williams AE, Rhudy JL. The influence of conditioned fear on human pain thresholds: Does preparedness play a role? *J Pain* 2007; **8**: 598–606.

22. Lattal KA, ed. Reflections on BF Skinner in psychology. *American Psychologist* 1992; **47**: 1269–533.

23. Bandura A. *Social Learning Theory* (Englewood Cliffs, NJ: Prentice Hall, 1977).

24. Bandura A. *Foundations of Thought and Action: A Social Cognitive Theroy* (Englewood Cliffs, NJ: Prentice Hall, 1986).

25. Galef BG, Laland KN. Social learning in animals: Empirical studies and theoretical models. *Bioscience* 2005; **55**: 489–99.

26. Vlaeyen JWS, Linton SJ. Fear-avoidance and its consequences and chronic musculoskeletal pain: A state-of-the-art. *Pain* 2000; **85**: 317–32.

27. Jolliffe CD, Nicholas MK. Verbally reinforcing pain reports: An experimental test of the operant model of chronic pain. *Pain* 2004; **107**: 167–75.

28. Thomas JS, France CR. Pain-related fear is associated with avoidance of spinal motion during recovery from low back pain. *Spine* 2007; **32**: 460–66.

29. Schwartz L, Jensen MP, Romano JM. The development and psychometric evaluation of an instrument to assess spouse responses to pain and well behavior in patients with chronic pain: The Spouse Response Inventory. *J Pain* 2005; **6**: 243–52.

30. Walker LS, Williams SE, Smith CA, *et al.* Parent attention versus distraction: Impact on symptom complaints by children with and without chronic functional abdominal pain. *Pain* 2006; **122**: 43–52.

31. Lousberg R, Vuurman E, Lamers T, *et al.* Pain report and pain-related evoked potentials operantly conditioned. *Clin J Pain* 2005; **21**, 262–71.

32. Giardino ND, Jensen MP, Turner JA, *et al.* Social environment moderates the association between catastrophizing and pain among persons with spinal cord injury. *Pain* 2003; **106**: 19–25.

33. Moseley GL, Arntz A. The context of noxious stimulus affects the pain it evokes. *Pain* 2007; **133**: 64–71.

34. Holzl R, Kleinbhl D, Huse E. Implicit operant learning of pain sensitization. *Pain*, 2005; **115**: 12–20.

35. McDonald RV, Siegel S. Intra-administration associations and withdrawal symptoms: morphine-elicited morphine withdrawal. *Exp Clin Psychopharmacol* 2004; **12**: 3–11.

36. Sokolowska M, Segal S, Kim JA. Intra-administration associations: Conditioned hyperalgesia elicited by morphine onset cues. *J Exp Psychol Anim Behav Processes* 2002; **28**: 319–320.

37. Taddio A, Shah V, Gilbert-MacLeod C, *et al.* Conditioning and hyperalgesia in newborns exposed to repeated heel lances. *JAMA* 2006; **295**: 793–800.

38. Goodman JE, McGrath PJ. Mothers' modeling influences children's pain during a cold pressor task. *Pain* 2003; **104**: 559–65.

39. Sullivan MJAO, Adams H, Sullivan ME. Communicative dimensions of pain catastrophizing: Social cueing effects on pain behavior and coping. *Pain* 2004; **107**: 220–6.

40. Raber P, Devor M. Social variables affect phenotype in the neuroma model of neuropathic pain. *Pain* 2002; **97**: 139–50.

41. Prkachin KM, Schultz IZ, Hughes E. Pain behavior and the development of pain-related disability: The importance of guarding. *Clin J Pain* 2007; **23**: 270–7.

42. Sanders SH. Risk factors in the development and management of low back pain in adults. In *Low Back*

Pain: A symptom based approach to diagnosis and treatment, eds. KS Rucker, AJ Cole and SM Weinstein. (Boston, MA: Butterworth Heinemann, 2000), pp. 299–311.

43. Sanders SH, Harden RN, Vicente PJ. Evidence-based clinical practice guidelines for interdisciplinary rehabilitation of chronic nonmalignant pain syndrome patients. *Pain Pract* 2005; **5**: 303–15.

44. Sanders SH. Operant conditioning with chronic pain: back to basics. In *Psychological Approaches to Pain Management: A practitioner's handbook,* 2nd edn., eds. DC Turk RJ Gatchel (New York: Guilford Press, 2002), pp. 128–37.

45. Andrasik F. The essence of biofeedback, relaxation, and hypnosis. In *Psychosocial Aspects of Pain: A handbook for health care professionals,* eds. RH Dworkin and WS Breitbart. (Seattle, WA: IASP Press, 2004), pp. 285–315.

46. Gatchel JR, Pulliam C, Maddrey AM. Biofeedback with pain patients: Evidence for its effectiveness. *Semin Pain Med* 2003; **1**: 55–66.

47. Vlaeyen JWS. Fear and musculoskeletal pain. In *Proceedings of the 10th World Congress on Pain,* eds. JO Dostrovsky, DB Carr and M Koltzenburg. (Seattle, WA: IASP Press, 2003), pp. 631–50.

48. Vlaeyen JWS, de Jong J, Siewben J, *et al.* Graded exposure in vivo for pain-related fear. In *Psychological Approaches to Pain Management: A practitioner's handbook,* 2nd edn. eds. DC Turk and RJ Gatchel. (New York: Guilford Press, 2002), pp. 210–33.

49. Kessler RS, Patterson RC, Dane J. Hypnosis and relaxation with pain patients: Evidence for its effectiveness. *Seminars in Pain Med* 2003; **1**: 67–78.

50. Keefe FJ, Beaupre PM, Gil KM, *et al.* Group therapy for patients with chronic pain. In *Psychological Approaches to Pain Management: A practitioner's handbook,* eds. DC Turk and RJ Gatchel. (New York: Guilford Press, 2002), pp. 234–55.

51. Liddle SD, Baxter GD, Gracey JH. Exercise in chronic low back pain: What works? *Pain* 2004; **107**: 176–90.

52. Turk DC, Wack JT, Kerns RD. An empirical examination of the "pain behavior" construct. *J Behav Med* 1985; **8**: 119–30.

53. Dworkin RH, Turk DC, Wyrwich KW, *et al.* Interpreting the clinical importance of treatment outcomes and chronic pain clinical trials: IMMPACT recommendations. *J Pain* 2008; **9**: 105–21.

54. Cleeland CS. Measurement of pain by subjective report. In *Advances in Pain Research and Therapy. Volume 12. Issues in Pain Measurement,* eds. CR Chapman and JD Loeser. (New York: Raven Press 1989), pp. 391–403.

55. Tan, G, Jensen, MP, Thornby, JI, *et al.* Validation of the Brief Pain Inventory for chronic nonmalignant pain. *J Pain* 2004; **5**: 133–37.

56. Beck, AJ, Steer, RA, *Beck Depression Inventory* (San Antonio, TX: Psychological Corp).

57. American Medical Association. *ICD-9 CM 2008* (Washington, DC: AMA, 2008).

58. Hare, BD Lipman, AG. Uses and misuses of medication in the management of chronic, noncancer pain. In *Problems in Anesthesia: Chronic Pain,* eds. BD Hare and PG Fine. (Hagerstown, MD: JB Lippincott, 1990), pp. 577–94.

59. NICE. *Drug Misuse: Opioid Detoxification*; 2007. www.nice.org.uk. [accessed June 2010].

60. Linton SJ, Boersma K, Jansson M, *et al.* The effect of cognitive-behavioral and physical therapy preventative interventions on pain-related sick leave: A randomized controlled trial. *Clin J Pain* 2005; **21**, 109–19.

61. Morley S. Relapse prevention: Still neglected after all these years. *Pain 2008*; **134**, 239–40.

62. Naylor MR, Keefe FJ, Brigidi B, *et al.* Therapeutic interactive voice response for chronic pain reduction and relapse prevention. *Pain* 2008; **134**: 335–45.

63. Malenbaum S, Keefe FJ, Williams AC, *et al.* Pain in its environmental context: Implications for designing environments to enhance pain control. *Pain* 2008; **134**: 241–4.

Cognitive behavioral therapy in pain management

John D. Otis, Donna B. Pincus and Mary E. Murawski

Cognitive-behavioral therapy (CBT) is a skills-based treatment approach that focuses on teaching patients ways to identify and change maladaptive thoughts, feelings, and behaviors, and to replace them with those that are more adaptive, with the ultimate goal of improving patients' overall quality of life and reducing psychological distress. In addition, cognitive-behavioral treatment approaches focus on changing certain target behaviors that appear to be problematic and teaching adaptive ways of coping. Cognitive-behavioral approaches have been shown to be highly effective in treating a range of disorders, from depression and other mood disorders to pain disorders in adults and in children. The application of the cognitive-behavioral model to the management of chronic pain is based on the understanding that pain is a complex experience that is not only influenced by the presence of underlying pathology, but also by an individual's thoughts, emotions and behaviors [1]. When applied to the treatment of chronic pain, the CBT approach targets patients' maladaptive cognitive and behavioral coping and promotes the adoption of perceptions of enhanced personal control related to pain and an adaptive and active problem-solving approach to pain management.

Cognitive and behavioral interventions have gained considerable empirical support for their efficacy in the management of chronic pain. In a study of 28 veterans with chronic pain, Kerns et al. found that relative to patients placed in a wait-list (WL) control condition, patients who received behavioral and cognitive behavioral treatments for their pain demonstrated significant reductions in their use of the healthcare system [2]. In addition, only patients receiving CBT showed significant improvements on multiple self-report measures of pain severity, affective distress, instrumental daily activity, and dependency. A study by Turner and Clancy demonstrated the efficacy of cognitive-behavioral (CB) and operant-behavioral

(OB) therapy in the treatment of chronic low back pain when compared to a WL control condition [3]. Their results indicated that participants assigned to the CB or OB conditions demonstrated significantly greater improvements in physical and psychosocial disability when compared to participants in the WL condition. While improvements reported by the CB and OB participants were not significantly different at 12-month follow-up, participants in the CB condition reported higher treatment satisfaction and rated their treatment as more helpful. Research also suggests that CB interventions can have the added benefit of decreasing the use of clinical services and costs associated with pain care [4]. As a more recent example, in a randomized controlled trial conducted by Turner et al., patients completing a four-session CB intervention for pain associated with temporomandibular disorder showed significantly greater improvements in adaptive coping with pain, lower pain interference, and greater clinically meaningful improvements in pain intensity, jaw function, and depression at 12-month follow-up when compared with patients assigned to an education/attention control condition [5]. This particular study has been praised for its methodological rigor and sophistication among randomized clinical trials evaluating cognitive-behavioral interventions for pain [6]. In a frequently cited meta-analysis, Morley et al. concluded from the examination of 25 randomized controlled trials that CBT for chronic pain is effective, as it resulted in significantly greater improvements in pain experience, cognitive coping and appraisal, and reductions in behavioral expressions of pain when compared with alternative active treatments [7]. Further, in a recent meta-analysis of 22 randomized controlled trials of psychological treatments for non-cancerous chronic low back pain, CB and self-regulatory treatments were found to be efficacious [8].

Behavioral and Psychopharmacologic Pain Management, ed. Michael H. Ebert and Robert D. Kerns. Published by Cambridge University Press. © Cambridge University Press 2011.

Structure of cognitive-behavioral therapy for chronic pain

Key components of CBT for pain management

The primary goal of CBT for pain management is to promote an active approach to tackling the many challenges associated with the experience of chronic pain. A shift from a perspective of helplessness with regard to these challenges to one of personal responsibility, self-control, and confidence is encouraged. The cognitive-behavioral approach is informed by the understanding that people generally do not stop being active because of pain, but because they have become adjusted to the idea that they are physically disabled. Thus, CBT for chronic pain involves challenging negative thinking, changing behaviors that are contributing to the experience of pain, and teaching patients ways of safely reintroducing enjoyable activities. This can be a particularly daunting task when pain-related thoughts and behaviors have been in place for many years.

While CBT for chronic pain may include a variety of skills and techniques, there are several components that may be considered "core elements" to this approach for chronic pain management. These elements include graded homework assignments, cognitive restructuring (i.e., teaching patients to challenge negative thinking), relaxation training (i.e., teaching diaphragmatic breathing, visual imagery, progressive muscle relaxation, etc.), and time-based activity pacing (i.e., teaching patients to pace themselves based on time rather than work accomplished).

Since individuals who experience chronic pain often report reduced activity levels and declines in social role functioning, graded task assignments that emphasize increased activity and productive functioning are essential for treatment and encourage the reintroduction of a healthy and more active lifestyle. Prior to the onset of treatment, a therapist should work with the patient to outline the specific overall treatment goals that will be worked towards over the course of therapy. These goals should be behavioral and quantifiable rather than goals such as "experiencing less pain" or "feeling better about myself". For example, a patient who has set an overall treatment goal of walking 1 mile per day by the end of the treatment program could begin by setting the goal of walking half a mile three times per week and gradually increasing the distance walked with each visit to the therapist. Goals do not have to focus on exercise; rather, goals can include performing activities such as having lunch with a friend, working on an art project or other hobby, or spending more time with family. Each therapy session would begin with a review of the goals assigned during the previous session and an evaluation by the patient and the therapist, using a weekly goal completion form, to determine the extent to which the patient achieved the assigned goals (See Figure 12.1). Making homework evaluation an expected part of treatment increases the likelihood of homework completion and builds into therapy an opportunity to positively reinforce the patient for goal accomplishment.

Cognitive restructuring is a process for teaching patients to recognize the thoughts that give rise to negative emotions, to evaluate the thoughts by gathering evidence for or against the thought, and then to change negative thoughts into more adaptive thoughts. One of the first steps in teaching this skill is to educate the patient on the power of "automatic thoughts." Automatic thoughts are thoughts that one has immediately after getting any kind of information. They occur very quickly, and without instruction to pay sufficient attention to them, patients may not even be aware of them. Automatic thoughts are often very adaptive. For example, a person arriving home late one evening to find his front door open and broken glass on his steps might immediately think that someone had broken in to his house. However, there are times when automatic thoughts are not based on logic, but instead are based on biases and faulty information. These thoughts can trigger even more negative thoughts that can have an impact on emotions and how patients feel physically, including the experience of pain. Patients can usually identify a time when they became emotionally worked up over an event only later to find out that their thoughts were not accurate and they had been unnecessarily upset. Using a cognitive restructuring worksheet is a helpful way to bring a patient through the process of how to identify and challenge negative thoughts. As practice continues, individuals gain skill in changing maladaptive thoughts and thus reducing negative emotions that can impact pain (see Figure 12.2).

When some people begin a project it is very hard for them to stop working on it before it's completed. They work on the project non-stop despite the onset of pain. As a result of "working through" the pain, the

Therapy Session Number: _____

Please rate goal accomplishment for the week by marking the scale below: 0 (not at all accomplished) to 10 (completely accomplished). Please complete for each established goal.

Goal 1.   Walk around the block twice a week_____

0   1   2   3   4   ⑤   6   7   8   9   10
Notes:_only walked around the block once_____

Goal 2.   Go to lunch with my friend_____

0   1   2   3   4   5   6   ⑦   8   9   10
Notes:_____

Goal 3.   _Work on an art project_____

0   1   2   3   4   5   6   7   8   ⑨   10
Notes:_____

Goal 4.   _____

0   1   2   3   4   5   6   7   8   9   10

Notes:_____

Goal 5.   _____

0   1   2   3   4   5   6   7   8   9   10

Notes:_____

Figure 12.1 Weekly goal completion form. Adapted from Fig. 4.1, p.30 from *Managing Chronic Pain by Otis, John D.* (2007) By permission of Oxford University Press, Inc.

level of pain increases as the patient continues working on the project. This can sometimes result in severe pain that requires rest for an extended period of time before a person is able to work again. Once the pain decreases, the person may feel the necessity of working extra hard in order to catch up on time lost, and does everything on the "to do" list on that day, only to end up in more pain for days afterwards. This cycle of work, pain, and rest is very common for individuals who have chronic pain. One method for breaking this cycle is called "time-based pacing." Time-based pacing is a process in which activity breaks are based on time intervals, not on how much of the job is completed. For example, a patient is asked to identify a job they frequently do that can result in increased pain. The patient is asked to estimate how long he can perform the job before his pain increases (active time) and how long he will need to rest before becoming active again (rest time). This active-rest schedule is then used when completing the entire project. Although different jobs will require different active-rest cycles, using a time-based pacing strategy will reduce time spent recovering from pain flare-ups due to over activity.

When placed in the proper sequence, the skills taught in each CBT session build on one another in a sequential manner, encourage confidence and self-efficacy, and help to promote increased control over the experience of chronic pain. There are a number of CBT-based treatment manuals available that can be useful treatment tools for therapist and patients (see Table 12.1).

Treatment modality: individual vs. group treatment

Cognitive-behavioral therapy for pain management can be facilitated in individual or group formats, both with potential benefits and challenges that are important to consider when choosing the optimal treatment modality for a new patient. While individual therapy

Situation	Emotion	Automatic thought	Evidence for	Evidence against	Positive coping thought
Describe the event that led to the unpleasant emotion	Specify sad, angry, etc. and rate the emotion from 0 to 100%	Write the automatic thought that preceded the emotion	What is the evidence that this thought is true?	What is the evidence that this thought is false?	What else can I say to myself instead of the automatic thought?
My pain increases for no apparent reason	Frustrated 100% depressed 70%	I cant take this, I cant cope with my pain	Sometimes it is hard to do the things I want to do because of my pain	There are times when the pain is not so bad, and I can have a good time doing activities I enjoy	Even though I may feel pain at times, I am still able to do many things, and I can cope well many times. I will focus on my positive abilities to cope with anything that comes my way
					Emotion
					Re-rate the emotion from 0 to 100% Frustrated 40% Depressed 30%

Figure 12.2 Cognitive restructuring worksheet adapted from Fig. 7.1 p. 62 from *Managing Chronic Pain* by Otis, John D. (2007) By permission of Oxford University Press, Inc.

is sometimes specifically requested by patients, there are several advantages to group treatment. First, group treatment is more time-efficient for the therapist, who is able to provide treatment to anywhere from 5 to 10 participants at the same time. Second, group treatment provides a mechanism for participants to learn coping skills from other group members who may have similar pain complaints or who have had to overcome similar hurdles in coping with a painful medical condition. Utilizing real-life examples from group members is helpful when illustrating the use of new skills (e.g., cognitive restructuring). Third, interacting with others in a group may enable patients to see that they are not alone in dealing with the distress and disability

that often accompany chronic pain. Further, conducting treatment in a group format allows patients who have chronic pain to gain valuable social support from other group members. However, there are times when individual therapy will be the treatment approach of choice. Individual therapy provides greater opportunity for patient-specific problem solving and goal setting. For example, in an individual format, a therapist can devote more time to directly addressing the issues and challenges most relevant to the patient and tailoring treatment to meet his needs. There is more flexibility in timing of sessions when providing individual therapy, as sessions can be scheduled to meet the needs of one person rather than a group. In addition, a patient

Table 12.1 Cognitive behavioral therapy (CBT)-based treatment manuals

Title	Author	Brief description
Managing Chronic Pain: A Cognitive-Behavioral Therapy Approach (Both Therapist Guide and Patient Workbook available)	John D. Otis, Ph.D.	CBT manual for the treatment of chronic pain, part of acclaimed Treatments That Work Series, helpful for both clinicians and patients
Cognitive Therapy for Chronic Pain: A Step-by-Step Guide	Beverly E. Thorn, Ph.D.	Cognitive therapy for pain management, helpful for clinicians working with patients living with chronic pain
Mastering Chronic Pain: A Professional's Guide to Behavioral Treatment (Both Therapist Guide and Patient Handbook available)	Robert N. Jamison, Ph.D.	CBT-based program for pain management, helpful for both clinicians and patients
Managing Pain Before it Manages You, 3rd edn.	Margaret A. Caudill, M.D., Ph.D., M.P.H.	Useful self-help reference for patients trying to manage chronic pain
The Pain Survival Guide: How to Reclaim Your Life	Dennis C. Turk, Ph.D and Frits Winter, Ph.D.	Self-help reference for patients trying to cope with the impact of chronic pain on daily life, part of APA Lifetools series

may report feeling uncomfortable sharing information with a group.

Important treatment issues

Several specific issues that can influence the effectiveness of treatment warrant further discussion, including access to care, engagement in treatment, and maintenance of treatment effects. While CBT approaches have been found to be highly effective, providers may need to continually work to reduce barriers and increase access to care. One way that therapists can facilitate access is by regularly communicating with other healthcare providers, such as primary care physicians, who frequently interact with patients with chronic pain. These providers can be encouraged to educate their patients regarding non-invasive treatment options such as CBT. Access can also be facilitated by offering treatment in accessible locations such as community-based clinics, or in office space within the primary care setting. In order for benefits to be obtained from CBT for pain management a patient will need to be engaged in the process of therapy and adhere to weekly treatment goals. This should be encouraged in the first session of therapy by giving the patient a simple and convincing rationale for investing time and effort in treatment. Providing the patient with a convincing rationale for coming to therapy, consistently practicing newly learned skills, and completing out-of-session homework is critical. Additionally, it is beneficial to assist the patient with maintaining motivation to adhere to treatment by acknowledging the

time and effort involved in making lifestyle changes while highlighting the numerous potential benefits of doing so. It is important that therapists acknowledge the limitations of treatment and set realistic expectations related to treatment outcomes (i.e., the pain may never go away). Lastly, to best facilitate maintenance of treatment effects, teaching relapse prevention and problem-solving skills is imperative.

Application of the CBT model to the primary care setting

A "stepped care" approach, which emphasizes care coordination among providers, can be used to assist primary care physicians when treating patients who have chronic pain. Using this approach, the level of care is guided by a patient's response to treatment and readiness to engage in self-care [9]. This approach has been used for a variety of medical conditions and health behaviors including alcohol use [10], cigarette use [11], and cholesterol level reduction [12]. The approach can be conceptualized as consisting of three successive steps that are guided by the patient's response to treatment in the preceding step.

Step 1 is appropriate for all patients seeking treatment for pain from their primary care provider; it involves identifying and addressing specific patient concerns about pain and enhancing patient readiness for self-care. For example, one common concern of patients is that pain is a symptom of underlying disease or pathology. Once this concern is identified, the primary care provider can address it by explaining how obtaining a detailed medical history and performing a diagnostic examination can exclude such conditions. A patient who has pain may also fear that exercise or activity will result in further injury. This concern can be addressed by explaining the benefits of remaining active and by creating a plan with the patient for gradually returning to a safe level of activity.

Techniques based on motivational interviewing can be employed by primary care providers to encourage patients' readiness to engage in self-care behaviors [13]. These techniques include addressing a patient's unrealistic expectations of the likelihood of a medical cure for pain, offering support for effective self-care strategies he/she is currently using, and developing a plan for managing pain flare-ups. Psychologists can facilitate this communication by educating and training primary care providers, medical residents, and interns in motivational interviewing to improve provider–patient communication.

Step 2 is appropriate for patients who continue to experience pain and disability several weeks after the initial primary care visit. These patients require a more active approach to pain management that may include identifying the specific difficulties they are experiencing (e.g., pain when lifting heavy objects at work), developing and implementing an individually tailored treatment plan, and providing support and follow-up. Given that implementing this intervention might require additional time, a consultation with a psychologist is an important option for a primary care provider. After a brief screening evaluation, the psychologist determines whether the patient's goals are more likely to be achieved through brief individual therapy or a more comprehensive program for pain management. Alternatively, the psychologist can encourage the patient's engagement in psychoeducational groups led by peers or healthcare professionals with expertise in pain management. Research studies investigating the efficacy of active psychoeducational programs for patients with pain have yielded positive results [14, 15].

Step 3 is appropriate for the patient who continues to experience a significant level of disability and emotional distress despite the efforts of the primary care provider or the availability of brief therapy or psychoeducational programs. Individuals in this stage may have complex medical and social histories and are often seen as very challenging cases to manage within the limitations of the primary care setting.

Interdisciplinary pain management programs are well suited for this type of patient care. For these patients, more extensive involvement of the psychologist or other mental health professionals may be indicated. Psychologists can teach providers to encourage and motivate patients to take advantage of the services that psychologists have to offer.

Application of the CBT model to different populations

Children

Brief episodes of acute pain related to routine injuries and illnesses are common throughout development, with 15% of healthy school-aged children reporting brief episodes of pain [16]. Children typically have short-lived responses to acute pain, and normal activity is often quickly resumed, as is typically observed with adults. However, chronic pain in children, often associated with an underlying disease, a traumatic injury, or an ongoing trauma causing sustained injury can result in a considerable amount of suffering in the child and family, disruption of the family routine, and restriction of the child's daily activities, thereby increasing the risk of long-term disability [17]. Chronic pain in childhood has been shown to interfere in children's quality of life, causes many missed days from school, and often causes the family to seek medical care for pain relief [18]. In fact, chronic pain in childhood can often result in somatic and psychiatric dysfunction, with studies showing that children experiencing chronic pain are more likely than other children to complain of anxiety, to demonstrate hypochondriacal beliefs, to engage less frequently in social activities, and to experience higher levels of generalized anxiety [19]. Chronic pain conditions in childhood may arise due to known injury (such as rheumatologic disease, sickle cell disease, or HIV infection), or to traumatic injury (due to burns, physical abuse, or motor vehicle accidents), while some chronic pain conditions in childhood may have less clear etiologies, e.g., chronic headache [16]. Due to increased research over the past 20 years on chronic pain in children, we now understand that children's pain, like adult's pain, is not simply directly related to the extent of physical injury or level of tissue damage, but is influenced by many psychological factors that can modify the neural signals for pain and increase or decrease a child's distress. Researchers have suggested that children's pain is more plastic than that of adults, such that psychosocial factors may exert an even more powerful influence on children's pain perception than on adults' pain perception [20]. For example, parents' response to children's expression of pain can either further exacerbate or reduce the child's perception or expression of pain. In addition, children's ongoing physical growth may also play a role in their ability to recover more quickly than adults from injury.

The presentation of chronic pain in children may also differ from that of adults, and there are numerous factors that may influence the child's experience of pain, including child factors (e.g., cognitive level, or temperament), behavioral factors (e.g., child's distress responses, avoidance of activities), cognitive factors (e.g., expectations about treatment efficacy), and emotional factors (e.g., anticipatory anxiety, depression [20]. While some of these factors are stable for a child (e.g., temperament), other factors change progressively, (e.g., age, cognitive level, physical state, and family learning). Child factors and situational factors (e.g., level of control over situation) may interrelate to shape how children generally interpret the various sensations caused by tissue damage. For example, as children grow, they learn ways to express pain and ways to cope with pain, and their experience is certainly shaped by their family, culture, and interactions with caregivers and peers. This notion is consistent with Melzack and Wall's gate control theory, which conceptualized pain as a multidimensional experience, characterized by physiologic, affective, cognitive, behavioral, and social dimensions [21]. Thus, even though the tissue damage for several children may be the same, certain factors specific to each child or to each child's environment can intensify pain and distress, trigger pain episodes, and prolong pain-related disability, while other factors may buffer the effects of the pain, and enable the child to engage in healthy coping, and lessen distress. Thus, a thorough assessment is crucial to determine the extent to which cognitive, behavioral, emotional, or situational factors contribute to or buffer the pain experience for a child, with the understanding that these factors are likely to vary between children and may even vary over time for the same child.

Pain behavior in children varies as a function of the child's developmental level. Older children are typically able to describe the location, intensity, duration, and sensation of pain, whereas younger children may not be able to distinguish pain from other negative affective states [22]. Pain behavior in children has also been found to differ depending on the presence or absence of a caregiver during a painful medical procedure, with some studies finding that children whose mothers were present were more distressed, but that children prefer parents or caregivers to be present [23]. Parents' attitudes and expectations, their anxiety levels, and whether they are overly protective and reinforcing of dependence are variables that may affect children's ability to successfully cope. Also, some parents may inadvertently cue and reinforce their child's distress, while others may promote coping by the child [24]. Due to the number of parental variables that may influence child coping, there is a need to assess characteristics of the parent, child, and parent–child interactions when assessing pain in children. Given the host of factors that may influence a child's experience of pain, it is not surprising that the treatment of pain in childhood requires an integrated approach, informed by the many factors that may influence a child's pain, including the family and cultural factors that might impact the child, and the child's current methods of coping with pain. Kozlowska *et al.* present a conceptual model and practice framework for managing chronic pain in children and adolescents, which includes an integrated family-based assessment and treatment approach [25]. The authors emphasize the need to identify the contribution of various systems on a children's subjective experience of pain, thereby avoiding the deleterious polarization of the pain as either "physical" or "psychogenic."

Cognitive-behavioral treatments for chronic pain in children provide children with concrete strategies to lessen their pain and distress and help them return to developmentally appropriate activities. Some CB strategies that have been utilized with child patients with pain include teaching children distraction techniques (such as counting) during painful medical procedures, or thinking about a favorite holiday. In addition, children have found it helpful to "throw away" negative thoughts about their ability to cope and instead utilizing positive coping thoughts such as "I can cope with anything that comes my way; I am very strong and brave." Children have also found relaxation techniques helpful for coping with painful procedures. Parents can also be taught such cognitive-behavioral strategies, so that children can be reminded to utilize them when participating in normal daily activities. The ultimate goal of CB strategies is to help children have concrete tools to cope with their experience of pain so that developmentally appropriate activities can resume.

Older adults

The human body is prone to physical changes related to the passage of time including the effects of use, neglect, or disease, all of which may result in impairments and disability. Surveys have estimated the prevalence of pain in the general population of older adults to be 20% to 50% [26]. Chronic pain may threaten independence by decreasing a person's ability to ambulate freely. The reduction in physical activity can hasten the development of disability, and, in itself can be a risk factor for many health problems. Research has documented a significant relationship between the presence of pain and disability in older adults [27, 28]. Additional pain related factors that may increase the risk for disability in this age group include pain intensity, number of pain locations, and pain duration [29, 30]. Some of the painful conditions experienced by older adults include musculoskeletal disorders, rheumatoid and osteoarthritis, and diabetic neuropathy [31]. Despite some changes that occur with age, research indicates that older adults with pain often report similar levels of pain intensity when compared to younger adults with chronic pain [32]. However, older adults tend to report less pain-related negative affect and suffering when compared with younger adults. One explanation for this observation may be that older adults' reaction to pain has been influenced by their socialization history [33]. For older adults, the presence of pain may be viewed as an expected part of growing older. In addition, the fact that a person is older may mean that they have had previous exposures and more experience with painful conditions and are less affected by their presence. These are important factors to consider because the older adult may be less likely to report significant pain complaints during a pain assessment, even though they may be experiencing discomfort.

There are several psychosocial factors that should be considered that could impact an older adult's ability to cope with pain. Physical and financial limitations often prevent older adults from engaging in outside activities that would provide opportunities to develop supportive emotional relationships with others. Social support networks have been found to help alleviate the effects of stress, promote effective health behaviors, and influence health outcomes [34, 35]. Older adults typically have family-linked relationships and few supports outside the family. As families become more geographically separated and spouses pass away, opportunities for social support may further decrease. For this reason, when providing pain management with older adults it may be beneficial for treatment to be held in a group format. Such a format would provide opportunities for adults to engage in positive social interactions and would promote the building of social networks that might not otherwise be available. While there have only been a few research studies demonstrating the efficacy of CBT for pain management for older adults [36, 37], their results have been supportive of this treatment approach.

Pain management and co-morbid conditions

Chronic pain affects more than just a person's back or knee, it can negatively impact their entire life and the lives of significant others. Pain can impact the activities they are able to do and the thoughts they have about themselves and the world. For these reasons, chronic pain is frequently associated with co-morbid mental health conditions that can exacerbate the experience of pain. It is important that therapists assess for the presence of these conditions, consider the manner in which these conditions may impact the pain experience, and modify treatment if necessary to best meet the needs of these individuals.

Depression

Numerous studies have documented a significant relationship between pain and depression [38, 39] with depression co-prevalence rates being estimated to be 20–54% in chronic pain samples [40, 41]. Depression is associated with significantly higher pain intensity and disability in patients with chronic pain [40, 42]. According to Robinson and Riley [43], the relationship between depression and pain is probably not direct, but mediated by biological or psychosocial variables such as somatization, catastrophizing, social factors, and perceptions of life control. A cognitive-neurobiological model of the interaction between pain and depression has also been proposed [44]. Studies reporting on the efficacy of CBT for chronic pain have documented improvements in mood as a result of treatment [8].

Anxiety

Relative to depression, anxiety disorders have received less attention in the chronic pain literature. In an effort to gain a greater understanding of the prevalence of anxiety in patients with chronic pain, McWilliams *et al.* analyzed data from 5877 individuals who participated in the National Comorbidity Survey (1994) [45]. Their analyses indicated that participants with chronic pain were significantly more likely to have a mood or anxiety disorder than individuals in the general population. It was noted that associations between pain and several of the anxiety disorders (i.e., panic disorder, agoraphobia, and post-traumatic stress disorder) were actually stronger than the relationship between pain and mood disorders (i.e., depression). One specific factor that may play a role in the relationship between anxiety and pain is called "anxiety sensitivity." Anxiety sensitivity refers to the fear of arousal-related sensations (e.g., increased heart rate, shortness of breath), arising from beliefs that these sensations have harmful consequences. Research has found that for patients who have chronic pain, higher anxiety sensitivity is associated with greater anxiety and fear of pain, more negative affect, and greater avoidance of activities [46, 47]. Thus, anxiety sensitivity may represent a vulnerability in the development and maintenance of pain-related anxiety and avoidance behaviors. To address this, therapists should consider providing opportunities for patients to gain exposure to and mastery of feared pain-related sensations and experiences. These exposures can serve as positive, corrective experiences that can help the patient to challenge unhealthy thinking, avoidant behaviors, and ultimately lead to improved management of both chronic pain and anxiety symptoms.

Post-traumatic stress disorder

Post-traumatic stress disorder (PTSD) can occur following exposure to an event that is, or is perceived to be, threatening to the well-being of oneself or another person. The estimated lifetime prevalence rate for PTSD in the general population is 6.8%; however, some studies have indicated that between 34–50% of patients with chronic pain have PTSD or significant PTSD symptomatology [48]. Patients with chronic pain and PTSD experience more intense pain and affective distress, higher levels of life interference, and greater disability than patients with either pain or PTSD alone [49, 50]. Given the symptoms often associated with PTSD (i.e., issues with trust and avoidance), these patients are at increased risk of not engaging in CBT for pain and for not receiving adequate care. It has been reported by some patients that the experience of pain and trauma interact with one another. For example, back pain can serve as a reminder of a traumatic accident, or conversely, thinking about a traumatic event can make pain

seem more intense. In some cases it may be beneficial for a therapist to recommend treatment by a provider who has expertise in the treatment of PTSD. Given the high rates of co-morbidity between chronic pain and PTSD in US Veterans, the Department of Veterans Affairs is funding research exploring the benefits of an integrated treatment for both conditions [51]. An integrated treatment has its advantages because it can address underlying issues that are influencing both conditions, can be more time and cost efficient than being in sequential treatment, and can be less burdensome on the patient.

Substance abuse

While the reported rates of substance abuse in patients with a chronic pain condition vary, a recent article estimated that 24–67% of patients with substance use disorders are also affected by chronic pain [52]. Substance abuse is an important treatment concern when attempting to engage a patient in self-management approaches, as patients who are abusing substances are often noncompliant with treatment recommendations. While it is often reported by patients abusing substances that they are doing so in an effort to cope with pain, it is more likely that even the complete resolution of the pain would not eliminate the substance abuse problem. For this reason, patients with chronic pain who are actively abusing substances should be treated for the abuse problem before the pain problem. In order to get the most benefit from pain treatment patients should agree to attend therapy sessions substance-free. In situations where parallel treatment is being considered for pain and substance abuse, regular communication between treatment providers is recommended.

Personality disorders

A relationship between chronic pain and personality disorders (PD) is well-established, with prevalence rates ranging from 31% to 81% in the research literature [53, 54]. In a recent study, Conrad et al. administered the Structured Clinical Interview for DSM-IV Personality Disorders (SCID-II) to 207 patients with chronic low back pain [55]. Their results indicated that 41% of the sample had at least one PD. According to Weisberg and Keefe, a diathesis-stress model may be used to explain the relationship between PD and chronic pain [56]. According to this model, personality patterns associated with poor coping styles are more likely to decompensate in the face of an injury, disability, and pain. However, this also suggests that if improvements in pain management or functioning are achieved the traits associated with the PD may not be as evident. While more research is needed in this area, the recognition of the high prevalence of PD in patients with chronic pain is important as the presence of a PD can have a significant impact on the quality of care a patient is likely to receive. The objectives of creating trust and alliance with the patient can more effectively be achieved when therapists can recognize the personality characteristics of their patients and consider how to effectively work with them.

Cognitive impairment

There are many conditions that can lead to cognitive impairments, from neurodegenerative conditions such as Alzheimer's disease, vascular conditions such as stroke, or traumatic events such as head or blast injury. Since pain is a subjective experience, cognitive and communication impairments can be significant obstacles when attempting to gain an accurate pain assessment [57]. Several techniques have been developed to gain a more accurate assessment of pain including behavioral monitoring and specialized pain assessment scales [58]; however, providers need to consider the limitations of each patient in order to choose the best assessment practices. The types of cognitive impairments experienced may also dictate the elements of CBT that can be effectively employed. For example, patients who have difficulty with abstract thinking might benefit from a more behavioral approach to treatment rather than an approach that requires the ability to think about one's own thoughts. Overall, it is important that therapists are flexible in the manner in which they deliver treatment, match the treatment to the needs of the patient, and regularly assess the effectiveness of pain interventions.

Clinical case example

Presenting problem/client description

Mrs. Anderson is a 60-year-old, married Caucasian female who was referred to a pain psychologist by her primary care physician for a comprehensive evaluation related to her chronic low back pain. Upon receiving the consultation request, the psychologist contacted the referring physician to discuss any specific concerns or issues that prompted the referral and which might be helpful to address during the pain assessment. The primary care provider described encouraging

Mrs. Anderson to increase her activity level and improve her overall health behaviors; however, the patient continued to maintain a sedentary lifestyle and was thus becoming increasingly disabled. Also of note, the provider indicated that Mrs. Anderson seemed to be reporting higher levels of pain than would be expected for her type of injury.

Mrs. Anderson's assessment began with a 45-minute clinical interview, with the goal of assessing the relationship among the dimensions of pain, distress, and disability and the social context in which they occur. Behavioral observations of Mrs. Anderson revealed a mild to moderate level of pain behaviors, such as: grimacing and occasionally bracing her back with her hand. During the interview, Mrs. Anderson reported that her back pain began approximately 3 years ago subsequent to falling on a patch of ice. She described, "I was rushing to work, and then suddenly I just slipped and fell onto my lower back." She reported continuing to work following this injury but described opting for early retirement, beginning approximately 2 years ago, due to her continued experience of pain. Furthermore, she described decreasing her participation in activities she previously enjoyed, such as spending time with friends or working in her garden, due to her experience of pain. She characterized the pain as a constant aching with intermittent "sharp, stabbing" pain that is exacerbated by engaging in any form of physical activity. She reported obtaining only minimal relief with the use of her current pain medication but indicated she did not want an increased dosage or stronger medication, as she preferred, "not to rely on medications to be able to function."

Mrs. Anderson is a college graduate who worked as a high-school history teacher for over 30 years. She and her husband of 35 years have four adult children. She described her husband as caring and supportive but reported encountering financial difficulties subsequent to her early retirement that have somewhat strained their marital relationship.

Mrs. Anderson denied any history of alcohol or illicit drug abuse. She reported a history of cigarette smoking since the age of 18. She expressed a desire to quit smoking but indicated being hesitant for fear she may gain weight, noting "I've already gained 20 pounds in the past 2 years." She denied a history of depression or mental health treatment; however, she reported feeling "worthless," "unmotivated," and "irritable and unhappy" almost every day for the past 8–10 months. She reported that she occasionally wonders if life is worth living but she denied any real plan or intent to harm herself. Mrs. Anderson's primary care provider had been managing her pain conservatively with recommendations of rest and light activity, and a referral to physical therapy where she received heat and massage to relax her back muscles. Her primary care provider also decided to prescribe a low-dose, non-narcotic analgesic. A recent MRI revealed a slight disc compression at L3–L4; however, a consulting neurologist documented that these findings could not fully account for Mrs. Anderson's current level of pain and disability. Mrs. Anderson's medical history was also significant for hypertension, psoriasis, and obesity.

Following the clinical interview, Mrs. Anderson was asked to complete several self-report questionnaires related to her experience of pain so as to supplement information gained from the interview. The results of the assessment indicated that Mrs. Anderson was experiencing a moderate level of depression associated with the onset of her chronic pain condition. Furthermore, her depressive symptoms were now likely contributing to increased disability and pain. Factors contributing to her depressive symptoms included adjustment to early retirement, arguments with her husband about economic difficulties, negative thoughts about herself (e.g., "I'm useless and miserable"), increased social isolation, and reduced pleasant activities. This was supported by her responses on several self-report questionnaires, which indicated she was experiencing a moderate level of depressive symptoms and a significant level of interference in her daily activities. Scores on a measure of coping strategies revealed Mrs. Anderson primarily utilized prayer as her strategy for managing her pain. She also secondarily employed catastrophizing (e.g., "This is never going to get better"). The initial assessment enabled the psychologist to conceptualize Mrs. Anderson's pain experience, including factors contributing to its development and maintenance. Her specific difficulties included her level of pain, poor coping strategies, significant number of depressive symptoms, marital strain, decreased participation in pleasant activities, and unhealthy lifestyle behaviors (i.e. smoking, decreased physical activity, poor nutrition).

Multidisciplinary pain management team

Following the completion of the pain assessment by the psychologist, Mrs. Anderson's case was presented to the multidisciplinary pain management team. The team agreed that surgical options were inappropriate at this time, but rather less invasive treatments would be preferable. Specifically, it was the opinion of the team that participation in individually based pain management therapy would be especially beneficial for Mrs. Anderson. Additional suggestions were provided by various team members. First, weight loss was considered an important long-term goal given that weight loss is often associated with reductions in pain. To facilitate healthy changes in nutrition and diet, one team member recommended that Mrs. Anderson meet with a dietician to learn helpful weight-management skills and develop an overall weight-loss plan. Next, the physical therapist on the team recommended that Mrs. Anderson engage in more active (e.g., muscle strengthening), rather than passive (e.g., heat packs) rehabilitation approaches to increase her strength and flexibility. The importance of increasing Mrs. Anderson's overall level of physical activity, so as to improve overall muscle strength and assist with weight loss efforts, was underscored. Lastly, no changes in Mrs. Anderson's current pain medications were recommended by the neurologist. The neurologist suggested re-evaluating the need for modifying Mrs. Anderson's medications subsequent to her participation in pain management therapy. All of these recommendations were communicated to the primary care provider following the meeting.

Mrs. Anderson was contacted by the psychologist, at which time the results of the assessment were reviewed and potential areas for intervention were highlighted. Mrs. Anderson agreed she could benefit from learning ways to more effectively manage her pain. Time was spent describing the therapy process and scheduling a time for the first session. Expectations for active participation in the treatment process (including practice and the completion of homework assignments) were emphasized and the psychologist's genuine interest to begin working with the patient was conveyed.

Course of treatment

Mrs. Anderson was seen by the psychologist for 11 sessions of weekly individual psychotherapy approximately 50 minutes in duration. Following the CBT model of pain management, the first session of treatment involved re-conceptualizing pain as a manageable, but not curable, condition that can be influenced by a person's thoughts and behaviors. Next, the psychologist demonstrated empathy by briefly discussing with Mrs. Anderson that her pain is most certainly a real and significant stressor in her life and is not "just in her head" as she sometimes believes others may imply. The psychologist explained, "Living with chronic pain is definitely effortful, that's why we're going to work together these next 10 sessions to find ways to help you decrease your level of pain and manage how much pain impacts your overall quality of life." Additionally, the psychologist recognized the importance of setting realistic expectations about treatment benefits. Specifically, the therapist addressed the issue that this 11-week therapy would not "cure" her pain but rather help lessen the impact of pain on daily functioning. Acceptance of this idea that pain will likely always be a part of her life was a key point because patients who are waiting for a cure for their pain are less likely to take responsibility for managing pain or to actively participate in psychotherapy related to pain. Next, the relationship between pain, negative thoughts, and disability was explained. Specific circumstances from Mrs. Anderson's own life were utilized as examples. Mrs. Anderson was able to offer examples of when feelings of sadness or anger precipitated increases in her pain. She was also able to articulate how her pain impacted all areas of her life, and was more than just a sensory experience confined to her lower back.

Mrs. Anderson worked with the psychologist to develop several overall treatment goals that she could work towards achieving by the end of the 11-week treatment. Goals were identified cooperatively with the patient, rather than set solely by the psychologist, so as to empower Mrs. Anderson to be an active participant in her own treatment and to engender an increased investment in the achievement of the goals. Goals that were behavioral and quantifiable in nature were developed, rather than vague goals (e.g., reduce pain, increase fitness), to facilitate measurement of progress over the course of treatment. Next, it was explained to Mrs. Anderson that each week she would establish small, "do-able" goals that successively approximate the overall treatment goals. The importance of "setting yourself up to succeed" was then discussed with the patient. Specifically, the psychologist explicated the benefits of increasing Mrs. Anderson's acceptance of "where she is currently at" and subsequently setting realistic goals that will be achievable from week to week, such that she can experience success in accomplishing her weekly goals and ultimately her overall treatment goals.

Mrs. Anderson expressed a desire to work on goals related to weight loss and increasing her participation in social activities. The psychologist validated the importance of each of these goals, utilizing her goals as concrete examples to further underscore the important interaction between physical/mental/social health and pain management. Ways in which to generate behavioral, quantifiable measures of the goals were then discussed. Ultimately, four treatment goals were identified. First, Mrs. Anderson indicated she was currently consuming approximately four cans of regular soda per day and two or three glasses of iced tea per day. To assist with weight loss, in accordance with recommendations made by the dietician, Mrs. Anderson set a goal to decrease her consumption of high-calorie, high-sugar drinks and increase her consumption of water and other no-calorie liquids (such as diet soda). Thus, her first treatment goal was identified: consume eight glasses of water/no-calorie liquids a day and fewer than two "regular"/high-calorie drinks per day. Next, Mrs. Anderson indicated she currently consumed approximately two servings of fruit per day and one or no servings of vegetables per day. Thus, to improve her overall nutrition, and again assist with weight loss (by substituting fruit/vegetables for higher-calorie snacks), Mrs. Anderson set her second treatment goal: increase consumption of fruits and vegetables to five servings a day. Mrs. Anderson's third goal, related to increasing her level of physical activity, was then identified: walk for a minimum of 30 minutes/day for a minimum of four times a week (in addition to practicing stretches/exercises recommended by the physical therapist). Mrs. Anderson initially expressed a desire to set a goal of walking 60 minutes every day; however, upon discussion with the psychologist, the patient recognized the importance of setting a more realistic goal given her current frequency of walking of approximately 10 minutes/day, twice a week. Lastly, Mrs. Anderson identified her fourth and final treatment goal: participate in at least two social activities per week. This goal targeted increasing the patient's social interaction from her current rate of only one or no social activity per 2 weeks.

In addition to building rapport during the first session, the psychologist also found it important to try to instill hope, noting to the patient, "I appreciate how difficult it will be to add another thing into your week, but I believe that through your participation in this treatment you will learn new strategies to better manage your pain and achieve your goals." While it is important to impart hopefulness and "sell" the treatment so as to promote patient participation, remaining realistic is essential. Patients beginning pain management therapy, especially those experiencing depression, may be exceedingly put off by "Pollyanna" claims purported by a therapist. Thus, the psychologist chose not to end the first session by speaking of hopes to "cure" or "drastically alleviate" the patient's pain; but rather, the psychologist opted to convey a more realistic message regarding the potential outcome of treatment, by articulating to the patient, "Ultimately, at the conclusion of these 11 weeks, you will hopefully have developed some new skills to effectively cope with pain, and reduce the impact of pain on your daily life."

Each session began with a review of the previous week's behavioral goals and an evaluation by the patient and the therapist of her success in achieving her goals. The psychologist positively reinforced the patient for completion of her goals and problem solved with the patient about challenges encountered when trying to accomplish goals. Goals were subsequently revised as needed to continue forward progress towards ultimate achievement of overall treatment goals. For example, Mrs. Anderson expressed encountering difficulties when trying to accomplish her goal of consuming water/no-calorie liquids. Specifically, the patient reported significant problems switching from drinking her regular soda to diet soda because of her dislike for the taste of diet sodas. The psychologist worked collaboratively with the patient to generate and discuss possible solutions. Mrs. Anderson indicated she was pleased by the idea of becoming a "detective" to figure out which diet sodas tasted best. Furthermore, she expressed motivation to continue her efforts to switch to no-sugar sodas given the important implications for both weight loss and diabetes prevention. Initially Mrs. Anderson modified her goals related to liquid consumption slowly (e.g., the first 3 weeks she remained at a goal of simply consuming four glasses of water/no-calorie liquids per day), but subsequently increased her weekly goals as she overcame barriers to success.

Following the review of goals and goal-setting, specific cognitive-behavioral coping skills were then introduced to help Mrs. Anderson manage her pain more effectively. Each session began with an outline of the major topics to be covered and subsequently consisted of educational information, a review of the skill to be taught, in-session practice of the skill, and homework designed to facilitate the acquisition of the skill. This was presented to Mrs. Anderson by explaining that each week a new pain management strategy or "tool" would be introduced and practiced so as to compile a "tool box" she could use even after treatment completion. Utilizing this analogy, the psychologist validated that while Mrs. Anderson may have found one or two ways, or tools, to use to manage her pain, it would be helpful to have a tool box filled with many different tools, rather than simply try to rely on "a screwdriver" for all situations. The analogy seemed to resonate with Mrs. Anderson, as she agreed that "sometimes life throws in a few nails, so you need a "hammer" or a "drill," alternate ways to cope with difficult situations. The psychologist also encouraged the patient to be open to learning all of the skills presented, noting that some people find some tools more helpful than others but that all of the tools have the potential to be beneficial.

The importance of practicing the techniques reviewed in each session and the completion of homework assignments was emphasized. The psychologist explained that the actual therapy session was only 50 minutes a week, which is such a small amount of time in relation to how many minutes are in a day or a whole week; thus, it was stressed, "to really learn a skill, out-of-session practice is key." Mrs. Anderson was also encouraged to "practice patience with yourself as much as possible" because "these are new skills; they'll take time to learn, just like anything new you've ever tried to learn before." Additionally, to reinforce realistic expectations, the psychologist noted, "You've spent years developing certain habits and patterns related to pain, it will take more than a few days to re-learn new habits and patterns."

Initial sessions focused on teaching skills related to relaxation, such as diaphragmatic breathing, visual imagery, and progressive muscle relaxation. Mrs. Anderson was receptive to learning these techniques and expressed satisfaction regarding her experiences of decreased pain subsequent to her at-home practice. This early success provided an opportunity for the psychologist to reinforce her active efforts to manage her pain.

Next, she was taught to identify and label her thoughts and emotions, to identify cognitive errors (e.g., errors in ways of thinking), and to challenge negative automatic thoughts using a process called "cognitive restructuring". Negative thoughts about herself and catastrophic ways of thinking were specifically addressed. Mrs. Anderson recognized that she often engaged in "unhelpful" thinking (i.e., "Life will never be the same now because of my back pain") that precipitated negative feelings. Furthermore, she recognized that her thoughts and negative feelings frequently prompted negative/unpleasant behaviors (i.e., isolating herself socially, experiencing increases in her pain). Mrs. Anderson was also taught ways to gradually reintroduce pleasant activities into her life. In a subsequent session, Mrs. Anderson expressed her excitement as she described attending an outdoor concert with her friends. She recounted feeling thrilled to share in such a pleasant event noting, "A year ago, I never would have thought I would actually enjoy an outing like that." Mrs. Anderson was also introduced to other "tools" to improve her pain management, such as: time-based pacing, assertive communication skills, and stress management skills. Education related to stress management seemed particularly valuable for Mrs. Anderson. She recognized that she often attempted to cope with stressful situations, such as arguments with her husband, by "leaving to go out for a smoke." Mrs. Anderson acknowledged that employing more adaptive coping strategies could help her improve her pain management as well as the management of other aspects of her life. The psychologist applauded the patient's awareness of her own behavioral patterns and positively reinforced her generalizing the utilization of a new skill to multiple areas of her life.

During the final session, the psychologist and Mrs. Anderson reviewed previously presented topics and addressed strategies for coping with future pain flare-ups or temporary increases in pain. The psychologist explained that even though Mrs. Anderson had successfully completed this program, it was likely that she would experience pain flare-ups in the future. Thus, the importance of preparing for flare-ups was emphasized. Mrs. Anderson and the psychologist discussed specific strategies including: preparing for a pain flare-up before it occurs (i.e., becoming aware of emotional and physical cues that pain is increasing), confronting pain flare-ups by using self-management strategies (i.e., relaxation strategies, restructuring negative thoughts), and using positive coping statements in place of negative thoughts (e.g., I've handled this much pain before, and I can do it again). Lastly, achievement of overall treatment goals was reviewed and post-treatment self-report questionnaires were assigned for completion. Mrs. Anderson was thanked for her time and significant efforts and was encouraged to continue working towards her goals.

Outcome and prognosis

Ultimately, Mrs. Anderson learned a number of techniques to help her lessen the impact of chronic pain on her overall quality of life. Exercises such as diaphragmatic breathing and progressive muscle relaxation helped her learn to relax her body and to identify when she was becoming tense. Mrs. Anderson recognized that her negative thoughts and increased isolation prior to initiating treatment contributed to her depressive symptoms and subsequently intensified her experience of pain. By practicing cognitive restructuring she became skilled at identifying her negative thoughts and replacing them with more adaptive, balanced cognitions. This, along with homework assignments designed to increase her engagement in pleasant activities and participation in social events, resulted in a significant decrease in her depressive symptoms.

Mrs. Anderson successfully accomplished all of her goals by the end of treatment. She was able to significantly modify her nutrition, such that she no longer consumed high-calorie sodas or iced teas and consumed five servings of fruits and vegetables almost every day. Additionally, she was able to attain a higher frequency of physical activity and greater overall fitness level by walking four or five times a week for 30 minutes or more and practicing stretching exercises recommended by her physical therapist. These changes in diet and physical activity helped facilitate a weight loss of 6 pounds by the end of treatment. Mrs. Anderson expressed she was extremely pleased by the weight loss and indicated she was motivated to continue maintaining these healthy lifestyle behaviors so as to lose additional weight. Mrs. Anderson was also able to successfully increase her frequency of social interaction, such that by the end of treatment she was regularly engaging in social events two or three times a week. Specifically, she expressed her delight regarding recently initiating membership in the local gardeners' club. She explained she was proud of herself for finding a way to return to her hobby of gardening while also discovering a venue to positively interact with others who shared a similar interest. Of particular note, Mrs. Anderson stated that she now had increased her enjoyment of life, and that pain was no longer such a significantly limiting factor. Furthermore, she reported that of all of the skills she learned in treatment, she found learning skills related to cognitive restructuring and stress management most helpful.

A brief follow-up assessment conducted several months later revealed that Mrs. Anderson had continued working towards her goals of weight loss and increased social interaction. She remained actively involved in her gardening group and joined a retirees' walking club as well. She had lost an additional 7 pounds since the end of treatment and noted her overall lifestyle had become healthier. She indicated she was even contemplating joining a smoking cessation group. Furthermore, Mrs. Anderson reported, "we're still very much financially strapped, but I deal with my stress better now and so my husband and I don't have to fight about the money all the time." She also indicated enjoying a more harmonious relationship with her husband as she was now less irritable and depressed. Lastly, Mrs. Anderson reported continued experiences of pain; however, she described she had learned helpful ways to cope with pain and was pleased that subsequent to her participation in treatment, she was able to manage her pain effectively and no increases in her pain medication were made. She concluded, "My pain hasn't gone away completely, but it's just more manageable now."

Summary and discussion

Research on the efficacy of psychological approaches to chronic pain management has burgeoned in the last decade, with substantial gains being made in our understanding of the various factors that contribute to the development and maintenance of chronic pain conditions. Cognitive-behavioral therapy is an effective treatment for a variety of chronic pain conditions. The CBT approach has been shown to help patients develop a healthier and more active lifestyle, reduce maladaptive thinking related to pain, and improve overall quality of life. In order to maximize the effectiveness of CBT, further research is needed on ways to tailor both the content and the method of delivery of CBT for patients with specific painful conditions. Providers should be encouraged to recognize the importance of treating the entire person – not just a particular pain disorder, and to prioritize the development of innovative and effective treatment approaches for chronic pain management.

References

1. Keefe FJ, Gill KM. Behavioral concepts in the analysis of chronic pain syndromes. *J Consult Clin Psychol* 1986; **54**: 776–83.

2. Kerns RD, Turk DC, Holzman AD, Rudy TE. Comparison of cognitive behavioral and behavioral approaches to the outpatient treatment of chronic pain. *Clin J Pain* 1986; **1**: 195–203.

3. Turner JA, Clancy S. Comparison of operant behavioral and cognitive behavioral group treatment for chronic low back pain. *J Consult Clin Psychol* 1988; **56**: 261–6.

4. Caudill M, Schnabel R, Zuttermeister P, *et al.* Decreased clinic use by chronic *Pain* 1991; **7**: 305–10.

5. Turner JA, Mancl L, Aaron LA. Short- and long-term efficacy of brief cognitive-behavioral therapy for patients with chronic temporomandibular disorder pain: A randomized, controlled trial. *Pain* 2006; **121**: 181–94.

6. Morley S. RCTs of psychological treatments for chronic pain: Progress and challenges. *Pain* 2006; **121**: 171–2.

7. Morley S, Eccleston C, Williams A. Systematic review and meta-analysis of randomized controlled trials of cognitive behaviour therapy and behaviour therapy for chronic pain in adults, excluding headache. *Pain* 1999; **80**: 1–13.

8. Hoffman BM, Papas RK, Chatkoff DK, Kerns RD. Meta-analysis of psychological interventions for chronic low back pain. *Health Psychol* 2007; **26**, 1–9.

9. Von Korff, M. Pain management in primary care: An individualized stepped care approach. In *Psychosocial Factors in Pain: Critical perspectives,* eds. RJ Gatchel and DC Turk. (New York: Guilford Press, 1999), pp. 360–73.

10. Sobell MB, Sobell LC. Stepped care as a heuristic approach to the treatment of alcohol problems. *J Consult Clin Psychol* 2000; **68**: 573–9.

11. Abrams DB, Orleans, CT, Niaura RS, *et al.* Integrating individual and public health perspectives for treatment of tobacco dependence under managed health care: A combined stepped-care and matching model. *Ann Behav Med* 1996; **18**: 290–304.

12. Oster G, Borok GM, Menzin J, *et al.* A randomized trial to assess effectiveness and cost in clinical practice: Rationale and design of the cholesterol reduction intervention study. *Control Clin Trials* 1995; **16**: 3–16.

13. Miller WR, Rollnick S. *Motivational Interviewing: Preparing people to change addictive behavior.* 2nd edn. (New York: Guilford Press, 2002).

14. Von Korff M, Moore J.E Lorig K, *et al.* A randomized trial of a lay person led self-management group intervention for back pain patients in primary care. *Spine* 1998; **23**: 2608–15.

15. Moore JE, Von Korff M, Cherkin D, Saunders K, Lorig K. A randomized trial of a cognitive-behavioral program for enhancing back pain self care in a primary care setting. *Pain* 2000; **88**: 145–53.

16. Chambliss CR, Heggen J, Copelan DN, Pettignano R. The assessment and management of chronic pain in children. *Pediatr Drugs* 2002; **4**: 737–46.

17. Caffo E, Belaise C. Psychological aspects of traumatic injury in children and adolescents. *Child Adolesc Psychiatr Clin N Am* 2003; **12**: 493–535.

18. Huguet A, Miro J. The severity of chronic pediatric pain: An epidemiological study. *J Pain* 2008; **9**: 226–36.

19. Campo JV, DiLorenzo C, Chiappetta L. Adult outcomes of pediatric recurrent abdominal pain: Do they just grow out of it? *Pediatrics* 2001; **108**: E1–7.

20. McGrath PA, Hillier LM. A practical cognitive behavioral approach for treating children's pain. In *Psychological Approaches to Pain Management: A practitioner's handbook*, 2nd edn, eds. DC Turk and RJ Gatchel. (New York: Guilford Press, 2002), pp. 534–52.

21. Melzack R, Wall PD. Pain mechanisms: A new theory. *Science* 1965; **50**: 971–9.

22. Tarnowski KJ, Brown RT. Burn injuries. In *Handbook of Pediatric and Adolescent Health Psychology*, eds. AJ Goreczny and M Hersen. (Needham, MA: Allyn Bacon, 1999), pp. 115–26.

23. Gonzalez JC, Routh DK, Saab, PG, *et al.* Effects of parent presence on children's reactions to injections: Behavioral, physiological, and subjective aspects. *J Pediatr Psychol* 1989; **14**: 449–62.

24. Blount RL, Landolf-Fritsche B, Powers SW, Sturges JW. Differences between high and low coping children and between parent and staff behaviors during painful medical procedures. *J Pediatr Psychol* 1991; **16**: 795–809.

25. Kozlowska K, Rose D, Khan R, *et al.* A conceptual model and practice framework for managing chronic pain in children and adolescents. *Harv Rev Psychiatry* 2008; **16**: 136–50.

26. Kendig H, Browning CJ, Young AE. Impacts of illness and disability on the well-being of older people. *Disabil Rehabil* 2000; **22**: 15–22.

27. Leveille SG, Ling S, Hochberg M, *et al.* Widespread musculoskeletal pain and the progression of disability in older disabled women. *Ann Intern Med*, 2001; **135**: 1038–46.

28. Al Snih S, Markides KS, Ray L, Goodwin JS. Impact of pain on disability among older Mexican Americans. *J Gerontol Med Sci* 2001; **56**: M400–M404.

29. Scudds RJ, Robertson JM. Pain factors associated with physical disability in a sample of community dwelling senior citizens. *J Gerontol Med Sci* 2000; **55**: 393–9.

30. Reid MC, Crone KT, Otis JD, Kerns RD. Differences in pain-related characteristics among younger and older veterans receiving primary care. *Pain Med* 2002; **3**: 102–7.

31. Berkow R, Talbott JH. *The Merck Manual of Diagnosis and Therapy* 13th edn. (Rahway, NJ: Merck Sharp Dohme Research Laboratories, 1995).

32. Harkins SW, Price DD. Assessment of pain in the elderly. In *Handbook of Pain Assessment*, eds. DC Turk and R Melzack. (New York: Guilford Press, 1992), pp. 315–31.

33. Whitbourne SK, Cassidy EL. Adaptation. In *Encyclopedia of Gerontology*, Vol. 1, ed. J Birren. (San Diego: Academic Press, 1996), pp. 65–9.

34. Berkman LF, Syme SL. Social network, host resistance, and mortality: A nine-year follow-up study of Alameda County residents. *Am J Epidemiol* 1979; **109**, 186–204.

35. Cohen, S. Social supports and physical health: Symptoms, health behaviors, and infectious disease. In *Life-span Developmental Psychology*, eds. EM Cummings, AL Greens, KH Karraker. (Hillsdale, NJ: Erlbaum, 1991), pp. 213–34.

36. Cook AJ. Cognitive-behavioral pain management for elderly nursing home residents. *J Gerontol B Psychol Sci Soc Sci* 1998; **53**: P51–9.

37. Reid MC, Otis J, Barry LC, Kerns RD. Cognitive-behavioral therapy for chronic low back pain in older persons: A preliminary study. *Pain Med* 2003; **4**: 223–30.

38. Gallagher RM, Marbach JJ, Raphael KG, Dohrenwend BP, Cloitre M. Is major depression comorbid with temporomandibular pain and dysfunction syndrome? A pilot study. *Clin J Pain* 1991; **7**: 219–25.

39. Gaskin ME, Greene AF, Robinson ME, Geisser ME. Negative affect and the experience of chronic pain. *J Psychosom Res* 1992; **36**: 707–13.

40. Banks SM, Kerns RD. Explaining high rates of depression in chronic pain: A diathesis-stress framework. *Psychol Bull* 1996; **119**: 95–110.

41. Wilson KG, Eriksson MY, D'Eon JL, Mikail SF, Emery PC. Major depression and insomnia in chronic pain. *Clin J Pain* 2002; **18**: 77–83.

42. Ericsson M, Poston WSC II, Linder J, *et al.* Depression predicts disability in long-term chronic pain patients. *Disabil Rehabil* 2002; **24**: 334–40.

43. Robinson ME, Riley J. The role of emotion in pain. In *Psychosocial Factors in Pain: Critical perspectice*, eds. R Gatchel and D Turk. (New York: Guildford Press, 1999).

44. Fields H. Depression and pain: A neurobiological model. *Neuropsychiat Neuropsychol Behav Neurol* 1991; **41**: 83–92.

45. McWilliams LA, Cox BJ, Enns MW. Mood and anxiety disorders associated with chronic pain: an examination in a nationally representative sample. *Pain* 2003; **106**: 127–33.

46. Asmundson GJ, Norton G. Anxiety sensitivity in patients with physically unexplained chronic back pain: A preliminary report. *Behav Res Ther* 1995; **33**: 771–7.

47. Zvolensky MJ, Eifert GH, Lejuez CW, Hopko DR, Forsyth JP. Assessing the perceived predictability of anxiety-related events: A report on the Perceived Predictability Index. *J Behav Ther Exp Psychiatry* 2000; **31**: 201–18.

48. Asmundson GJ, Norton G, Allerdings M, Norton P, Larson D. Post-traumatic stress disorder and work-related injury. *J Anxiety Disord* 1998; **12**: 57–69.

49. Turk DC, Okifuji A. Perception of traumatic onset, compensation status, and physical findings: Impact on pain severity, emotional distress, and disability in chronic pain patients. *J Behav Med* 1996; **19**: 435–53.

50. Sherman JJ, Turk DC, Okifuji A. Prevalence and impact of posttraumatic stress disorder-like symptoms on patients with fibromyalgia syndrome. *Clin J Pain* 2000; **16**: 127–34.

51. Otis JD, Keane T, Kerns RD, Monson C, Scioli E. The development of an integrated treatment for veterans with comorbid chronic pain and post-traumatic stress disorder. *Pain Med* 2009; **10**: 1300–11.

52. Olsen Y, Alford D. Chronic pain management in patients with substance use disorders. *Adv Stud Med* 2006; **6**: 111–23.

53. Gatchel RJ, Garofalo JP, Ellis E, Holt, C. Major psychological disorders in acute and chronic TMD: An initial examination. *J AmDent Assoc* 1996; **127**: 1365–74.

54. Burton K, Polatin PB, Gatchel RJ. Psychosocial factors and the rehabilitation of patients with chronic work-related upper extremity disorders. *J Occup Rehabil* 1997; **7**: 139–53.

55. Conrad R, Schilling G, Bausch C, *et al.* Temperament and character personality profiles and personality in chronic pain patients. *Pain* 2007; 197–209.

56. Weisbeg JN, Keefe F J. Personality, individual differences and psychopathology in chronic pain. In *Psychosocial Factors in Pain: Critical perspectives,* eds. RJ Gatchel and DC Turk. (New York: Guilford Press, 1999), pp. 56–73.

57. Buffum MD, Hutt E, Chang VT, Crame MH, Snow AL. Cognitive impairment and pain management: Review of issues and challenges. *J Rehabil Res Rev* 2007; **44**: 315–30.

58. Shega JW, Rudy T, Keefe FJ, *et al.* Validity of pain behaviors in persons with mild to moderate cognitive impairment. *J AmGeriat Soc* 2008; **56**: 1631–7.

13

Non-pharmacologic neuromodulatory approaches to pain management

Gabriel Tan, Mark P. Jensen, Tam K. Dao, Brenda Stoelb and Jay Gunkelman

The field of non-pharmacological neuromodulation has a rich history and its course has been influenced by developments in behavioral learning theories, psycho-physiology, behavioral medicine, bio-medical engineering, and cybernetics. Recent resurgence in interest can be attributed to three simultaneously emerging trends [1]. The first is the emergence of technology and algorithms that allow the near simultaneous recording, analysis, and response to neuronal depolarization/ repolarization (that is, EEG). The second converging trend is the increased skepticism with many pharmacological treatments given the side effects and long-term toxic effects to the human body. The third is the development of a strong popular interest and a commitment to safe, non-toxic, non-invasive, and self-regulatory ways of dealing with symptoms and the achievement of well-being which transcends the achievement of a symptom-free state.

Prior to the middle of the twentieth century, pain was viewed primarily as a simple reflexive response to physical or tissue damage wherein nociceptive information is transmitted directly from the damaged tissue to a "pain center" in the brain. In this view, the intensity of "real" pain was believed to be related to the amount of physical or structural damage that occurred in the periphery, and the brain was accorded the role of a relatively passive recipient of sensory information. The advent of the gate-control theory marked an important turning point in our understanding of pain [2]. In brief, this theory provided a model of how nociceptive input can be influenced and modulated in the spinal cord before it reaches the brain, where it is further processed to produce the "experience" of pain. More recent advances in neuroimaging technology in pain research have shifted some focus away from the periphery and spinal cord to the supraspinal levels (the brain), and have greatly advanced our understanding of the multiple integrative and interlocking neurophysiological

mechanisms that modulate nociceptive information at many levels, including the cortex (Figure 13.1).

This research, demonstrating an important role for cortical activity in the processing and experience of pain, provides a neurophysiological basis for treatments that are designed to affect pain by altering cortical activity. The focus of this chapter is on selected non-pharmacological approaches that (purportedly) do just that. The chapter begins with a brief review of the neurophysiology and anatomy of pain. The remainder, and bulk, of the chapter describes, and reviews, the available evidence supporting the efficacy of interventions that target the cortical networks associated with pain.

Neurophysiology and anatomy of pain

Physiology of pain

Before proceeding to imaging studies, a brief overview of the physiology of pain is in order. At the peripheral nervous system, myelinated alpha-delta fibers transmit sharp pain while slower, unmyelinated C-fibers transmit dull or burning pain sensations. Pain signals travel along a combination of these fibers and enter the central nervous system at the dorsal horn of the spinal column where pain signals are modified before ascending to the different brain regions [2]. Pain signals travel via several tracts to the brain. Spinothalamic tract neurons project onto the thalamus which, in turn, projects onto the primary (SI) and secondary (SII) somatosensory cortices. Other pathways have been identified. For instance, the affective–motivational dimension of pain appears to correspond with the pathways in which ascending nerve fibers project onto the thalamus, the hypothalamus, and the limbic system. The limbic system with its projections to the prefrontal cortex plays a major role in

---

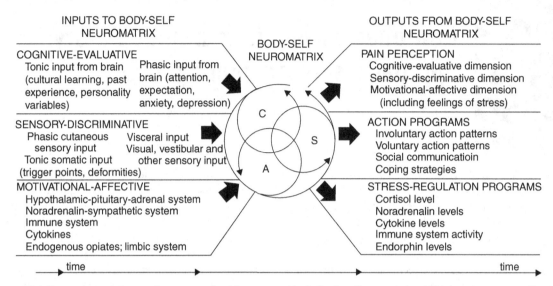

Figure 13.1 Factors that contribute to the patterns of activity generated by the body-self neuromatrix, which comprises sensory, affective, and cognitive neuromodules. The output patterns from the neuromatrix produce the multiple dimensions of pain experience as well as concurrent homeostatic and behavioral responses. Permission to use this figure has been kindly granted by Ronald Melzack via electronic communication.

emotions, memory, and attention. The anterior cingulate cortex (ACC) is connected to several cortical areas including the prefrontal cortex, parietal cortex, and the motor system. Additional pathways include projections from the dorsal horn in the spinal column to other areas of the brain including the medulla, reticular formation, and periaquaductal grey matter.

Imaging studies on pain

It is well accepted that pain is complex with multiple central representations – emotional, anticipatory, affective, and cognitive components in addition to the sensory component – making the task of imaging quite challenging [3].

The identification of the anatomical structures in the brain that are involved in pain processing and modulation has been carried out primarily by using the positron emission tomography (PET) and functional magnetic resonance imaging (fMRI) technologies. These investigations are relatively recent and have been completed mostly within the last 15–20 years. Functional activation of brain regions is thought to be reflected by increases in the regional cerebral flow (rCBF) in PET studies and in the blood oxygen level dependent (BOLD) signal in fMRI. Both methods have significant limitations and drawbacks, although fMRI is believed to have several advantages over PET, including better temporal resolution, a non-radioactive

environment, no required injection, and the possibility of doing individual analysis. It should also be pointed out that imaging studies using fMRI are limited to activation studies and are not able to provide information on resting state or on specific neurotransmitter or receptor involvement. Keeping these limitations in mind, pain responses based on PET and fMRI studies have produced fairly similar results.

In a review and meta-analysis of the functional imaging of brain responses to pain, Peyron *et al.* reported that rCBF increases to noxious stimuli are almost always observed in the SII and insular regions and in the ACC, and with less consistency in the contra-lateral thalamus and the SI [4]. Furthermore, the sensory-discriminative aspects of pain processing appear to involve the lateral thalamus, SI, SII, and insula whereas the ACC appears to be involved more in the affective and intentional concomitants of pain sensation and selective responding. In addition to the ACC, attentional and memory impact of pain appears to also involve the posterior parietal and prefrontal cortices.

Two phenomena associated with chronic pain are hyperalgesia (increased sensitivity to pain) and allodynia (pain from stimuli which are not normally painful). Chronic spontaneous pain is associated with decreased resting rCBF in the contralateral thalamus and this may be reversed by analgesic procedures. Allodynia has been shown to be associated with amplification of the thalamic, insular, and SII responses, concomitant to a paradoxical CBF decrease in the ACC. Peyron and colleagues concluded that available data would suggest that hemodynamic responses to pain reflect simultaneously the sensory, cognitive, and affective dimensions of pain, and that the same structures may both respond to pain and participate in pain modulation [4].

In summary, the following areas of the brain appear to be related to the perception of pain: primary and secondary somatosensory cortex, anterior cingulate cortex, amygdala (A1), thalamus, insular cortex, prefrontal cortex and posterior cortex [5]. Furthermore, fMRI studies have identified the following factors to be related to the experience of pain: attention/distraction, anticipation/fear, depression, anxiety, placebo, and pleasure [5]. Finally, pain affect appears to be encoded differently than pain sensation [6].

Electroencephalography and pain

While fMRI measures changes in cerebral blood flow and PET focuses on changes in localized brain metabolites, Electroencephalography (EEG) measures changes in brain electrical field activities. In a recent review, Jensen and colleagues summarized the existing evidence for a relationship between brain EEG activity and the experience of pain; specifically, data suggest that in otherwise healthy individuals, the subjective experience of pain is associated with relatively lower amplitudes of slower wave (delta, theta and alpha) activity and relatively higher amplitudes of faster wave (beta) activity [7]. Furthermore, the review noted that although a causal link between experience of pain and brain activity as measured by EEG has not been established, there is a potential for altering EEG rhythms, and therefore the experience of pain, via operant conditioning in a treatment modality referred to as EEG biofeedback or neurofeedback (see below).

Interventions/treatments that target cortical network associated with pain

Recent advances and thinking in the understanding of pain suggest that pain transmission and pain modulation are related but separate processes. Pain transmission involves transduction, primary afferent, dorsal horn, ascending pathways and cortical projections, while pain modulation involves peripheral modulation, gate mechanisms, descending inhibition, and higher cortical modulation. Both peripheral and central processes are involved when pain becomes "out of control" as in many chronic pain conditions. Central processes include glial activation, wind-up (central desensitization), de-afferentation, and cortical reorganization. Neuromodulatory pain interventions are often designed to target one or more of these processes.

It could be argued that ultimately, many if not all pain interventions, would influence the experience of pain at the central and/or autonomic nervous system, particularly the cortical level. This chapter is limited to discussing approaches aimed primarily at pain modulation at the cortical level. Medications, surgeries, behavioral and cognitive behavioral interventions, which presumably also impact cortical processing of nociceptive information, are presented elsewhere in this book. For this chapter, three categories of interventions will be discussed: cortical stimulation, hypnosis, and neurofeedback/biofeedback.

Cortical stimulation

The use of electrical and magnetic energy for therapeutic purposes can be traced back for thousands of years to when necklaces, bracelets, and amulets were used for their healing powers. In antiquity, for example, women would wear magnetic amulets on their foreheads to preserve their youth while men wore amulets as protection. The power of the amulet was thought to be transmitted by electrical and magnetic energy. It has been written that Galen, a prominent physician and philosopher who was born around 129 A.D, used electric energy in the form of electric shocks as a treatment for a number of ailments including epilepsy, melancholia, and depression (as cited by Kneeland and Warren [8]). Similarly, Scribonius Largus, a Roman physician, used the electric current found in torpedo fish to treat headaches and gout (as cited by Kneeland and Warren [8]). From these pioneers and others came the idea that physical and mental ailments were related, at least in part, to electrical currents.

Despite a long history of individuals using electrical and magnetic currents for therapeutic purposes, only within the last few centuries have there been experiments conducted to investigate the relationships between neurophysiology and electrical currents. One of the first of these was conducted in 1786 by a physician and a physicist by the name of Luigi Galvani. Galvani discovered that he was able to induce muscular contractions in the legs of frogs by applying a pair of scissors along the trajectory of the sciatic nerve during an electric storm (cited in Kipnis [9]).

Clinically, the use of electrical stimulation to treat pain or induce a state of analgesia began in earnest around the 1960s with the publication of the gate control theory of pain [2]. Using the gate control model as a theoretical basis, investigators began to study the impact of electrical stimulation on the central nervous system and on the modulation of pain, particularly the spinal cord and certain regions of the brain such as the cerebral cortex and the thalamus [10, 11]. Since then, knowledge of electrical and magnetic energy, human physiology, and the neurophysiological correlates of pain have advanced greatly, leading to the development of additional electrical stimulation approaches to managing pain.

In general, the use of electrical stimulation as a therapeutic process on activities of the central, peripheral, and autonomic nervous system is labeled as *neuromodulation*. The modern era of neuromodulation consists of a variety of techniques and operations ranging from invasive (e.g., sacral nerve stimulation) to non-invasive (e.g., cranial electrotherapy stimulation) procedures.

Recent findings suggest that pain in certain neuropathic pain syndromes (e.g., complex regional pain syndrome, fibromyalgia, and phantom-limb pain) correlates with functional reorganization of the somatosensory and motor cortex [12–14]. Cortical reorganization typically involves two main phenomena: changes in somatotopic organization and changes in excitability of the somatosensory motor cortex [15]. Furthermore, there is some evidence to indicate a relation between the degree of the cortical reorganization and pain, and that the reversal of cortical reorganization in patients with spontaneous or provoked pain is accompanied by pain relief [16, 17].

Modulation of cortical excitability for pain relief can be accomplished by both invasive and non-invasive techniques. Deep brain stimulation is performed by implanting electrodes in selected structures within the brain or over the motor cortex. Non-invasive techniques include repetitive transcranial magnetic stimulation, transcranial direct current stimulation on the scalp, and micro-current cranial electrotherapy stimulation. While deep brain and other invasive electrical stimulation appears promising, clinical use of this technique has been limited and the number of research studies remains small, possibly due the invasive nature, risk and relative expense of the procedures [18–20].

Transcranial magnetic stimulation

Repetitive transcranial magnetic stimulation (rTMS) uses the principle of electromagnetic induction to focus induced currents in the brain. Single pulses of current are applied to depolarize neurons transiently while repetitive pulses from the rTMS equipment induce excitability that lasts beyond the duration of the stimulation. The technique has been studied in healthy volunteers, as well as in patients with several painful and non-painful disorders including trigeminal neuralgia, post-stroke pain, spinal cord injury, brachial plexus or trigeminal nerve lesion, complex regional pain syndromes, fibromyalgia, and phantom limb pain. The efficacy of rTMS is "parameters-dependent," meaning that the effect depends on the parameters selected to carry out the intervention. The outcomes are homogeneous with overall mean pain relief in the range of 20–45% [21]. However, there is no published evidence yet concerning its long-term efficacy.

This technique can also be used to repetitively stimulate an area of the cortex, though with little spatial specificity, thus making it a poor tool to affect deeper areas of the cortex known to be involved in the processing of pain, such as the cingulate. Nonetheless, stimulation of the somatosensory areas associated with the pain perception (see a homunculus depiction for localization diagrams) can fatigue those areas, thus influencing the perception of pain at least for a short refractory period. This procedure has been performed with phantom pain and tinnitus [22]. When these procedures result in improvements in pain, stimulators are surgically implanted for longer lasting results [23].

A typical rTMS protocol consists of about 20 sessions, each lasting about 15 minutes; an hour is used for a depression protocol (combined with 45 minutes of cognitive behavior therapy). A cortical activation protocol would use 10 Hz stimulation while a decreasing activation protocol would use 1 Hz stimulation; the stimulation strength being set associated with levels that trigger the motor response threshold (for the thumb/hand)[1].

Transcranial direct current stimulation

Transcranial direct current stimulation involves applying a low amplitude direct current on the scalp using two electrodes. The direct stimulation is intended to influence neuronal excitability and to modulate the firing rates of individual neurons in the treated areas of the brain. There is less empirical evidence for the use of tDCS compared to rTMS;

---

[1] Information courtesy of Martjin Arns, Director, Brainclinics Treatment B.V, Bijleveldsingel 34, 6524 AD Nijmegen, The Netherlands.

however, mean pain relief of up to 58%, at least in the short term, has been reported [24]. Furthermore, tDCS has also been shown to be capable of increasing and decreasing the cortical function of localized areas by 30–40%, and in chronic pain, it may be applied over the somatosensory area to down-modulate the function of this area. This technique is also being used experimentally at this time in many application areas to modulate cortical function; its long-term effect on chronic pain is currently not known.

In a typical protocol for tDCS, the stimulation is generally in the range of one milliamp of direct current. Sessions are 10–20 minutes of stimulation of either the anodal (plus) or cathodal (minus) pole of the battery over the active site. The other lead has to be placed either over another active site, or on a non-cephalic location like the shoulder. The electrodes are large rubber with saline pads, or carbon pads in most modern devices.

Smaller surfaces used in smaller electrode assemblies can cause skin irritation, and in rare cases even electrolytic "burns" if too small an area is prepared.

Cranial electrotherapy stimulation

Cranial electrotherapy stimulation (CES) involves the delivery of a low-level electrical current that is transmitted via external, skin surface electrodes (usually placed on the ears). The low-level current is ordinarily sub-threshold for sensory detection, and appears to engage electrical and neurochemical mechanisms that affect network electrophysiological activity of brain systems mediating arousal, sensory processing, and thus, pain and pain modulation.

Several well-designed studies of CES treatment have been conducted utilizing a variety of patient populations. In one double-blind study, CES (active and sham) was tested for its ability to produce dental anesthesia. Although the results were variable, favorable outcomes were generally reported [25]. In another study, Heffernan examined EEG spectra and pain relief, employing a two-part, double-blind approach that compared CES to control and other forms of central stimulation (i.e., Liss Stimulator) [26]. In this study, results were also variable, yet the authors were able to conclude that CES produced EEG spectral smoothing and pain relief that was superior to sham control or comparison treatment. Naveau and colleagues utilized a randomized, double-blind protocol to evaluate the capacity of CES to reduce the required analgesic dose of fentanyl in rectal cancer

patients undergoing nd-YAG laser treatment [27]. The authors reported that CES treatment enabled a 31% decrease in the dose of fentanyl required to elicit pain relief.

A double blind, placebo-control study of 60 patients indicated that CES, as compared to sham treatment or wait list control, was effective in reducing tender points by 28% and self-rated pain by 27% [28]. More recently, a double-blind control study comparing CES to sham treatment for 38 patients suffering from pain associated with spinal cord injury concluded that it is efficacious in reducing pain and pain interference [29]. Although published research to date indicates that treatment with CES is promising for short-term pain relief, further research is needed to document its long-term effects on chronic pain.

Hypnotic analgesia for chronic pain

In recent years, the use of hypnosis to treat chronic pain in clinical settings has experienced resurgence in popularity due in part, perhaps, to the "treatment resistant" nature of many chronic pain conditions and the adverse effects often experienced following pharmaceutical interventions. The definition of hypnosis provided by the American Psychological Association's Division 30 (Society of Psychological Hypnosis) states that "hypnosis typically involves an introduction to the procedure during which the subject is told that suggestions for imaginative experiences will be presented" and that following such an introduction, "one person (the subject) is guided by another (the hypnotist) to respond to suggestions for changes in subjective experience, alterations in perception, sensation, emotion, thought, or behavior" [30]. Similarly, hypnotic treatment for chronic pain generally begins with an induction, which consists of one or more suggestions for alterations in the patient's behavior or perception (e.g., focused attention and/or relaxation), and is typically followed by specific suggestions for modifying how the patient perceives or experiences pain. Post-hypnotic suggestions, which might include the suggestion that any benefits experienced by the patient during the session will last beyond the end of the session, or that the patient can recreate a state of comfort and relaxation outside of the session by using a specified cue (e.g., taking a deep breath, holding it for a moment, and then releasing it), are also considered to be an integral part of the treatment.

In hypnotic analgesia for the treatment of chronic pain, the training is usually not just in hypnosis, but in the use of *self-hypnosis*. Self-hypnosis emphasizes teaching the patient how to use hypnosis outside of the treatment sessions and encourages regular practice. The goal, therefore, is not only to alter the patient's experience of pain during the sessions, but to give the patient the skills to modify the experience of pain in his/her daily life. To achieve this aim, post-hypnotic suggestions can be given which address how frequently the patient will practice the skills taught outside of session (e.g., "for a minute or two every hour, or for several minutes, a few times a day") and how continued practice will improve both how the patient feels and the automaticity with which he/she can use these skills.

A typical hypnosis session for chronic pain management consists of: (1) initial discussion of response to self-hypnosis practice since the most recent session (i.e., response to the inductions used and suggestions included); (2) discussion of possible goals for the current hypnosis session (e.g., improved sleep quality, pain reduction, increased pain acceptance); (3) presentation of a 20–40 minute induction followed by hypnotic suggestions (including post-hypnotic suggestions, as appropriate; see a more detailed description below) with an audio recording made of the session for the patient to listen to during home practice; (4) careful observation of patient response during the session (e.g., indications of depth of relaxation and response to suggestions); (5) discussion of patient response to the induction and suggestions; and (6) discussion of goals for the next session. Clinical research studies usually provide 4 to 10 sessions of hypnosis [31], although many clinicians choose to begin with four sessions, and then determine if more are indicated following these. The two most common reasons for treatment discontinuation after four sessions include (1) such significant treatment gains that additional sessions are not deemed necessary by the client and clinician, and (2) so little benefit that additional sessions are deemed to be a waste of the patient's resources. Additional treatment sessions, usually up to ten (but sometimes more if additional gains are being made) are provided when the client and clinician see some progress, and determine that additional hypnosis sessions may provide even more benefit.

In a typical treatment session the patient is first instructed to get comfortable and invited to close his/her eyes. Then the hypnotist begins the induction. A common induction involves the hypnotist counting from 1 to 10 while the patient is told to imagine descending an elevator or staircase, and that for each level the patient descends, he/she is becoming more and more deeply relaxed. Another common induction is simple progressive muscle relaxation – inviting the patient to experience different muscle groups as "heavy, comfortable, and relaxed." Prior to the induction, the patient is asked to describe, in detail, a "special place" – a place, real or imagined, where he/she feels safe and comfortable. These details are written down by the hypnotist and then relayed back to the participant following the induction, as the suggestion is made that the patient use all of his/her senses to fully experience being in this special place. At this point, if the patient has indicated that a body of water is present in his/her special place, the hypnotist can ask if the patient might receive any benefit from sitting/laying/floating in the "healing" water whose temperature is "just right."

After the patient has been guided through the special place imagery, the hypnotist may suggest a classic hypnotic experience (e.g., heavy hand, hands pulled together, head pulled to side, heavy arm). This is done to help increase confidence in both the patient and the experimenter for hypnotic responding, and to help induce a deeper trance. Following this, a number of suggestions are given to alter the patient's experience or perception of pain. These may include suggestions for decreased unpleasantness of sensations, decreased intensity of sensations (direct pain diminution), imagined anesthesia (hypno-anesthesia), a global sense of deep relaxation and comfort, or substituting uncomfortable sensations with "neutral" sensations (sensory substitution). If the patient has indicated prior to the session that he/she has experienced problems with "breakthrough pain" (significant increases in pain that occur on top of background chronic pain) or with pain "flare-ups" that occur in response to specific activities or situations, the hypnotist can further administer suggestions for modifying this type of pain experience. Suggestions might also be targeted for other pain-related issues, such as improved sleep, enhanced well-being, and improved ability to engage in an active life-style, as appropriate. Post-hypnotic suggestions are then given for self-hypnosis, i.e., suggestions for the use of hypnosis outside of the session, signaled by a cue (e.g., deep breath), or suggestions for ongoing practice of the skills learned during session. At the end of the session, the hypnotist brings the patient out of hypnosis, typically by counting backwards from 10 to 1 and suggesting that the patient is becoming more and more awake and alert, while staying relaxed, as the count approaches "1."

The hypnotist also assesses the patient's pain characteristics (e.g., intensity and unpleasantness), often on an 11-point numerical rating scale (NRS; 0 = no pain to 10 = worst pain imaginable) both at the beginning and the end of each treatment session. This information about changes in the patient's pain experience are thus used to determine what modifications, if any, need to be made to the hypnosis script prior to the next session. Depending on the treatment protocol, the hypnotist may also assess some of these characteristics during the session, typically at transitions between different suggestions, to assess what effect the specific suggestions are having on the patient's perception of pain. Additionally, recordings or CDs of one or more sessions are provided to the patient for continued practice on his/her own of the hypnotic skills taught.

In recent years, several reviews of controlled randomized trials of hypnotic analgesia for the treatment of chronic pain have been conducted [31–35]. The studies summarized in these reviews have included a wide variety of chronic pain conditions including migraine headache [36, 37], fibromyalgia [38]; osteoarthritis [39]; low back pain [40–42], cancer pain [43, 44], and pain secondary to physical disability [45]. Based on the findings from these studies, the reviews have concluded that (1) hypnosis results in significant reductions in pain compared to no treatment; (2) hypnosis is often more effective than non-hypnotic interventions such as attention, physical therapy, and education; (3) when hypnosis is compared to hypnosis-like treatments (e.g., progressive muscle relaxation training, autogenic training), pain reduction outcomes are often similar; and (4) reductions in chronic pain associated with hypnosis treatments tend to be maintained over time, even up to 12 months post-treatment.

Another common finding from the hypnosis literature is the high degree of variability of treatment response. The average pre- to post-treatment decrease in pain intensity, on a 0–10 scale, for example, has been reported to be in the 0.94 to 1.20 range [45]. This is not a substantial decrease; perhaps even barely noticeable to the average person. However, this average change hides the fact that some patients report marked (a 30% or greater reduction) decreases in average daily pain intensity following hypnosis treatment, while others show much less or even no improvement. Responder analyses provide rates of response, and can tell the clinician more regarding the expected effects of treatment than can reports of average changes in pain. Using a 30% reduction as an indication of a clinically meaningful response, responder analyses yield response rates ranging from 37% to 47% in patients with chronic pain who participate in hypnosis treatment [45].

Mechanism of action of hypnosis

Although the mechanism of action of hypnosis is not fully understood, several fMRI studies have suggested that the ACC plays a prominent role in modulating the effect of hypnosis over pain, particularly when suggestions focus on reducing the affective or "unpleasantness" component of pain [46, 47]. Hypnosis has also been shown to attenuate the magnitude of activation in the anterior basal ganglia and left ACC in the case of thermal pain [48]. It has also been shown that hypnosis activates cortical sites that are distinctively different from distraction and counter-stimulation, suggesting that different mechanisms underlie these different treatment approaches [48]. Finally, there is some evidence to suggest the possibility that hypnotic susceptibility could be raised by increasing the theta/beat ratio via EEG biofeedback training [49].

Case example

To illustrate the administration and the effectiveness of hypnotic analgesia for chronic pain, a brief synopsis of a case study will be presented here; for a detailed description, see Stoelb, et al. [50]. The patient was a 27-year-old male Army Sergeant who had sustained a spinal cord injury (SCI) at the level of the 6th cervical vertebrae (C6) from a gunshot wound to the neck while stationed in Iraq. He was completely paralyzed from the chest down, but had maintained some movement in his arms. The patient, who was cared for at a Veteran's Administration hospital, had a number of SCI-related pain problems which were interfering substantially with his rehabilitation and care. For example, the patient's occupational therapist (OT) reported that the patient's pain level, both during and following therapy, was "around a 10" on a 0–10 NRS, and that the patient's hands had become "claw-like" and almost non-functional due to contractures (an abnormal, often permanent shortening of the muscle, that results in distortion or deformity). Both the patient and his OT endorsed that the patient's hands – particularly his left – were incredibly sensitive and even a light touch on these areas would cause the patient to experience a great deal of pain. Each time the staff attempted to provide range-of-motion to the patient's hands, he became irate and often demanded that care providers leave the room and turn out the lights. As the patient had experienced a number of untoward side effects from pain medications, instruction in self-hypnosis was presented to him as an alternate treatment option, which he agreed to try.

The patient received ten sessions of the self-hypnosis training treatment protocol detailed above [45]. Prior to beginning treatment, the patient described his primary pain site as his hands, with the pain in his left hand being worse. He also rated a number of pain sensations (e.g., sharp, aching, throbbing, shooting) as a "10" on a 0–10 NRS. Each treatment session followed the typical order previously outlined (induction, special place imagery, classic hypnotic suggestion, analgesic suggestions, post-hypnotic suggestions, coming out of hypnosis), and pain was assessed by the hypnotist before, during, and after each session, based on the protocol.

During both the first and second session, the patient's current pain intensity dropped from moderate levels (6/10 and 5/10, respectively) to 0s immediately after the hypnotic induction. He continued to show a great deal of improvement in both his pain intensity and pain affect levels throughout the remainder of the treatment sessions. Among the many improvements the patient reported, three of the most notable were: (1) between sessions 6 and 7, the patient's OT reported that during therapy, he was now able to move the patient's fingers into a straight, horizontal position, without any bend in the joints, which was previously not possible because it had been "incredibly painful" for the patient; (2) in the week prior to session 10, the patient's pain medication (methadone) had been reduced from 10 mg two times per day, to 5 mg two times per day; and (3) the patient's pain intensity and pain affect ratings at the end of each hypnosis session were never greater than a 2 on the 11-point NRS. During a 6-month telephone follow-up, the patient reported that his pain intensity level and sensitivity to pain had continued to decrease substantially. At its worst, he stated his pain intensity level was a 5 or 6, and at best, it was a 1.5/2. He endorsed continued use of the practice CD (which was given to him during treatment) and the self-hypnotic skills he had learned during the treatment sessions, particularly the "special place" imagery.

Neurofeedback/biofeedback for pain management

Biofeedback

The field of biofeedback has a rich history and its course has been influenced by developments in behavioral learning theories, psychophysiology, behavioral medicine, bio-medical engineering, and cybernetics. Recent resurgence in interest can be attributed to three simultaneously emerging trends [1]. The first is the emergence of technology and algorithms that allow the near simultaneous recording, analysis, and response to neuronal depolarization / repolarization (that is, EEG). The second converging trend is the increased skepticism with many pharmacological treatments given the side effects and long-term toxic effects to the human body. The third is the development of a strong popular interest and a commitment to safe, non-toxic, non-invasive, and self-regulatory ways of dealing with symptoms and the achievement of well-being which transcends the achievement of a symptom-free state.

Although all biofeedback involves learning improved self-regulation of the physiology that is purported to "cause" or relate to the pain condition in question via the principals of operant conditioning, biofeedback may be divided into somatic (or peripheral) and central (or neurofeedback or EEG-related) biofeedback. The former has been used extensively for psycho-physiological disorders such as neuromuscular pain conditions, migraine, bruxism and tempero-mandibular point disorders, Raynaud's disease, and a host of other mechanically mediated pain disorders attributable to dysregulated sympathetic tone. In neurofeedback (or EEG biofeedback), the target organ is the brain.

Several definitions of biofeedback have been proposed. Some emphasize the processes or procedures; others stress the goal or objectives of biofeedback, while others attempt to combine both elements. On May 18, 2008, three primary organizations associated with biofeedback (the Association for Applied Psychophysiology and Biofeedback – AAPB; the Biofeedback Certification Institute of America – BCIA; and the International Society for Neurofeedback and Research – ISNR) reached an agreement on a universal definition of biofeedback as:

> "Biofeedback is a process that enables an individual to learn how to change physiological activity for the purposes of improving health and performance. Precise instruments measure physiological activity such as brainwaves, heart function, breathing, muscle activity, and skin temperature. These instruments rapidly and accurately "feed back" information to the user. The presentation of this information – often in conjunction with changes in thinking, emotions, and behavior – supports desired physiological changes. Over time, these changes can endure without continued use of an instrument."

Table 13.1 Outline/content of a typical biofeedback session

a. Pre-session assessment (progress since last visit, if applicable)

b. Review of the goal for this session

c. Pre-session rating of pain and other important outcome measures

d. Decision concerning the biofeedback modality/ protocol to use

e. Instruction to patient (if applicable)

f. Implement the training/protocol (a session usually takes 30–50 minutes, depending on the protocol)

g. Record observations

h. Post-session rating of pain and other outcomes, as appropriate

i. Feedback from patient regarding the session

j. End session with instruction for next session, if applicable

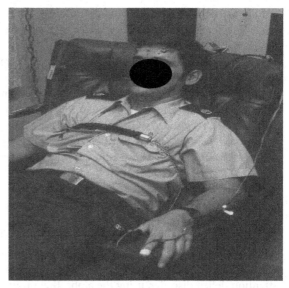

Figure 13.2 A patient wearing biofeedback recording sensors.

Table 13.1 shows the outline/content of a typical biofeedback session.

Minimal instruction is usually provided to the patient regarding specific strategies to use during the biofeedback session. Usually, the patient is instructed to simply bring on a tone or to move a bar past a preset threshold on the screen. In short, the patient is asked to use the feedback (visual or audio) to move towards the target such as lower sEMG, higher alpha amplitude, etc. All biofeedback procedures are based on operant-conditioning principles.

A typical patient wearing psychophysiological recording sensors can be seen in Figure 13.2. In this picture, the patient can be seen wearing muscle tension sensors on his forehead, a respiration belt around his chest to record breathing, a temperature sensor (for near surface blood flow) on his pointer finger, and a heart rate sensor on his thumb. He would also have sensors for sweating mounted on his palm or fingers and sensors for brain waves on his scalp.

Peripheral biofeedback

The selection of modality/protocol is based on the presenting problems, clinical interviews, review of medical chart, psychometric testing data, goals of training/ treatment, and in selected cases, physiological stress profiling.

Several reviews on the efficacy of biofeedback therapies for pain management are available [51, 52, 53]. In a recent review of complementary and alternative medicine (CAM) modalities/therapies to pain management, Tan *et al.* [52] utilized the treatment efficacy guidelines of the Clinical Psychology Division of the American Psychological Association [54] where level 1 is "not empirically supported," level 5 is "efficacious and specific (the highest level of efficacy)," and levels 2 to 4 are inbetween. The review concluded that biofeedback is efficacious for the following pain conditions:

Level 4: Migraine, tension headaches, and muscle-related orofacial pain.

Level 3: Stress and muscle tension-related incontinence, cramping and burning phantom pain, irritable bowel syndrome, Raynaud's disease, posture related pain, stress-induced chest pain.

Level 2: Premenstrual syndrome and dysmenorrhea, pain from spastic muscles and muscle spasms, pelvic floor pain, carpel tunnel syndromes, myofascial/trigger point related pain, fibromyalgia.

Central biofeedback (neurofeedback)

As previously mentioned, neurofeedback (NF; also referred to as EEG biofeedback) may be defined as a form of biofeedback where the target of change is the brain (specifically, the EEG). Changes in brain electrical field activities are measured by EEG, and modifying the EEG pattern of rhythms to alter/modulate pain experience via operant conditioning is the basis of NF.

For a more detailed discussion on neurofeedback, the reader is referred to the text book edited by Evans and Abarbanel [55].

Neurofeedback is a new and constantly evolving field. There are probably as many practitioners who advocate that all NF requires a quantitative assessment of the brain's EEG (referred to as quantitative EEG or QEEG for short) prior to starting NF as there are those who would view QEEG as an unnecessary and costly burden for the patient. Those who advocate for and use QEEG assess EEG activity in the patient prior to treatment, and compare the results to one of several normative data bases. They then develop NF interventions based on the QEEG analysis. Those who do not use QEEG normally apply one of several general NF protocols based on the nature of the presenting complaints (e.g., up-training C3 SMR or C4 beta for attention deficit disorder, using the alpha-theta training protocol for addiction, or addressing frontal alpha asymmetry for depression). Neurofeedback can focus on a number of aspects of EEG-assessed cortical activity, including altering: (1) the power (or amplitude) of specific frequencies; (2) specific ratios of amplitudes; and (3) the coherence, phase and synchrony among different areas or parts of the brain. For more details, the reader is again referred to the book on NF and conference proceedings of the ISNR and AAPB, as well as the journals published by the two professional organizations (*Applied Psychophysiology and Biofeedback*, and *Journal of Neurotherapy*).

Recent research findings indicate several possible targets for neurofeedback interventions for pain management. The first entails failure modes in the anterior cingulate. As has been previously discussed, the anterior cingulate plays a major role in pain perception. When the anterior cingulate is not functioning properly, there is a lack of normal cognitive and emotional flexibility, and the brain can be "stuck" on pain sensation [56]. When the cingulate fails to function normally, awareness can over-focus, as seen in generalized anxiety disorder and obsessive compulsive disorder/oppositional defiant, as well as in cases of chronic pain [57]. There are three failure modes of the anterior cingulate: (1) an excess of alpha (the most prevalent), (2) an excess of slow wave activity; and (3) beta spindling. The latter pattern is reported by Johnstone *et al.*, and Arns *et al.* [58, 59]. The two initial patterns were originally identified by cluster analysis in work done by NYU's Brain Research Laboratory by Dr. Leslie Prichep and colleagues [60, 61].

Other potential targets for neurofeedback include the somatosensory areas for modulating pain perception, the thalamic relays for modulating pain sensation (e.g., in "central pain" syndromes, where there is no peripheral stimuli involved), and cortical reorganization (a type of neural plasticity, resulting in loss of sensory input such as in phantom limb pain, where the adjacent cortical areas "invade" due to decreased lateral inhibition; [13]).

Despite the wide variations on how to approach and carry out NF, the general procedure to NF bears close resemblance to the biofeedback procedure previously described, although one distinction, discussed above, concerns the degree to which one relies on using QEEG assessment to guide and/or determine the selection of the intervention protocol.

Efficacy of neurofeedback

Much of the activities in NF have focused on areas other than pain. In the area of NF as applied to chronic pain, there are mainly case reports and few controlled research studies. Because efficacy cannot be concluded based solely on this level of support, more research is needed before a claim of efficacy for NF for pain management can be made. This does not necessarily mean that clinical applications in chronic pain cannot be effective on an individual case basis, or that NF cannot be used in clinical research to explore its effects. However, this does mean that we are not yet able to conclude that NF necessarily has a specific beneficial effect on pain or the impact of pain in persons presenting with chronic pain conditions.

Despite the limitation on efficacy research, several studies do show some promising results. In a study involving 40 patients suffering from fibromyalgia, Caro and Winter found significant improvement in measures of self-reported pain, attention, tender points, and fatigue [62]. Similarly, another group of 30 fibromyalgia patients who were treated with EEG-driven NF (in combination with surface electromyography biofeedback) significantly improved in pain, perceived mental clarity, mood, and sleep [63]. Sime reported a case of trigeminal neuralgia which was treated with a combination of BF and NF and led to the abortion/avoidance of a major planned surgery to sever the trigeminal nerve [64]. The protocol consisted of ten peripheral BF sessions, NF training at C3 (to improve sleep), and low reward frequency training at T3–T4 (to decrease pain). More recently, Jensen *et al.* reported some success with NF for treating 18 patients diagnosed with complex regional pain syndrome (CRPS) type I [65]. These were patients with severe long-standing CRPS type I who were enrolled in a 20-day comprehensive CRPS treatment. Partialing out the effects of the other treatments in the program, the individualized NF protocols were shown to reduce pain intensity at the primary site with half of the study participants showing meaningful change of 30% or more. Improvements were also found in five of the seven secondary measures including muscle tension, aches and spasms, sense of well-being, pain at second site, and skin sensitivity. Finally, deCharms *et al.* combined fMRI technology with NF to demonstrate that patients were able to learn to control relative activation on the rostral anterior cingulate cortex (associated with the processing of the experience of pain), resulting in a significant reduction in pain [66].

Mechanism of action for biofeedback

The mechanism of action for biofeedback in pain management has not been fully established. However, there is increasing evidence that for chronic muscle or myofascial pain syndrome, pain modulation with biofeedback is achieved via both de-catastrophizing (changes in beliefs about pain) and by learning lowered arousal techniques that keep sympathetic pathways to trigger points from being maintained [67, 68]. For pain conditions such as fibromyalgia, phantom, or other centrally mediated pain, biofeedback may counter the effect of central sensitization through decreasing sympathetic overload, parasympathetic withdrawal, and stress hormones. There is also some evidence that changing improper muscle contraction and blood flow patterns has a direct effect on pain caused by these problems [69, 70]. Biofeedback (at least in the case of cultivated lowered arousal) has also been shown to decrease the stress response, which in turn, leads to decreased activation of the ACC, insular cortex, SI and SII, and the amygdala, all areas activated by pain [71].

Summary and conclusion

Pain is experienced when complex neurophysiological networks, involving peripheral, spinal, and cortical neurons are engaged, and can be relieved when these processes are interrupted. A number of interventions, broadly labeled as "non-pharmacological neuromodulation" approaches, have been examined as potential treatments for chronic pain. These approaches specifically target the neurological processes involved in the processing and experience of pain. They include electrical stimulation, self-hypnosis training, and biofeedback

and/neurofeedback approaches. There is varying evidence supporting the short- and long-term efficacy of these approaches. Although no intervention has yet been demonstrated to be ineffective, at present, some (e.g., self-hypnosis training) have greater evidence than others (e.g., neurofeedback training). Randomized clinical trials of all of these approaches are needed, especially with respect to their long-term efficacy. In the meantime, clinicians may wish to try any one of these treatments, especially those that are minimally invasive, to explore their efficacy on an individual basis.

References

1. Laibow, R. Medical applications of neurobiofeedback. In *Quantitative EEG and neurofeedback*, eds. JR Evans and A Abarbanel. (CA: Academic Press, 1999), pp. 93–101.

2. Melzack R, Wall PD. Pain mechanisms: A new theory. *Science* 1965; **150**: 971–9.

3. Stephenson DT, Arneric SP. Neuroimaging of pain: Advances and future prospects. *J Pain* 2008; **9**: 567–79.

4. Peyron R, Laurent B, Garcia-Larrea L. Functional imaging of brain reponses to pain. A review and meta-analysis. *Neurophysiol Clin* 2000; **30**: 263–88.

5. Mackey, S. *Biofeedback: Past, present, and future. Presented at American Pain Society 27th Annual Scientific Conference.* (Tampa, FL, 2008).

6. Rainville P, Duncan GH, Price DD, Carrier B, Bushnell MC. Pain affect encoded in human anterior cingulate but not somatosensory cortex. *Science* 1997; **277**: 968–71.

7. Jensen MP, Hakimian S, Sherlin L H, Fregni F. New insights into non-pharmacological and noninvasive neuromodulatory approaches for the treatment of pain. *J Pain* 2008; **9**: 193–9.

8. Kneeland TW, Warren CAB. *Pushbutton Psychiatry: A history of electroshock in America* (Westport, CT: Praeger, 1994).

9. Kipnis N. Luigi Galvani and the debate on animal electricity, 1791–1800. *Ann Sci* 1987; **44**: 107–42.

10. Benabid A, Wallace B, Mitrofanis J, *et al.* Therapeutic electrical stimulation of the central nervous system. *CR Biology* 2005; **328**: 177–86.

11. Ranck JB. Which elements are excited in electrical stimulation of mammalian central nervous system: a review. *Brain Res* 1975; **98**: 417–40.

12. Eisenberg E, Chistyakov AV, Yudashkin M, *et al.* Evidence for cortical hyperexcitability of the affected limb representation area in CRPS: A psychophysical and transcranial magnetic stimulation study. *Pain* 2005; **113**: 99–105.

13. Flor H, Elbert T, Knecht S, *et al.* Phantom limb pain as a perceptual correlate of cortical reorganization. *Nature* 1995; **357**: 482–4.

14. Maihofner C, Handwerker HO, Neundorfer B, Birklein F. Patterns of cortical reorganization in Complex Regional Pain Syndrome. *Neurology* 2003; **61**: 1707–15.

15. Knotkova, H. Cortical stimulation for persistent pain syndromes: novel strategies. *Presented at American Pain Society 27th Annual Scientific Conference.* (Tampa, FL, 2008).

16. Birbaumer N, Lutzenberger W, Montoya P, *et al.* Effects of regional anaesthesia on phantom limb pain are mirrored in changes in cortical reorganization. *J Neurosci* 1997; **17**: 5503–8.

17. Pleger B, Tegenthoff M, Ragert P, *et al.* Sensorimotor returning in complex regional pain syndrome parallels pain reduction. *Annal Neurol* 2005; **57**: 425–9.

18. Brown JA, Pilitsis JG. Motor cortex stimulation for central and neuropathic facial pain: A prospective study of 10 patients and observations of enhanced sensory and motor function during stimulation. *Neurosurgery* 2005; **56**: 290–7.

19. Nguyen JP, LefaucherJP, Le Guerinel C, *et al.* Motor cortex stimulation in the treatment of central and neuropathic pain. *Arch Med Res* 2000; **31**: 263–5.

20. Brown JA, Barbaro NM. Motor cortex stimulation for central and neuropathic pain: current status. *Pain* 2003; **104**: 431–5.

21. Fregni F, Pascual-Leone A. Technology insight: noninvasive brain stimulation in neurology-perspectives on the therapeutic potential of rTMS and tDCS. *Nat Clin Pract Neurol* 2007; **7**: 381–90.

22. De Ridder D, De Mulder G, Sunaert S, Moller A. Somatosensory cortex stimulation for deafferentation pain. *Neuromodulation* 2006; **9**: 149.

23. De Ridder, D, Ryu H, Moller A, *et al.* Functional anatomy of the human cochlear nerve and its role in microvascular decompressions for tinnitus. *Neurosurgery* 2004; **54**: 381–90.

24. Fregni F, Boggio PS, Lima MC, *et al.* A sham-controlled, phase II trial of transcranial direct current stimulation for the treatment of central pain in traumatic spinal cord injury. *Pain* 2006; **122**: 197–209.

25. Clark MS, Silverstone LM, Lindenmuth J, *et al.* An evaluation of the clinical analgesia/anesthesia efficacy on acute pain using the high frequency neural modulator in various dental settings. *Oral Surg Oral Med Oral Pathol Oral Radiol Endod* 1987; **63**: 501–5.

26. Heffernan M. The effect of variable microcurrents on EEG spectrum and pain control. *Can J Clin Med* 1997; **4**: 4–11.

27. Naveau S, Barritault L, Zourabichvili O, *et al.* Analgesic effect of transcutaneous cranial electrostimulation in patients treated by Nd: YAG laser for cancer of the rectum. A double-blind randomized trial. *Gastroenterol Clin Biol* 1992; **16**: 8–11. [In French.]

28. Lichtbroun AS, Raicer MC, Smith RB. The treatment of fibromyalgia with cranial electrotherapy stimulation. *J Clin Rheumatol* 2001; **7**: 72–8.

29. Tan G, Rintala DH, Thornby JI, Yang J. Using cranial electrotherapy stimulation to treat pain associated with spinal cord injury. *J Rehabil Res Dev* 2006; **43**, 461–74.

30. Green JP, Barabasz AF, Barrett D, Montgomery GH. Forging ahead: The 2003 APA Division 30 definition of hypnosis. *Int J Clin Exp Hypn* 2005; **53**: 259–64.

31. Patterson DR, Jensen MP. Hypnosis and Clinical pain. *Psychol Bull* 2003; **29**: 495–521.

32. Elkins G, Jensen MP, Patterson DR. Hypnotherapy for the management of chronic pain. *Int J Clin Exp Hypn* 2007; **55**: 275–87.

33. Jensen MP, Patterson DR. Hypnotic treatment of chronic pain. *J Behav Med* 2006; **29**: 95–124.

34. Montgomery GH, DuHamel KN, Redd WH. A meta-analysis of hypnotically induced analgesia: How effective is hypnosis? *Int J Clin Exp Hypn* 2000; **48**: 138–53.

35. Patterson DR, Jensen MP. Hypnosis and clinical pain. *Psychol Bull* 2003; **129**: 495–521.

36. Andreychuk T, Skriver C. Hypnosis and biofeedback in the treatment of migraine headache. *Int J Clin Exp Hypn* 1975; **33**: 172–83.

37. Friedman H, Taub HA. Brief psychological training procedures in migraine treatment. *Am J Clin Hypn* 1984; **26**: 187–200.

38. Hannen HC, Hoenderdos HT, van Romunde LK, *et al.* Controlled trial of hypnotherapy in the treatment of refractory fibromyalgia. *J Rheumatol* 1991; **18**: 72–5.

39. Gay M, Philipport P, Luminet O. Differential effectiveness of psychological interventions for reducing osteoarthritis pain: A comparison of Erikson hypnosis and Jacobson relaxation. *Eur J Pain* 2002; **6**: 1–16.

40. McCauley JD, Thelen MH, Frank RG, Willard RR, Callen KE. Hypnosis compared to relaxation in the outpatient management of chronic low back pain. *Arch Phys Med Rehabil* 1983; **64**: 548–52.

41. Spinhoven P, Linssen ACG. Education and self-hypnosis in the management of low back pain: A component analysis. *British J Clin Psychol* 1989; **28**: 145–53.

42. Tan G, Fukui T, Jensen MP, Thornby JI, Waldman K. Using hypnosis to treat chronic low back pain. *Int J Clin Exp Hypn* 2010; **58**: 53–61.

43. Elkins GR, Cheung A, Marcus J, Palamara L, Rajab H. Hypnosis to reduce pain in cancer survivors with advanced disease: A prospective study. *J Cancer Integr Med* 2004; **2**: 167–72.

44. Spiegel D, Bloom JR. Group therapy and hypnosis reduce metastatic breast carcinoma pain. *Psychosom Med* 1983; **45**: 333–9.

45. Jensen MP, Hanley MA, Engel JM, *et al.* Hypnotic analgesia for chronic pain in persons with disabilities: A case series. *Int J Clin Exp Hypn* 2005; **53**: 198–228.

46. Faymonville ME, Boly M, Laureys S. Functional neuroanatomy of the hypnotic state. *J Physiol* 2006; **99**: 463–9.

47. Faymonville ME, Laureys S, Degueldre C, *et al.* Neural mechanisms of antinociceptive effects of hypnosis. *Anesthesiology* 2000; **92**: 1257–67.

48. Chen AC. New perspective in EEG/MEG brain mapping and PET/fMRI neuroimaging of human pain. *Int J Psychophysiol* 2001; **42**: 147–59.

49. Batty M, Bonnington S, Tang B, Hawken M, Gruzelier J. Relaxation strategies and enhancement of hypnotic susceptibility: EEG neurofeedback, progressive muscle relaxation, and self-hypnosis. *Brain Res Bull* 2006; **71**, 83–90.

50. Stoelb BL, Jensen MP, Tackett MJ. Hypnotic analgesia for combat-related spinal cord injury pain: A case study. *Am J Clin Hypn* 2009; **51**: 273–80.

51. Tan G, Sherman R, Shanti B. Biofeedback pain interventions. *Pract Pain Manage* 2003; **3**: 12–18.

52. Tan G, Craine MH, Bair MJ, *et al.* Efficacy of selected complementary and alternative medicine (CAM) interventions for chronic pain. *J Rehabil Res Dev* 2007; **44**: 195–222.

53. Sherman RA. Pain assessment and intervention from a psychological perspective. (Association of Applied Psychophysiology and Biofeedback, 2003).

54. Chambless DL, Baker MJ, Baucom DH, *et al.* Update on empirically validated therapies, II. *Clinical Psychol* 1998; **51**: 3–16.

55. Evans JR, Abarbanel A (eds.). *Introduction to Quantitative EEG Neurofeedback* (California: Academic Press, 1999).

56. Shafritz KM, Kartheiser P, Belger A. Dissociation of neuronal systems mediating shifts in behavioral response and cognitive set. *Neuroimage* 2005; **25**: 600–6.

57. Woodward TS, Ruff CC, Ngan TC. Short- and long-term changes in anterior cingulate activation during resolution of task-set competition. *Brain Res* 2006; **1068**: 161–9.

58. Johnstone J, Gunkelman J, Lunt J. Clinical database development: Characterization of EEG phenotypes. *Clinical EEG and Neurosci* 2005; **36**: 99–107.

59. Arns M, Gunkelman J, Breteler M, Spronk D. EEG phenotypes predict treatment outcome to stimulants in children with ADHD. *J Integr Neurosci* 2008; **7**: 421–38.

60. Bolwig TG, Hansen ES, Hansen A, Merkin H, Prichep LS. Toward a better understanding of the pathophysiology of OCD SSRI responder: QEEG source localization. *Acta Psychiatr Scand* 2007; **115**: 237–46.

61. Hansen ES, Prichep LS, Bolwig TG, John ER. Quantitative electroencephalography in OCD-patients treated with paroxetine. *Clinical EEG* 2003; **34**: 70–4.

62. Caro XJ, Winter EF. Attention measures improve in fibromyalgia patients receiving EEG biofeedback training: A pilot study. *Arthritis Rheum* 2001; **44**: S71.

63. Mueller H, Donaldson S, Nelson D, Layman, M. Treatment of fibromyalgia incorporating EEG-driven stimulation: A clinical outcomes study. *J Clin Psychol* 2001; **57**: 933–52.

64. Sime A. Case study of trigeminal neuralgia using biofeedback and peripheral biofeedback. *J Neurother* 2004; **71**: 59–71.

65. Jensen MP, Griesen C, Tracy-Smith V, Bacigalupi SC, Othmer S. Neurofeedback treatment for pain associated with complex regional pain syndrome type I: A case series. *J Neurother* 2007; **11**: 45–53.

66. deCharms C, Christoff K, Glover G.H, *et al.* Learned regulation of spatially localized brain activation using real-time fMRI. *Neurolmage* 2004; **21**: 436–43.

67. Crider A, Glaros AG, Gevirtz RN. Efficacy of biofeedback-based treatments for temporomandibular disorders. *Appl Psychophysiol Biofeedback* 2005; **30**: 333–45.

68. McNulty WH, Gevirtz RN, Hubbard DR, Berkoff GM. Needle electromyographic evaluation of trigger point response to a psychological stressor. *Psychophysiology* 1994; **31**: 313–16.

69. Nestoriuc Y, Martin A. Efficacy of biofeedback for migraine: A meta-analysis. *Pain*, 2007; **128**: 111–27.

70. van Haselen RA, Fisher PA. A randomized controlled trial comparing topical piroxicam gel with a homeopathic gel in osteoarthritis of the knee. *Rheumatology* 2000; **39**: 714–19.

71. Critchley HD, Melmed RN, Featherstone E, *et al.* Volitional control of autonomic arousal: A functional magnetic resonance study. *Neuroimage* 2002; **16**: 909–19.

14 Cognitive coping strategies in pain management

Laura E. Pence, Beverly E. Thorn and Amber M. Davis

Although there is a large literature on the efficacy of cognitive pain coping strategies, it has been difficult to synthesize in a meaningful way. It is evident from previous reviews that the use of cognitive coping techniques can be associated with reductions in acute, chronic, and laboratory-induced pain [1–5]. However, it is difficult to draw conclusions regarding the efficacy of *specific* cognitive coping strategies due to the way the research literature is organized and the different terminology used across studies. These barriers frequently leave the reader with more questions than answers.

The purpose of the current chapter is to provide an update on prior reviews and book chapters [2, 4], and, more importantly, to offer a different approach. First, we elaborate on the problems associated with evaluating specific coping techniques. Next, we review the literature on discrete strategies rather than composites of strategies. Finally, we seek to identify individual differences that affect the efficacy of these coping strategies. The role of individual differences in coping efficacy has not been previously reviewed, and although these potential moderators have not been thoroughly examined, there is some current evidence that merits discussion.

Description and criticisms of available literature

Typically, pain researchers have categorized coping strategies into rationally derived composites such as emotion-focused vs. problem-focused [6] and passive vs. active [7]. These rationally derived composites group together various discrete coping techniques that may influence pain via different processes. Empirically derived composite categories of coping strategies have also been reported, combining specific techniques into statistically correlated meta-categories or factors [8–10]. There are statistical and methodological

advantages to studying composites rather than discrete coping strategies because it decreases the overall number of variables under examination. However, research that uses coping composites may have limited clinical utility, rendering only broad conclusions such as identifying those that are generally considered adaptive (e.g., problem focused, active) vs. maladaptive (e.g., emotion-focused, passive). Studies using coping composites do not provide information regarding the efficacy of a specific strategy, nor do they allow exploration of potential moderating variables on the efficacy of specific strategies. Researchers have suggested that examining individual coping strategies may be more useful than studying coping composites when attempting to identify the conditions under which coping efforts have the greatest effect [11]. Moreover, research has shown that individual coping scales are better than coping composites at explaining variance in pain intensity and activity interference [12].

In addition to the problems posed by using coping composites, there are a variety of issues related to the terminology used in coping research that hinder the ability of readers to understand and make generalizations from the literature. One problem is that cognitive coping terms used in the literature are often described using imprecise definitions. For example, "attention to pain" could refer to focusing on the sensory aspects of pain or focusing on one's emotional response to pain. Although both involve attention towards pain, they are associated with different pain related outcomes [13, 14]. Researchers also use different labels for coping techniques that seem to refer to the same cognitive strategy. For example, one study used the term "stoic distancing" to refer to attempts to avoid acknowledging, dwelling upon, or expressing the extent of pain [15], while other authors use the term "ignoring" or "denying" when referring to this strategy [16, 17]. Furthermore, the

Behavioral and Psychopharmacologic Pain Management, ed. Michael H. Ebert and Robert D. Kerns. Published by Cambridge University Press. © Cambridge University Press 2011.

reinterpretation of pain sensations (e.g., "I don't think of it as pain, but rather a dull or warm feeling," and "If my pain feels shooting, I try and pretend that it is only tingling") has been variously referred to as "emotional distancing from pain," "dissociation," "focused sensory attention," and "somatization" [2, 3, 18]. Other studies use coping terms with an operational definition that is atypical, for example, one study used the term "imagery" when participants were instructed to imagine they feel happy, comfortable, and content or to imagine they feel uncomfortable, terrible, and mean [19]. Since most studies using the term "imagery" are referring to visualization of relaxing scenes or other pleasant visual images, using the same term to refer to a different type of strategy may add confusion to an already complex literature. In general, there is a lack of clarity in the literature as to the terminology used to describe cognitive coping strategies.

The coping literature is also complicated by inconsistent findings. For example, the literature on the use of distraction for chronic pain includes reports of significant positive associations between use of distraction and pain severity ratings [20, 21]. However, there are also reports of a significant inverse relation between use of distraction and chronic pain [22] as well as nonsignificant associations between use of distraction and pain severity [16, 23–25]. Possible explanations for inconsistent findings include procedural differences across studies, terminology inconsistencies, and use of composite coping strategies. It is also difficult to track null findings regarding discrete coping strategies when as many as seven or more different coping strategies may be examined in a single study and statistically significant findings are generally emphasized.

Additionally, there are some complications associated with studying pain in general. Pain is a multidimensional construct, including physical sensations, cognitive evaluation, and affect. Researchers have found that coping strategies may be differentially efficacious for the sensory vs. the affective domains of pain [13, 14]. Moreover, the efficacy of cognitive coping strategies may be different for chronic pain and acute or experimentally induced pain.

Finally, the cognitive coping literature has typically focused on the efficacy of cognitive coping strategies for broad groups of people, without attention to individual difference variables (e.g., pain factors, personality factors, sex) that may moderate the efficacy of particular strategies. These individual differences are important to consider as we determine the clinical utility of various coping strategies. A better understanding of individual differences is needed in order to draw reliable conclusions regarding the efficacy of discrete cognitive coping strategies.

Methodology and organization of review

For the current review, multiple electronic databases (PsychLit, Pubmed, Cochrane data base, Sumsearch) were used and several citation lists were searched for relevant literature. We sought to obtain unpublished research (e.g., dissertations, conference presentations) as well as published studies, but we limited our review to studies published in English. Eligible literature included correlational examinations of self-reported coping strategies and pain indicators (both cross sectional and longitudinal), as well as empirical studies. The included empirical studies either measured self-reported coping in regards to an experimental pain task or manipulated at least one cognitive coping strategy in comparison to a control condition or an alternative strategy condition (e.g., distraction vs. focused attention). Studies involving pediatric participants were not reviewed. Other eligibility requirements included: (1) operationally defined discrete cognitive strategies (i.e., not composites of multiple coping strategies or empirical factors) as independent variables; (2) report of number of participants and specific pain stimulus utilized (if laboratory-induced pain) or pain condition (e.g., mixed chronic pain); and (3) quantifiable dependent variables related to the experience of pain. For clinical acute or chronic pain studies, dependent variables of interest included pain severity or frequency, activity levels, disability, mood, and quality of life. For experimental pain studies, outcome variables of interest included pain severity, threshold, or tolerance, as well as other indicators such as muscle tension. Inconsistent comparison groups and the large number of potential moderating variables prevented statistical pooling and meta-analyses of the data.

The most recent comprehensive review of the pain coping literature was conducted by Boothby et al. [2], with a focus on coping and adjustment to chronic pain. For cognitive coping strategies reviewed as discrete techniques by Boothby et al. (i.e., distraction/diverting attention, ignoring pain, reinterpreting pain, and coping self-statements), we summarize previous conclusions and focus on the literature published after the 1999 chapter. We also review studies of acute or experimental pain, which were generally not addressed by

Boothby *et al.* The experimental pain literature was reviewed because it is likely that the best evidence regarding the efficacy of discrete coping strategies will be established through experimental pain studies. This is because experiments allow for the ability to manipulate and isolate specific coping attempts, control for confounding variables, and determine cause and effect. For discrete coping strategies not previously reviewed (i.e., imagery, sensory focus/focused attention, dissociation, and emotional disclosure), we offer a more comprehensive review of research published since 1980.

Discrete cognitive coping strategies were organized into two broad categories used by Turk *et al.* [26]: (1) strategies used primarily to remove one's attention from pain or pain-avoidant strategies (i.e., mental suppression, distraction, and imagery); and (2) strategies used primarily to change one's appraisal or emotional processing of the pain without avoiding the pain (i.e., sensory focus, reinterpretation of sensations, dissociation, coping self-statements, and emotional disclosure). The literature on each coping strategy is organized as follows: correlational studies, longitudinal studies, treatment outcome studies, experimental studies, and moderating variables. It is notable that most of the studies involving chronic pain are correlational, while most of the experimental studies are with laboratory-induced pain.

Strategies used to remove one's attention from the pain stimulus

This group of coping techniques consists of strategies that are designed to help the individual cope with pain by removing one's attentional focus from the pain, either through ignoring or denying the pain completely, or through replacing thoughts about pain with other thoughts, stimuli, tasks (distraction), or pleasant imagery. These strategies do not directly address the emotional aspects of pain.

Stoic distancing/ignoring/avoidance/ thought suppression

Strategies like stoic distancing, ignoring, or thought suppression are defined as inhibiting an unwanted thought or as attempts to avoid acknowledging, dwelling upon, or expressing the extent of pain [15, 27]. Research on thought suppression in general (i.e., not specific to pain) has suggested that attempts to suppress thoughts ironically cause unwanted thoughts to become more accessible in consciousness. Therefore,

attempts to suppress awareness of pain may actually increase awareness of pain [28]. Indeed, ignoring pain during debridement procedures for burn treatment has been positively associated with subsequent intrusive thoughts regarding the procedure [29].

Boothby *et al.* [2] noted that ignoring pain was occasionally associated with higher levels of functioning in persons with chronic pain, evidenced by an increased ability to work, greater activity levels, or lesser pain intensity ratings. However, ignoring pain was much more frequently shown to be unrelated to variables such as pain interference, ability to work, psychological functioning, or pain severity in correlational and longitudinal research on persons with chronic pain. The authors suggested that ignoring pain has little influence on adjustment in persons with chronic pain.

More recent correlational research has continued to demonstrate the lack of meaningful relations between ignoring pain and adjustment to chronic pain in a host of outcome variables, including: pain severity [15, 16, 20, 21, 30–33]; pain interference [31]; physical disability [21, 31–34] ; activity levels [21, 31]; depressive symptoms [21, 31, 33]; psychosocial disability [21]; anxiety symptoms [16] and work status [21]. However, there are a small minority of studies that have reported significant associations with ignoring pain. In these few studies, ignoring pain has been associated with reductions in pain interference and psychosocial disability [24], inactivity [20], and analgesic use [30]. Furthermore, there have been several other reports of positive correlations between ignoring pain and improved mood [16, 20], as well as less pain-related anxiety [21]. Conversely, one study found that ignoring pain was associated with less perceived control over pain [35]. There are fewer studies examining self-reported thought suppression during acute pain, but they indicated conflicting results: one study reported higher levels of worst pain in post-surgical patients [22] but another study reported lower levels of pain severity during mammography [23] .

There was only one recent study addressing longitudinal effects of ignoring pain. Haythornthwaite *et al.* found that ignoring pain did not prospectively predict pain intensity, pain interference, or activity levels 8 weeks later in post-herpetic neuralgia patients [31]; however, ignoring pain was predictive of greater depressive symptoms 8 weeks later. This study is important not only because it reports longitudinal data, but in that it also uses multiple outcome measures over several pain-related domains.

There are several experimental studies examining the effect of trait avoidance or specific instructions to engage in thought suppression using the cold pressor experimental pain task in college students. Most studies reported that high general experiential avoidance (not specific to pain) or instructions to suppress pain-related thoughts are associated with significantly lower pain tolerance and poorer recovery from experimental pain [27, 36–39]. Only one unpublished study failed to find these associations [40]. Experiential avoidance or instructions to suppress thoughts show variable results with pain intensity and pain distress, sometimes associated with higher reported pain intensity and pain distress ratings [36, 38, 41] and sometimes unrelated to pain threshold or intensity rating [27, 37, 39]. Feldner *et al.* suggested that avoidance is more strongly related to how long the pain will be tolerated than to how quickly an individual notices pain or the perceived severity of the stimulus [37]. The authors suggest this association may have important implications for persons with chronic pain, such as their willingness to participate in reconditioning programs.

In a novel experiment measuring muscle tension as well as cardiovascular response to cold pressor pain in low back pain patients, Burns compared the impact of a variety of cognitive coping strategies (including mental suppression) during which participants were also given a mental stressor (mental arithmetic) [28]. Participants with low back pain instructed to suppress pain sensations showed greater increases in muscle tension and prolonged increases in blood pressure compared to the other conditions (low back pain participants or healthy controls assigned to sensory focus, distraction, or a control condition). There were no effects of coping strategy on self-reported pain or negative affect.

In regards to individual difference variables that might relate to the efficacy of ignoring/avoidant coping, personality, race, education, sex, satisfaction with social support, pain severity and catastrophizing have been examined. It has been reported that neither the big five personality factors nor race (Caucasian vs. African-American) moderate the effects of stoic distancing or ignoring pain, although Caucasians reported greater use of ignoring pain in some [15, 20], but not all studies. In a study exploring race and education differences in coping, Cano *et al.* found that although African-Americans reported using ignoring pain strategies more frequently than Caucasians, when education was added as a covariate the race difference disappeared [24]. This finding adds to a growing body of literature that race differences in pain and coping are at least partially mediated by education. These authors note that people with low education may be less likely to seek out and use more cognitively challenging coping skills (such as cognitive restructuring) and instead rely on less complex (and more maladaptive) coping skills, such as ignoring or attempting to mentally suppress pain.

Regarding sex differences in ignoring pain, both females and males with chronic pain generally report utilizing ignoring pain at similar rates [42]. In an experimental study researchers found that males reported greater sensory pain when instructed to avoid sensations, thoughts, and feelings related to the cold pressor task (avoidance) than when instructed to concentrate on sensations from the cold water (sensory focus), although females did not demonstrate this difference [43].

Other moderators explored include perceived social support, pain severity, and catastrophizing. Holtzman *et al.* found that when patients with rheumatoid arthritis (RA) reported satisfaction with their social support, greater use of stoic distancing was related to lower levels of pain severity [32]. However, when participants did not perceive helpful support, stoic distancing was associated with higher levels of pain across the day. Reported pain severity has also been shown to moderate the association between ignoring pain and activity levels. Specifically, as pain severity increases, any positive associations between ignoring pain and activity levels become even less robust [4], although pain intensity levels do not seem to moderate previously reported relations between ignoring pain and perceived control over pain [35]. Finally, level of catastrophizing has been shown to be related to specific increases in paraspinal muscle activity in low back pain participants instructed to suppress pain in a cold pressor task [44]. The authors concluded that for those who catastrophize, efforts to suppress pain awareness caused exaggerated muscular tension near the site of injury.

Overall, although some adaptive relations with ignoring pain, thought suppression, or stoic distancing have been reported [20], the majority of the literature indicates that avoidance or suppression of pain is a strategy that is ineffective or even counterproductive for coping with both chronic and acute or experimental pain. This may be particularly true for persons who catastrophize, have lower education, less social support, and/or more severe pain.

Distraction/diverting attention

These techniques are defined as directing attention away from pain to another stimulus or task, without explicit instructions to mentally suppress thoughts regarding the pain [16, 45]. Studies also sometimes use the term "avoidant coping" to refer to distracting thoughts or activities [46, 47]. Previous studies have explored a variety of types of distraction: cognitive tasks (e.g., search & find letter task on a computer, counting backwards by 3s, verbal repetition of letters), performance tasks (e.g., playing a pocket video game, tracking a traveling light), or focusing thoughts on topics unrelated to pain without a task (e.g., generating fantasies, watching neutral picture slides). There is a large literature on distraction, both before and subsequent to the Boothby *et al.* review [2].

Boothby *et al.* reported that relations between distraction and functioning in patients with chronic pain were inconsistent, with distraction sometimes associated with lesser disability and better mood, sometimes with greater pain severity and psychological distress, and sometimes unrelated to a variety of pain related variables such as pain severity, disability, ability to work, and psychological functioning [2].

Subsequent correlational research has continued to reveal inconsistent associations between diverting attention and pain-related variables in persons with chronic pain. In numerous studies distraction has been shown to be unrelated to various pain-related variables: pain severity [16, 23–25, 30, 33]; pain interference [24]; physical disability [24, 33, 34]; psychosocial disability [24]; depression, or activity levels [48]. Although atypical, in one study distraction was found to be inversely related to current pain in persons undergoing knee or hip replacement surgery [22], and in another study, distraction was inversely associated with analgesic medication use [30]. Conversely, in some studies, greater use of distraction has been associated with greater pain among patients with RA [20] and mixed chronic pain patients [21, 46]. Furthermore, distraction has been correlated with greater physical disability, psychosocial disability, pain-related anxiety [21], and depressive symptoms [21, 33], and lower activity levels and likelihood of working [21].

There has been only one longitudinal study examining distraction. Haythornthwaite *et al.* found that use of distraction at baseline did not prospectively predict post-herpetic neuralgia pain severity, pain interference, activity levels or depression at 8-week follow-up [48].

There are few clinical treatment studies related to distraction. In one study, patients utilizing distraction while undergoing a painful medical procedure reported greater subjective ratings of pain control, but similar anxiety ratings, compared to no treatment controls [49]. A series of studies of burn patients undergoing wound dressing changes who were randomly assigned to one of three groups (distraction, sensory focus, or no treatment control) found that distraction was not associated with pain severity or tension during burn dressing changes [25, 29]. However, distraction was associated with lower perceptions of relief from pain during burn dressing changes relative to sensory focus [25]. Burn pain may be somewhat unique in the category of "acute" pain in that during the treatment phase debridement interventions cause recurrent acute pain episodes.

There have been a large number of studies examining the efficacy of distraction as a coping technique for laboratory-induced pain in healthy participants. Distraction has been found to be the most frequently reported spontaneous coping strategy in these types of studies [50]. Most studies of healthy experimental pain subjects find distraction techniques to be associated with a variety of adaptive pain-related variables when compared to controls and/or those instructed to use some other cognitive strategy. Such associations include higher pain tolerance [51–55]; higher pain threshold [53, 56]; and lower pain severity [54, 55, 57–64]. However, there have also been a number of experimental studies using pain-free participants that failed to find an effect of distraction on similar pain variables, including pain tolerance [40, 56, 61]; pain severity [27, 28, 40, 65–68]; pain discomfort [67]; recovery from pain [40]; or negative affect [28]. Two studies reported that although distraction had a positive or neutral effect on some outcome variables, distraction also had disadvantageous effects on other pain related outcomes, including slower recovery from pain [27] and greater psychological distress during experimental pain [53].

There are a small number of studies examining the efficacy of distraction for persons with chronic pain while undergoing an experimental pain task, and these have inconsistent results. In one study, distraction was equally efficacious in reducing pain severity reports during the cold pressor task for both healthy controls and persons with low back pain [67], but in another study, distraction used by persons with chronic pain resulted in shorter cold pressor pain tolerance times and higher reported pain severity relative to healthy controls [69]. Studies of distraction and exercise persistence in persons with chronic low back pain have also yielded inconsistent results. One study found that distraction improved performance in terms of time spent exercising and number of steps taken without increases in pain severity following the task [69]; however, a more recent study found that, compared to no-distraction controls, participants in the distraction condition reported greater pain following the task and performance was not improved [70]. A third study found that a distraction task resulted in increased persistence on a painful task for chronic pain patients, but not for healthy controls [71].

A number of moderating variables have been studied related to distraction or diverting attention. Although it makes intuitive sense that complexity (e.g., more complex verbal arithmetic compared to less complex verbal arithmetic) or type of the distraction task (e.g., a cognitive distraction compared to a performance distraction) would moderate the efficacy of distraction, the majority of available studies have not found differential efficacy based on these factors [3, 61, 65, 72]. However, one study reported that participants in a "high load" distraction condition (i.e., a visual search task with a large number of non-target stimuli in the search field) reported lower pain intensity than participants in a "low load" distraction task (i.e., a visual search task with a low number of non-target stimuli in the search field) [73], and a second study found that a performance distraction task (playing a video game) was related to increases in pain tolerance but not pain severity relative to a cognitive distracter (counting backwards, imagining pleasant imagery, and disassociating from pain) [55]. It is interesting to note that absorption or involvement in the distracting task is positively associated with the effect of distraction on pain severity and tolerance [54, 59]. Thus, overall, it appears that the specific type of distraction utilized in managing acute pain is not important, although involvement in the distracting task is important to maximize the efficacy of distraction.

Females with chronic pain report more frequent use of diverting attention than males [42]. Although some research indicates that distraction is not differentially efficacious for males and females in terms of experimental pain threshold, tolerance, and severity [59, 74], other research has found that distraction-based coping is associated with improvements in experimental pain severity, pain tolerance, and affective pain relative to controls or an acceptance based alternative strategy for women but not for men [74, 75, 76].

Race has also been examined as a moderator of diverting attention. In one study, African-Americans reported utilizing diverting attention more frequently than Caucasian Americans, but this difference was mediated by education level, such that when education level was controlled, there was no longer a racial difference in use of diverting attention [24]. Additionally, the efficacy of diverting attention has been shown to be independent of race [20, 24], demonstrating that race is not related to use or efficacy of diverting attention.

Various characteristics of pain have been examined as moderators of the efficacy of distraction. In one experimental pain study distraction was equally effective at low and high pain intensities in students undergoing a cold pressor trial (CPT) [59]. However, one correlational study reported that the positive association between diverting attention and activity levels was stronger in persons reporting less severe pain [4].

Duration of pain may also moderate the efficacy of distraction. The literature as a whole implies that distraction is not efficacious for chronic or acute clinical pain, but is often efficacious for experimental pain. One study has demonstrated that diverting attention (termed "avoidant coping" in this study) was associated with less depression, less anxiety, and more social activity in persons with recent onset pain (less than 4 weeks), while the opposite relation was found for persons with chronic pain (greater than 6 months) [47]. Studies have also demonstrated that the efficacy of distraction decreases as the duration of the experimental pain stimulus increases [61, 77]. Further, the presence of a pre-existing chronic pain condition may [69] or may not [67] reduce the efficacy of distraction for coping with acute or experimental pain. These results indicate that the effectiveness of distraction may decrease as pain intensity or duration increases.

Multiple cognitive variables that moderate the efficacy of distraction have also been identified including expectancies, fear of pain, catastrophizing, and anxiety. Significantly greater pain reductions were reported by experimental pain participants who were provided with positive feedback from a sham "personality test" about their ability to use the strategies than participants who were provided negative feedback [63]. This finding, however, may speak less to the efficacy of distraction and more to the influence of social contingencies on coping in general. Along similar lines, other researchers have found that the pain reductions reported by college students using distraction to cope with experimental pain were correlated with their expectancies regarding the efficacy of the technique [54, 59].

Fear of pain has been shown to increase attention to pain during distraction tasks and to moderate the efficacy of distraction [70]. Distraction was associated with lower pain only in persons low on fear of pain, while highly fearful individuals showed a slight increase in pain relative to baseline while utilizing distraction [78]. Similarly, catastrophizing has also been found to increase attention to pain during a distraction task [70] and to moderate the efficacy of distraction. Distraction was associated with improved pain tolerance for lower catastrophizers but not higher catastrophizers [51].

Some research on anxiety and coping efficacy have reported no differences between high and low anxiety groups (general anxiety and experimentally induced pain specific anxiety) on pain severity ratings or pain tolerance when using cognitive distraction [52, 57]. However, another study found that health-related anxiety moderated the efficacy of distraction during physical therapy such that for highly health-anxious patients, distraction was associated with greater affective pain, but also with greater perceived ability to decrease pain in general, compared to those lower on health-related anxiety [79]. It is interesting to note that this study also reported that, while distraction was more efficacious than a sensory focus manipulation for persons low on health-related anxiety, the opposite was true for the highly health-anxious persons. Taken together, there are mixed results regarding the impact of anxiety on the effectiveness of coping techniques, though there is more support for the importance of pre-existing health-related anxiety in chronic pain patients than for generalized anxiety or experimentally induced pain-related anxiety. Combined, these studies on cognitive moderators of distraction suggest that cognitive variables are associated with the efficacy of distraction. In particular negative pain related cognitions or cognitions that make disengagement from pain more difficult appear to decrease the efficacy of distraction.

Overall, the research suggests that distraction is not helpful, and possibly even detrimental, for chronic pain and, perhaps, acute clinical pain (e.g., burn pain). However, there is evidence to suggest that distraction can be useful in managing acute experimental pain, particularly in those participants who are not particularly anxious and do not engage in other negative pain-related cognitions such as catastrophizing.

Imagery

Imagery, also known as guided imagery, has been defined as "the production of particular images with pain-attenuating potential" [80]. Imagery might involve imagining a scene that is compatible with the pain stimulus, e.g., imagining a winter scene while undergoing cold pressor pain [56]; imagining a scene incompatible with pain, e.g., imagining a warm pleasant scene while undergoing cold pressor pain; imagining a safe or pleasant place or activity [81], or visualizing images of healing [82].

Boothby et al. did not review the imagery literature [2]. Although now dated, a meta-analysis of cognitive strategies used for managing pain found use of imagery was related to lesser pain severity compared to controls or those given alternative cognitive strategies [3]. No correlational cross-sectional or longitudinal studies examining imagery and chronic pain were found. However, there have been a large number of treatment studies examining the efficacy of imagery for coping with acute clinical pain (e.g., medical procedural pain, post-surgical pain) and chronic pain (e.g., cancer pain, headache, interstitial cystitis, fibromyalgia, phantom limb pain, or regional pain syndrome), several of which included follow-ups.

Most treatment studies have shown that, relative to controls or use of an alternative strategy, use of imagery is associated with a variety of adaptive pain-related variables, including: lower reported pain severity [82–89]; less pain related distress or anxiety [83, 87]; less use of analgesic medication [84, 87, 89, 90]; greater perceived ability to cope with pain [91]; improvements in headache activity [92, 93] ; less additional bodily pain [93]; less impact of pain [94]; improved mental health [93]; and shorter hospital stays [83, 90, 95]. Those studies including follow-up reported that these gains were maintained 8–10 weeks later [88, 92, 94]. A few studies have failed to find significant differences between imagery and control groups on pain severity [81, 94–96], pain related disability [93], migraine activity [91], medication use [91, 95], fatigue [81, 95], recovery of physical function [88], anxiety [95], or length of hospital stay [89]. However, no studies have reported maladaptive effects of imagery (e.g., increased pain severity).

Experimental studies examining the efficacy of imagery for healthy participants undergoing experimental pain tasks have shown that, compared to controls, use of imagery results in lesser reported pain severity [59, 63, 97], greater pain tolerance [56, 97, 98], higher pain threshold [56, 99], and lower heart rate during the experimental pain task [98]. Only one experimental study failed to find an association between use of imagery and pain discomfort relative to controls [56], and only two studies reported that imagery was equally or less efficacious than an alternative strategy (distraction, reinterpretation) on affecting pain severity [59] or threshold [99].

Several potential moderators of imagery have been examined, and some have been shown to be unimportant. The most frequently examined moderator of imagery is the type or focus of imagery. Many comparisons have demonstrated that different types of imagery are equally efficacious, including imagining pleasant scenes compared to imagining scenes with many details [92], reinterpretative imagery (imagining cold pressor pain as having one's hand in an oasis in a desert) compared to a pleasant activity (riding a carnival ride) [59], and pain compatible imagery compared to pain incompatible imagery [56, 98, 99]. It is also notable that "dosage" (the frequency with which imagery is used) is generally not associated with any pain-related outcomes [93, 94], with the exception that more frequent use of imagery was related to better mental health in one study [93]. The ability of imagery to affect pain has also been shown to be independent of sex [59, 86], race, and type of cancer diagnosis [86]. However, similar to distraction, the efficacy of imagery has been related to expectancy and absorption in the imagery task: greater positive expectancy about one's ability to successfully employ the imagery technique and greater absorption in the imagery task are associated with greater improvements in pain [59, 63].

In summary, there is sufficient evidence to suggest that imagery is efficacious for coping with chronic, acute, and experimental pain. Imagery appears to be efficacious regardless of the focus of the imagery (e.g., pleasant scene, detailed scene, pain incompatible experience), frequency of practice, or demographic characteristics of the participant, although positive expectancies and absorption in the task are important.

Strategies used to change one's appraisal or emotional processing of the pain stimulus

An important point about the next general category of strategies is that, rather than directing one's attention away from the pain stimulus, these strategies are used to directly or indirectly help the individual reinterpret the pain stimulus itself (e.g., as sensory patterns occurring within the body) and/or reduce the emotional impact of the pain stimulus. The strategies to be reviewed under this category include focusing on the sensory aspects of the pain stimulus, reinterpretation of the sensations, dissociation, coping self-statements, and emotional disclosure. These cognitive strategies are fundamentally different from those strategies teaching individuals to avoid the pain experience via mental suppression, distraction, or pain-incompatible imagery.

Sensory focus/focused attention

Strategies used to focus one's attention toward the pain have included focusing on the sensory aspects of the pain experience (sensory focus) as well as focusing on one's emotional reactions to the pain experience (emotion focus). Sensory focus involves instructing individuals to focus on the objective sensations of the stimulus [100, 101]. In addition to being labeled sensory focus, these strategies have also been labeled "somatization" and "distancing" [18]. Implied in the sensory focus strategy is that in attending to the sensory qualities of the stimulus, one is less likely to be fixated on emotional (affective) and cognitive (evaluative) reactions to the stimulus. On the other hand, emotion focus directs individuals to attend to their emotional reactions to the pain stimulus, rather than to the pain stimulus itself. In most cases, neither sensory focus nor emotion focus strategies attempt to change one's sensory or emotional response to the pain experience, but rather, the strategies attempt to differentially direct one's attention toward certain aspects of the pain experience.

Some of the research on focused attention failed to make a distinction between sensory focus and emotion focus, which has proven quite problematic in making meaningful interpretations regarding outcome. In an early meta-analysis of both experimental and clinical pain studies examining cognitive coping strategies [13], it was initially concluded that when considered together, strategies focusing one's attention toward pain were less effective than distraction strategies focusing one's attention away from the pain experience. However, when attentional strategies were further classified as involving attention to the objective physical qualities of pain (sensory focus) vs. attending to the emotional aspects (emotion focus), sensory focus was more efficacious than avoidance of pain, whereas attention to the pain with no specific focus or emotion focused monitoring were inferior to avoidance strategies. Thus, it is important to make a distinction between these two types of attentional strategies.

A comprehensive discussion of the research findings related to attention focus is found below. In this section, we are specifically aiming toward evaluating the potential efficacy of sensory focus, although some of the studies do not clearly delineate the type of focused attention studied, possibly explaining some of the discrepant findings. At first glance, it seems counter-intuitive that cognitive strategies used to focus one's attention toward the pain stimulus would increase one's ability to cope with the pain. Available research, however, suggests that certain types of attentional focus may serve as useful pain coping strategies. Furthermore, exploration of individual difference variables offers additional clarification about the moderators of efficacy of these techniques.

There are no correlational or longitudinal research studies specifically examining the relationship between the use of sensory focus or emotion focus strategies and pain-related outcome, although the literature consistently reports that emotion-focused attention to pain is correlated with negative outcomes [2].

In an effort to examine the relation of attention to pain with other pain-related variables, McCracken constructed a measure of pain vigilance and awareness of pain and then correlated it with other pain-related variables in a sample of patients with chronic pain [102]. It is important to note that the measure of attention to pain used in this study focused largely on one's perceived sensitivity to changes in the experience of pain, and did not specifically examine attention to the sensory or affective dimensions of pain. Awareness of changes in pain and vigilance associated with the pain experience were found to be positively related to pain anxiety, pain severity, physical disability and physician visits due to pain. It was also found that the level of pain awareness and vigilance significantly predicted distress, disability, and doctors visits independent of pain intensity, pain duration, and demographics such as gender, age, and education [102]. It may be that when one is very sensitive to changes in pain levels, and moreover, vigilant for such changes, such fixated attention toward pain sensation is maladaptive. On the other hand, the literature examining sensory focus seems to be examining a different sort of pain awareness – one in which one attends to the objective sensory qualities of the experience without necessarily becoming vigilant for sensations or changes in sensations.

Treatment outcome studies using sensory focus have reported generally favorable results. In a study by Logan *et al.*, sensory focus during an endodontic procedure was found to significantly reduce sensory pain compared to an information control condition, but there were no differences in ratings of pain unpleasantness or in the amount of control over pain participants reported experiencing [103]. In another study with healthy women during childbirth, instructions to monitor the sensory features of labor contractions resulted in lower pain reports during labor compared to controls, although women in the sensory focus condition did not differ from women who had attended LaMaze Childbirth classes on sensory pain reports [101]. Further, a study exploring the use of sensory focus in burn patients reported greater pain relief in the sensory focus group compared to a music distraction technique and a reduction in remembered pain in the sensory focus group compared to a usual medical care group [25]. However, a follow-up analysis of the data controlling for spontaneous use of coping strategies labeled ignoring, catastrophizing, and reinterpretation of pain revealed that, although there were no group differences in tension experienced during the procedure, participants in the sensory focus condition experienced more intrusive thoughts during the 30 minutes after the procedure compared to those in the music distraction group [29].

In most of the available experimental pain studies, sensory focus manipulations have been found to result in one or more positive pain-related outcomes. For example, in a very early experiment, Johnson found that instructing participants to focus on specific expected sensations during an ischemic pain test resulted in a trend toward sensation ratings leveling off over repeated trials, whereas participants instructed to use a mathematical distraction test reported significant increases in pain sensation ratings over time [104]. In other studies, sensory focus resulted in significantly higher tolerance time, lower pain intensity, and lower pain unpleasantness than no-intervention control or those instructed to focus on their emotional response to the pain [54, 105, 106], but not pain threshold or intensity in one study [105]. It has also been reported that sensory focus instructions result in faster recovery from experimental pain in comparison to other strategies such as mental suppression of the pain or distraction, although pain intensity ratings at the end of the cold pressor task did not differ across groups [27]. Reporting discrepant findings, Miron and colleagues found that when participants focused their attention on the pain stimulus itself they perceived pain as more intense and more unpleasant than when their attention was diverted away from the pain [64].

Several studies have not designated and/or separated sensory vs. emotional focus, making it difficult to interpret the results. For example, in a study by Keogh and Mansoor it was found that participants who were instructed to focus on sensory *and* emotional aspects of CPT pain experience showed greater pain tolerance than participants in an avoidance condition instructed to ignore the cold water sensations and think about something else [41]. The issue of confounding sensory focus and emotion focus is further illustrated in studies reporting that, compared to those in distraction or control conditions, use of focused attention, without specification of sensory or emotion focus, resulted in higher pain intensity ratings as well as lower tolerance times [52, 53, 67, 107]. The lack of distinction between sensory and emotion focus may account for these findings since participants may have been focusing on either the sensory or emotional aspects of the pain experience, or they may have been focusing on both.

It is interesting to note that mindfulness-based strategies teach individuals to be aware of, note, and not suppress stimuli that come into consciousness. There is a growing literature of treatment studies on mindfulness-based pain and stress-reduction. A meta-analysis of controlled studies of mindfulness for a wide range of clinical populations (including, but not limited to chronic pain) reported significant, moderate effect size improvements on standardized measures of physical and mental well-being [108]. Regarding meditation treatments specific to chronic pain, two randomized controlled treatment studies [109, 110] and three non-randomized controlled trials found meditation to be more beneficial than standard care with respect to pain perception, pain coping and measures of affect immediately post-treatment and also at follow-up [111, 112, 113]. While mindfulness techniques involve considerably more than sensory focus strategies, the principle of acknowledging stimuli (and emotions) rather than suppressing or avoiding such thoughts and feelings certainly shares some similarities with sensory focus and other strategies that acknowledge the stimulus, rather than mentally suppress or avoid it.

A variety of moderating variables, including sex and several cognitive/affective variables, have been examined and offer additional information regarding the conditions under which sensory focus may or may not be efficacious. In many cases, these have been experimental pain studies with pain-free volunteers, although there are some studies in which participants had clinical acute or chronic pain.

In experimental pain studies, sensation monitoring produced tolerance gains in males but not females [14], and males reported less sensory pain compared to females when they were instructed to focus on pain sensation [43].

In another experimental cold pressor study, fear of pain was examined as a moderator of the efficacy sensory focus strategies [78]. The sensory focus task was more efficacious in reducing pain intensity in those individuals scoring higher on a measure of fear. Similar findings were reported in a study with chronic pain patients, in which health anxiety was found to moderate the efficacy of sensory focus used during physical therapy. In those patients scoring higher on health anxiety, attention to sensations resulted in lower anxiety and pain ratings compared to suppression type instructions (labeled distraction instructions in this study). In non-health anxious patients, attention to sensations increased anxiety compared to those non-health anxious patients given the distraction/mental suppression instructions [79].

On the other hand, manipulated threat expectancy appears to have a different effect on the impact of attentional strategies. In a cold pressor study in which pain-free volunteers received either a threat or reassurance message prior to the cold pressor, the efficacy of instructing participants to focus on sensory pain-related words vs. focusing on affective pain-related words was explored [114]. A significant interaction for pain threshold and tolerance time revealed that affective word focus was superior to sensory word focus for participants in the threat condition, whereas sensory word focus was superior to affective word focus in the non-threat condition. Thus, attending to the sensory components of pain was only related to increased pain threshold and tolerance when pain threat expectancy was low, which is seemingly discordant with Hadjistavropoulos *et al.* [79] and Roelofs *et al.* [78]. It is possible that the different results obtained from the two studies could be explained by the fact that neither Roelofs *et al.* nor Hadjistavropoulos *et al.* manipulated anxiety or threat, but rather measured the psychosocial state of the participant, whereas Boston and Sharpe actually attempted to manipulate level of threat [114].

Another cognitive/affective variable that has received a great deal of research attention is catastrophizing. Michael & Burns [115] investigated the effects of sensory focus, affective focus, and a control condition on chronic pain patients assessed as high or low catastrophizers. In the sensory focus condition, low catastrophizers showed increased pain thresholds and tolerance times on a cold pressor task, whereas high catastrophizers showed no appreciable change following sensory focus instruction. Furthermore, while low catastrophizers showed no significant changes in pain threshold or tolerance times following affective focus, high catastrophizers showed reduced pain threshold and lower tolerance times. Thus, sensory focus was efficacious for low catastrophizers, but not for high catastrophizers, whereas affective focus was found to be maladaptive for those who were high on catastrophizing. Again, this finding seems at odds with the Hadjistavropoulos et al. [79] and Roelofs et al. [78] studies finding that participants high on fear or health anxiety seemed to benefit from sensory focus instructions. It may be that catastrophizing, as a negative cognitive state, is different from fear and anxiety which are negative affective states and thus their moderating effect on sensory focus is separable. Obviously, more research is needed to clarify the moderating effect of negative cognitions and affect as they relate to sensory focus strategies.

Desire for control has also been found to be a unique contributing variable to the effects of sensory focus. In a study of participants undergoing a root canal procedure, those in the sensory focus condition classified as having a high desire for control but low perceived control reported lower pain intensity than those in a no-intervention control condition immediately following the procedure and one week thereafter [103]. These results extended previous research in which patients with low felt control as well as low desire for control reported greater pain with sensory focus instructions over emotion focus instructions [116]. Both of these studies point to the clinical importance of considering the patients' coping preferences, which moderate efficacy.

Overall, there is moderate support for the use of sensory focus strategies, particularly in participants who have relatively high negative affect (health anxiety or fear), or, interestingly, for those with relatively low negative cognitive appraisals (pain-related catastrophizing). Certainly, given the body of research reviewed here, it is clear that sensory focus holds more promise than emotion focus strategies. It is important to note that the available research explores only a very limited period of instruction (usually one trial) and does not explore the efficacy of an extended period of instruction in sensory focus strategies. It may be that there is a cumulative effect of learning to be aware of, and observe the sensory qualities of the stimulus that eventually reduces affective reactivity. Further research will help clarify this issue, particularly longitudinal studies with more extensive treatment interventions.

Reinterpretation/cognitive reframing

Reinterpretation is defined by changing one's thoughts about the pain experience [117]. For example, one might refer to sensations in a benign or less threatening manner (e.g., "a dull feeling" or "tingling") rather than thinking about sensations in a way that is more threatening or has negative connotations (e.g., "pain" or "shooting") [2]. Similarly, the term "redefinition" has been used to describe the attempt to see the pain in a different light that makes it seem more bearable [1, 118]. Based on the existing correlational research yielding primarily non-significant relations between reinterpretation and chronic pain outcomes, Boothby et al. suggested that reinterpretation is only minimally related to adjustment to chronic pain, but potentially useful for coping with acute pain [2].

The more recent correlational research has continued to find primarily non-significant associations between reinterpretation and a wide variety of pain-related variables. These include pain severity[16, 20, 24, 30, 31, 33], pain interference [24], physical disability [10, 24, 33, 34], mood [16, 20, 31, 33], anxiety [16], activity levels [20, 31], and exercise persistence [10] in persons with chronic pain. Non-significant relations have also been found between reinterpretation and pain severity in persons undergoing mammography as well as those undergoing experimental pain [23, 50]. Some correlational studies have found significant inverse associations between reinterpretation and pain severity, physical disability [21], psychosocial disability [21, 24] and analgesic use [30] in persons with chronic pain, as well as positive relations between reinterpretation and perceived tension during burn wound debridement [29] and perceived control over pain [35]. Thus, in correlational research with chronic pain populations as well as acute clinical and laboratory experimental pain, reinterpretation of pain sensations has been found to either have no significant relationship to pain variables, or to mainly have an adaptive relation with pain outcome variables.

One study examined the longitudinal associations of reinterpretation and found that use of reinterpretation did not prospectively predict pain severity, pain interference, depression, or activity levels 8 weeks later [48]. There has been one treatment study (an unpublished dissertation) utilizing reinterpretation. In this study, amputee patients instructed in reinterpretation and relaxation reported less severe pain than patients taught relaxation alone [117].

The few existing experimental pain studies examining reinterpretation have produced inconsistent findings. In one study instruction in reinterpretation resulted in higher pain threshold and lower pain severity relative to controls [59, 119, 120]; however, another found no difference on pain tolerance between the reinterpretation group and controls [119]. Additionally, each experimental pain study reported that use of reinterpretation produced comparable results in terms of pain threshold, tolerance, and severity compared to alternative coping strategies including distraction, imagery, dissociation, and positive expectancies [59, 119, 120].

Several variables, including pain severity, sex, race, and education level, have been examined as moderators of the efficacy of reinterpretation. One unpublished dissertation reported a weak interaction between reinterpretation and pain severity. In this study, use of reinterpretation was associated with lower pain severity only in persons with low levels of average pain [121]. Another correlational study found that the positive relation between self-reported use of reinterpretation and perceived control over pain was the same at varying levels of pain severity [35].

The evidence regarding sex and the efficacy of reinterpretation is inconsistent. Some studies reported that the efficacy of reinterpretation was not different for males and females in terms of pain threshold [120], tolerance [119], and pain ratings [59]. However, one study reported that males increased pain threshold more than females after learning reinterpretation [119], while a different series of studies reported that reinterpretation resulted in higher pain tolerance and lower pain severity for women only [75, 76]. Females and males have been shown to report similar frequency of use of spontaneous reinterpretation strategies [42].

Race has been shown to have moderate associations with reinterpretation. In one study, reinterpretation was positively associated with pain severity and negative affect for African-Americans, but was inversely associated with pain severity and negative affect for White-Americans [20]. The role of education

may be an important confound unexamined in the previous research as another study reported that the association between reinterpretation and physical disability is mediated by education. Thus, persons (both African-American and White-American) with low education levels exhibit a positive association between reinterpretation and physical disability, while persons with high education levels exhibit an inverse relation between reinterpretation and physical disability [24].

Based on the available literature, there is no support for the use of reinterpretation as a method of coping with chronic pain. Reinterpretation may potentially be useful for coping with acute pain, but the only current supporting evidence is in experimental pain studies rather than acute clinical pain studies. Demographic variables such as sex, race, and education also seem to be important factors in the efficacy of reinterpretation, and more research will be necessary to understand the role of these moderators.

Cognitive reframing is a concept that is similar to reinterpretation in that it also involves changing thoughts regarding pain. In the pain coping literature, cognitive reframing refers to perceiving one's situation positively via reappraisal and downward social comparison. Greater use of cognitive reframing has been associated with lower pain levels in RA patients [15, 32]. Furthermore, reframing was more strongly associated with lower pain in persons higher on extraversion relative to persons lower on extraversion [15]. Additionally, patients more satisfied with their social support were more likely to report using reframing as a pain coping strategy [32]. The utility of reframing as a coping strategy has not been examined with acute or experimental pain. More research is needed regarding cognitive reframing in order to form conclusions regarding its utility in coping with pain.

Dissociation

Dissociation refers to separating feelings of pain and other sensations (i.e., cold) with a focus on the feeling other than pain. This technique requires an awareness of pain sensations but allows for a different focus of attention [119]. Although there have been several laboratory studies exploring the use of dissociation, there is no research regarding using this strategy with chronic pain, and there appears to be no current clinical research on dissociation. In the early studies, dissociation was reported to be related to increases in pain threshold during the cold pressor task to a greater degree than controls, and relatively equal to those using reinterpretation [119]. Other studies have defined dissociation as imagining that the painful body part is detached from the rest of the body or is made of wood [55]. In the Williams and Kinney study, it is hard to determine the effectiveness of dissociation because it was used in combination with distraction and imagery for cold pressor pain. It is interesting to note that participants who used this combination of coping strategies had similar pain intensities to controls, suggesting that the combination of dissociation, distraction, and imagery was not particularly effective in reducing pain reports in experimental pain study participants [55]. The only relevant study regarding potential moderators of dissociation reported that the strategy was equally efficacious for males and females in terms of experimental pain tolerance, but that males showed greater increases in pain threshold than females [119]. Overall, dissociation appears to be a potentially promising coping strategy, but it has lost attention in the research literature.

Coping self-statements

Coping self-statements are affirming self-statements that can be used in a variety of situations to facilitate adaptive coping responses [18]. Boothby *et al.* reported that the existing correlational and treatment literature suggested that coping self-statements were generally unrelated to pain or functioning, but that, when significant relations were found between self-statements and outcomes, they were generally adaptive rather than maladaptive [2].

Correlational research on coping self-statements and chronic pain since the Boothby *et al.* review has produced similar results [2]. Most associations with coping self-statements have been non-significant. These non-significant associations include the following variables: pain severity [20–24, 31, 33, 122, 123]; pain interference [24, 123]; fibromyalgia impact [124]; depression [31, 33]; physical disability [21, 33, 122, 123]; psychosocial disability [21, 24]; work status [21]; activity levels [21, 123]; fatigue, anxiety [124]; and pain-related anxiety [21].

Occasionally the use of coping self-statements has been found to have maladaptive associations such as greater functional disability [34] and greater depression [33] in patients with chronic pain. Two studies examined how self-reported use of coping self-statements correlated with acute clinical pain (mammography and electrodiagnostic testing). Both studies found

that use of coping self-statements positively correlated with reported pain severity [23, 125]. However, at least for the correlational studies involving acute medical procedures (mammography, electrodiagnostic testing), it is possible that the use of spontaneously generated coping self-statements are employed only when one judges a situation to be stressful. This is a disadvantage of correlational research, as it does not determine cause–effect relationships.

In a number of studies, however, the use of coping self-statements has been shown to be inversely related to pain severity, analgesic use [30], physical disability [24], negative affect, and depression [20, 21, 122–124]. Furthermore, the use of coping self-statements is positively correlated with perceived control over pain [35], activity levels [20, 31] and quality of life [124, 126]. It is notable that results regarding coping self-statements may differ based on the measure of coping self-statements. For example, in one study, both the Cognitive Strategies Questionnaire (CSQ) and the Chronic Pain Coping Inventory (CPCI) were used to predict pain-related outcomes. In multiple regression models, the CSQ coping self-statement subscale was predictive of depression, while the CPCI subscale was not predictive of depression [33].

One study examining the efficacy of coping self-statements longitudinally found that self-reported use of coping self-statements at baseline did not prospectively predict pain severity, pain interference, activity levels or depression 8 weeks later in multivariate models [48]. A treatment study for patients with fibromyalgia found that increases in positive self-statements over the course of treatment were correlated with greater improvements in psychological distress, both at post-treatment and 6-month follow-up, but changes in coping self-statements were not significantly associated with pain severity, pain interference, or activity levels [127]. Only one experimental pain study has examined coping self-statements. The authors found that instructions to use positive self-statements and task relevant statements affirming the ability to cope with the cold pressor task were associated with higher pain tolerance and threshold compared to cognitive distraction tasks and controls [56].

There is limited research available examining individual difference variables related to coping self-statements. Three correlational studies also examined potential moderators. Haythornthwaite *et al.* reported that the association between coping self-statements and perceived control over pain is independent of pain severity [35]. It has been reported that race was not a moderating factor of the positive association between self-reported use of coping self statements and activity level in patients with chronic pain [20]. Cano *et al.* found more complex relations concerning coping self-statements, race, and education [24]. The researchers found that, for both African-Americans and White Americans, greater use of coping self-statements was associated with lesser physical disability and psychosocial disability, but only for persons of lower education. For persons of higher education, use of coping self-statements was associated with slightly greater physical and psychosocial disability. No interactions between coping self-statements and pain severity or interference were found in this study. In the single experimental study available examining the efficacy of coping self-statements, Beers & Karoly assessed individual coping styles (repression, sensitization) prior to manipulating cognitive strategies, and found that pre-existing coping style was not a moderator of the efficacy of coping self-statements on pain threshold or tolerance times [56].

In summary, it is important to note that the vast majority of research regarding coping self-statements is correlational, and thus definitive conclusions regarding its efficacy are not possible. But, correlational research continues to suggest that use of coping self-statements is neither particularly efficacious nor maladaptive for a wide variety of pain-related outcomes in patients with chronic pain. One possible exception is that coping self-statements are more consistently associated with improved mood than not. There is a paucity of experimental and treatment research available on this strategy, and therefore, although we cannot conclude that coping self-statements are efficacious, there is enough promise in the available research to continue examining the issue. In particular, experimental and treatment outcome studies are needed.

Emotional disclosure/expressive writing

Recently, there has been a large body of research generated about the effects of emotional disclosure, also commonly referred to as expressive writing, on pain and other psychological and physiological outcomes. Emotional disclosure typically involves writing about one's thoughts and feelings regarding stressful events, although the writing aspect can be substituted with speaking into an audio recorder. The disclosures are not usually shared with others [18]. The suggested topic of emotional disclosures (e.g., pain related experiences and emotions vs. non-pain related experiences and emotions) often varies from study to study, which makes conclusions about the strategy more difficult.

The efficacy of emotional disclosure for pain has not been reviewed previously; however, there are more general published meta-analyses on emotional disclosure. These studies have reported that, for healthy participants, emotional disclosure is generally associated with improvements in physical health, psychological well-being, physiological functioning, and general well-being [128]. Furthermore, for persons with existing medical and psychiatric conditions, emotional disclosure is associated with improvements in physical functioning but not with significant improvements in psychological outcomes [129].

No correlational studies or studies of emotional expression and experimental pain were found. However, there are a large number of randomized treatment studies available, many including follow-up data, addressing the efficacy of emotional disclosure for persons with chronic pain conditions such as fibromyalgia, RA, cancer, or mixed chronic pain. Many studies have found that, immediately following the expressive writing task, persons practicing emotional disclosure report more negative emotions such as sadness, anger, or fear [130–133], but the negative impact on affect generally disappears by follow-up [128, 130, 131].

Shortly after expressive writing (e.g., 1–4 weeks later), a few studies have reported beneficial differences between emotional disclosure groups and controls including lower reported pain [133], and better sleep [130]. However, most studies report non-significant differences between emotional disclosure groups and controls at short term follow-up. Outcome variables measured in these studies reporting non-significant findings include pain severity [130, 132–137]; pain interference [137]; disease activity or impact [130, 135, 138]; physical disability or dysfunction [130, 132, 134]; mood or psychological well-being [130, 132, 135, 137, 138]; sleep disturbance [137]; fatigue [134, 135]; healthcare utilization, social support [130]; and general well-being [136].

Comparisons at more long-term follow-up (ranging from 10 weeks post treatment to 15 months post treatment) have produced more promising results. Many studies have reported that emotional disclosure is associated with a variety of adaptive pain-related outcomes. These include lower pain severity ratings [130, 133, 139, 140], and less disease activity or impact

[130, 138, 140], physical dysfunction [132], mood disturbance [132, 135, 138], healthcare utilization [130], sleep disturbance [130], and fatigue [130, 134, 135]. However, some studies continue to report non-significant results in terms of pain severity [131, 132, 133, 134], disability, mood [131–134], disease impact [135], activities, or social contacts [140].

There is relevant research available on the influence of individual differences on the efficacy of expressive writing based on pain populations, as well as the previously mentioned meta-analysis which also examined possible moderators of the efficacy of emotional disclosure in healthy adults [128]. The efficacy of emotional disclosure has been shown to be unrelated to patient variables such as age, sex, disability status, number of stressful life events, or a mean stress rating [128, 132, 141]. It has also been shown that for specific outcomes of psychological and physiological function, the efficacy of emotional disclosure tends not to be related to aspects of the emotional disclosure process (including the number of emotional disclosure sessions, the length of emotional disclosure sessions, or the time between emotional disclosure sessions) [128]. However, in terms of an overall effect size that includes general well-being and physical functioning, it was reported that longer times between sessions are associated with a greater overall effect size. One study reported comparable efficacy of emotional disclosure for persons with chronic pain regardless of whether or not the content of the emotional disclosure was pain related [132]; however, Smyth [128] reported some benefits of writing about current, as opposed to past, traumatic experiences. Outcomes of emotional disclosure have also been shown to be unrelated to the personal nature of emotion expressed or to the degree of emotion expressed during writing [132]. However, two studies found that some limited outcomes were associated with the degree of anger expressed during disclosure [141, 142], but the amount of anxiety or depression expressed were unrelated to pain and mood outcomes [141].

There is evidence to suggest that the efficacy of emotional disclosure is related to interpersonal relationships. One study found differences between the emotional disclosure and control groups on outcomes including pain, psychological well-being and fatigue only for persons classified as interpersonally distressed (e.g., receiving low support from their spouse) [143]. Further, multiple studies have found that the efficacy of expressive writing is dependent on social constraints (e.g., the spouses inhibit emotional expression), such that emotional disclosure was associated with less distress in patients with high social constraints, but was associated with higher distress in patients with low social constraints [137, 144].

Several emotional variables, including ambivalence over emotional expression, skillfulness in emotional expression, and negative affect, have also been examined as moderators of emotional disclosure. Ambivalence over emotional expression was associated only with improvements in sleep but no other outcomes in one study [142], and with only disability in another study such that greater ambivalence was associated with lower disability [133]. The inability to express emotion with words was not related to outcomes associated with emotional disclosure in one study [142], while another study reported that people with limited motivation or ability to process and express emotions benefited less from emotional disclosure [145]. Baseline negative affect was positively associated with improvements in mood and disability in the disclosure group [133]. Additionally, Kelley et al. found that larger increases in negative mood during the emotional disclosure task were associated with greater improvements in joint condition in RA patients, but were unassociated with other outcomes [132].

Pain catastrophizing has also been identified as an important moderator of the efficacy of emotional disclosure. For example, expressive writing instructions applied during dental treatment eliminated pre-existing differences between catastrophizers and non-catastrophizers on pain intensity and emotional distress. Furthermore, the intervention was efficacious in reducing pain intensity and emotional distress only for higher catastrophizers. One session of expressive writing/emotional disclosure lowered pain intensity ratings and emotional distress, but did not change participant's trait catastrophizing scores [146]. Similarly, in another study on chronic pain, catastrophizing was predictive of reductions in disability in the disclosure group, but not controls [133].

Finally, in terms of possible mechanisms of the efficacy of emotional disclosure, heart rate habituation has been shown to mediate treatment effects of emotional disclosure, with greater heart rate habituation associated with fewer somatic complaints in cancer patients undergoing emotional disclosure [147]. Use of negative emotion words also partially mediates the treatment effects, with greater use of negative emotion words associated with fewer subsequent somatic complaints [147]. The researchers have suggested that improvements associated with emotional disclosure may be linked to the extent to which autonomic arousal is decreased as patients process negative memories.

Although there are some inconsistencies in the research, there is adequate support for the use of emotional expression in persons with pain. In general, the beneficial effects are not observed until several months after the intervention. Further, although emotional disclosure has been shown to produce initial increases in negative mood, these increases dissipate over time and appear to be related to increased benefits resulting from the intervention. It is also notable that the time spent participating in emotional disclosure (e.g., 20 minutes for three sessions) is short compared to the duration of positive effects observed in these studies. The evidence suggests that emotional disclosure is especially useful for persons with pain who experience little emotional support from others, high negative affectivity, or frequent pain related catastrophic thinking.

Summary and conclusion

The purpose of this chapter was to provide an update on prior reviews and book chapters [2, 4], and to provide a more comprehensive review by including the acute clinical pain and laboratory-experimental pain literature. Furthermore, we focused our review on the efficacy of discrete coping strategies rather than coping composites, and sought to identify important moderators of efficacy of these coping strategies. The role of individual differences in coping efficacy has not been previously reviewed.

This is a difficult literature to synthesize and review for a variety of reasons, including a lack of clarity in terminology used to describe cognitive coping strategies; inconsistent findings based on procedural differences between studies, terminology inconsistencies and frequent use of composite coping strategies; complexities involved in studying a multidimensional construct such as pain; and a lack of attention to possible moderators of efficacy.

In summary, the cognitive coping literature as a whole continues to suggest that specific cognitive coping can result in improved pain, functional adjustment, and mood. A summary of the findings for each of the individual strategies, separated by type of pain, is found in Table 14.1. Although the literature was organized into two broad categories: (1)

strategies used primarily to remove one's attention from pain or pain-avoidant strategies (i.e., avoidance/suppression, distraction, imagery); and (2) strategies used primarily to change one's appraisal or emotional processing of the pain without avoiding the pain (i.e., sensory focus, reinterpretation of the sensations, dissociation, coping self-statements, emotional disclosure), there were no broad conclusions to be drawn regarding these categories of strategies as a whole. Furthermore, specific moderating variables appear to differentially affect the efficacy of cognitive strategies. This complicates the picture, but offers interesting potential insights into the mechanisms through which individual coping strategies may have their efficacy.

Imagery is the single cognitive coping strategy that has good evidence for efficacy across experimental, acute pain, and chronic pain, whereas mental suppression/ignoring is reliably associated with poor outcome across all reviewed categories of pain. Distraction has shown substantial efficacy for experimental pain, but it does not appear to be clinically useful, since it is not associated with positive outcomes for acute clinical pain or chronic pain. Sensory focus has moderate support in the experimental and acute pain literature, but its efficacy in chronic pain has not been explored. Dissociation has received little recent research attention, although it has shown some promise in experimental pain studies. It is likely that both sensory focus and dissociation strategies would have to be adapted for use with patients with chronic pain, since experimental strategies are usually one trial instructions. It is possible that mindfulness strategies, which are practiced on a daily basis and have been shown to be efficacious with chronic pain conditions, share some common mechanisms with sensory focus strategies. Emotional disclosure and, to some extent, reinterpretation of pain have shown efficacy for coping with chronic pain, and the use of coping self-statements appears to enhance mood, but is otherwise unrelated to pain outcomes.

Some themes can be gleaned by examining the role of individual difference variables across all the reviewed coping strategies. Race generally does not seem to moderate coping efficacy; rather, racial differences can be accounted for by education level. It is difficult to determine whether sex is a meaningful moderator of coping. Specific procedural aspects of the methods of coping (e.g., number of sessions, frequency of sessions, complexity of tasks) do not seem to

Table 14.1 Summary of relations between cognitive coping strategies and experimental, acute, and chronic pain

Category	Description	Experimental pain	Acute clinical pain	Chronic pain
Suppression/ignoring	Avoiding, ignoring, or denying thoughts about the pain	–	–	–
Distraction/diverting attention	Directing attention away from pain to another stimulus or task	+	0/–	0/–
Imagery	Producing images with pain-attenuating potential	+	+	+
Sensory focus/focused attention	Focusing on the sensory aspects of pain	+	+	?
Reinterpretation	Changing thoughts about the pain experience	0	?	0/+
Dissociation	Separating feelings of pain and other sensations (i.e., cold) with a focus on the feeling other than pain	+	?	?
Coping self-statements	Affirming self-statements	?	?	+ (mood) 0 (all other outcomes)
Emotional disclosure/ expressive writing	Expressing feelings regarding stressful events or pain	?	?	+

+: adaptive association; –: maladaptive association; 0: no association; ?: current research does not allow for a conclusion.

be important, which may indicate that slight variants in procedure should not impact the efficacy of most strategies. However, absorption in the assigned coping strategy and expectancies regarding the efficacy of a particular strategy do seem to be important. Finally, cognitive and affective variables including anxiety, fear of pain, pain catastrophizing, and negative affect appear to be important in the efficacy of most coping strategies, although the way in which each of these variables impacts efficacy varies somewhat across coping strategies.

In conclusion, when one considers the available literature including experimental pain, acute clinical pain, and chronic pain, there is evidence of differential efficacy for individual cognitive strategies. Moreover, key moderators, such as level of absorption in the task, education, negative affect, and negative cognitions have been identified as important moderators for further study. Future studies can expand our understanding of the efficacy of cognitive coping strategies by carefully defining the strategies examined, investigating specific strategies rather than rationally or empirically derived composites, and by including and further examining potentially important moderators of the efficacy of specific cognitive strategies.

References

1. Affleck, G, Urrows, S, Tennen, H, Higgins, P. Daily coping with pain from rheumatoid arthritis: Patterns and correlates. *Pain* 1992; **51**: 221–9.

2. Boothby JL, Thorn BE, Stroud MW, Jensen MP. Coping with pain. In *Psychosocial Factors in Pain: Critical perspectives,* eds. RJ Gatchel and D. Turk. (New York: Guilford Press, 1999), pp. 343–59.

3. Fernandez E, Turk DC. The utility of cognitive coping strategies for altering pain perception: A meta-analysis. *Pain* 1989; **38**: 123–35.

4. Jensen MP, Karoly P. Control beliefs, coping efforts, and adjustment to chronic pain. *J Consult Clin Psychol* 1991; **59**: 431–8.

5. Niven CA, Gijsbers K. Coping with labor pain. *J Pain Symptom Manage* 1996; **11**, 116–25.

6. Lazarus RS, Folkman S. *Stress, Appraisal, and Coping* (New York: Springer, 1984).

7. Brown KG, Nacassio PM. Development of a questionnaire for the assessment of active and passive coping strategies in chronic pain patients. *Pain* 1987; **31**: 53–64.

8. Geisser ME, Robinson ME, Henson CD. The coping strategies questionnaire and chronic pain adjustment: A conceptual and empirical reanalysis. *Clin J Pain* 1994; **10**: 98–106.

9. Keefe FJ, Crisson J, Urban BJ, Williams DA. Analyzing chronic low back pain: The relative contribution of pain coping strategies. *Pain* 1990; **40**: 293–301.

10. Rapp SR, Rejeski WJ, Miller MR. Physical function in older adults with knee pain: The role of pain coping skills. *Arthritis Care Res* 2000; **13**: 270–9.

11. Jensen MP, Romano JM, Turner JA. Chronic pain coping measures: individual vs. composite scores. *Pain* 1992; **51**: 273–80.

12. Lester N, Lefebvre JC, Keefe FJ. Pain in young adults: III. Relationships of three pain-coping measures to pain and activity interference. *Clin J Pain* 1996; **12**: 291–300.

13. Suls J, Fletcher B. The relative efficacy of avoidant and non-avoidant coping strategies: A meta-analysis. *Health Psychol* 1985; **4**: 249–88.

14. Keogh E, Herdenfeldt M. Gender, coping and the perception of pain. *Pain* 2002; **97**: 195–201.

15. Newth S, Delongis A. Individual differences, mood, and coping with chronic pain in rheumatoid arthritis: A daily process analysis. *Psychol Health* 2004; **19**: 283–305.

16. Grant L, Long B, Willms J. Women's adaptation to chronic back pain: Daily appraisals and coping strategies, personal characteristics and perceived spousal responses. *J Health Psychol* 2002; **7**: 545–64.

17. Turner JA, Clancy S. Strategies for coping with chronic low back pain: Relationships to pain and disability. *Pain* 1986; **24**: 355–64.

18. Thorn BE. *Cognitive Therapy for Chronic Pain* (New York: Guilford Press, 2004).

19. Alden AL, Dale JA, DeGood, DE. Interactive effects of the affect quality and directional focus of mental imagery on pain analgesia. *Appl Psychophysiol Biofeedback* 2001; **26**: 117–26.

20. Jordan M, Lumley M, Leisen J. The relationships of cognitive coping and pain control beliefs to pain and adjustment in African-American and Caucasian woman with rheumatoid arthritis. *Arthritis Care Res* 1998; **11**: 80–8.

21. McCracken L, Eccleston C. Coping or acceptance: What to do about chronic pain? *Pain* 2003; **105**: 197–204.

22. Pellino T, Gordon DB, Engelke ZK, *et al.* Use of nonpharmacologic interventions for pain and anxiety after total hip and total knee arthroplasty. *Orthop Nurs* 2005; **24**: 182–90.

23. Asghari A, Nicholas MK. Pain during mammography: The role of coping strategies. *Pain* 2004; **108**: 170–9.

24. Cano A, Mayo A, Ventimiglia M. Coping, pain severity, interference, and disability: The potential mediating roles of race and education. *J Pain* 2006; 7: 459–68.

25. Haythornthwaite JA, Lawrence JW, Fauerbach JA. Brief cognitive interventions for burn pain. *Ann Behav Med* 2001; **23**: 42–9.

26. Turk D, Miechenbaum D, Geist M. *Pain and Behavioral Medicine. A Cognitive-Behavioral Perspective* (New York: Guilford Press, 1983).

27. Cioffi D, Holloway J. Delayed costs of suppressed pain. *J Pers Soc Psychol* 1993; **64**: 274–82.

28. Burns JW. The role of attentional strategies in moderating links between acute pain induction and subsequent psychological stress: Evidence for symptom-specific reactivity among patients with chronic pain versus healthy nonpatients. *Emotion* 2006; **6**: 180–92.

29. Fauerbach JA, Lawrence JW, Haythornthwaite JA, Richter L. Coping with stress of a painful medical procedure. *Behav Res Ther* 2002; **40**: 1003–15.

30. Gustafsson M, Gaston-Johansson F, Aschenbrenner D, Merboth M. Pain, coping and analgesic medication usage in rheumatoid arthritis patients. *Patient Educ Couns* 1999; **37**: 33–41.

31. Haythornthwaite JA, Clark MR, Pappagallo M, Raja SN. Pain coping strategies play a role in the persistency of pain in post-herpetic neuralgia. *Pain* 2003; **106**, 453–60.

32. Holtzman S, Newth S, Delongis A. The role of social support in coping with daily pain among patients with rheumatoid arthritis. *J Health Psychol* 2004; **9**: 677–95.

33. Tan G, Jensen MP, Robinson-Whelen S, Thornby JI, Monga TN. Coping with chronic pain: A comparison of two measures. *Pain* 2001; **90**: 127–33.

34. van Vuuren BJ, van Heerden HJ, Becker PJ, Zinzen E, Meeusen R. Fear-avoidance beliefs and pain coping strategies in relation to lower back problems in a South African steel industry. *Eur J Pain* 2006; **10**: 233–9.

35. Haythornthwaite JA, Menefee LA, Heinberg LJ, Clark MR. Pain coping strategies predict perceived control over pain. *Pain* 1998; 77: 33–9.

36. Elfant E, Burns JW, Zeichner A. Repressive coping style and suppression of pain-related thoughts: Effects on responses to acute pain induction. *Cognition and Emotion* 2007; **22**: 671–96.

37. Feldner MT, Hekmat H, Zvolensky MJ, *et al.* The role of experiential avoidance in acute pain tolerance: A laboratory test. *J Behav Ther Exp Psychiatry* 2006; **37**: 146–58.

38. Masedo AI, Esteve R. Effects of suppression, acceptance, and spontaneous coping on pain tolerance, pain intensity and distress. *Behav Res Ther* 2007; **45**: 199–209.

39. Zettle R D, Hocker TR, Mick KA, *et al.* Differential strategies in coping with pain as a function of level of experiential avoidance. *Psychol Rec* 2005; **55**: 511–24.

40. Grundt AM. Dismantling instruction to distract from a painful stimulus: Approach/avoidance functions of distracting instructions. (Doctoral dissertation, University of Nevada, Nevada). *Dissert Abstr Int Sec B Sci Eng* 2000; **61**(*2-B*): 1082.

41. Keogh E, Mansoor L. Investigating the effects of anxiety sensitivity and coping on the perception of cold pressor pain in healthy women. *Eur J Pain* 2001; **5**: 11–22.

42. Grossi, G, Soares JJF, Lundberg U. Gender differences in coping with musculoskeletal pain. *Int J Behav Med* 2000; **7**: 305–21.

43. Keogh E, Hatton K, Ellery D. Avoidance versus focused attention and the perception of pain: Differential effects for men and women. *Pain* 2000; **85**: 225–30.

44. Quartana PJ, Burns JW, Lofland KR. Attentional strategy moderates effects of pain catastrophizing on symptom-specific physiological responses in chronic low back pain patients. *J Behav Med.* 2007; **30**: 221–31.

45. Rosentiel AK, Keefe FJ. The use of coping strategies in chronic low back pain patients: Relation to patient characteristics and current adjustment. *Pain* 1983; **17**: 33–44.

46. Endler NS, Corace KM, Summerfeldt LJ, Johnson JM, Rothbart P. Coping with chronic pain. *Pers Individ Diff* 2003; **34**: 323–46.

47. Holmes JA, Stevenson CAZ. Differential effects of avoidant and attentional coping strategies on adaptation to chronic and recent-onset pain. *Health Psychol* 1990; **9**: 577–84.

48. Haythornthwaite JA, Clark MR, Pappagallo M. Pain coping strategies play a role in the persistence of pain in post-herpetic neuralgia. *Pain* 2003; **106**: 453–60.

49. Diette GB, Lechtzin N, Haponik E, Devrotes A, Rubin HR. Distraction therapy with nature sights and sounds reduces pain during flexible bronchoscopy: A complementary approach to routine analgesia. *Chest* 2003; **123**: 941–8.

50. Sullivan MJ, Tripp DA, Santor D. Gender differences in pain and pain behavior: The role of catastrophizing. *Cognit Ther Res* 2000; **24**: 121–34.

51. Heyneman NE, Fremouw WJ, Gano D, Kirkland F, Heiden L. Individual differences and the effectiveness of different coping strategies for pain. *Cognit Ther Res* 1990; **14**: 63–77.

52. James JE, Hardardottir D. Influence of attention focus and trait anziety on tolerance of acute pain. *Br J Health Psycho* 2002; **7**: 149–62.

53. McCaul KD, Haugtvedt C. Attention, distraction, and cold-pressor pain. *J Pers Soc Psychol* 1982; **43**: 154–62.

54. Stevens MJ, Terner JL. Moderators of cognitive coping derived from attentional and parallel processing models of pain. *Imagination Cogn Pers* 1992; **12**: 341–53.

55. Williams SL, Kinney PJ. Performance and nonperformance strategies for coping with acute pain: The role of perceived efficacy, expected outcomes, and attention. *Cognit Ther Res* 1991; **15**: 1–19.

56. Beers TM, Karoly P. Cognitive strategies, expectancy, and coping style in the control of pain. *J Consult Clin Psychol* 1979; **47**: 179–80.

57. Arntz A, De Jong P. Anxiety, attention and pain. *J Psychosom Res* 1994; **37**: 423–32.

58. Bishop SR. Attention mediates the relation between catastrophizing and pain. (Doctoral dissertation, Dalhousie University, Canada, 1998). *Dissert Abstr Int Sec B Sci Eng* 1999; **60**(*3-B*): 1321.

59. Devine DP, Spanos P. Effectiveness of maximally different cognitive strategies and expectancy in attenuation of reported pain. *J Pers Soc Psychol* 1990; **58**: 672–8.

60. Farthing GW, Venturion M, Brown, S. Suggestion and distraction in the control of pain: A test of two hypotheses. *J Abnorm Psychol* 1984; **93**: 266–76.

61. Hodes RL, Howland EW, Lightfoot N, Cleeland CS. The effects of distraction on responses to cold pressor pain. *Pain* 1993; **41**: 109–14.

62. Janssen SA, Arntz A, Bouts S. Anxiety and pain: Epinephrine-induced hyperalgesia and attentional influences. *Pain* 1998; **76**: 309–16.

63. Marino J, Gwynn MI, Spanos, NP. Cognitive mediators in the reduction of pain: The role of expectancy, strategy use, and self-presentation. *J Abnorm Psychol* 1989; **98**: 256–62.

64. Miron D, Duncan GH, Bushnell MC. Effects of attention on the intensity and unpleasantness of thermal pain. *Pain* 1989; **39**: 345–52.

65. Christenfeld, N. Memory for pain and delayed effects of distractiton. *Health Psychol* 1997; **16**: 327–30.

66. Duker PC, van den Bercken J, Foekens M. Focusing versus distraction and the response to clinical electrical shocks. *J Behav Ther Exp Psychol* 1999; **30**: 199–204.

67. Nouwen A, Cloutier C, Kappas A, Warbrick T, Sheffield D. Effects of focusing and distraction on cold pressor-induced pain in chronic back pain patients and control subjects. *J Pain* 2006; **7**: 62–71.

68. Spanos NP, Stam HJ, Brazil K. The effects of suggestion and distraction on coping ideation and reported pain. *J Ment Imagery* 1981; **5**: 75–90.

69. Johnson MH, Petrie SM. The effects of distraction on exercise and cold-presser tolerance for chronic low back pain sufferers. *Pain* 1997; **69**: 43–8.

70. Goubert L, Crombez G, Eccleston C, Devulder J. Distraction from chronic pain during a pain-inducing activity is associated with greater post-activity pain. *Pain* 2004; **110**: 220–7.

71. Rode S, Salkovskis PM, Jack T. An experimental study of attention, labeling and memory in people suffering from chronic pain. *Pain* 2001; **94**: 193–203.

72. McCaul KD, Monson N, Maki RH. Does distraction reduce pain-produced distress among college students? *Health Psychol* 1992; **11**: 210–17.

73. Veldhuijzen D, Kenemans J, de Bruin C, Olivier B, Volkerts E. Pain and attention: Attentional disruption or distraction? *J Pain* 2006; **7**: 11–20.

74. Keogh E, Bond FW, Hanmer R, Tilston J. Comparing acceptance and control-based coping instructions on the cold-pressor pain experiences of healthy men and women. *Eur J Pain* 2005; **9**; 591–8.

75. Jackson T. Interpersonal transactions and responses to cold pressor pain among Australian women and men. *Sex Roles* 2007; **56**: 55–62.

76. Jackson T, Iezzi T, Chen H, Ebnet S, Eglitis K. Gender, interpersonal, transactions, and the perception of pain: An experimental analysis. *J Pain* 2005; **6**: 228–36.

77. Barber TX, Cooper BJ. Effects of experimentally induced and spontaneous distraction. *Psychol Rep* 1972; **31**, 647–51.

78. Roelofs J, Peters ML, van der Zijden M, Vlaeyen J. Does fear of pain moderate the effects of sensory focusing and distraction on cold pressor pain in pain-free individuals? *J Pain* 2004; **5**: 250–6.

79. Hadjistavropoulos HD, Hadjistavropoulos T, Quine A. Health anxiety moderates the effects of distraction versus attention to pain. *Behav Res Ther* 2000; **38**: 425–38.

80. Fernandez, E. A classification system of cognitive coping strategies for pain. *Pain* 1986; **26**: 141–51.

81. Haase O, Schwenk W, Hermann C, Muller JM. Guided imagery and relaxation in convention colorectal resections: A randomized, controlled, partially blinded trial. *Dis Colon Rectum* 2005; **48**: 1955–63.

82. Carrico DJ, Peters KM, Diokno AC. Guided imagery for women with interstitial cystitis: Results of a prospective, randomized controlled pilot study. *J Altern Complement Med* 2008; **14**: 53–60.

83. Antall GF, Kresevic D. The use of guided imagery to manage pain in an elderly orthopedic population. *Orthop Nurs* 2004; **23**: 335–40.

84. Daake DR, Geuldner SH. Imagery instruction and the control of post-surgical pain. *Appl Nurs Res* 1989; **2**: 114–20.

85. Fors EA, Gotestam KG. Patient education, guided imagery and pain related talk in fibromyalgia coping. *Eur J Psychiatry* 2000; **14**: 233–40.

86. Kwekkeboom KL, Kneip J, Pearson L. A pilot study to predict success with guided imagery for cancer pain. *Pain Manag Nurs* 2003; **4**: 112–23.

87. Manyande A, Berg S, Gettins D, *et al*. Preoperative rehearsal of active coping imagery influences subjective and hormonal responses to abdominal surgery. *Psychosom Med* 1995; **57**: 177–82.

88. Moseley GL. Graded motor imagery for pathologic pain: A randomized controlled trial. *Neurology* 2006; **67**: 2129–34.

89. Tusek DL, Church JM, Strong SA, Grass JA, Fazio VW. Guided imagery: A significant advance in the care of patients undergoing elective colorectal surgery. *Dis Colon Rectum* 1997; **40**: 172–8.

90. Halpin LS, Speir AM, CapoBianco P, Barnett SD. Guided imagery in cardiac surgery. *Outcomes Manag* 2002; **6**: 132–7.

91. Ilacqua GE. Migraine headaches: Coping efficacy of guided imagery training. *Headache* 1994; **34**: 99–102.

92. Brown JM. Imagery coping strategies in the treatment of migraine. *Pain* 1984; **18**: 157–67.

93. Mannix L, Chandurkar R, Rybicki L, Tusek D, Solomon, G. Effect of guided imagery on quality of life, for patients with chronic tension type headaches. *Headache* 1999; **39**: 326–34.

94. Menzies V, Taylor AG, Bourguignon C. Effects of guided imagery on outcomes of pain, functional status, and self-efficacy in persons diagnosed with fibromyalgia. *J Altern Complement Med* 2006; **12**: 23–30.

95. Deisch, P, Soukup, SM, Adams P, Wild MC. Guided imagery: Replication study using coronary artery bypass graft patients. *Nurs Clin North Amer* 2000; **35**: 417–25.

96. Danhauer SC, Marler B, Rutherfod CA, *et al*. Music or guided imagery for women undergoing colposcopy: A randomized controlled study of effects on anxiety, perceived pain, and patient satisfaction. *J Low Genit Tract Dis* 2007; **11**: 39–45.

97. Worthington EL, Shumate M. Imagery and verbal counseling methods in stress inoculation training for pain control. *J Counsel Psychol* 1981; **28**: 1–6.

98. Neumann W, Kugler J, Pfand-Neumann P, *et al*. Effects of pain incompatible imagery on tolerance of pain, heart rate and skin resistance. *Percept Mot Skills* 1997; **84**: 939–43.

99. Johnson MH, Breakwell G, Douglas W, Humphries S. The effects of imagery and sensory detection distractors on different measures of pain: How does distraction work? *Br J Clin Psychol* 1998; **37**: 141–54.

100. Leventhal H, Bron D, Shacham S, Engquist G. Effects of prepatory information about sensations, threat of pain, and attention on cold pressor distress. *J Pers Soc Psychol* 1979; **37**: 688–714.

101. Leventhal EA, Leventhal H, Shacham S, Easterling DV. Active coping reduces reports of pain from childbirth. *J Consult Clin Psychol* 1989; **57**: 365–71.

102. McCracken LM. Attention to pain in persons with chronic pain: A behavioral approach. *Behav Ther* 1997; **28** 271–84.

103. Logan HL, Baron RS, Kohout F. Sensory focus as therapeutic treatments for acute pain. *Psychosom Med* 1995; **57**: 475–84.

104. Johnson JE. Effects of accurate expressions about sensations on the sensory and distress components of pain. *J Pers Soc Psychol* 1973; **27**: 261–75.

105. Ahles TA, Blanchard EB, Leventhal H. Cognitive control of pain: Attention to the sensory aspects of the cold presser stimulus. *Cognit Ther Res* 1983; 7: 159–177.

106. Dar R, Leventhal H. Schematic processes in pain perception. *Cognit Ther Res* 1993; **17**: 341–57.

107. Arntz A, Dreessen L, De Jong P. The influence of anxiety on pain: Attentional and attributional mediators. *Pain* 1994; **56**: 307–14.

108. Grossman P, Niemann L, Schmidt S, Walach H. Mindfulness-based stress reduction and health benefits. A meta-analysis. *J Psychosom Res* 2004; **57**: 35–43.

109. Carson JW, Keefe FJ, Lynch TR, *et al*. Loving-kindness meditation for chronic low back pain: Results from a pilot trial. *J Holist Nurs* 2005; **23**: 287–304.

110. Plews-Ogan M, Owens JE, Goodman M, Wolfe P, Schorling J. A pilot study evaluating mindfulness-based stress reduction and massage for the management of chronic pain. *J Gen Intern Med* 2005; **20**: 1136–38.

111. Grossman P, Tiefenthaler-Gilmer U, Raysz A, Kesper U. Mindfulness training as an intervention for fibromyalgia: Evidence of postintervention and 3-year follow-up benefits in well-being. *Psychother Psychosom* 2007; **76**: 226–33.

112. Kabat-Zinn J. An outpatient program in behavioral medicine for chronic pain patients based on the practice of mindfulness meditation: Theoretical considerations and preliminary results. *Gen Hosp Psychiatry* 1982; **4**: 33–47.

113. Sagula D, Rice KG. The effectiveness of mindfulness training on the grieving process and emotional well-being of chronic pain patients. *J Clin Psychol Med Settings* 2004; **11**: 333–42.

114. Boston A, Sharpe L. The role of threat-expectancy in acute pain: Effects of attentional bias, coping strategy effectiveness and response to pain. *Pain* 2005; **199**, 168–75.

115. Michael E, Burns JW. Catastrophizing and pain tolerance among chronic pain patients: Moderating effects of sensory and affect focus. *Ann Behav Med* 2004; **27**: 185–94.

116. Baron RS, Logan H, Hoppe S. Emotional and sensory focus as mediators of dental pain among patients differing in desired and felt dental control. *Health Psychol* 1993; **12**: 381–9.

117. Levine RB. Treatment efficacy of a combined relaxation/reinterpretation of pain strategy to control stump pain. (Doctoral dissertation). *Diss Abstr Int Sec B Sci Eng* 1991; **51**: 5579.

118. Keefe FJ, Affleck G, Lefebvre JC, *et al*. Pain coping strategies and coping efficacy in rheumatoid arthritis: A daily process analysis. *Pain* 1997; **69**: 35–42.

119. Blitz B, Dinnerstein AJ. Role of attentional focus in pain perception: Manipulation of response to noxious stimulation by instructions. *J Abnorm Psychol* 1971; **77**: 42–5.

120. Scott DS, Leonard CF. Modification of pain threshold by the covert reinforcement strategy and a cognitive strategy. *Psychol Record* 1978; **28**: 49–57.

121. Grant LD. The relationship between pain appraisals and coping strategy use and adaptation to chronic low back pain: A daily diary study. (Doctoral dissertation, University of British Columbia, Canada). *Dissert Abstr Int Sec B Sci Eng* 1997; **59(2-B)**: 872.

122. Ersek M, Turner JA, Kemp, CA. Use of the Chronic Pain Coping Inventory to assess older adults' pain coping strategies. *J Pain* 2006; 7: 833–42.

123. Tan G, Nguyen Q, Anderson KO, Jensen M, Thornby J. Further validation of the Chronic Pain Coping Inventory. *J Pain* 2005; **6**: 29–40.

124. Garcia-Campayo J, Pascual A, Alda M, Ramirex MTG. Coping with fibromialgia: Usefulness of the Chronic Pain Coping Inventory-42. *Pain* 2007; **132**: S68–S76.

125. Buckelew SP, Conway RC, Shutty MS, *et al*. Spontaneous coping strategies to manage acute pain and anxiety during electrodiagnositc studies. *Arch Phys Med Rehabil* 1992; **73**: 594–98.

126. Van Lankveld W, Bosch P, Van De Putte L, Naring G, Van der Saak C. Disease-specific stressors in rheumatoid arthritis: Coping and well-being. *Br J Rheumatol* 1994; **33**: 1067–73.

127. Nielson WR, Jensen MP. Relationship between changes in coping and treatment outcome in patients with fibromyalgia syndrome. *Pain* 2004; **109**: 233–41.

128. Smyth JM. Written emotional expression: Effect sizes, outcome types, and moderating variables. *J Consult Clin Psychol* 1998; **66**: 174–84.

129. Frisna PG, Borod JC, Leopre S J. A meta-analysis of the effects of expressive written emotional disclosure on the health outcomes of clinical populations. *J Nerv Ment Dis* 2008; **192**: 629–34.

130. Gillis ME, Lumley MA, Mosley-Williams A, Leisen JC, Roehrs T. The health effects of at-home written emotional disclosure in fibromyalgia: a randomized trial. *Ann Behav Med* 2006; **32**: 135–46.

131. Keefe FJ, Anderson T, Lumley M, *et al.* A randomized, controlled trial of emotional disclosure in rheumatoid arthritis: Can clinician assistance enhance the effects? *Pain* 2008; **137**: 164–72.

132. Kelley JE, Lumley MA, Leisen JCC. The health effects of emotional disclosure in rheumatoid arthritis. *Health Psychol* 1997; **16**: 331–40.

133. Norman SA, Lumley, MA, Dooley JA, Diamond MP. For whom does it work? Moderators of the effects of written emotional disclosure in a randomized trial among women with chronic pelvic pain. *Psychosom Med* 2004; **66**, 173–83.

134. Danoff-Burg S, Agee JD, Romanoff NR, Kremer JM, Strosberg JM. Benefit finding and expressive writing in adults with lupus or rheumatoid arthritis. *Psychol Health* 2006; **21**: 651–65.

135. Broderick JE, Junghaenel DU, Schwartz JE. Written emotional expression produces health benefits in fibromyalgia patients. *Psychosom Med* 2005; **67**: 326–34.

136. Cepeda MS, Chapman CR, Miranda N, *et al.* Emotional disclosure through patient narrative may improve pain and well-being: Results of a randomized controlled trial in patients with cancer pain. *J Pain Symptom Manage* 2008; **35**: 623–31.

137. De Moor JS, Moye L, Low MD, *et al.* Expressive writing as a presurgical stress management intervention for breast cancer patients. *J Soc Integr Oncol* 2008; **6**: 59–66.

138. Wetherell MA, Byrne-Davis L, Dieppe P, *et al.* Effects of emotional disclosure on psychological and physiological outcomes in patients with rheumatoid arthritis: An exploratory home-based study. *J Health Psychol* 2005; **10**: 277–85.

139. Rosenburg HJ, Rosenburg SD, Ernstoff MC, *et al.* Expressive disclosure and health outcomes in a prostate cancer population. *Int J Psychiatry Med* 2002; **32**: 37–53.

140. Smyth JM, Stone AA, Hurewitz A, Kaell A. Effects of writing about stressful experiences on symptom reduction in patients with asthma or rheumatoid arthritis: A randomized trial. *JAMA* 1999; **281**: 1304–9.

141. Graham JE, Lobel M, Glass P, Lokshina I. Effects of written anger expression in chronic pain patients: Making meaning from pain. *J Behav Med* 2008; **31**: 201–12.

142. Gillis ME. The effects of written emotional disclosure on adjustment in Fibromyalgia syndrome. Unpublished doctoral dissertation. (Wayne State University, Detroit, Michigan 2002).

143. Junghaenel DU, Schwartz JE, Broderick JE. Differential efficacy of written emotional disclosure for subgroups of fibromyalgia patients. *Br J Health Psychol* 2008; **13**: 57–60.

144. Zakowski SG, Ramati A, Morton C, Johnson P, Flanigan R. Written emotional disclosure buffers the effects of social constraints on distress among cancer patients. *Health Psychol* 2004; **23**: 555–63.

145. Kraft CA, Lumley MA, S ' Souza PJ, Dooley JA. Emotional approach coping and self-efficacy moderate the effects of written emotional disclosure and relaxation training for people with migraine headaches. *Br J Health Psychol* 2008; **13**: 67–71.

146. Sullivan MJ, Neish N. The effects of disclosure on pain during dental hygiene treatment: the moderating role of catastrophizing. *Pain* 1999; **79**: 155–63.

147. Low CA, Stanton AL, Danoff-Burg S. Expressive disclosure and benefit finding among breast cancer patients: Mechanisms for positive health effects. *Health Psychol* 2006; **25**: 181–9.

Couple and family psychotherapeutic approaches to pain management

Annmarie Cano, Jaclyn Heller Issner and Courtney L. Dixon

Introduction

Pain does not occur in isolation but is expressed within an interpersonal context. Indeed, research has demonstrated that there is a consistent association between marital distress and physiological and immune processes that affect physical health and pain [1]. Furthermore, marital dissatisfaction, behaviors during interaction, and spouse responses to pain behaviors are associated with a variety of pain adjustment variables [2]. Healthy family members are often affected by chronic pain and can also contribute to patients' adjustment [2, 3]. A meta-analytic review of 70 studies of family-based interventions for chronic illness showed that 54% of interventions focused on relationship issues and most of these interventions focused on spousal relationships [4]. Martire *et al.* concluded that family-based treatments for chronic illnesses are promising interventions for both patients and family members [4]. Thus, when considering pain treatments, it is essential that clinicians consider involving family members as active members of the treatment team.

The purpose of this chapter is to provide an overview of theory and research concerning family factors in chronic pain. A theoretical overview of how pain impacts and is impacted by the family is presented first. Then, various treatment methods that incorporate families are described and a case study is presented. We conclude by offering recommendations for further research and treatment innovation that might contribute to the quality of life of both patients and their families.

Theoretical conceptualizations of the social context of pain

The operant model of pain was one of the first models to advance the theory that family members have an active role in pain patients' behavior [5]. According to the operant model, spouses may respond to patients' pain behaviors by reinforcing (e.g., providing help or attention) or punishing (e.g., expressing negative affect) pain behaviors. Family members may also ignore pain behaviors, leading to their extinction or reinforce well behaviors, encouraging activity. In a series of observational studies with couples in which one partner had chronic pain, Romano and colleagues demonstrated that solicitous spouse responses (e.g., getting the patient something to eat or drink when they are in pain) are positively associated with verbal and non-verbal pain behaviors, and that punishing spouse responses (e.g., expressing irritation or anger at the patient) are inversely associated with non-verbal pain behaviors [6, 7]. These data provide the most direct evidence for the operant model to date. The operant model has also found some support in pediatric samples. For instance, daughters reported more pain when their mothers were reassuring and provided empathy than daughters of mothers who distracted their child during a cold pressor experiment [8].

Cognitive-behavioral models of pain argue that in addition to behaviors, perceptions of those behaviors can affect pain adjustment [9, 10]. Indeed, researchers have found that patient reports of spouses' negative or hostile responses to pain such as anger and irritability are related to increased pain severity and depressive symptoms [11–17]. Solicitous spouse responses including getting the patient medication or something to eat or drink when they are in pain, are related to increased pain severity, physical disability, and depression [2].

Recent research has also examined the reinforcement of well behaviors. Facilitative responses to well behaviors are negatively related to physical disability whereas negative responses to well behavior are positively related to pain behaviors and physical disability in chronic musculoskeletal pain and headache patient samples [18, 19]. In both studies, facilitative responses

---

Behavioral and Psychopharmacologic Pain Management, ed. Michael H. Ebert and Robert D. Kerns. Published by Cambridge University Press. © Cambridge University Press 2011.

to well behavior were positively correlated with solicitous responses to pain behavior. Interestingly, facilitative responses to well behavior and solicitous responses were also negatively related to punishing spouse responses to pain. However, punishing spouse responses to pain and negative responses to well behaviors were not significantly correlated. Taken together, these studies suggest more complex behavioral repertoires in which spouses engage. Additional research is needed to determine how the dynamic interplay between these various responses influence pain and disability in significant others.

With regard to pediatric pain, parental solicitousness is related to a child's pain disability [20]. The child's reports of parental solicitousness are also related to a child's reported somatic complaints if the child reported greater depressive or anxiety symptoms. However, some data do not support a relationship between children's reports of parental solicitousness and somatic complaints [21]. Children's perceptions of their illnesses can create difficulties in family adaptation. Lipani and Walker found that child-reported pain severity and perceived threat was related to maternal worry and limitations in family activities [22]. Both the severity of children's pain and children's beliefs about their pain were independently related to family functioning.

Family systems models have also been developed to explain how family functioning variables such as cohesion and conflict might impact pain adjustment [23]. Such models propose that the functioning of each individual family member is dependent on the functioning of the family as a whole [16, 24]. It has been suggested by some systems models that physical symptoms like pain may serve to maintain homeostasis or stability in the family [13, 16, 24]. In addition, family interaction may be adversely impacted by persistent illness. Research on adults has shown that headache families report less openness in expressing feelings in comparison to backpain and pain-free groups [25, 26]. Other research has shown that patients with pain report more family conflict and control and less cohesion than healthy controls [27]. While there is some evidence supporting family systems models of pain, more recent interest has focused on cognitive-behavioral-interpersonal perspectives.

One such model that is receiving increasing amounts of attention is the communal coping model of pain catastrophizing [28, 29]. Pain catastrophizing is a negative outlook on pain that consists of rumination, magnification, and helplessness [30]. According to the communal coping model, patients may engage in catastrophizing

because it allows them to convey their pain-related distress to close others who might be able to provide help. Catastrophizing might translate into particular kinds of pain behaviors or other interaction strategies that might elicit social support. Research has provided some support for this model. For instance, pain behavior during a cold pressor task mediates the association between pain catastrophizing and observers' ratings of participants' pain severity [31]. Sullivan et al. found that greater catastrophizing was associated with longer displays of communicative pain behaviors such as facial expressions of pain when someone was present during the cold pressor task than when the participant was alone in the room [32]. In a study of pain patients and their spouses, pain adjustment variables were correlated with the spouses' ability to infer patients' pain during a lifting task, providing evidence that spouses may attend to characteristics of the patient in making their estimations [33]. However, patients' pain behaviors during the task were not related to empathic accuracy. Thus, the next step in this research is to determine how spouses determine pain levels in their partners.

Also in support of the communal coping model, researchers have shown that pain catastrophizing is related to social support. For instance, pain catastrophizing is positively correlated with solicitous responses from significant others in samples of patients with spinal cord injuries and chronic musculoskeletal pain [34, 35]. The duration of the pain syndrome also matters. Cano found that at shorter pain durations, greater catastrophizing was associated with greater solicitous spouse responses, suggesting that spouses may provide pain-specific support in response to patient catastrophizing [34]. On the other hand, at longer pain duration, greater catastrophizing was associated with less social support from the spouse, suggesting that chronic catastrophizing may spur a loss of intimacy in couples. Buenaver et al. found similar results, with pain catastrophizing related more strongly to perceived solicitous responses at shorter pain durations [36]. They also found that catastrophizing was related to greater punishing spouse responses when patients reported lower levels of social support. Thus, the associations between catastrophizing and support may depend on a variety of patient factors.

The communal coping model has also received support in child samples. In healthy children experiencing laboratory-induced pain, catastrophizing is predictive of increased pain intensity and unpleasantness and seeking social support was predictive of lower pain tolerance [37]. In a sample of children with and without clinical pain, Vervoort *et al.* found that greater pain catastrophizing was associated with a higher self-reported tendency of the child to verbally share their pain experience with others, and catastrophizing was also associated with paternal and maternal perceptions of the verbal and non-verbal communicative pain behaviors of their children [38]. However, the clinical sample had fewer verbal communications about their pain. Perhaps, the relationship between the child and caregiver changes in the context of chronic pain, with parents engaging in less reinforcing communication about pain over time.

Models have also been developed to explain the role of empathy in pain. According to Goubert *et al.*, the pain empathy process involves several components [39]. First, there are top-down characteristics of the observer that contribute to the observer's understanding or "sense of knowing" about the patient's pain. These characteristics could include the observer's personal experience with pain and the observer's own levels of pain catastrophizing. Second, patient characteristics, i.e., bottom-up variables, also contribute to the observer's understanding of pain. Bottom-up variables include the patient's facial expressions or verbal expressions of pain. A variety of behavioral and emotional responses are likely once observers have a sense of knowing about the patient's pain. Behavioral responses could include validation of the patient's experience or withdrawal. Emotional responses could include feeling distressed for oneself or for the patient.

Leonard and Cano found that spouse catastrophizing about their partners' pain problems was associated with spouse psychological distress for those spouses who also reported chronic pain but not for spouses without chronic pain [40]. These results demonstrate that particular top-down characteristics of the observer, i.e., their own pain experiences, are important in contributing to their emotional distress. In another study, emotional responses of parents were examined in response to vignettes about their child in painful or stressful situations [41]. Imagining children in pain produced other-oriented emotional responses (e.g., understanding, compassion, and sympathy) and personal emotional distress in parents. Parents with high dispositional empathy and who catastrophized reported more self-oriented and other-oriented emotions. In a study of parents and their children, children's facial expressions of pain and parental catastrophizing about their

children's pain during a pain pressure task led parents to give higher estimates of their children's pain [42]. Furthermore, parents and children were more likely to agree about the pain experienced by the child when parents catastrophized about their child's pain.

In sum, a great deal of research suggests that the social context is extremely influential in the development and maintenance of pain. Family members may reinforce pain and well behaviors and perceptions of these relationships may also contribute to pain adjustment and psychological well-being. Furthermore, patients' and family members' thoughts about the pain, including pain catastrophizing, can influence social support and empathic understanding, and distress among patients and their family members. Given the importance of close others in the pain process, researchers have developed a variety of treatments to test the value of including family members in treatments.

Treatments for children with pain

Family-based treatments for pain conditions in childhood have primarily developed along behavioral or cognitive-behavioral lines. Degotardi *et al.* evaluated an 8-week cognitive-behavioral intervention for 67 children with juvenile primary fibromyalgia syndrome (JPFS) and their parents [43]. The intervention included psychoeducation about sleep and pain for children and parents, cognitive restructuring of children's maladaptive pain cognitions, behavioral analysis of parents' reinforcement of pain behaviors, instruction in coping skills (i.e., distraction, relaxation, and self-reinforcement), and instruction in improving daily activities (e.g., postural changes, attitudes, and factors that maintain the sick role).

Most of the children (67%) completed the program. Children reported fewer physical symptoms (i.e., pain, fatigue, sleep disturbance, headaches, and gastric disturbances) after treatment. Children's anxiety, somatization, and internalizing as well as their quality of life and perceived control over JPFS improved after the intervention. Parents also reported that their children had fewer pain complaints and engaged in their social and school activities. However, the dropout rate (33%) was problematic. Families reported that they could not continue treatment because of scheduling conflicts, dissatisfaction with treatment, accessibility to the clinic, and problems with insurance coverage. Because a control group was not included, it is not clear if this treatment would be beneficial for all children with fibromyalgia or if other modes of treatment would be just as effective.

Kozlowska *et al.* integrated behavioral and family systems models into their multidisciplinary intervention for children with somatoform pain disorder [44]. The treatment team consisted of a pain physician, nurse practitioner, medical fellow, physical therapist, and two psychologists. Forty children were referred to the clinic, and 28 were treated with the intervention. The referred children reported chronic pain experiences from 1 month to 6.5 years, with an average of 14.6 months. Attendance of the family was a requirement at the initial session, which involved assessment and psychoeducation of the physical, emotional and behavioral, and social factors contributing to the child's pain experience. The treatment occurred over a 6-month period and was tailored to each unique case. A case example involved breathing, muscle-relaxation, visualization exercises, identifying worry and anxiety symptoms, discussing parental experiences of the medical system, cognitive-behavioral and problem-solving strategies, and meeting with the school. After treatment, 82% of the children reported significant reductions in pain intensity, 71% returned to school full time, and 29% part time. Additionally, 71% of the children returned to premorbid levels of activities of daily living such as sporting and other extracurricular activities. Again, the lack of a control group limits the strength of conclusions that could be made about such treatment.

Two studies have compared family-based pediatric pain treatments to control groups. Allen and Shriver investigated the role of parents in biofeedback treatment for childhood migraine [45]. Inclusion criteria included at least two migraine headaches a month with a minimum 6-month history of headache. Children ($n = 27$) were assigned to a thermal biofeedback intervention combining home and clinic biofeedback practice, or the same biofeedback intervention plus parental pain management guidelines. Children participated in six weekly treatment sessions lasting approximately 40 minutes each. Daily home biofeedback practices were also included in the treatment. The clinic treatment sessions consisted of four phases: a 10-minute habituation period, a 10-minute period of biofeedback training, a 5-minute rest period, and a second 10-minute biofeedback practice session. Parents in the parental pain management group were given a handout that instructed parents to minimize their responses to pain behavior, to insist upon active participation in normal daily activities, and to praise and support the practice of biofeedback. At the end of each session of biofeedback, parents were asked to review and report on their implementation of the guidelines. Parents in the biofeedback only group were not given specific instructions to modify their responses to their children's pain.

Although children in both groups experienced significant reductions in headache activity, children in the parent management group experienced greater reductions in headache frequency, were more likely to experience clinically significant improvements, were more likely to be headache-free, and experienced significantly greater improvements in adaptive functioning. The differences between the groups were maintained through the first 3 months following treatment, but were not significant at 1-year follow-up because the biofeedback only group continued to improve. Overall, the findings suggest that the involvement of parents in the behavioral treatment of the children relates to a number of favorable outcomes in the short-term.

Cognitive-behavioral techniques have also been tested in children with recurrent abdominal pain. Robins *et al.* investigated whether the combination of standard medical care (SMC) and short-term cognitive-behavioral family therapy (CBT) in the treatment of recurrent abdominal pain was more efficacious than SMC alone [46]. Effectiveness was defined as reductions in the sensory aspects of pain, and efficacy was defined as reductions in school absences and utilization of healthcare services.

Eighty-six parent–child dyads, with children ranging in age from 6 to 16 years old, were recruited for this study. Dyads were randomly assigned to the two treatment conditions. The SMC condition entailed "usual and customary" medical treatment, consisting of follow-up office visits, education, support, and information about high fiber diets, oral medications, and supplements. The CBT condition included five 40-minute sessions that were scheduled bimonthly. The first and last two sessions included the parent and child whereas the second and third sessions included the child alone. The CBT objectives included increasing children's repertoire of pain management techniques (e.g., breathing, imagery, and relaxation techniques), increasing understanding of connection between stress and pain perception, encouraging active coping (e.g., positive self-talk, discourage catastrophizing), and increasing parent–child collaboration in pain management (e.g., reframe role of parent from "protector" to "coach"). The child had homework assignments between each session to practice the learned skills.

After 3–12 months, the SMC + CBT group had fewer school absences, less abdominal pain, and lower pain frequency, duration, and severity than the SMC only group. However, significant group differences were not found for somatization, functional disability levels, and medical care utilization. Nonetheless, this research suggests the benefit of adding CBT to usual medical regimens for children with persistent pain.

Across these studies, the extent to which parents were involved in the studies was variable. There were also several similarities across studies. Each study included an educational component so that parents and children learned about the nature and course of the chronic pain syndrome. Parents and children were taught to take control of the pain by learning effective behavioral and coping strategies. Parents were also taught to coach their children and encourage activity. The treatments had varying levels of success, which is to be expected given the diversity of age, diagnoses, and treatment modalities included.

Treatments involving couples and spouses

More studies have been conducted to test the benefits of partner involvement in pain treatment. Spouse-assisted coping skills training (S-CST), which is a cognitive-behavioral treatment for chronic pain that actively involves spouses, has been developed and tested [47–49]. The training is typically conducted in a group setting with ten to twelve 2-hour weekly sessions. Behavioral rehearsal is used in a variety of pain-related and non-pain-related situations to teach couples how to improve communication skills aimed at developing and enhancing coping skills including relaxation, imagery, and distraction techniques. Teaching dyadic coping is essential as research shows that collaboration between partners is needed if chronic illness results in daily physical limitations [50]. In addition, spouses are encouraged to provide feedback to each other about the effectiveness of coping efforts. Couples are also encouraged to practice their new skills during joint activities at home that might elicit pain. Such practice is expected to maintain gains over time.

In a study of patients with persistent knee pain due to osteoarthritis, S-CST was compared to coping skills training without spouse involvement (CST) and a control group that involved education about arthritis and spousal support [47, 48]. There were few differences between the two CST groups; however, post-treatment and follow-up results suggested that better treatment outcomes (i.e., pain severity, psychological disability, pain behavior, marital adjustment, coping) were experienced by the S-CST group followed by the CST group. Both CST groups experienced better outcomes than the control group. Although the CST and S-CST groups did not differ on outcomes, they may differ in terms of mechanisms. Initial improvement in marital satisfaction was related to better pain adjustment at 12-month follow-up in the S-CST group [48]. In contrast, initial improvement in marital satisfaction in the other two groups was related to some indicators of poor pain adjustment. A more recent study of patients with osteoarthritic knee pain showed that S-CST with or without an exercise component was shown to be related to greater self-efficacy and coping than exercise training alone or standard care [49]. However, there were no significant group differences on marital satisfaction, pain, or psychological disability. These results suggest that teaching communication and behavior change skills are essential in pain treatment. However, additional work needs to be conducted to determine the mechanisms that might account for improvement in S-CST.

An adaptation of S-CST has also been tested as a brief intervention for cancer pain [51]. Partner-guided pain management involved three home-based sessions over the course of approximately 2 weeks. Sessions included educating couples about cancer pain management and teaching couples pain coping skills including relaxation training and imagery. Couples were also taught how to pace activity and maintain skills over time. Behavioral rehearsal was used in sessions to train the spouses on how to coach the patients in the coping skills. This intervention was compared against a usual care condition. There were no significant differences between groups in terms of patients' pain ratings. However, partners in the partner-guided condition reported significantly greater self-efficacy in assisting patients with pain and other symptoms. In addition, there was a trend for partners to report less caregiver burden in the partner-guided group.

Treatment approaches that focus on couples' coping skills have also been used with older adults. A couple-oriented education and support intervention was tested against patient-oriented education and support and usual care groups in a sample of 242 older adults with osteoarthritis [52]. Participants in the education and support interventions attended six weekly group sessions that lasted 2 hours each. The education and support conditions included information about arthritis etiology and treatment, exercises designed to manage pain and increase strength, the importance of communication, and information regarding effective coping skills. Participants in these conditions set goals at the end of each session and reported their ability to meet their goals at the next session. Finally, participants were encouraged to rely on each other for support. The couple intervention also presented this information from a couple's perspective rather than the individual perspective offered in the patient-oriented group. Furthermore, the goals a t the end of each session involved both spouses.

There were few differences among the three groups from pre-intervention to 6-month follow-up. When comparing the two education and support groups, participants in the patient-oriented group experienced greater improvements in arthritis severity, physical function, and pain severity. In contrast, the couple-oriented group experienced lower levels of perceived stress and critical attitudes than the patient-oriented group. Additional analyses demonstrated that change over time in the spouses of patients depended on gender and marital satisfaction. That is, spouses with high marital satisfaction experienced decreases in depressive symptoms if they were in the couple-oriented group whereas spouses with low marital satisfaction experienced increases in depression if they participated in the couples approach. Furthermore, wives of patients reported lower stress over time if they participated in the couple-oriented group. The fact that the patient-oriented group experienced greater improvement in pain adjustment whereas the couple-oriented treatment group reported better psychological adjustment suggests that the couples approach is more appropriate for patients who experience distress. Furthermore, distressed spouses and wives may benefit from couple-oriented treatments.

In addition to coping skills training with couples, insight-oriented therapy has been tested as a treatment for chronic pain. Insight-oriented therapy explores relationship processes rather than teaching pain coping skills. In one study, couples attended five monthly sessions of insight-oriented couple therapy or were included in a no-treatment control group [53]. Both groups experience declines in marital satisfaction over the 12-month follow-up but the decline was significantly smaller in the couple therapy group. Furthermore, couples in the couple therapy group reported that their communication improved whereas the control group reported communication declines. There were no significant group differences on pain or disability at the 12-month follow-up [54]. At 5-year follow-up, the therapy group reported significantly better psychological health than the control group. However, the groups were similar on marital satisfaction, pain, or disability [55]. Insight-oriented therapy may be appropriate to treat psychological distress and possibly marital satisfaction in couples with pain, but it does not appear to relate to improvement in pain adjustment.

In sum, the vast majority of research on couples-based treatments for chronic pain have been grounded in cognitive-behavioral theory. Effective interventions with couples focus on skills building, communication training, and behavioral rehearsal to improve marital, psychological, and pain adjustment. However, interventions based on coping skills training have mixed results and it is unclear what aspects of relationships are being changed that might result in improved pain adjustment. Treatments based on increasing insight into relationship dynamics do not appear to directly impact pain adjustment, although they lead to some improvements in psychological and marital well-being. Next, recommendations are made for choosing family-based treatments for chronic pain and directions for the development of other interventions are made.

Recommendations and future directions

At this time, cognitive-behavioral interventions (e.g., S-CST, parent involvement in pediatriac biofeedback) appear to be best suited to treating chronic pain in families. Family members can be enlisted as important members of the treatment team who can support patients in pain management goals. These cognitive-behavioral treatments include components aimed at educating patients and family members about the illness and teaching and practicing coping skills that are effective in managing pain. Family-based treatments for chronic pain also encourage effective communication skills so that patients can request support from family members and provide feedback about their assistance. Such treatments are effective for chronic illness in general and pain problems specifically. Across studies, supportive and collaborative strategies to manage illness are associated with positive adjustment whereas unsupportive behaviors such as criticism and control are associated with poor adjustment [50]. Research has also shown that family-based treatments for chronic illness that include illness education and coping skills training appear to be more effective than patient-oriented treatments [50, 52, 56]. Thus, it makes sense to incorporate partners and other family members in treatments for chronic illnesses such as pain. Research also suggests that children of family members with pain should receive referrals to programs that could enhance their coping skills and build social support.

While cognitive-behavioral family-based treatments appear to be effective in managing psychological disability and distress in patients and family members, these interventions do not consistently outperform cognitive-behavioral treatments that focus solely on patients. This is intriguing given that operant and cognitive-behavioral theories place such importance on the role of family members in patient's adjustment to pain. Perhaps other approaches to chronic pain treatment should be investigated to enhance the efficacy of family-based interventions. One such approach for adults is insight-oriented therapy, which was related to good relationship and psychological health outcomes [53], yet additional research is needed to determine whether such treatment is effective in reducing pain and disability. For pediatric pain, recommends new family-based interventions that help children learn to manage important tasks concerning their illness through education and advocacy as well as coping and emotional support [57]. According to this model, parents play an active role in facilitating children's coping efforts that are directed toward the illness as well as social relationships within and outside of the family. Thus, parents may need explicit training in providing instrumental and emotional support to their children.

Therapy based on emotion regulation and empathy models may also be promising because these models identify aspects of relationships that have not been sufficiently addressed in traditional cognitive-behavioral interventions for families with pain. According to emotion regulation models of couples' interaction, emotional validation is thought to enhance the emotion regulation process for both partners because such behaviors allow each person to process stressful or aversive stimuli [58, 59]. Indeed, self-disclosure of emotions, partner responsiveness, and empathy predict intimacy and satisfaction in couples [60–64]. In contrast, interactions characterized by invalidation, such as hostility or ignoring partner's emotional responses, indicate rejection and disregard for the partner, in turn, disrupting emotion regulation attempts.

Applied to couples and families experiencing pain, good interaction skills including empathy may promote healthy emotion regulation attempts when dealing with the affective distress associated with pain and disability. In contrast, invalidation may contribute to distress and poor coping efforts. Research with pain couples provides preliminary support for these hypotheses. Johansen and Cano investigated the role of intimacy-based marital interaction during a 15-minute marital problem-solving task [65]. In this study of community couples with at least one partner having chronic musculoskeletal pain, approximately half of the sample displayed anger/contempt, a form of emotional invalidation, during interaction. Anger and contempt were negatively related to marital satisfaction. Anger was associated with greater depressive symptoms when only the patient reported chronic pain (as opposed to when the spouse also reported chronic pain). These results held when controlling for marital satisfaction as well as other demographic variables. Thus, invalidation in the context of interacting about marital problems appears to be related to relationship and psychological problems in some patients.

There has also been some work on the affective properties of pain-related interaction. Newton-John and Williams conducted a qualitative self-report study of chronic pain couples and found that solicitous spouse responses are not always received favorably as evidenced by a hostile-solicitous category [66]. In addition, Newton-John and Williams argue that talking about pain may actually be beneficial to patients. These ideas are in line with emotion regulation models of interaction [58, 59] and intimacy research [61]. Models of pain empathy also suggest that talking about pain may be a form of emotional self-disclosure that fosters the spouse's understanding of pain-related distress so that empathy and validation can be provided [39]. However, such a conceptualization of self-disclosure and empathic responses by family members is in sharp contrast to the operant model's conceptualization of verbal pain behavior and solicitous responses.

Preliminary work suggests that solicitous spouse responses and validation are distinct types of interaction. Cano *et al.* argue that empathic responses should not be confused with solicitousness [67]. In this study, couples discussed the impact of pain on their lives. Each partner's behaviors were coded for validating (i.e., empathic) and invalidating (i.e., non-empathic) behaviors. A factor analysis showed that validation and invalidation expressed by each spouse loaded with each partner's reports of punishing spouse responses on a Non-empathic Responding factor. Both partners' reports of solicitous and distracting spouse responses loaded on a different factor that was labeled Solicitous Responding. The Non-empathic Responding factor was more strongly associated with patients' marital quality than the Solicitous Responding factor. Thus, validating responses do not appear to be just another form of solicitous spouse responses. Furthermore, punishing responses appear to be highly invalidating to patients. This study suggests that examining responses from a variety of theoretical perspectives might aid in expanding theory and identifying other treatments from the marital and family therapy literature that might be appropriate for persons with pain.

One such treatment, integrative behavioral couple therapy (IBCT), recommended for couples dealing with chronic pain [68], was developed from the cognitive-behavioral marital therapy tradition in which behavior change is encouraged for both partners [69, 70]. Therapists specializing in IBCT use a combination of behavioral strategies (e.g., behavior exchange, communication training) and emotional acceptance techniques. Emotional acceptance involves changing the way each spouse perceives their partner's undesirable behaviors. For example, personality or behavior patterns (e.g., extraversion) that were once irritating to the partner may become acceptable or valued by the partner.

Integrative behavioral couple therapy is an efficacious treatment for psychological and marital distress [71, 72], and may be appropriate for chronic pain for several reasons. First, depression and anxiety as well as marital discord, problems that are addressed by IBCT, are reported by many couples with pain [73]. Second, spouses have difficulty understanding the pain and disability experienced by their partners [74, 75]. This incongruence in pain and disability ratings may be due to a poor understanding of the emotional consequences of pain. In fact, patients believe that significant others do not understand their pain and emotional suffering [76]. The contention of IBCT is that emotional acceptance or empathy is needed along with behavior change otherwise changes cannot be sustained or may even be perceived as insincere attempts to change behavior. Third, patients may be afraid to talk about their pain because they have been rejected or invalidated [77]. Porter et al. also found that low self-efficacy and greater holding back in talking about cancer pain were associated with distress and pain catastrophizing

[78]. Furthermore, self-efficacy in talking about pain appeared to mediate the association between holding back and distress and catastrophizing. Thus, both partners' fears can be addressed with emotional acceptance and communication training techniques. Because IBCT combines behavior change with emotional acceptance, couples may experience greater or longer lasting treatment responses with IBCT.

Another promising technique that has been tested with adults and children is emotionally focused therapy (EFT) [79, 80]. According to this model of therapy, emotions are critical in close relationships, interactions, and in forming attachment bonds because they communicate motivations and needs to others and affect others' responses. The therapist targets rigid patterns of interaction and negative affect that might contribute to distress in the individual and the family. The goals of this empirically supported treatment are to foster more secure attachments with relationship partners by validating and accepting each partner's emotions and interactional styles, identifying negative interaction patterns including unacknowledged feelings about interactions, and practicing new interaction skills that adequately address each partner's needs for emotional expression and healthy attachments [81].

Kowal et al. suggest that EFT may be an effective treatment for couples dealing with chronic illness because creating secure attachment bonds can serve to improve physical health as well as the relationship [80]. The studies in their review suggest that insecure attachment is related to poorer health outcomes and insecurely attached individuals might be less likely to seek support needed to improve health. Although EFT has not been tested directly with couples with pain, it has been tested with parents of ill children. Walker et al. recruited 32 couples with a chronically ill child [82]. Couples were randomly assigned to EFT or a wait-list control that was offered EFT treatment when the study was completed. The treatment group experienced significantly greater marital adjustment than the control group upon treatment completion, which was maintained at 5-month follow-up. These results suggest that treatment focusing on attachment needs and emotional processes is particularly useful for helping partners support each other in the face of the stress and threatened loss of a child. However, it is unclear how children are indirectly affected by the treatment. Additional research with IBCT and EFT is needed to determine the extent to which each intervention aids in pain management. Nevertheless, it appears that these treatments, both of which more directly target the emotion regulation properties of interaction, offer promising new directions for clinicians and researchers. We now present a hypothetical case example in which elements of S-CST and IBCT are applied.

Case example

Mr. and Mrs. S. are a couple in their late fifties. They have three adult children who do not live with them. Mr. S. recently retired from his job as a foreman at an automotive company. Mrs. S. continues to work as an elementary school teacher. Mr. S. has experienced back pain for 15 years and has tried a variety of treatments for his pain including medications, nerve blocks, and surgery. He is currently taking oral analgesics (NSAIDS) for his pain, which he rates as a 5 on a 0–10 scale. Mr. S. reported that his wife does not understand his pain and that she criticizes him often for not being able to keep up with housework. The couple reportedly gets into arguments once a week and will sometimes go for a day or two without speaking to each other. At times, one partner will recruit their children to be their spokespeople to the other partner. Mr. S. told his physician that he's at "his wit's end" in knowing how to handle this and that the arguments leave him feeling exhausted, irritable, and with more pain. Mr. S's physician referred the couple for therapy, explaining to Mrs. S. that it must be stressful for her to be married to someone with chronic pain and that perhaps therapy would be beneficial for easing the tension that both partners were experiencing.

At the first therapy visit, Dr. T., a clinical psychologist, conducted an assessment with both partners to explain the purpose of the initial visits: to determine each spouse's concerns about the relationship, including concerns about the pain problem, and to identify areas in which each partner would like to see improvements. Dr. T. began by obtaining a relationship history from the couple (e.g., "How did the couple meet? What attracted them to each other?"). This line of questioning often builds intimacy between partners as they recall the initial stages of their relationship. Dr. T. then asked when they began to notice problems and to what they attribute those problems. During the session, Dr. T. observed how the couple interacted with one another. Did they use humor? Was the couple respectful or contemptuous toward each other? Did Mr. S. engage in pain behaviors and if so, how did Mrs. S. respond? At the end of this session, Dr. T. provided some feedback

to the couple about their strengths and positive qualities including the couple's determination to remain together despite pain, their attempts to use humor to cope with stressful circumstances, and their close relationship with their children and grandchildren. Dr. T. also suggested some areas to address including the couple's communication skills, pain coping attempts, and perspective taking. The couple agreed with Dr. T.'s assessment and agreed that they should try therapy to alleviate some of the distress they were experiencing.

Once the initial assessment period was completed, Dr. T. met weekly with the couple for eight sessions. Initially, Dr. T. used examples from the couple's everyday life to engage Mr. and Mrs. S. in discussions about how their lives had been transformed by pain. For instance, Dr. T. would ask about how the couple got along since the previous session. Invariably, there was a disagreement or some tension about pain. Dr. T. used these instances to ask pointed questions about how each partner felt about the situation: "What did it feel like, Mr. S., when your wife seemed disappointed in your not doing the chores?" Dr. T. also made interpretations about the couples' thoughts and feelings when it would aid in building empathy and perspective-taking: "So, Mrs. S., you were not necessarily angry at Mr. S. for not doing the chores but you were angry because you could not do anything to get rid of his pain." At times, Dr. T. taught appropriate communication skills. For instance, when it became clear that Mrs. S.'s genuine suggestions for making housework more manageable were perceived by Mr. S. as criticism, Dr. T. engaged the couple in an open discussion about how to talk about housework in a constructive manner. Dr. T. assigned behavioral homework for the couple including engaging in one shared activity per week that the couple enjoyed. Eventually, Dr. T. took a less active role in negotiating conflict and was able to provide favorable feedback to the couple about their improved communication and empathy skills.

Once improvements in the relationship were observed, Dr. T. decided to train both partners in S-CST skills for another four sessions. This part of treatment included training in relaxation skills and activity pacing. Because the couple had improved in taking each other's perspectives, they were able to engage in these activities without feeling resentful of the other partner's role. The couple was able to see the pain as a "project" and was able to consider the other partner's point of view. Upon treatment completion Mr. S. reported to his physician that the couple argued less and that his wife, while still not fully knowing what chronic pain was like, at least attempted to understand his pain. He reported that he rarely had flare-ups due to relationship stress and that he was also walking more because the couple regained enjoyment in each other's company while exercising. Mrs. S. also accompanied her husband to his appointments and was more interested in being involved in treatment decisions as a supportive partner. Although he still experiences pain, Mr. S. was less distressed and fatigued.

Conclusion

In sum, a variety of couple and family-based treatments are available to address pain in adults and children. To date, the most effective family-based treatments are ones that enlist the support of family members, provide information about chronic pain, teach effective coping skills to deal with maladaptive cognitions and behaviors, and encourage activity. However, couple and family treatments have not always resulted in clear benefits over patient-only treatment. Furthermore, recent evidence suggests that addressing empathy and emotion regulation may offer additional improvements, especially for distressed patients and their family members. It may be most appropriate to refer patients to cognitive-behavioral approaches when the family is relatively well-adjusted, which would be indicated by relationship satisfaction and healthy interaction skills. However, when the clinician judges that the family relationships are strained or there is a lack of empathy for the pain problem, interventions targeting these relationship dynamics (e.g., IBCT, EFT) may need to be considered.

Acknowledgment

The first author was supported by K01 MH66975 while working on this chapter.

References

1. Kiecolt-Glaser J, Newton T. Marriage and health: His and hers. *Psychol Bull* 2001; **127**: 472–503.

2. Leonard MT, Cano A. Pain affects spouses too: Personal experience with pain and catastrophizing as correlates of spouse distress. *Pain* 2006; **126**: 139–46.

3. Coyne JC, Fiske V. Couples coping with chronic and catastrophic illness. In *Family Health Psychology*, eds. TJ Akamatsu, MAP Stephens, SE Hobfoll, JH Crowther. (Washington: Taylor and Francis, 1992), pp. 129–49.

4. Martire LM, Lustig AP, Schulz R, Miller GE, Helgeson VS. Is it beneficial to involve a family member? A meta-analysis of psychosocial interventions for chronic illness. *Health Psychol* 2004; **23**: 599–611.

5. Fordyce WE. *Behavioral Methods for Chronic Pain and Illness* (St. Louis, MO: C.V. Mosby, 1976).

6. Romano JM, Turner JA, Friedhman LS, *et al.* Sequential analysis of chronic pain behaviors and spouse responses. *J Consult Clin Psychol* 1992; **60**: 777–82.

7. Romano JM, Jensen MP, Turner JA, Good AB, Hops H. Chronic pain patient-partner interactions: Further support for a behavioral model of chronic pain. *Behav Ther* 2000; **31**: 415–40.

8. Chambers CT, Craig KD, Bennett SM. The impact of maternal behavior on children's pain experiences: An experimental analysis. *J Pediatr Psychol* 2002; **27**: 293–301.

9. Turk DC, Meichenbaum D, Genest M. *Pain and Behavioral Medicine: A cognitive-behavioral perspective* (New York: Guilford Press, 1983).

10. Gatchel RJ, Peng YB, Peters M, Fuchs PN, Turk DC. The biopsychosocial approach to chronic pain: Scientific advances and future directions. *Psychol Bull* 2007; **133**: 581–624.

11. Cano A, Weisberg J, Gallagher M. Marital satisfaction and pain severity mediate the association between negative spouse responses to pain and depressive symptoms in a chronic pain patient sample. *Pain Med* 2000; **1**: 35–43.

12. Cano A, Gillis M, Heinz W, Foran H. Marital functioning, chronic pain, and psychological distress. *Pain* 2004; **107**: 99–106.

13. Flor H, Turk DC, Rudy TE. Pain and families. II. Assessment and treatment. *Pain* 1987; **30**: 29–45.

14. Kerns RD, Haythornwaite J, Southwick S, Giller EL. The role of marital interaction in chronic pain and depressive symptom severity. *J Psychosom Res* 1990; **34**: 401–8.

15. Paulsen JS, Altmaier EM. The effects of perceived versus enacted social support on the discriminative cue function of spouses for pain behaviors. *Pain* 1995; **60**: 103–10.

16. Turk DC, Kerns RD, Rosenberg R. Effects of marital interaction on chronic pain and disability: Examining the down side of social support. *Rehabil Psychol* 1992; **37**: 259–74.

17. Williamson D, Robinson ME, Melamed B. Pain behavior, spouse responsiveness, and marital satisfaction in patients with rheumatoid arthritis. *Behav Modif* 1997; **21**: 97–118.

18. Pence LB, Thorn BE, Jensen MP, Romano JM. Examination of perceived spouse responses to patient well and pain behavior in patients with headache. *Clin J Pain* 2008; **24**: 654–61.

19. Schwartz L, Slater MA, Birchler GR. The role of pain behaviors in the modulation of marital conflict in chronic pain couples. *Pain* 1996; **65**: 227–33.

20. Peterson CC, Palermo TM. Parental reinforcement of recurrent pain: The moderating impact of child depression and anxiety on functional disability. *J Pediatr Psychol* 2004; **29**: 331–41.

21. Jellesma FC, Rieffe C, Terwogt MM, Westenberg PM. Do parents reinforce somatic complaints in their children? *Health Psychol* 2008; **27**: 280–85.

22. Lipani TA, Walker LS. Children's appraisal and coping with pain: Relation to maternal ratings of worry and restriction in family activities. *J Pediatr Psychol* 2006; **31**: 667–73.

23. Kerns RD, Otis JD. Family therapy for persons experiencing pain: Evidence for its effectiveness. *Seminars in Pain Med* 2003; **1**: 79–89.

24. Scholevar GP, Perkel R. Family systems intervention and physical illness. *Gen Hosp Psychiatry* 1990; **12**: 363–72.

25. Ehde DM, Holm JE, Metzger DL. The role of family structure, functioning, and pain modeling in headache. *Headache* 1991; **31**: 35–40.

26. Kopp M, Richter R, Rainer J, *et al*. Difference in family functioning between patients with chronic headache and patients with chronic low back pain *pain* 1995; **63**: 219–24.

27. Feuerstein M, Sult S, Houle M. Environmental stressors and chronic low back pain: Life events, family, and work environment. *Pain*, 1985; **22**: 295–307.

28. Sullivan MJL, Thorn BE, Haythornthwaite JA, *et al*. Theoretical perspectives on the relation between catastrophizing and pain. *Clin J Pain* 2001; **17**: 52–64.

29. Thorn BE, Ward LC, Sullivan MJL, Boothby JL. Communal coping model of catastrophizing: Conceptual model building. *Pain* 2003; **106**: 1–2.

30. Sullivan MJL, Bishop S, Pivik J. The Pain Catastrophizing Scale: Development and validation. *Psychol Assess* 1995; **7**: 524–32.

31. Sullivan MJL, Martel MO, Tripp D, Savard A, Crombez G. The relation between catastrophizing and the communication of pain experience. *Pain* 2006; **122**: 282–8.

32. Sullivan MJL, Adams H, Sullivan ME. Communicative dimensions of pain catastrophizing: Social cueing effects on pain behaviour and coping. *Pain* 2004; **107**: 220–6.

33. Gauthier N, Thibault P, Sullivan MJL. Individual and relational correlates of pain-related empathic accuracy in spouses of chronic pain patients. *Clin J Pain* 2008; **24**: 669–77.

34. Cano A. Pain catastrophizing and social support in married individuals with chronic pain: The moderating role of pain duration. *Pain* 2004; **110**: 656–64.

35. Giardino ND, Jensen MP, Turner JA, *et al*. Social environment moderates the association between catastrophizing and pain among persons with spinal cord injury. *Pain* 2003; **106**: 19–25.

36. Buenaver LF, Edwards RR, Haythornthwaite JA. Pain-related catastrophizing and perceived social responses: Inter-relationships in the context of chronic pain. *Pain* 2007; **127**: 234–42.

37. Qian L, Tsao JC, Myers CD, Kim S, Zeltzer LK. Coping predictors of children's laboratory-induced pain tolerance, intensity, and unpleasantness. *J Pain* 2007; **8**: 707–17.

38. Vervoort T, Craig KD, Goubert L, Dehoorne J, Joos R *et al*. Expressive dimensions of pain catastrophizing: A comparative analysis of school children and children with clinical pain. *Pain* 2008; **134**: 59–68.

39. Goubert L, Craig KD, Vervoort T, *et al*. Facing others in pain: The effects of empathy. *Pain* 2005; **118**: 285–8.

40. Leonard MT, Cano A. Pani effects spouses too: Personal experience with pain and catastrophizing as corrolates of spouse distress. *Pain* 2006; **126**: 137–46.

41. Goubert L, Vervoort T, Sullivan MJL, Verhoeven, Crombez G. Parental emotional responses to their child's pain: The role of dispositional empathy and catastrophizing about their child's pain. *J Pain* 2008; **9**: 272–9.

42. Goubert L, Vervoort T, Cano A, Crombez G. Catastrophizing about their children's pain is related to higher parent-child congruency in pain ratings: An experimental investigation. *Eur J Pain*. 2009; **13**: 196–201.

43. Degotardi PJ, Klass ES, Batya SR, *et al*. Development and evaluation of a cognitive-behavioral intervention for juvenile fibromyalgia. *J Pediatr Psychol* 2006; **31**: 714–723.

44. Kozlowska K, Rose D, Khan R, *et al*. A conceptual model and practice framework for managing chronic pain in children and adolescents. *Harv Rev Psychiatry* 2008; **16**: 136–50.

45. Allen KD, Shriver MD. Role of parent-mediated pain behavior management strategies in biofeedback treatment of childhood migraines. *Behav Ther* 1998; **29**: 477–90.

46. Robins PM, Smith SM, Glutting JJ, Bishop CT. A randomized controlled trial of a cognitive-behavioral family intervention for pediatric recurrent abdominal pain. *J Pediatr Psychol* 2005; **30**: 397–408.

47. Keefe F, Caldwell D, Baucom D, Salley A. Spouse-assisted coping skills training in the management of osteoarthritic knee pain. *Arthritis Care Res* 1996; **9**: 279–91.

48. Keefe F, Caldwell D, Baucom D, *et al.* Spouse-assisted coping skills training in the management of knee pain in osteoarthritis: Long-term followup results. *Arthritis Care Research* 1999; **12**: 101–11.

49. Keefe F, Blumenthal J, Baucom D, *et al.* Effects of spouse-assisted coping skills training and exercise training in patients with osteoarthritic knee pain: A randomized controlled study. *Pain* 2004; **110**: 539–49.

50. Berg CA, Upchurch R. A developmental-contextual model of couples with chronic illness across the adult life span. *Psychol Bull* 2007; **133**: 920–54.

51. Keefe FJ, Ahles TA, Sutton L, *et al.* Partner-guided cancer pain management at the end of life. *J Pain Symptom Manage* 2005; **29**: 263–72.

52. Martire LM, Schulz R, Keefe FJ, Rudy TE, Starz T. Couple-oriented education and support intervention: Effects on individuals with osteoarthritis and their spouses. *Rehabil Psychol* 2007; **52**: 121–32.

53. Saarijarvi S. A controlled study of couple therapy in chronic low back pain patients: Effects on marital satisfaction, psychological distress and health attitudes. *J Psychosom Res* 1991; **35**: 265–72.

54. Saarijarvi S, Rytokoski U, Alanen E. A controlled study of couple therapy in chronic low back pain patients: No improvement of disability. *J Psychosom Res* 1991; **35**: 671–77.

55. Saarijarvi S, Alanen E, Rytokoski U, Hyyppa M. Couple therapy improves mental well-being in chronic low back pain patients: A controlled, five year follow up study. *J Psychosom Res* 1992; **36**: 651–6.

56. Campbell TL. The effectiveness of family interventions for physical disorders. *J Marital Fam Ther* 2003; **29**: 263–81.

57. Drotar D. Integrating theory and practice in psychological intervention with families of children with chronic illness. In *Family Health Psychology*, eds. TJ Akamatsu, MAP Stephens, SE Hobfoll, JH Crowther. (Washington: Taylor and Francis, 1992), pp. 175–92.

58. Fruzzetti AE, Iverson KM. Mindfulness, acceptance, validation, and "individual" psychopathology in couples, In *Mindfulness and Acceptance: Expanding the cognitive-behavioral tradition*, eds. SC Hayes, VM Follette, MM Linehan. (Guilford Press: New York, 2004), pp. 168–91.

59. Fruzzetti AE, Iverson KM Intervening with couples and families to treat emotion dysregulation and psychopathology, In *Emotion Regulation in Couples and Families: Pathways to dysfunction and health*, eds. DK Snyder, JN. Hughes. (Washington, DC: American Psychological Association, 2006) pp. 249–67.

60. Angera JJ, Long ECJ. Qualitative and quantitative evaluations of an empathy training program for couples in marriage and romantic relationships. *J Couple Relatsh Ther* 2006; **5**: 1–26.

61. Laurenceau J, Feldman Barrett L, Pietromonaco PR. Intimacy as an interpersonal process: The importance of self-disclosure, partner disclosure, and perceived partner responsiveness in interpersonal exchanges. *J Pers Soc Psychol* 1998; **74**: 1238–51.

62. Laurenceau JP, Feldman Barrett L, Rovine MJ. The interpersonal process model of intimacy in marriage: A daily diary and multilevel modeling approach. *J Fam Psychol* 2005; **19**: 314–23.

63. Long ECJ, Angera JJ, Carter SJ, Nakamoto M, Kalso M. Understanding the one you love: A longitudinal assessment of an empathy training program for couples in romantic relationships. *Fam Relat* 1999; **48**: 235–42.

64. Mitchell AE, Castellani AM, Herrington RL, *et al.* Predictors of intimacy in couples' discussions of relationship injuries: An observational study. *J Fam Psychol* 2008; **22**: 21–9.

65. Johansen A, Cano A. A preliminary investigation of affective interaction in chronic pain couples. *Pain* 2007; **132**: S86–S95.

66. Newton-John TR, Willams AC. Chronic pain couples: Perceived marital interactions and pain behaviours. *Pain* 2006; **123**: 53–63.

67. Cano A, Barterian J, Heller J. Empathic and nonempathic interaction in chronic pain couples. *Clin J Pain* 2008; **24**: 678–84.

68. Cano A, Leonard MT. Integrative behavioral couple therapy for chronic pain: Promoting behavior change and emotional acceptance. *J Clin Psychol* 2006; **62**: 1409–18.

69. Christensen A, Jacobson N, Babcock J. Integrative behavioral couple therapy. In *Clinical Handbook of Marital Therapy* 2nd edn. eds. N Jacobson Gurman (New York: Guilford Press, 1995), pp. 31–64.

70. Jacobson N, Christensen A. *Acceptance and Change In Couple Therapy: A therapist's guide to transforming relationships* (New York: Norton, 1998).

71. Christensen A, Atkins D, Berns S, *et al.* Traditional versus integrative behavioral couple therapy for significantly and chronically distressed married couples. *J Consult Clin Psychol* 2004; **72**: 176–91.

72. Jacobson N, Christensen A, Prince S, Cordova J, Eldridge K. Integrative behavioral couple therapy: An acceptance-based, promising new treatment for couple discord. *J Consult Clin Psychol* 2000; **68**: 351–5.

73. Leonard M, Cano A, Johansen A. Chronic pain in a couples context: A review and integration of

theoretical models and empirical evidence. *J Pain* 2006; **7**: 377–90.

74. Cano A, Johansen A, Franz A. Multilevel analysis of spousal congruence on pain, interference, and disability. *Pain*, 2005; **118**: 369–79.

75. Cano A, Johansen A, Geisser M. Spousal congruence on disability, pain, and spouse responses to pain. *Pain*, 2004; **109**: 258–65.

76. Herbette G, Rime B. Verbalization of emotion in chronic pain patients and their psychological adjustment. *J Health Psychol* 2004; **9**: 661–76.

77. Morley S, Doyle K, Beese A. Talking to others about pain: Suffering in silence. In *Proceedings of the Ninth World Congress on Pain: Progress in pain research and management*, eds. M. Devor, M. Rowbothan, Z. Wiesenfeld-Hallin. (Seattle: IASP Press, 2000), pp. 1123–9.

78. Porter LS, Keefe FJ, Wellington C, de Williams A. Pain communication in the context of osteoarthritis: Patient and partner self-efficacy for pain communication and holding back from discussion of pain and arthritis-related concerns. *Clin J Pain* 2008; **24**: 662–8.

79. Johnson SM, Greenberg LS. Emotionally focused couples therapy: An outcome study. *J Marital Fam Ther* 1985; **11**: 313–17.

80. Kowal J, Johnson SM, Lee A. Chronic illness in couples: A case for emotionally focused therapy. *J Marital Fam Ther* 2003; **29**: 299–310.

81. Johnson S. *The Practice of Emotionally Focused Couple Therapy: Creating connection* (New York: Brunner-Routledge, 2004).

82. Walker JG, Johnson S, Manion I, Cloutier P. Emotionally focused marital intervention for couples with chronically ill children. *J Consult Clin Psychol* 1996; **64**: 1029–36.

Psychopharmacologic and psychotherapeutic approaches to pain management

Raphael J. Leo and Wendy J. Quinton

Introduction

In the past, pain had been conceptualized by clinicians as a purely sensory phenomenon emanating from a pathophysiologic state, e.g., tissue injury generating pain transduction through the activity of peripheral or visceral nociceptors. The treating physician would then be proactive in undertaking pharmacologic and other interventions to treat the underlying disease state or relieve pain. In ambiguous cases for which the source of pain was unclear, there would often be an exhaustive search for biomedical causes and treatment. Taken from this perspective, there was an implicit mind-body dualism of pain, distinguishing it as either somatic (physical in origin) or psychogenic (psychological in origin). Consequently, there was a tendency to attribute to psychic factors any pain process in which the physical causes could not be fully delineated, when pain complaints seem disproportionate to the underlying disease, or when the pain failed to respond to treatment as expected [1]. Patients deemed to have psychogenic pain were dismissed from medical care and instead relegated to the province of psychiatry and psychology.

Concurrently, in an attempt to delineate diagnostic criteria to assist in the classification of patients for whom psychological disturbances "masquerade" as somatic preoccupations such as pain, early versions of the Diagnostic and Statistical Manual of Psychiatric Disorders (DSM) required that clinicians infer whether psychological underpinnings or conflicts precipitated pain complaints. Thus, if it were evident from physical examination and diagnostic evaluation that a physical cause could not fully account for the pain, psychiatric labels were invoked reflecting the psychological origins of the pain – for example, psychogenic pain disorder from DSM-III [2] and somatoform pain disorder from DSM-III-R [3]. Borrowing from psychodynamic conceptualizations, early DSM diagnostic criteria

perpetuated the prevailing mind-body dualism characteristic of medical treatment at the time.

It has long been observed that differences exist in perceived pain severity and perceived level of impairment among individuals with comparable disease. Such observations have led to a paradigm shift, viewing pain as a perceptual phenomenon. From this perspective, it is recognized that pain is not only a sensory experience, but also that one's perception of pain intensity is influenced by cognitive, affective and social variables. In contrast to the step-wise care of the biomedical approaches whereby psychological and psychiatric care is reserved as the treatment of last resort for the recalcitrant patient, there has been an alteration in approaches to pain management, encompassing the collaborative efforts of psychiatrists, psychologists and other mental health practitioners. This chapter will attempt to address the evolution in the conceptualizations of chronic non-malignant pain conditions, as well as the prevailing research assessing the efficacy of psychotherapeutic and psychopharmacologic approaches to pain management.

Current conceptualization of pain disorder

There is a continuum of somatic distress and symptom preoccupation along which patients may fall. Some patients with recurrent and enduring pain are reasonably well-adjusted whereas others notably display pain preoccupation and associated distress, citing it as the source of all of their misery. The DSM taxonomy was modified to assist in the classification of patients for whom pain has become the predominant focus of clinical attention and for whom psychological factors are implicated and believed to have a significant contributory role in the pain. For many of those with pain

Behavioral and Psychopharmacologic Pain Management, ed. Michael H. Ebert and Robert D. Kerns. Published by Cambridge University Press. © Cambridge University Press 2011.

disorder, marked disability might be alleged, and the patient's life becomes centered around pain.

There was a transition in the thinking underlying diagnosis of pain disorder from earlier DSM versions. The terms somatoform and psychogenic were dropped [4]. There is no longer a requirement for exclusion of a physical cause for the pain, and the primacy of psychological factors (i.e., conflicts and emotional states) underlying and accounting for pain was de-emphasized. The current DSM-IV-TR [5] leaves open the possibility that psychological factors can contribute to the pain experience by precipitating, exacerbating, or maintaining pain but do not necessarily have to fully account for it. This approach is more consistent with current views of the interrelationships between pain and psychological factors.

The following five criteria need to be met for a patient to be appropriately diagnosed with pain disorder: (1) pain in one or more anatomic sites of sufficient severity to warrant clinical attention; (2) the pain causes significant distress, or results in impairments in social or occupational functioning; (3) psychological factors play a significant role in the onset, exacerbation or maintenance of pain; (4) the symptoms are not fabricated or feigned and the person is not malingering; (5) the pain is not better accounted for by another psychiatric disorder, e.g., depression, anxiety or psychosis [5]. Theoretically, such diagnostic criteria may assist clinicians with identification of those individuals with chronic pain who have higher levels of distress and dysfunctional psychological attributes, and thus may benefit most from psychotherapeutic and psychopharmacologic treatment endeavors.

Although improved over previous versions, there are several criticisms of the DSM-IV-TR taxonomy. In contrast to many other psychiatric disorders, the criteria of pain disorder often are perceived as insufficiently defined, lacking a checklist of symptoms that collectively delineate the syndrome. An inference is still required on the part of the clinician to determine whether and to what extent psychological factors are involved in the patient's plight. Similarly, there are no guidelines allowing one to ascertain whether pain is "not better accounted for" by a mood disorder [6]; in fact, this can be quite undecipherable given the high co-morbidity of mood disturbances with pain (discussed in Chapter 7).

By being grouped under the rubric of somatoform disorders, pain disorder may still connote the implied mind-body dualism of other somatoform disorders, i.e., somatic preoccupation occurring in the absence of,

or in excess of what would be expected, given objective findings. As a result, the nosology of pain disorder is likely to be misunderstood by non-psychiatric clinicians [7]; the potential pejorative implication may be that the patient is disingenuous or faking. Ironically, in redefining pain disorder in DSM-IV-TR, the intent was to overcome this archaic dualism.

Lastly, the diagnostic criteria for pain disorder do not, in and of themselves, assist clinicians with arriving at treatments to effectively manage the condition. The criteria do not help clinicians identify the unique attributes of those with the condition, and as a result, do not facilitate customizing interventions more closely to patients' needs and circumstances, thereby optimizing treatment benefits [8].

The biopsychosocial model of pain

The ubiquity of pain and the fact that enduring and intractable pain syndromes are common has prompted the question whether, and to what extent, factors other than those which are purely physical/sensory contribute to the perception of pain and its associated impairments. Such differences have prompted efforts to establish theoretical models that serve to unveil the complexities underlying, and otherwise explicate, how psychological (both cognitive and emotional factors), social and physical factors interact to influence how chronic painful conditions are experienced. One such model, the biopsychosocial model [9], has gained significant appeal, emphasizing the bidirectional influences of psychological states and nd their associated symptoms, including pain. Rather than dichotomizing between physical vs. psychological origins, the biopsychosocial perspective maintains that the experience of pain, i.e., one's presentation and response to treatment, are determined by the interaction of biological factors, the patient's psychological makeup, the presence of psychological co-morbidities, and the extent of social support and extenuating environmental circumstances [1, 10].

The biomedically based conceptualizations described earlier viewed pain as a static entity, either pathophysiologically determinable or not. The biopsychosocial model offered a more expanded and dynamic approach to pain. The range of biopsychosocial factors relevant to a particular patient can change throughout the various phases of pain response [11]. Following tissue injury, trauma, and inflammation, there is an acute pain phase, where treatment is centered on pain relief, identification and, if possible, remediation of the underlying medical condition. During this initial phase, it is common for patients to experience fear and anxiety, e.g., alarm about what the pain might signal or indicate, and concerns regarding the ability to take steps to relieve it, etc. Psychological and social factors play a relatively limited role in precipitating, maintaining, or exacerbating pain during this phase; therefore, psychiatric and/or psychological involvement may not be necessary, or at most, would likely be minimal. Focused, short-term psychopharmacologic and psychotherapeutic efforts may be necessary to address mood disturbances, adjustment disorders, maladaptive coping, etc., until the pain is alleviated and the patient's condition improves. Recovery is the typical response for most patients.

For patients in whom pain persists, i.e., those entering subacute and subsequent chronic pain phases, however, psychological and social covariates start to play a more significant role in the overall pain experience [12]. The stress of unrelenting pain can unearth a variety of premorbid, semidormant characteristics and aspects of personality [13]. These factors, in turn, can influence one's construal of the pain. It is not uncommon for patients to become preoccupied with pain and perceived disability. Protracted pain can affect mood, thought patterns, perceptions, coping abilities, and personality. Psychological vulnerabilities may develop into psychiatric disorders. Regular activities and interests may be avoided due to fear of increasing pain or furthering injury. Social and interpersonal relationships may be profoundly affected. For example, restriction in the types of work activity and job loss, the resultant restrictions in income, financial hardships imposed by medical treatment, and changes in role responsibilities and support needs within the home can cumulatively adversely affect the patient and contribute to strained relationships. The patient may experience impatience with treatment measures, intolerance for adverse effects, and lack of follow through with rehabilitative efforts. Beset with multiple psychosocial stressors and sequelae, the needs of the chronic pain patient can overwhelm the solo practitioner. The psychologist and/or psychiatrist may be enlisted, working with practitioners in other disciplines to develop coordinated efforts to help the patient manage pain and improve adaptive function.

Components of the biopsychosocial model

The psychological components of pain can be subcategorized into those that reflect underlying pathological states, as well as subsyndromal cognitive and emotional factors augmenting the distress and discomfort of patients with enduring pain. Chronic pain is not a unitary condition, rarely presenting alone; any focus on somatic concerns should prompt the clinician to consider psychiatric co-morbidities in which pain or other related somatic concerns might be a feature or focus and which warrant medical attention [14]. Physicians and medical personnel enlisted to care for the patient with chronic pain will have to consider an extensive psychiatric differential diagnosis, discussed in Chapter 6.

Subsyndromal cognitive variables are of particular importance in understanding psychological covariates of pain, including one's belief systems and cognitive appraisals. The beliefs held by the patient about the meaning of the pain, expectations about future pain, and interpretation of the impact the pain has on his or her life, functioning, and relationships are relevant to understanding the cognitive components of pain. Cognitive appraisal of pain depends on the individual's perspective on the consequences of pain for his or her well-being, the importance he or she assigns to the pain, and his or her view of the measures available to cope with the pain and its ramifications.

Specifically, negative pain-related cognitions, e.g., catastrophizing, helplessness, and lack of perceived control over pain and related stressors, are robust predictors of pain and disability, and significantly impede one's adaptation in the face of chronic painful conditions [15, 16]. In fact, such cognitions can feed and even serve as ineffective coping strategies, which may have adverse influences exceeding those of other variables, e.g., biomechanical deformities and pathophysiological disease status [17–20]. Catastrophizing, i.e., the tendency to exaggerate the perceived threat associated with pain and to negatively evaluate one's ability to deal with it [21], for example, has been associated with higher rates of self-reported pain and increased levels of perceived pain-related disability [22]. In addition, individuals prone to catastrophizing demonstrate higher rates of analgesic usage as well as greater healthcare utilization [23, 24].

Cognitive processes and emotional states have a reciprocal relationship. Thus, negative cognitive approaches, e.g., catastrophizing, helplessness, are likely to reduce self-efficacy, hamper development of effective coping, drain one's support systems, accentuate unpleasant emotional states (e.g., anger, anxiety, and depression), and exacerbate pain. For example, using a daily diary methodology to assess the relationship between pain and depression, it was observed that depression severity on a given day predicted the subsequent day's pain rating [25]. Further, research has shown that difficulties in identification, management and expression of unpleasant affective states have been linked with pain and associated pain-related distress [26].

Identification of problematic emotions and cognitive patterns should signal a need for inquiry into the coping strategies used by the individual to self-soothe, reduce distress, and modulate unpleasant states. An extensive body of literature has demonstrated a relationship between coping and adjustment among persons with chronic pain [27, 28]. Coping with a chronic illness requires the individual to adopt new strategies for coping with pain and other unpleasant symptoms. To do so effectively, patients need to believe that they possess the repertoire of skills necessary and develop confidence in their ability to efficaciously implement those strategies. Evidence suggests that patients invoking active coping strategies, i.e., activity, exercise, distraction, and other measures whereby one takes control over one's pain management, experience improved adjustment, functioning, and less depression and disability than individuals relying on passive coping strategies, i.e., maladaptive strategies to abdicate responsibility for pain management such as resting, reliance on analgesic use, deferring to physicians [28].

Relatively little has been unveiled about the social/interpersonal underpinnings of chronic pain syndromes. It is pertinent to consider the significant persons in the patient's life, how the pain has influenced relationships with those persons, how the patient's pain influences the behaviors of others, and the extent to which one's adaptation in the context of pain may be shaped or reinforced by the responses of others in one's life [29]. For example, solicitousness on the part of a spouse or significant other toward the patient with chronic pain has been linked with heightened pain intensity, frequency of overt pain behaviors as well as perceived disability and reported life interference from pain [30–32]. The basis for such influences is likely rooted in social contingencies, e.g., positive attention from one's family member. At the same time, the experience of chronic pain may have a profound negative impact on marital and familial relationships, e.g., affecting perceived marital satisfaction, intimacy, and financial stability, among other factors [1].

Another social factor impacting the experience of chronic pain and resultant disability is interpersonal distress. High levels of interpersonal distress, whereby pain-afflicted individuals perceive significant others in their lives to be essentially non-supportive, has been linked with perceived pain severity and disability [33–35]. Individuals with irritable bowel syndrome (IBS), for example, have been shown to display difficulties with non-assertiveness and social inhibition [36]. It appears intuitive that pain-afflicted individuals who perceive others in their lives as unsupportive and those who are unable to make their needs known to others are likely to experience difficulties in the appropriate discharge of emotional distress and in soliciting needed support when their repertoire of coping skills wane.

Empirical endeavors into the reciprocal relationships between social factors and pain, i.e., contributing to pain and/or affected by pain, have been fraught with issues common to much of the research on factors influencing the pain experience. The existing studies are often cross-sectional and correlational in nature thereby limiting the ability to make inferences regarding causal relationships. In addition, other factors, e.g., patient gender, selection bias of samples assessed, types of instrumentation and assessment measures utilized to ascertain social components of pain, can influence the outcomes of such investigations [33, 37]. Despite the potential limitations, greater empirical attention to the variety of biopsychosocial derivatives impacting upon the experience of the chronic pain patient is needed.

Neuromatrix theory and the biopsychosocial model

Advances in the neuroscience of pain processing have provided support for the role of higher brain centers, i.e., those responsible for emotion and cognition, in influencing pain transmission from the periphery [38]. Rather than construing the spinal cord (dorsal horns) and brain as passive recipients of pain information from the periphery, the neuromatrix model of pain acknowledges that the brain is dynamically involved in the processing (inhibition, modulation, or excitation) of pain. This is thought to involve the sensory, thalamic, limbic, hypothalamic-pituitary axis, and cortical pathways [38, 39].

Stress (both physical and psychological) triggers mechanisms attempting to restore homeostasis. When stress persists, e.g., in the form of ongoing pain, psychological distress, inadequate coping with environmental stressors, persisting depression, multiple processes are set in motion that exceed the delicately balanced regulatory homeostatic mechanisms initially intended to effectively manage stress, and instead generate destructive processes perpetuating pain. Several lines of research have pointed to plausible mechanisms underlying the reciprocal relationships between pain, affective distress, and stress: (1) the amygdala (a limbic structure) acts as the interface between pain and emotional states; chronic negative affective states can influence the amygdala to enhance the response to pain [40]; (2) exposure to stress can heighten cytokine reactivity, i.e., inflammatory processes, and heighten cortisol secretion, leading to destructive processes (immune dysregulation, bone demineralization and muscle atrophy), enhancing the propensity toward pain, increasing pain sensitivity and predisposing one toward depression; (3) stress and pain can alter the mechanisms by which the brain functions in its own maintenance [41, 42]. Presumably through heightened glucocorticoid activity, stress and pain can alter the expression of neurotrophic factors, e.g., brain derived neurotrophic factor (BDNF), reducing dendritic branching within hippocampal structures and predisposing one toward depression. Down-regulation of BDNF is preventable with antidepressant medication and, in the course of depression treatment, antidepressants can restore normal serum BDNF levels [43]. Together, these lines of evidence begin to delineate the complex interactions of central nervous system (CNS) mechanisms involved in pain and emotional processing, stress regulation, and cognitive processes. In the composite, such evidence, and related emerging research, lend support for theoretical conceptualizations, such as that of the biopsychosocial approach, that intuitively reflect the challenges faced when dealing with patients with unrelenting pain.

Treatment approaches

The biopsychosocial approach to pain challenges clinicians to think about integrated care. In the biopsychosocial perspective, stratified care is suggested, whereby psychiatric and psychological care is introduced earlier in the course of treatment, to address psychiatric co-morbidities and subsyndromal psychological states, thereby mitigating those factors that can contribute to, maintain, and exacerbate later stages of pain. Given the inherent complexities involved in the pain experience, it is essential that one keep in mind that the goals of treatment include the provision of

pain relief, maximizing one's functioning and quality of life while at the same time keeping to a minimum risks of iatrogenic harm. The issues discussed herein will focus on the utility of psychotherapeutic and psychopharmacological approaches in pain management strategies.

Education approaches

Comprehensive treatment approaches for pain management often include an emphasis on patient education. Patient education programs consist of planned activities/curricula that serve to enhance patient awareness about their illness, and the utility of measures such as pharmacological and surgical approaches, and exercise. Information may be provided in several didactic sessions, or in a home-based self-instructional format. Employed in a number of chronic pain conditions, e.g., osteoarthritis, rheumatoid arthritis, fibromyalgia, acute and chronic back pain, such programs are designed to impart information, foster treatment adherence, and empower patients with problem-solving skills and maintenance of self-care activities without incurring additional injury so as to encourage patients to become proactive in their care [44–46]. The goals of educational programs are summarized in Table 16.1.

Taken in the composite, meta-analyses of the effectiveness of educational programs in a number of pain conditions indicate that educational approaches promote knowledge, but are limited with regard to reducing pain or functional disability [47–51]. For example, in a meta-analysis of randomized controlled trials assessing the effectiveness of patient education interventions among patients with rheumatoid arthritis, small but positive effects on physical functioning (disability, number of painful joints) and psychological status (depression and anxiety severity) were demonstrated immediately post-intervention [52]; however, the influence on pain was not found to be significant. Similarly, educational programs for low back pain patients fostered knowledge and led to improvements in posture and back movement but did not appear to influence pain intensity or functional status [51].

Furthermore, the positive effects of patient education programs were not sustained. As regards to educational programs for recurrent back pain, a meta-analysis of randomized controlled trials suggests that these programs produce only short-term influences [51–53].

Table 16.1 Goals of educational programs employed in chronic pain conditions

Educate patients about their underlying condition, etiologies, and longitudinal course

Educate patients about psychiatric co-morbidities, e.g., depression

Discuss the possibilities that exist within the realm of pharmacological and non-pharmacologic treatment approaches

Establish realistic expectations about "cure" vs. recovery/recovery of function

Encourage patients to participate in their own illness management

Provision of information regarding flexibility and strengthening exercises

Educate patients about self-management techniques that can be utilized in dealing with pain and depression, e.g., pain control techniques, relaxation techniques, guided imagery, among other strategies[a]

[a] Techniques used in psycho-educational interventions.

Several reasons have been offered as to why education programs produce disappointing results, i.e., fail to produce significant effects on pain or sustained improvements in other physical and psychological parameters. First, the provision of disease information does not naturally generalize to the development and refinement of disease management skills and behavioral strategies with which to cope with the disease. Among patients with arthritis and back pain, studies invoking combinations of treatment approaches, e.g., cognitive-behavioral arthritis education programs that incorporated didactic instruction with coping strategies training, stress management and reinforcement of health promoting behaviors, produced significant positive effects for physical and psychological outcome measures, whereas purely didactic (information-only) programs failed to do so [54, 55]. In addition, when educational programs for back pain are linked with the workplace, i.e., specific occupational requirements, moderate effects are observed in subjective (e.g., perceived pain and functional status) and objective criteria (e.g., return to work latencies) [53].

Second, the utility of educational programs may vary with the natural course, i.e., duration and extensiveness, of underlying disease. Thus, questions arise as to whether physical and/or psychological improvements may depend on intervening with patients early in the course of illness rather than later when patients have become entrenched with chronic disease [49, 52].

Lastly, compliance with principles taught in educational interventions appear to wane over time [56]. As a result, a greater emphasis in recent years has been devoted to recognition of patient preparedness for change and motivation-enhancing strategies to employ with chronic pain patients [57]. Those patients adhering to a biomedical orientation to pain are less inclined to accept self-management approaches to pain whereas those perceiving only limited attainable assistance from medical interventions are more inclined to pursue self-management approaches. To optimize outcomes of educational interventions, such programs will need to be tailored to the individual patient's readiness to change and address psychiatric co-morbidities and psychological covariates that may be undermining the goals of educational endeavors.

Psychotherapeutic modalities

The aim of various psychotherapeutic approaches is to modify the behavior, cognitions, and physiological reactivity associated with pain [1]. Although a number of psychotherapeutic and adjunctive techniques can be employed to address the biological, psychological, and social features associated with and contributing to pain (see Table 16.2); these are not mutually exclusive interventions but complement each other to effectively address a particular patient's needs. The varied psychotherapies differ with regard to their approach, perspectives, and goals. The focus of the discussion that follows is on cognitive-behavioral therapy use in chronic nonmalignant pain, as empirical investigation into the utility of psychotherapeutic approaches in recent years has been principally dominated by application of this modality.

Cognitive-behavioral therapy: key components

Cognitive-behavioral therapy (CBT) is focused on modification of the thoughts, beliefs and expectations that play a key role in pain perception as well as one's ability to adjust to pain. The types of thoughts and appraisals one has regarding the pain experienced or of related stressors can predict one's sense of self-efficacy and perceived control over pain and choices of coping options with which to deal with the pain and associated stressors. The components of CBT include cognitive restructuring, coping skills training, and maintenance training with rehearsal of learned techniques [1, 15, 58].

Table 16.2 Psychotherapeutic modalities employed in pain management

Modality	Techniques	Uses
Operant	Use of contingencies to promote exercise quotas & self care, activity scheduling; pacing & graded activity; desensitization	Increase exercise & activity levels; overcome fear that activity will precipitate pain
Cognitive-behavioral	Collaborative process to identify cognitive appraisals & assess utility of coping strategies; cognitive restructuring & coping skills training[a]	Reduce depression and anxiety; reduce problematic cognitive styles; develop effective coping strategies
Interpersonal	Role-playing, analysis of communication patterns	Address role transitions due to pain, relationship difficulties & interpersonal conflicts
Self-regulatory therapies		
Biofeedback	Physiologic parameters are measured & fed back to patient to facilitate gaining mastery over them	Muscle relaxation, control of physiologic parameters contributing to pain
Guided imagery	Talking patient through pleasant scenarios to produce vivid, distracting and relaxing images	Relaxation, distraction from pain
Hypnosis	Focused attention and dissociation is directed at altering pain experiences	Reduce pain, relaxation, distraction
Progressive muscle relaxation	Systematic, sequential muscle tightening & subsequent relaxation	Muscle relaxation, distraction from pain

[a] Can include self-regulatory approaches.

Cognitive restructuring, an interactive process involving the Socratic method, is used to teach patients to identify maladaptive and distorted thoughts that may lead them to avoid activities and to experience negative feelings, such as depression, anxiety, and anger. Patients are encouraged to reappraise irrational and self-defeating thoughts and reframe them, replacing them with those that are more rational and objective. Coping skills training is aimed at assisting patients with developing a repertoire of skills for managing pain as well as problem-solving strategies that may be useful in a wide range of situations that induce pain. Using homework completed by the patient and issues discussed in sessions, the therapist assists the patient in identifying situations that are likely to tax coping abilities, assessing the utility of the existing strategies, developing alternatives when existing strategies fail to produce relief, and rehearsing newly developed coping strategies when those situations re-occur.

Previous investigations have supported the notion that cognitive misinterpretations, such as, catastrophizing and fear-avoidance (i.e., the tendency to avoid activity for fear of precipitating or exacerbating pain) are predictive of subsequent disability [22, 59–61]. Additionally, research indicates that patients' expectations regarding their treatment and their ability to work influence adherence to treatment [62] and return to work [63]. The modification of distorted cognitions and expectations as occurs in CBT may, therefore, help restore adaptive functioning and foster adherence with rehabilitation and other treatment measures.

Consistent with the neuromatrix theory, the presumption is that as a result of cognitive restructuring and coping skills training, patients will experience less physiological arousal and less intense pain. In a study employing positron emission tomography, improvement in symptoms following CBT treatment was found to correspond with changes in baseline limbic activity, i.e., in the amygdala and anterior cingulate cortex [64]. Although the sample size was small and solely consisted of patients with chronic IBS, the preliminary evidence gleaned from this investigation suggests that CBT may have a role in modification of brain circuitry in a manner that decreases painful symptoms, specifically by altering the activity of those brain areas mediating both pain perception and emotional self-regulation.

The effectiveness of CBT as a treatment for pain

Cognitive-behavioral therapy has been used as a treatment for a diverse array of chronic pain problems, having been applied to patients with headache [65, 66]; facial pain, e.g., temporomandibular disorders (TMD) [67–70]; arthritis, e.g., osteo- and rheumatoid arthritis [15, 71]; fibromyalgia [72]; and low back pain [73, 74]. Investigations of the effectiveness of CBT have been done both across and within various pain conditions. Across conditions, i.e., grouping different pain conditions together, CBT has been shown to significantly reduce pain severity and increase coping and social role functioning compared to wait-listed control conditions [75]. Further, after reviewing the evidence across a number of painful medical conditions, a National Institutes of Health (NIH) technology conference concluded that there was moderate evidence to support the use of CBT in reducing chronic pain [76]. Analysis of the efficacy of CBT within specific pain conditions, however, paints a more complex picture than general across-condition comparisons.

In some conditions, CBT has been shown to be an effective treatment. For example, meta-analyses have found a moderate and significant effect of CBT in reducing headache frequency, severity, and/or duration [66], and a greater percentage of headache index improvement among patients treated with CBT than wait-listed controls [65]. Among patients with arthritis, meta-analysis has demonstrated that CBT produced reductions in pain severity ratings and perceived disability, as compared with wait-list, usual treatment, or attention-placebo controls [71].

In other conditions, CBT is best described as a treatment that is probably effective. It is recommended as an empirically validated treatment for fibromyalgia [72], having been shown to reduce pain severity and improve function compared to wait-listed or other (e.g., education, discussion group) controls. Contradictory evidence and differences in sets of studies being compared, however, have led to disagreements among empirical reviews regarding the treatment value of CBT in fibromyalgia [58, 72]. Research investigating the efficacy of CBT in the treatment of pain and related symptoms of IBS has yielded mixed results. It has been shown to be superior to inactive, e.g., wait-listed, controls but it has not been shown to be consistently effective in IBS when compared to active, e.g., attention-placebo, controls [77]. Systematic review of randomized control trials of CBT as a treatment for non-specific/non-cardiac chest

pain found that CBT resulted in a modest to moderate short-term (up to 9 months) improvement relative to standard care, wait-listed, attention placebo, or no intervention controls [78].

Research has shown CBT to be potentially useful in the treatment of TMD and chronic low back pain. The extant body of work on TMD is small and has yet to be comprehensively reviewed or meta-analyzed but has generally yielded somewhat inconsistent support for the efficacy of CBT in relieving pain and related symptoms [67–70]. In the treatment of patients with low back pain, evidence stemming from meta-analyses and systematic reviews suggests that the utility of CBT is variable. It resulted in significantly lower back pain intensity but no difference in health-related quality of life compared to wait-listed controls [73]. In addition, controversy attends the effectiveness of CBT on pain-related variables when such treatment is compared to alternative active treatments for low back pain [73–75]. Further, the efficacy of CBT in chronic low back pain is dependent on the outcome variables assessed. The benefits of CBT found on self-report measures are not always seen when observational outcome measures are employed, e.g., vocational functioning [79, 80]. Thus, for these pain conditions, the existing evidence suggests the more conservative conclusion that CBT may be an effective treatment.

Empirical investigations of the efficacy of CBT in a variety of other chronic pain conditions are notably sparse. It has not been systematically studied as a treatment for interstitial cystitis, chronic pelvic pain, or neuropathy. Studies that have investigated the role of CBT or related psychotherapeutic approaches in these pain disorders [81–87] are too few and/or of insufficient methodological quality, hence preventing definitive conclusions from being drawn. It is important to point out that CBT has been recommended as a treatment of chronic pain conditions for which its efficacy has not been systematically studied, e.g., chronic pelvic pain [88] and neuropathic pain [89]. Of course, it is imperative to highlight that the dearth of empirical research does not constitute evidence of a lack of efficacy in these conditions.

In addition to the summary of efficacy in addressing pain severity outlined above, it should be pointed out that CBT has also been demonstrated to influence psychological functioning (e.g., reduced catastrophizing [90]), physical functioning, and leisure activity [79], and the ability of patients to cope and more effectively self-manage symptoms [28]. In the effort to address multiple components of the pain experience, it seems reasonable to invoke CBT as part of an integrated, collaborative, and multidisciplinary treatment of several chronic pain conditions.

Considerations when assessing the efficacy of CBT

One factor limiting the ability to evaluate and summarize empirical investigations of CBT effectiveness is that in many studies there is significant heterogeneity in the constituents of the components of CBT treatments employed. Investigations have often relied on multiple, concurrent therapies to reduce pain severity and improve quality of life; e.g., educational interventions as well as adjunctive self-regulatory techniques, e.g., relaxation training, guided imagery, biofeedback, are often incorporated into CBT trials. Unfortunately, employing such multimodal approaches renders it difficult to determine the independent or comparative effects of specific components of treatment.

Data on outcomes of CBT trials both across and within pain conditions has been particularly limited in areas such as medication utilization, healthcare utilization, return to work, and reduction in sick leave/absences [75, 91]. These outcome measures would be of particular interest to insurers, third party payers, and workers' compensation boards. In fact, one of the purported short-comings of CBT trials is the over-reliance on self-reported measures, e.g., assessments of coping, cognitive misattributions, rather than more objective, observational measurements conducted by blind assessors, e.g., frequencies of overt pain behaviors, number of absences from school or work related to pain, frequency or analgesic use or analgesic requirements [75].

In addition, questions arise regarding the effectiveness of CBT over time. Some studies have found that patients with different pain conditions continue to maintain improvements in outcome measures at various longer-term follow-up periods [68, 77, 92, 93]. In contrast, other studies have found that the treatment benefits of CBT deteriorate over time [71, 94, 95]. Thus, there is considerable variability in the retention of positive outcomes among CBT-treated patients over the course of chronic painful conditions.

There are several factors that can undermine the long-term effectiveness of CBT. First, disease progression in chronic debilitating conditions may contribute to reduction in the long-term outcome of interventions such as CBT. Second, the stage in the course of

illness when CBT was implemented may influence long-term effects. Intervening with patients early in the course of illness may yield greater benefits from CBT as compared with interventions directed at those individuals with late stage disease [71, 96]. In the latter patients, maladaptive patterns of thinking, coping, and behaviors exacerbating pain and disability may become entrenched and may render patients recalcitrant to psychotherapeutic intervention [97]. Third, patients may fail to complete homework assignments or fail to implement the strategies acquired during therapy, i.e., cognitive structuring and coping skills, at home when they are no longer in session [98]. Not surprisingly, research has supported the notion that those patients who frequently employ techniques cultivated in the CBT training are those with the best long-term outcomes [99]. It would seem plausible that the provision of booster sessions or maintenance treatment would enhance treatment effects longitudinally; however, there is research that suggests such maintenance attempts do not increase long-term treatment effectiveness [100]. Investigations have found that the effects of CBT training can be enhanced by including spouses/family members in the training [101–103], thereby increasing the likelihood that implementation of coping strategies will be encouraged at home.

Psychopharmacologic agents

An array of psychopharmacologic agents are available for use in a number of painful conditions [1], summarized in Table 16.3. Empirical investigations of the utility of these psychoactive agents as adjunctive agents in chronic non-malignant pain management have largely focused on antidepressants and anticonvulsants; the discussion below focuses on these two classes of medications.

Antidepressants

Over the years, the pain-mitigating effects of antidepressants have been a focus of intensive investigation. Several lines of evidence suggest that the neuromodulatory and analgesic properties of antidepressants appear to be independent of their influences on mood. For example, antidepressant-induced analgesia has been demonstrated among non-depressed pain patients. Additionally, among depressed pain patients, antidepressant analgesia occurs faster and at doses far lower than those required for antidepressant effects [104–106]. Thus, antidepressants may be appropriately

Table 16.3 Uses of psychoactive adjuvant medications for pain management

Class of medication	Uses in pain management
Antidepressants	Neuropathic pain; tension and migraine headache; FM, functional GI disorders, facial pain, chronic pelvic pain; co-morbid depression/anxiety
Anticonvulsants	Neuropathic pain; migraine headache; central pain; phantom limb pain
Benzodiazepines	Muscle relaxation; anxiety associated with acute pain and procedures/interventions; insomnia
Lithium	Cluster headache (CH) prophylaxis; not effective for episodic CH
Stimulants	Opiate analgesia augmentation; opiate-induced fatigue and sedation
NMDA antagonists	Opiate analgesia augmentation; neuropathic pain

FM: fibromyalgia; GI: gastrointestinal; CH: cluster headache; NMDA: N-methyl-D-aspartate receptor.

utilized for patients with selected chronic pain syndromes, regardless of whether or not the patient is depressed. However, this is not to imply that antidepressant uses for pain are a panacea, but rather, the usefulness of antidepressant pharmacotherapy may depend upon the type of pain conditions for which they are being invoked, the neuromodulatory properties of the particular antidepressant, and perhaps, the timing in the course of illness when the antidepressant is employed.

The effectiveness of antidepressants as a treatment for pain

Several meta-analyses and evidence-based reviews suggest that antidepressants are useful in mitigating pain associated with neuropathy [107, 108], headache [109], fibromyalgia [110, 111] and IBS [112, 113]. Interestingly, antidepressants are advocated for use in other chronic pain syndromes, e.g., rheumatologic pain conditions, chronic pelvic pain, interstitial cystitis, and oro-facial pain [114–116]. However, these assertions are not often based on a solid foundation of empirical work; in fact, in some of these conditions, e.g., chronic pelvic pain and interstitial cystitis, there are few randomized controlled trials with small sample sizes upon which such recommendations are based [115, 117–119].

Differences in the efficacy of antidepressants exist with respect to specific types of pain conditions. For example, antidepressants are robustly efficacious in treating neuropathic pain [108]. However, despite substantial evidence that tricyclic antidepressants (TCAs) are effective in mitigating pain associated with diabetic neuropathy and post-herpetic neuralgia, they appear to lack pain-mitigating effects in burning mouth syndrome and HIV-related neuropathies [108]. Similarly,

analyses of antidepressant efficacy in IBS reveal inconsistencies; whereas some suggest that TCAs are effective in mitigating chronic, severe abdominal pain [112, 113], others concluded that TCAs failed to demonstrate a significant analgesic benefit [120]. These inconsistencies may be due to variations in responsiveness of subsets of IBS patients, i.e., the utility of TCAs appeared to be best among those persons with diarrheal-type as opposed to those with constipation-type disorder [112, 113]. Lastly, although antidepressants were efficacious in alleviating several symptoms of fibromyalgia [111], the symptoms for which they are effective can vary. Fibromyalgia patients treated with antidepressants demonstrated moderate improvements in sleep, pain as well as assessments of overall well-being; however, effects were mild for fatigue and number of trigger points.

The types of painful conditions amenable to treatment with antidepressants suggest that there are unique elements that underlie their effectiveness. The pain-mitigating effects of antidepressants are thought to involve a number of neuromodulatory influences within the nervous system. Analgesia produced by antidepressants is thought to be primarily mediated by enhancing the inhibitory neurotransmitters (e.g., noradrenergic (NE) and serotonergic (5-HT) present within descending pain-mediating pathways extending down the spinal cord from axons emanating from the dorsolateral pontomesencephalic tegmentum and rostral ventromedial medulla [121, 122]. Additional analgesic effects of antidepressants may be mediated by: (1) reduction in the synthesis and release of pain-promoting neurotransmitters, e.g., glutamate in the spinal cord [123], (2) antagonism of N-methyl-D-aspartate (NMDA) receptor effects, (3) blockade of sodium channels with resultant diminution of painful afferent inputs from the peripheral and central nervous

Table 16.4 Classification of predominant neurotransmitter influences of antidepressants

Serotonergic	Noradrenergic	Dual mechanism
SSRIs	TCAs	SNRIs
Citalopram	Desipramine	Duloxetine
Escitalopram	Other	Venlafaxine [a]
Fluoxetine	Reboxetine [b]	Milnacipran [b]
Fluvoxamine		TCAs
Paroxetine		Amitriptyline
Sertraline		Imipramine
TCAs		Nortriptyline
Clomipramine		Other
		Mirtazapine

[a] Combined NE and 5-HT effects are dose dependent;
[b] Unavailable in the USA.
  SSRI: Selective serotonin re-uptake inhibitor.
  TCA: tricyclic antidepressant; SNRI: serotonin and norepinephrine inhibitor.

systems [124], (4) augmentation of opioid effects within the CNS [125, 126], and lastly (5) reduction of the extent of limbic output, which might otherwise contribute to depression and anxiety that exacerbate underlying pain.

Differences in antidepressant neuromodulatory effects and efficacy in pain treatment

Evidence gathered from clinical trials and meta-analyses suggests that antidepressants influencing both NE and 5-HT transmission exert analgesic effects that are greater than those antidepressants with more specific effects, e.g., influencing 5-HT re-uptake or NE re-uptake alone [127–132]. Thus, TCAs exerting both NE and 5-HT influences demonstrated robust reductions in neuropathic pain and headache burden as well as analgesic requirements [109]. Antidepressants commonly employed in pain management are presented in Table 16.4 according to their primary neuromodulatory effects.

The serotonin and norepinephrine re-uptake inhibitors (SNRIs), i.e., venlafaxine and duloxetine (milnacipran discussed below), have likewise demonstrated utility as analgesic agents. Both agents have been demonstrated to have pain-mitigating effects in randomized controlled trials of patients with neuropathy [133–135] and fibromyalgia [136, 137], with and without co-morbid depression. Duloxetine has received

Food and Drug Administration (FDA) approval for treatment of diabetic neuropathy. Simultaneous NE and 5-HT influences are achieved at low doses with duloxetine; doses as low as 20 mg/d may be sufficient [133]. Unlike duloxetine, the 5-HT effects are predominant at low doses for venlafaxine. To achieve pain mitigating effects, antidepressant level dosing may be required [137].

However, the pain-mitigating effects of selective serotonin re-uptake inhibitors (SSRIs) appear to be less certain; as a class the SSRIs have not been demonstrated to be as consistently analgesic as the TCAs or SNRIs [127, 138]. There is some question whether the reduced efficacy of the SSRIs as compared with TCAs and SNRIs is related to the 5-HT selectivity of the SSRIs. In one study, fluoxetine was less effective than amitriptyline and desipramine and fared no better than placebo [129]. Clinical trials assessing efficacy of SSRIs for addressing pain associated with neuropathy and fibromyalgia have yielded conflicting results [107, 127–130, 132, 138–142]; there is limited data suggesting that paroxetine and citalopram may be effective in alleviating symptoms of diabetic neuropathy [143, 144] and that fluoxetine is useful in fibromyalgia [140].

Efficacy of antidepressants as a function of duration of illness

The mechanisms by which the antidepressants, and TCAs in particular, produce analgesia invoke a number of CNS effects modulating the process by which acute pain becomes chronic. It has long been observed that failure to mitigate pain early in the course of illness may lead to the development of an enduring and refractory pain state, through the process of central sensitization. Central sensitization is a time-dependent physiological event, whereby repetitive pain signals from the periphery leads to activation of higher order (CNS) neurons. The sensitization of the higher order neurons continues, producing what is interpreted by the brain as pain, even when peripheral nociceptive input ceases or is reduced. It appears, therefore, that antidepressant use might be best invoked earlier, rather than later, in the course of a pain-inducing condition, so as to mitigate the potential of central sensitization from developing. Although not extensively investigated, there is evidence to suggest that the earlier antidepressants are introduced in an illness, the better the response to their analgesic effects. For example, when amitriptyline is initiated within 3 months of developing the rash of herpes zoster infection, patients are less likely to develop the complications of post-herpetic neuralgia [145]. Restriction of and delays in the efficacy of TCAs in producing analgesia would be expected if administered after significant peripheral and central pathophysiologic mechanisms have set in place. It is best to initiate treatment at low doses; gradual dose increases are possible approximately every 3–7 days. If pain relief is inadequate, optimization of doses should be undertaken unless side effects supervene.

Practical matters related to antidepressant selection in pain management

Unfortunately, the adverse effects of TCAs, e.g., anticholinergic and alpha-adrenergic influences, limit their utility in pain treatment. Amitriptyline and imipramine have more troublesome side effects than the secondary amine TCAs (e.g., nortriptyline and desipramine). Tricyclic antidepressants are contraindicated in some patients: those with closed-angle glaucoma, recent myocardial infarction, cardiac arrhythmias, poorly controlled seizures, or severe benign prostatic hypertrophy.

Both the SSRIs and SNRIs offer the advantages of greater tolerability of side effects and relative safety in overdose as compared with TCAs. Side effects associated with SSRI use include nausea, diarrhea, insomnia or sedation, tremors, and sexual dysfunction; their use has been associated with, and may potentially exacerbate, restless legs syndrome [146]. Adverse effects of SNRIs (venlafaxine and duloxetine) can include nausea, dry mouth, nervousness, constipation, and somnolence. Venlafaxine may be associated with weight loss and elevations in diastolic blood pressure. If TCAs are intolerable, however, these agents may prove to be workable alternatives for the patient.

Other antidepressants in pain management

Few double-blind, randomized controlled studies have suggested the utility of antidepressants other than those which have been previously mentioned in pain management. Sustained-release bupropion, an antidepressant with a broad spectrum of activity, including NE, 5-HT, and dopamine, was found to reduce pain severity ratings among 70% of patients with chronic neuropathic pain [147]. Mirtazapine reduced headache frequency, duration, and severity/intensity among patients with recurrent, chronic daily tension headache [148]. Although not currently marketed in the USA as an antidepressant, milnacipran (an SNRI) has been demonstrated to reduce

baseline pain severity ratings as well as improve global assessments of well-being, e.g., fatigue and functional capacity among treated fibromyalgia patients [149]. One double-blind trial comparing amitriptyline with trazodone demonstrated that both agents led to reduced pain ratings among patients with deafferentation pain; however, the effects of amitriptyline were appreciated sooner than those in the trazodone treated groups [150]. Although anticholinergic side effects were more problematic among patients treated with amitriptyline, more subjects withdrew from trazodone treatment due to unpleasant side effects. Given the limited number of randomized controlled trials and small sample sizes, definitive statements regarding the utility of these agents and the generalizability of results are not possible. Additional randomized controlled trials investigating the role of these antidepressants in chronic pain management appear to be warranted.

Anticonvulsant drugs

Anticonvulsant drugs (ACDs) have efficacy in mitigating neuropathic pain, including trigeminal neuralgia and phantom limb pain [151], as well as migraine [152, 153]. Carbamazepine is FDA approved for the treatment of trigeminal neuralgia; gabapentin, for treatment of post-herpetic neuralgia; pregabalin, for post-herpetic neuralgia and diabetic neuropathy and more recently, fibromyalgia [154]; and divalproex sodium and topiramate have both been indicated for migraine prophylaxis. As with the antidepressants, analgesic differences exist among the ACDs with regard to utility across types of pain conditions. Thus, it appears as though those ACDs most useful for neuropathic pain treatment are least effective in migraine prophylaxis, whereas those that are useful in migraine prophylaxis are less effective in mitigating neuropathy. Nonetheless, older studies suggested that valproate was efficacious in chronic neuropathic pain [155–157].

As noted previously, neuronal hyperexcitability predisposes patients to central sensitization and chronic pain. Although the neuromodulatory mechanisms underlying analgesia produced by ACDs are varied, the mechanisms of action are thought to influence several of the physiologic changes contributing to neural hyperexcitability. Thus, pregabalin and gabapentin are thought to influence central pro-neuropathic processes, i.e., glutamate release, through alterations of voltage-gated calcium channels [158–160]. By contrast, the mechanisms underlying the utility of carbamazepine, lamotrigine, and oxcarbazepine, are presumed to be related to inhibition of voltage-gated sodium channels, thereby slowing peripheral nerve conduction of primary afferent fibers and dampening the painful sensory information relayed to the CNS [152]. Divalproex sodium and topiramate act through modulation of sodium channel activity and may increase inhibitory gamma–aminobutyric acid (GABA) mechanisms thereby inhibiting pain processes within the CNS.

Emerging evidence suggests the potential analgesic roles of newer ACDs, e.g., lamotrigine, oxcarbazepine, and tiagabine [152, 155, 161, 162]. Although these agents demonstrate some promise with regard to mitigating neuropathic states [163–165], their utility and safety among pain patients requires further investigation. They may offer better tolerability over other ACDs (e.g., carbamazepine) and may be useful for patients with intractable pain or pain that is poorly responsive to other agents.

Some data suggest that ACDs, i.e., pregabalin and gabapentin, may have a pre–emptive analgesic role [166]. Therefore, treatment efficacy may be best if initiated early in the course of illness.

Adverse effects common to ACDs include sedation, fatigue, gastrointestinal and motor side effects (tremor, ataxia, and nystagmus). Rash and Stevens-Johnson syndrome are possible with carbamazepine and lamotrogine [152]. Patients taking gabapentin or pregabalin do not require serum drug, hematologic, electrolyte, or hepatic enzyme monitoring as is often required with other ACDs, e.g., carbamazepine or divalproex sodium. Both agents are eliminated through renal excretion; dose reductions are required in patients with impaired renal function. Sedative effects can be accentuated when combined with alcohol, benzodiazepines, or barbiturates. Carbamazepine, oxcarbazepine, phenytoin, and topiramate can reduce the efficacy of oral contraceptives, increasing the risk of pregnancy. Fetal malformations are associated with carbamazepine, valproate, and phenytoin use during pregnancy [167].

Considering treatment options: anticonvulsant vs. antidepressants

Given that both antidepressants and ACDs have demonstrated efficacy in a number of chronic pain conditions, e.g., migraine headache and neuropathic pain, it is important to consider when to invoke either or both classes of agents in the treatment of patients with pain. The effectiveness of ACDs and anticonvulsants appear to be comparable. In a review of randomized controlled trials in which TCAs and anticonvulsants were employed to treat pain associated with diabetic and post-herpetic neuropathies, it was found that one-third of patients achieved at least 50% pain relief with either antidepressants or anticonvulsants [107, 138, 141]. However, adverse effects were slightly more common with antidepressant use, particularly TCAs, as compared with anticonvulsants [107, 141].

Considerations of medication selection include tolerability of side effects and safety of use of particular medications in the context of the patient's co-morbid medical and psychiatric conditions [168]. For the neuropathic pain patient or migraneur with co-morbid depression and/or anxiety, selection of an antidepressant might be most prudent. In addition, antidepressants might be a consideration when there is a desire to simultaneously address sleep and appetite disturbances accompanying painful conditions. On the other hand, ACDs have mood-stabilizing effects and may be ideal for patients with bipolar disorder, schizoaffective disorder, and impulsivity arising from dementia [169, 170]. Thus, patients with mood disturbances, impulsivity, and unpredictable aggression along with coexistent chronic pain may be ideal candidates for ACD selection.

Selection of ACDs or antidepressants for pain requires careful consideration of the risks and benefits for any given patient, e.g., the presence of certain medical co-morbidities may preclude the use of selective agents. Heart block, arrhythmias or severe cardiac disease prohibit use of TCAs. In the event of renal dysfunction, doses of venlafaxine, carbamazepine, oxcarbazepine, gabapentin, pregabalin and topiramate would need to reduced, and if severe enough, may preclude use of these agents. For patients with hepatic disease, doses of carbamazepine, oxcarbazepine and lamotrigine should be reduced. Tricyclic antidepressants can conceivably exacerbate encephalopathy associated with hepatic disease.

Because of the differences in presumed mechanisms of action between ACDs and antidepressants, it is plausible that ACDs would be viable alternatives for patients with persisting pain despite optimal antidepressant use or for whom antidepressant use proved intolerable. Alternatively, simultaneous administration of antidepressants and ACDs may be employed, capitalizing on complimentary mechanisms of action. When co-administered, lower doses of either or both agents may be sufficiently analgesic, perhaps making it possible to avoid doses that produce adverse effects.

Integrated psychopharmacologic and psychotherapeutic treatment: the lack of evidence-based research

It appears that optimal treatment of chronic pain, and efforts to optimize functioning, will require multi-modal treatment approaches involving psychiatric and psychological consultation and collaborative treatment. In the literature reviewed here, very few trials attempted to assess the differential benefits of, as well as the potential interactive effects of, combined pharmacological and psychological treatment interventions. In many cases, interventions assessing psychological therapies attempted to control for the influences of pharmacologic co-interventions, e.g., restricting or maintaining stable drug regimes during clinical trials. Direct comparisons of antidepressants vs. CBT (or other psychotherapy modalities) were seldom conducted to compare their relative effectiveness in improving pain or mood complicating chronic pain conditions. In one meta-analysis, CBT was found to be more effective than pharmacotherapy with antidepressants in patients with fibromyalgia [171]. One study found that CBT alone was not more effective than the combination of CBT with cyclobenzaprine, i.e., an antispasmodic with a tricyclic-like chemical structure, in reducing fibromyalgia severity symptoms; however, the number of tender points was significantly reduced at post-treatment only when the combination of CBT and pharmacologic treatment was employed [172]. In another study, CBT treatment did not add to the therapeutic effectiveness of antidepressant therapy in the treatment of depression associated with rheumatoid arthritis [173]. The extensive literature reviewed in this chapter suggests that both psychological and psychopharmacological treatment interventions have a significant role to play in the management of a diverse array of chronic pain conditions. Thus, it appears that future endeavors should be devoted to ascertaining the efficacy, utility, and potential improvements derived from combination treatments (both pharmacologic and psychotherapeutic) and determining if the yield is greater than with either treatment approach alone.

Problems with existing clinical research in pain

A number of important issues arise when evaluating clinical investigations of psychopharmacologic and psychotherapeutic treatment modalities in pain. First, although meta-analyses and evidence-based reviews provide the clearest comprehensive picture of the efficacy of a particular treatment, differences in study inclusion criteria for a particular analysis and differences in outcome variables of interest can lead to divergent conclusions between analyses of the same body of work. For example, as previously noted, there is a lack of agreement among meta-analyses and/or evidence-based reviews of the effectiveness of CBT in fibromyalgia as well as the utility of antidepressants in IBS. Consequently, despite an ample empirical research base, consensus regarding the value of a particular treatment sometimes remains elusive.

Second, it is essential to critically evaluate the meaningfulness of the comparisons being made in such studies. Generally, comparisons in clinical trials are undertaken between treated and control subjects (or comparisons of two different treatment conditions); efficacy is often based upon demonstration of a statistically significant difference between comparator groups. Statistical significance, however, can be contingent on several factors, i.e., reflecting not only the magnitude of the treatment effect but the variability within comparison groups in terms of the dependent measures and the sample size. It is conceivable therefore that demonstration of a statistically significant difference between treatment and comparator conditions may nonetheless fail to be clinically meaningful. For example, investigations with mean differences between comparator groups may be sufficiently powerful for the results to reach statistical significance, yet the impact of such changes for individual subjects may be negligible. Even trials with large group differences may be misleading. Significant group differences may be attributable to a few individuals within the active treatment group who demonstrate significant improvements, whereas many other patients within the treatment group may demonstrate little improvement or even worsening in the outcome measure. Thus, the average outcome differences between groups may bear little relationship to clinically relevant improvement for many persons with pain. As a result, efforts have been directed at identifying clinically significant outcome parameters for assessments of treatment efficacy in chronic pain trials [174].

Third, it is fallacious to assume that any treatment, because of its demonstrated utility in addressing pain in some conditions, would therefore be equally useful in other chronic pain conditions. It is intuitive that there would be marked heterogeneity among patients with differing chronic pain conditions, e.g., the psychological, social, and biological covariates of the patient with chronic pelvic pain are likely to differ from those of the patient with neuropathy or back pain. Thus, investigations that delineate the extent to which certain aspects of psychotherapeutic and/or psychopharmacological treatment are better suited for patients with one particular type of chronic pain condition vs. another are particularly valuable.

A final issue, related to the latter two, is that it may be pointless to attempt to assess the effectiveness of any specific psychological or psychopharmacological approach in the abstract. There is likely to be a substantial amount of inter-individual variability in responsiveness to any treatment. For example, evidence suggests that patients with similar conditions and ostensibly similar degrees of impairment respond differentially to the same treatment [175]. It is not, therefore, physical condition alone that determines responsiveness to an intervention but the psychosocial covariates of subgroups of patients with the same condition that are also likely to predict responsiveness to a treatment [175]. Thus, even among individuals with comparable disease, distinct identifiable subgroups of patients corresponding to differences in psychological profiles and biological response to pain are determinable [176–178]. Such observations suggest that treatment interventions may be differentially effective in individual patients. The key challenge may be one of customizing psychological and psychopharmacological treatment approaches to a patient's unique needs and circumstances [179]. In fact, consistent with the biopsychosocial approach, it is expected that some chronic pain patients are reasonably well adjusted whereas others manifest higher levels of distress (i.e., cognitive and behavioral dysfunction), and still others may be beset with significant and disabling psychiatric co-morbidities. Accordingly, generic application of any treatment approach may be relevant to some patients but ineffective for others [175, 178].

Taken together, the issues raised above highlight the importance of considering individual differences in the treatment of patients with chronic pain. Variations in personality traits, psychosocial profiles, psychiatric status, emotional and cognitive functioning, coping capabilities, and patients' preparedness for implementing changes necessitate pain treatments that are tailored to the individual [57, 178, 180]. Each of these components must be considered to arrive at a treatment designed to reduce pain and foster rehabilitative efforts necessary to optimize functioning despite pain. Ideally, selection of treatment should be supported by research evidence, clinical experience, and an ongoing assessment of efficacy and tolerability of treatment efforts.

Summary

Effective management of chronic non-malignant pain necessitates the consideration of biological as well as psychological and social covariates that influence the experience and manifestation of such chronic conditions. Evolving research in neuroscience continues to reveal the physiological substrates for interactions among these factors. Rather than relegating psychiatric and psychological interventions to treatments of last resort, it appears that such interventions may be warranted sooner rather than later and may help to mitigate the CNS processes that may beget persisting and disabling chronic pain states. A multi-modal approach, i.e., employing psychotherapeutic and psychopharmacologic treatments, may therefore be necessary to address the complex interactions among the covariates accompanying pain conditions. Although advances have been made in developing effective treatments, further investigation is required to determine under what circumstances and for whom such interventions prove effective.

References

1. Leo RJ. *Clinical Manual of Pain Management in Psychiatry* (Washington, DC: American Psychiatric Publishing, Incorporated, 2007).

2. American Psychiatric Association. *Diagnostic and Statistical Manual of Mental Disorders,* 3rd edn. (Washington, DC: American Psychiatric Association, 1980).

3. American Psychiatric Association. *Diagnostic and Statistical Manual of Mental Disorders,* 3rd edn, revised. (Washington, DC: American Psychiatric Association, 1987).

4. American Psychiatric Association. *Diagnostic and Statistical Manual of Mental Disorders,* 4th edn. (Washington, DC: American Psychiatric Association, 1994).

5. American Psychiatric Association. *Diagnostic and Statistical Manual of Mental Disorders,* 4th edn. *Text* Revision. (Washington, DC: American Psychiatric Association, 2000).

6. Sullivan MD. DSM - IV pain disorder: a case against the diagnosis. *Int Rev Psychiatry* 2000; **12**: 91–8.

7. Mayou R, Levenson J, Sharpe M. Somatoform disorders in DSM-V. *Psychosomatics* 2003; **44**: 449–51.

8. Gatchel RJ. A biopsychosocial overview of pretreatment screening of patients with pain. *Clin J Pain* 2001; **17**: 192–9.

9. Engel GL. The clinical application of the biopsychosocial model. *Am J Psychiatry* 1980; **137**: 535–44.

10. Gallagher RM. Treatment planning in pain medicine – integrating medical, physical, and behavioral therapies. *Med Clin North Am* 1999; **83**: 823–49.

11. Gatchel RJ. Early development of physical and mental deconditioning in painful spinal disorders. In *Contemporary Conservative Care For Painful Spinal Disorders*, eds. TG Mayer, V Mooney, RJ Gatchel. (Philadelphia: Lea Febiger, 1991).

12. Banks SM, Kerns RD. Explaining high rates of depression in chronic pain: a diathesis-stress framework. *Psychol Bull* 1996; **119**: 95–110.

13. Dersh J, Polatin PB, Gatchel RJ. Chronic pain and psychopathology: research findings and theoretical considerations. *Psychosom Med* 2002; **64**: 773–86.

14. Fishbain DA. Approaches to treatment decisions for psychiatric comorbidity in the management of the chronic pain patient. *Med Clin North Am* 1999; **83**: 737–60.

15. Keefe FJ, Abernethy AP, Campbell LC. Psychological approaches to understanding and treating disease-related pain. *Annu Rev Psychol* 2005; **56**: 601–30.

16. Sullivan MJ, Thorn B, Haythornthwaite JA, *et al.* Theoretical perspectives on the relation between catastrophizing and pain. *Clin J Pain* 2001; **17**: 52–64.

17. Hagglund KJ, Haley WE, Reveille JD, Alarcon GS. Predicting individual differences in pain and functional impairment among patients with rheumatoid arthritis. *Arthritis Rheum* 1989; **32**: 851–8.

18. Parker J, Frank R, Beck N, *et al.* Pain in rheumatoid arthritis: relationship to demographic, medical, and psychological factors. *J Rheumatol* 1988; **15**: 433–7.

19. Vlaeyen JWS. *Chronic Low Back Pain: Assessment and treatment from a behavioral rehabilitation perspective* (Amsterdam: Swets and Zeitlinger, 1991).

20. Young LD. Psychological factors in rheumatoid arthritis. *J Consult Clin Psychol* 1992; **60**: 619–27.

21. Rosenstiel AK, Keefe FJ. The use of coping strategies in chronic low back pain patients: relationship to patient characteristics and current adjustment. *Pain* 1983; **17**: 33–44.

22. Sullivan MJ, Stanish W, Waite H, Sullivan M, Tripp DA. Catastrophizing, pain, and disability in patients with soft-tissue injuries. *Pain* 1998; **77**: 253–60.

23. Gil KM, Thompson RJ, Jr, Keith BR, *et al.* Sickle cell disease pain in children and adolescents: change in pain frequency and coping strategies over time. *J Pediatr Psychol* 1993; **18**: 621–37.

24. Jacobsen PB, Butler RW. Relations of cognitive coping and catastrophizing to acute pain and analgesic use following breast cancer surgery. *J Behav Med* 1996; **19**: 17–29.

25. Affleck G, Tennen H, Urrows S, Higgins P. Neuroticism and the pain-mood relation in rheumatoid arthritis: insights from a prospective daily study. *J Consult Clin Psychol* 1992; **60**: 119–26.

26. Keefe FJ, Lumley M, Anderson T, *et al.* Pain and emotion: new research directions. *J Clin Psychol* 2001; **57**: 587–607.

27. Boothby JL, Thorn BE, Stroud MW, Jensen MP. Coping with pain. In *Psychosocial Factors in Pain*, eds. RJ Gatchel, DC Turk. (New York: Guilford Press; 1999), pp. 343–59.

28. Jensen MP, Turner JA, Romano JM, Karoly P. Coping with chronic pain: a critical review of the literature. *Pain* 1991; **47**: 249–83.

29. Turk DC, Okifuji A. Psychological factors in chronic pain: evolution and revolution. *J Consult Clin Psychol* 2002; **70**: 678–90.

30. Flor H, Kerns RD, Turk DC. The role of spouse reinforcement, perceived pain, and activity levels of chronic pain patients. *J Psychosom Res* 1987; **31**: 251–9.

31. Kerns RD, Haythornthwaite J, Southwick S, Giller EL, Jr. The role of marital interaction in chronic pain and depressive symptom severity. *J Psychosom Res* 1990; **34**: 401–8.

32. Kerns RD, Southwick S, Giller EL, *et al.* The relationship between reports of pain-related social interactions and expressions of pain and affective distress. *Behav Ther* 1991; **22**: 101–11.

33. Romano JM, Schmaling KB. Assessment of couples and families with chronic pain. In *Handbook of Pain*

Assessment, eds. DC Turk and R Melzack. (New York: Guilford, 1992), pp. 346–61.

34. Turk DC, Okifuji A, Sinclair JD, Starz TW. Differential responses by psychosocial subgroups of fibromyalgia syndrome patients to an interdisciplinary treatment. *Arthritis Care Res* 1998; **11**: 397–404.

35. Turk DC, Rudy TE. The robustness of an empirically derived taxonomy of chronic pain patients. *Pain* 1990; **43**: 27–35.

36. Lackner JM, Gurtman MB. Patterns of interpersonal problems in irritable bowel syndrome patients: a circumplex analysis. *J Psychosom Res* 2005; **58**: 523–32.

37. Kerns RD. Family therapy for adults with chronic pain. In *psychosocial factors in pain – critical perspectives*, eds. RJ Gatchel, DC Turk. (New York: The Guilford Press, 1999), pp. 445–56.

38. Melzack R. From the gate to the neuromatrix. *Pain* 1999; **82**(Suppl): S121–S126.

39. Rome HP Jr, Rome JD. Limbically augmented pain syndrome (LAPS): kindling, corticolimbic sentization, and the convergence of affective and sensory symptoms in chronic pain disorders. *Pain Med* 2000; **1**: 7–23.

40. Neugebauer V, Li W, Bird GC, Han JS. The amygdala and persistent pain. *Neuroscientist* 2004; **10**: 221–34.

41. Duman RS, Monteggia LM. A neurotrophic model for stress-related mood disorders. *Biol Psychiatry* 2006; **59**: 1116–27.

42. Duric V, McCarson KE. Hippocampal neurokinin-1 receptor and brain-derived neurotrophic factor gene expression is decreased in rat models of pain and stress. *Neuroscience* 2005; **133**: 999–1006.

43. Gonul AS, Akdeniz F, Taneli F, *et al*. Effect of treatment on serum brain-derived neurotrophic factor levels in depressed patients. *Eur Arch Psychiatry Clin Neurosci* 2005; **255**: 381–6.

44. Brady TJ, Kruger J, Helmick CG, Callahan LF, Boutaugh ML. Intervention programs for arthritis and other rheumatic diseases. *Health Educ Behav* 2003; **30**: 44–63.

45. Hayne CR. Back schools and total back care programmes – a review. *Physiotherapy* 1984; **70**: 14–17.

46. Schenk RJ, Doran RL, Stachura JJ. Learning effects of a back education program. *Spine* 1996; **21**: 2183–9.

47. Barlow JH, Turner AP, Wright CC. A randomized controlled study of the Arthritis Self-Management Programme in the UK. *Health Educ Res* 2000; **15**: 665–80.

48. Hammond A. Joint protection behavior in patients with rheumatoid arthritis following an education program: a pilot study. *Arthritis Care Res* 1994; **7**: 5–9.

49. Hawley DJ. Psycho-educational interventions in the treatment of arthritis. *Baillieres Clin Rheumatol* 1995; **9**: 803–23.

50. Helliwell PS, O' Hara M, Holdsworth J, *et al*. A 12-month randomized controlled trial of patient education on radiographic changes and quality of life in early rheumatoid arthritis. *Rheumatology* 1999; **38**: 303–8.

51. Maier-Riehle B, Harter M. The effects of back schools – a meta-analysis. *Int J Rehab Res* 2001; **24**: 199–206.

52. Riemsma RP, Taal E, Kirwan JR, Rasker JJ. Systematic review of rheumatoid arthritis patient education. *Arthritis Rheum* 2004; **51**: 1045–59.

53. Heymans MW, van Tulder MW, Esmail R, Bombardier C, Koes BW. Back schools for nonspecific low back pain: a systematic review within the framework of the Cochrane Collaboration Back Review Group. *Spine* 2005; **30**: 2153–63.

54. Keefe FJ, Van Horn Y. Cognitive-behavioral treatment of rheumatoid arthritis pain: maintaining treatment gains. *Arthritis Care Res* 1993; **6**: 213–22.

55. Turner JA. Educational and behavioral interventions for back pain in primary care. *Spine* 1996; **21**: 2851–7.

56. Linton SJ, van Tulder MW. Preventive interventions for back and neck pain problems: what is the evidence? *Spine* 2001; **26**: 778–87.

57. Kerns RD, Rosenberg R, Jamison RN, Caudill MA, Haythornthwaite J. Readiness to adopt a self-management approach to chronic pain: the Pain Stages of Change Questionnaire (PSOCQ). *Pain* 1997; **72**: 227–34.

58. Bradley LA, McKendree-Smith NL, Cianfrini LR. Cognitive-behavioral therapy interventions for pain associated with chronic illnesses. *Semin Pain Med* 2003; **1**: 44–54.

59. Leeuw M, Goossens ME, Linton SJ, *et al*. The fear-avoidance model of musculoskeletal pain: current state of scientific evidence. *J Behav Med* 2007; **30**: 77–94.

60. Vlaeyen JW, Kole-Snijders AM, Boeren RG, van Eek H. Fear of movement/(re)injury in chronic low back pain and its relation to behavioral performance. *Pain* 1995; **62**: 363–72.

61. Vlaeyen JW, Linton SJ. Fear-avoidance and its consequences in chronic musculoskeletal pain: a state of the art. *Pain* 2000; **85**: 317–32.

62. Mondloch MV, Cole DC, Frank JW. Does how you do depend on how you think you'll do? A systematic review of the evidence for a relation between patients'

recovery expectations and health outcomes. *CMAJ* 2001; **165**: 174–79.

63. Cole DC, Mondloch MV, Hogg-Johnson S. Listening to injured workers: how recovery expectations predict outcomes – a prospective study. *CMAJ* 2002; **166**: 749–54.

64. Lackner JM, Coad ML, Mertz HR, *et al.* Cognitive therapy for irritable bowel syndrome is associated with reduced limbic activity, GI symptoms, and anxiety. *Behav Res Ther* 2006; **44**: 621–38.

65. Andrasik F. What does the evidence show? Efficacy of behavioural treatments for recurrent headaches in adults. *Neurol Sci* 2007; **28**(Suppl 2): 70–7.

66. Campbell JK, Penzien DB, Wall EM. Evidenced-based guidelines for migraine headache: behavioral and physical treatments. The US Headache Consortium. www.aan.com/professionals/practice/pdfs/gl0089.pdf. [Accessed May 2010].

67. Dworkin SF, Turner JA, Mancl, L, *et al.* A randomized clinical trial of a tailored comprehensive care treatment program for temporomandibular disorders. *J Orofac Pain* 2002; **16**: 259–76.

68. Dworkin SF, Turner JA, Wilson L, *et al.* Brief group cognitive-behavioral intervention for temporomandibular disorders. *Pain* 1994; **59**: 175–87.

69. Turner JA, Mancl L, Aaron LA. Brief cognitive-behavioral therapy for temporomandibular disorder pain: effects on daily electronic outcome and process measures. *Pain* 2005; **117**: 377–87.

70. Turner JA, Mancl L, Aaron LA. Short- and long-term efficacy of brief cognitive-behavioral therapy for patients with chronic temporomandibular disorder pain: a randomized, controlled trial. *Pain* 2006; **121**: 181–94.

71. Astin JA, Beckner W, Soeken K, Hochberg MC, Berman B. Psychological interventions for rheumatoid arthritis: A meta-analysis of randomized controlled trials. *Arthritis Rheum* 2002; **47**: 291–302.

72. Goldenberg DL, Burckhardt C, Crofford L. Management of fibromyalgia syndrome. *JAMA* 2004; **292**: 2388–95.

73. Hoffman BM, Papas RK, Chatkoff DK, Kerns RD. Meta-analysis of psychological interventions for chronic low back pain. *Health Psychol* 2007; **26**: 1–9.

74. Ostelo RW, van Tulder MW, Vlaeyen JW, et al. Behavioural treatment for chronic low-back pain. *Cochrane Database Syst Rev* 2005; (1): CD002014.

75. Morley S, Eccleston C, Williams A. Systematic review and meta-analysis of randomized controlled trials of cognitive behaviour therapy and behaviour therapy for chronic pain in adults, excluding headache. *Pain* 1999; **80**: 1–13.

76. NIH Technology Assessment Panel on Integration of Behavioral and Relaxation Approaches into the Treatment of Chronic Pain and Insomnia. Integration of behavioral and relaxation approaches into the treatment of chronic pain and insomnia. *JAMA* 1996; **276**: 313–8.

77. Blanchard EB. A critical review of cognitive, behavioral, and cognitive-behavioral therapies for irritable bowel syndrome. *J Cogn Psychother* 2005; **19**: 101–23.

78. Kisely S, Campbell LA, Skerritt P. Psychological interventions for symptomatic management of non-specific chest pain in patients with normal coronary anatomy. *Cochrane Database Syst Rev* 2005; (1): CD004101.

79. Alaranta H, Rytokoski U, Rissanen A, *et al.* Intensive physical and psychosocial training program for patients with chronic low back pain. A controlled clinical trial. *Spine* 1994; **19**: 1339–49.

80. Scheer SJ. Watanabe TK. Radack KL. Randomized controlled trials in industrial low back pain. Part 3. Subacute/chronic pain interventions. *Arch Phys Med Rehabil* 1997; **78**: 414–23.

81. Albert H. Psychosomatic group treatment helps women with chronic pelvic pain. *J Psychosom Obstet Gynaecol* 1999; **20**: 216–25.

82. Chaiken DC, Blaivas JG, Blaivas ST. Behavioral therapy for the treatment of refractory interstitial cystitis. *J Urol* 1993; **149**: 1445–8.

83. Ehde DM, Jensen MP. Feasibility of a cognitive restructuring intervention for treatment of chronic pain in persons with disabilities. *Rehabil Psychol* 2004; **49**: 254–8.

84. Evans S, Fishman B, Spielman L, Haley A. Randomized trial of cognitive behavior therapy versus supportive psychotherapy for HIV-related peripheral neuropathic pain. *Psychosomatics* 2003; **44**: 44–50.

85. Farquhar CM, Rogers V, Franks S, *et al.* A randomized controlled trial of medroxyprogesterone acetate and psychotherapy for the treatment of pelvic congestion. *Br J Obstet Gynaecol* 1989; **96**: 1153–62.

86. Norrbrink Budh C, Kowalski J, Lundeberg T. A comprehensive pain management programme comprising educational, cognitive and behavioral interventions for neuropathic pain following spinal cord injury. *J Rehabil Med* 2006; **38**: 172–80.

87. Webster DC, Brennan T. Use and effectiveness of psychological self-care strategies for interstitial cystitis. *Health Care Women Int* 1995; **16**: 463–75.

88. Jarrell JF, Vilos GA, Allaire C, *et al.* Consensus guidelines for the management of chronic pelvic pain. *J Obstet Gynaecol Can* 2005; **27**: 781–826.

89. Haythornthwaite JA, Benrud-Larson LM. Psychological assessment and treatment of patients with neuropathic pain. *Curr Pain Headache Rep* 2001; **5**: 124–9.

90. Smeets RJ, Vlaeyen JW, Kester AD, Knottnerus JA. Reduction of pain catastrophizing mediates the outcome of both physical and cognitive-behavioral treatment in chronic low back pain. *J Pain* 2006; **7**: 261–71.

91. Meijer EM, Sluiter JK, Frings-Dresen MH. Evaluation of effective return-to-work treatment programs for sick-listed patients with non-specific musculoskeletal complaints: a systematic review. *Int Arch Occup Environ Health* 2005; **78**: 523–32.

92. Thieme K, Flor H, Turk DC. Psychological pain treatment in fibromyalgia syndrome: efficacy of operant behavioural and cognitive behavioural treatments. *Arthritis Res Ther* 2006; **8**: R121.

93. Turner JA, Clancy S. Comparison of operant behavioral and cognitive-behavioral group treatment for chronic low back pain. *J Consult Clin Psychol* 1988; **56**: 261–6.

94. McCracken LM. Cognitive-behavioral treatment of rheumatoid arthritis: a preliminary review of efficacy and methodology. *Ann Behav Med* 1991; **13**: 57–65.

95. Redondo JR, Justo CM, Moraleda FV, *et al.* Long-term efficacy of therapy in patients with fibromyalgia: a physical exercise-based program and a cognitive-behavioral approach. *Arthritis Rheum* 2004; **51**: 184–92.

96. Gatchel RJ, Stowell AW, Wildenstein L, Riggs R, Ellis E. Efficacy of an early intervention for patients with acute temporomandibular disorder-related pain: a one-year outcome study. *J Am Dent Assoc* 2006; **137**: 339–47.

97. Sinclair VG, Wallston KA. Predictors of improvement in a cognitive-behavioral intervention for women with rheumatoid arthritis. *Ann Behav Med* 2001; **23**: 291–7.

98. Parker JC, Frank R, Beck N, *et al.* Pain management in rheumatoid arthritis: a cognitive-behavioral approach. *Arthritis Rheum* 1988; **31**: 593–601.

99. Parker JC, Smarr KL, Buescher KL, *et al.* Pain control and rational thinking: implications for rheumatoid arthritis. *Arhritis Rheum* 1989; **32**: 984–90.

100. Carson JW, Keefe FJ, Affleck G, *et al.* A comparison of conventional pain coping skills training and pain coping skills training with a maintenance training component: a daily diary analysis of short- and long-term treatment effects. *J Pain* 2006; **7**: 615–25.

101. Keefe FJ, Caldwell DS, Baucom D, *et al.* Spouse-assisted coping skills training in the management of knee pain in osteoarthritis: long-term followup results. *Arthritis Care Res* 1999; **12**: 101–11.

102. Keefe FJ, Caldwell DS, Baucom D, *et al.* Spouse-assisted coping skills training in the management of osteoarthritic knee pain. *Arthritis Care Res* 1996; **9**: 279–91.

103. Radojevic V, Nicassio PM, Weisman MH. Behavioral intervention with and without family support for rheumatoid arthritis. *Behav Ther* 1992; **23**: 13–30.

104. Ansari A. The efficacy of newer antidepressants in the treatment of chronic pain: a review of current literature. *Harv Rev Psychiatry* 2000; **7**: 257–77.

105. Egbunike IG, Chaffee BJ. Antidepressants in the management of chronic pain syndromes. *Pharmacotherapy* 1990; **10**: 262–70.

106. Fishbain DA. Evidence-based data on pain relief with antidepressants. *Ann Med* 2000; **32**: 305–16.

107. Collins SL, Moore RA, McQuay HJ, Wiffen P. Antidepressants and anticonvulsants for diabetic neuropathy and postherpetic neuralgia: a quantitative systematic review. *J Pain Symptom Manage* 2000; **20**: 449–58.

108. Saarto T, Wiffen PJ. Antidepressants for neuropathic pain. *Cochrane Database Syst Rev* 2007, (4) Art No: CD005454, DOI: 10.1002/14651858. CD005454. pub2

109. Tomkins GE, Jackson JL, O'Malley PG, Balden E, Santoro JE. Treatment of chronic headache with antidepressants: a meta-analysis. *Am J Med* 2001; **111**: 54–63.

110. Arnold LM, Keck PE, Welge JA. Antidepressant treatment of fibromyalgia. A meta-analysis and review. *Psychosomatics* 2000; **41**: 104–13.

111. O'Malley PG, Balden E, Tomkins G, *et al.* Treatment of fibromyalgia with antidepressants: a meta-analysis. *J Gen Intern Med* 2000; **15**: 659–66.

112. Jackson JL, O'Malley PG, Tomkins G, *et al.* Treatment of functional gastrointestinal disorders with antidepressant medications: a meta-analysis. *Am J Med* 2000; **108**: 65–72.

113. Lesbros-Pantoflickova D, Michetti P, Fried M, Beglinger C, Blum AL. Meta: analysis: the treatment of irritable bowel syndrome. *Aliment Pharmacol Ther* 2004; **20**: 1253–69.

114. Kelada E, Jones A. Interstitial cystitis. *Arch Gynecol Obstet* 2007; **275**: 223–9.

115. Onghena P, Van Houdenhove B. Antidepressant-induced analgesia in chronic non-malignant pain: a

meta-analysis of 39 placebo-controlled studies. *Pain* 1992; **49**: 205–19.

116. Reiter RC. Evidence-based management of chronic pelvic pain. *Clin Obstet Gynecol* 1998; **41**: 422–35.

117. Sharav Y, Singer E, Schmidt E, Dionne RA, Dubner R. The analgesic effect of amitriptyline on chronic facial pain. *Pain* 1987; **31**: 199–209.

118. Stones W, Cheong YC, Howard FM. Interventions for treating chronic pelvic pain in women. *Cochrane Database Syst Rev* 2007; (4): CD000387.

119. Van Ophoven A, Pokupic S, Heinecke A, Hertle L. A prospective, randomised, placebo-controlled, double-blind study of amitriptyline for the treatment of interstitial cystitis. *J Urol* 2004; **172**: 533–6.

120. Quartero AO, Meineche-Schmidt V, Muris J, Rubin G, de Wit N. Bulking agents, antispasmodic and antidepressant medication for the treatment of irritable bowel syndrome. *Cochrane Database Syst Rev* 2005; (2): CD003460.

121. Fields HL, Basbaum AI. Central nervous system mechanisms of pain modulation. In *Textbook of Pain,* 4th edn., eds PD Wall and R Melzack. (Edinburgh: Churchill Livingstone, 1999), pp. 309–29.

122. Yokogawa F, Kiuchi Y, Ishikawa Y, *et al.* An investigation of monoamine receptors involved in antinociceptive effects of antidepressants. *Anesth Analg* 2002; **95**: 163–8.

123. Kawasaki Y, Kumamoto E, Furue H, Yoshimura M. Alpha 2 adrenoceptor-mediated presynaptic inhibition of primary afferent glutamatergic transmission in rat substantia gelatinosa neurons. *Anesthesiology* 2003; **98**: 682–9.

124. Gerner P, Mujtaba M, Sinnott CJ, Wang GK. Amitriptyline versus bupivacaine in rat sciatic nerve blockade. *Anesthesiology* 2001; **94**: 661–7.

125. Lee RL, Spencer PS. Effect of tricyclic antidepressants on analgesic activity in laboratory animals. *Postgrad Med J* 1980; **56**(suppl 1): 19–24.

126. Taiwo YO, Fabian A, Pazoles CJ, Fields HL. Potentiation of morphine antinociception by monoamine reuptake inhibitors in the rat spinal cord. *Pain* 1985; **21**: 329–37.

127. Lynch ME. Antidepressants as analgesics: a review of randomized controlled trials. *J Psychiatry Neurosci* 2001; **26**: 30–6.

128. Max MB. Treatment of post-herpetic neuralgia: antidepressants. *Ann Neurol* 1994; **35**(suppl): 50–3.

129. Max MB, Lynch SA, Muir J, *et al.* Effects of desipramine, amitriptyline, and fluoxetine on pain in diabetic neuropathy. *N Engl J Med* 1992; **326**: 1250–6.

130. McQuay HJ, Tramer M, Nye BA, *et al.* A systematic review of antidepressants in neuropathic pain. *Pain* 1996; **68**: 217–27.

131. Mochizucki D. Serotonin and noradrenaline reuptake inhibitors in animal models of pain. *Hum Psychopharmacol Clin Exp* 2004; **19**(suppl 1): 15–19.

132. Sussman N. SNRIs versus SSRIs: mechanisms of action in treating depression and painful physical symptoms. *Primary Care Companion J Clin Psychiatry* 2003; **5**(suppl 7): 19–26.

133. Goldstein DJ, Lu Y, Detke MJ, Lee TC, Iyengar S. Duloxetine vs. placebo in patients with painful diabetic neuropathy. *Pain* 2005; **116**: 109–18.

134. Rowbotham MC, Goli V, Kunz NR, Lei D. Venlafaxine extended release in the treatment of painful diabetic neuropathy: a double-blind, placebo-controlled study. *Pain* 2004; **110**: 697–706.

135. Sindrup SH, Bach FW, Madsen C, Gram LF, Jensen TS. Venlafaxine versus imipramine in painful polyneuropathy – A randomized, controlled trial. *Neurology* 2003; **60**: 1284–9.

136. Arnold LM, Lu Y, Crofford LJ, *et al.* A double-blind, multicenter trial comparing duloxetine with placebo in the treatment of fibromyalgia patients with or without major depressive disorder. *Arthritis Rheum* 2004; **50**: 2974–84.

137. Zijlstra TR, Barendregt PJ, van de Laar MAF. Venlafaxine in fibromyalgia: results of a randomized, placebo-controlled, double-blind trial (abstract). *Arthritis Rheum* 2002; **46**(suppl 9): 105.

138. Sindrup SH, Jensen TS. Efficacy of pharmacological treatments of neuropathic pain: an update and effect related to mechanism of drug action. *Pain* 1999; **83**: 389–400.

139. Anderberg UM, Marteinsdottir I, von Knorring L. Citalopram in patients with fibromyalgia – a randomized, double-blind, placebo-controlled study. *Eur J Pain* 2000; **4**: 27–35.

140. Arnold LM, Hess EV, Hudson JI, *et al.* A randomized, placebo-controlled, double-blind, flexible-dose study of fluoxetine in the treatment of women with fibromyalgia. *Am J Med* 2002; **112**: 191–7.

141. McQuay HJ. Neuropathic pain: evidence matters. *Eur J Pain* 2002; **6**(suppl A): 11–18.

142. Norregaard J, Volkmann H, Danneskiold-Samsoe B. A randomized controlled trial of citalopram in the treatment of fibromyalgia. *Pain* 1995; **61**: 445–9.

143. Sindrup SH, Bjerre U, Dejgaard A, *et al.* The selective serotonin reuptake inhibitor citalopram relieves the symptoms of diabetic neuropathy. *Clin Pharmacol Ther* 1992; **52**: 547–52.

144. Sindrup SH, Gram LF, Brosen K, Eshoj O, Mogensen EF. The selective serotonin reuptake inhibitor paroxetine is effective in the treatment of diabetic neuropathy symptoms. *Pain* 1990; **42**: 135–44.

145. Bowsher D. The effects of pre-emptive treatment of postherpetic neuralgia with amitriptyline: a randomized, double-blind, placebo-controlled trial. *J Pain Symptom Manage* 1997; **13**: 327–31.

146. Ohayon MM, Roth T. Prevalence of restless legs syndrome and periodic movement disorder in the general population. *J Psychosom Res* 2002; **53**: 547–54.

147. Semenchuk MR, Sherman S, Davis B. Double-blind, randomized trial of bupropion SR for the treatment of neuropathic pain. *Neurology* 2001; **57**: 1583–8.

148. Bendtsen L, Jensen R. Mirtazapine is effective in the prophylactic treatment of chronic tension-type headache. *Neurology* 2004; **62**: 1706–11.

149. Leo RJ, Milnacipran, a serotonin and nonpinephrine reuptake inhibition: a novel treatment for fibromyalgia. *Int J Clin Rheumatol*, 2009; **4**: 507–17.

150. Ventafridda V, Caraceni A, Saita L, *et al*. Trazodone for deafferentation pain: comparison with amitriptyline. *Psychopharmacology* (Berl) 1988; **95**(suppl): S44–S49.

151. McQuay H, Carroll D, Jadad AR, Wiffen P, Moore A. Anticonvulsant drugs for management of pain: a systematic review. *Br Med J* 1995; **311**: 1047–52.

152. Pappagallo M. Newer antiepileptic drugs: possible uses in the treatment of neuropathic pain and migraine. *Clin Ther* 2003; **25**: 2506–38.

153. Snow V, Weiss K, Wall EM, Mottur-Pilson C, American Academy of Family Physicians. Pharmacologic management of acute attacks of migraine and prevention of migraine headache. *Ann Intern Med* 2002; **137**: 840–9.

154. Crofford LJ, Rowbotham MC, Mease PJ, *et al*. Pregabalin for the treatment of fibromyalgia syndrome. *Arthritis Rheum* 2005; **52**: 1264–73.

155. Galer BS. Neuropathic pain of peripheral origin: advances in pharmacologic treatment. *Neurology* 1995; **45**(suppl 9): 17–25.

156. Maciewicz R, Bouckoms A, Martin JB. Drug therapy of neuropathic pain. *Clin J Pain* 1985; **1**: 39–49.

157. Swerdlow M. Anticonvulsant drugs and chronic pain. *Clin Neuropharmacol* 1984; **7**: 51–82.

158. Frampton JE, Scott LJ. Pregabalin in the treatment of painful diabetic neuropathy. *Drugs* 2004; **64**: 2813–20.

159. Guay DR. Oxcarbazepine, topiramate, zonisamide, and levetiracetam: potential use in neuropathic pain. *Am J Geriatr Pharmacother* 2003; **1**: 18–37.

160. Vinik A. Use of antiepileptic drugs in the treatment of chronic painful diabetic neuropathy. *J Clin Endocrinol Metab* 2005; **90**: 4936–45.

161. Khoromi S, Patsalides A, Parada S, *et al*. Topiramate in chronic lumbar radicular pain. *J Pain* 2005; **6**: 829–36.

162. Novak V, Kanard R, Kissel JT, Mendell JR. Treatment of painful sensory neuropathy with tiagabine: a pilot study. *Clin Auton Res* 2001; **11**: 357–61.

163. Remillard G. Oxcarbazepine and intractable trigeminal neuralgia. *Epilepsia* 1994; **35**: 528–29.

164. Solaro C, Uccelli MM, Brichetto G, Gaspperini C, Mancardi G. Topiramate relieves idiopathic and symptomatic trigeminal neuralgia. *J Pain Symptom Manage* 2001; **21**: 367–8.

165. Zakrzewska JM, Chaudhry Z, Nurmikko TJ, Patton DW, Mullens EL. Lamotrigine (lamictal) in refractory trigeminal neuralgia: results from a double-blind placebo controlled crossover trial. *Pain* 1997; **73**: 223–30.

166. Dahl JB, Mathiesen O, Moiniche S. 'Protective premedication': an option with gabapentin and related drugs? A review of gabapentin and pregabalin in the treatment of post-operative pain. *Acta Anaesthesiol Scand* 2004; **48**: 1130–6.

167. Yerby MS. Special considerations for women with epilepsy. *Pharmacotherapy* 2000; **20**(suppl 8): 159–70.

168. Leo RJ. Treatment considerations in neuropathic pain. *Curr Treat Options Neurol* 2006; **8**: 389–400.

169. Chandramouli J. Newer anticonvulsant drugs in neuropathic pain and bipolar disorder. *J Pain Palliat Care Pharmacother* 2002; **16**: 19–37.

170. Leo RJ, Narendran R. Anticonvulsant use in the treatment of bipolar disorder: a primer for primary care physicians. *Primary Care Companion J Clin Psychiatry* 1999; **1**: 74–84.

171. Rossy LA, Buckelew SP, Dorr N, *et al*. A meta-analysis of fibromyalgia treatment interventions. *Ann Behav Med* 1999; **21**: 180–91.

172. Garcia J, Simon MA, Duran M, Canceller J, Aneiros FJ. Differential efficacy of a cognitive-behavioral intervention versus pharmacological treatment in the management of fibromyalgic syndrome. *Psychol Health Med* 2006; **11**: 498–506.

173. Parker JC, Smarr KL, Slaughter JR, *et al*. Management of depression in rheumatoid arthritis: a combined pharmacologic and cognitive-behavioral approach. *Arthritis Rheum* 2003; **49**: 766–77.

174. Dworkin RH, Turk DC, Wyrwich KW, *et al.* Interpreting the clinical importance of treatment outcomes in chronic pain clinical trials: IMMPACT recommendations. *J Pain* **2008**; **9**: 105–21.

175. Turk DC, Okifuji A. Matching treatment to assessment of patients with chronic pain. In *Handbook of Pain Assessment*, eds. DC Turk and R Melzack. (New York: Guilford, 1992), pp. 400–14.

176. Jensen MP, Nielson WR, Turner JA, Romano JM, Hill ML. Readiness to self-manage pain is associated with coping and with psychological and physical functioning among patients with chronic pain. *Pain* 2003; **104**: 529–37.

177. Turk DC, Okifuji A, Sinclair JD, Starz TW. Pain, disability, and physical functioning in subgroups of patients with fibromyalgia. *J Rheumatol* 1996; **23**: 1255–62.

178. Turk DC, Okifuji A, Starz TW, Sinclair JD. Differential responses by psychosocial subgroups of fibromyalgia syndrome patients to an interdisciplinary treatment. *Arthritis Care Res* 1998; **11**: 397–404.

179. Nielson WR, Weir R. Biopsychosocial approaches to the treatment of chronic pain. *Clin J Pain* 2001; **17**(suppl 4): 114–27.

180. Keefe FJ, Lumley MA, Buffington AL, *et al.* Changing face of pain: evolution of pain research in psychosomatic medicine. *Psychosom Med* 2002; **64**: 921–38.

Integrative approaches to the management of painful
medical conditions
Management of spinal pain

Gerald W. Grass

Incidence and epidemiology of spinal pain

Few medical problems are more complex in nature and perplexing to effectively manage than pain. Of all pain syndromes, spinal pain represents one of the most common reasons why patients seek medical treatment. Seventy percent of all adults experience back or neck pain at some point in their lives, resulting in more than 15 million outpatient physician visits for back pain alone in a given year [1, 2]. Over 30 million people will suffer with spinal pain this year alone and almost two-thirds of all adults suffer from neck or back pain at some time during their lives [3]. Studies suggest that low back pain is second only to upper respiratory problems as a symptom related reason for visits to physicians [1, 4]. The costs of this problem, in both human suffering and dollars, are staggering. In the USA, back and neck problems are the second leading cause of disability and the leading cause of job-related disability, costing Americans more than $50 billion each year [3].

Many patients have self-limited episodes of acute low back pain and do not seek medical care. Among those who do seek medical care, it is often claimed that 90% of patients with acute low back pain improve within a short period of time [5], although clinical experience and recent epidemiological studies have called that prognosis into question. The literature in this area is confusing due to considerable variations regarding the exact definitions of low back pain as well as recovery. In an extensive review of the literature conducted by Hestbaek *et al.*, the reported proportion of patients who still experienced pain after 12 months after onset ranged from 42–75% and the risk of developing a recurrent episode of low back pain was consistently twice as high for those with a prior history of low back pain [6].

Although many options are available for evaluation and management of spinal pain, there has been little consensus regarding what constitutes appropriate evaluation and management of spinal pain. Unfortunately, clinical and experimental studies indicate that spinal pain may originate from many spinal structures, including ligaments, facet joints, vertebral periostium, the paravertebral musculature, the annulus fibrosis, and the spinal nerve roots. Physical signs and symptoms are often non-specific and the association between symptoms and imaging results is weak. It therefore becomes problematic determining the origin of pain resulting in the use of non-specific terms such as strain, sprain, or degenerative processes in describing the origins of spinal pain.

Often, the initial diagnosis and treatment of spinal pain occurs within the context of a primary care setting and it is not surprising then that up to 85% of patients with spinal pain seen in primary care cannot be given a precise diagnosis as to the origin or nature of their pain [5]. This often becomes a very challenging situation for the clinician and a frustrating encounter for the patient [7].

It is important that all specialties involved in evaluating patients who present with chronic spinal pain understand some of the basic reasons for developing pain-related problems including basic spinal anatomy, the underlying spine pathologies, pathophysiology of pain and available therapies. This will allow closer partnerships among physicians and other clinicians involved in the multidisciplinary treatments of patients presenting with chronic spinal pain.

Acute vs. chronic spinal pain

Low back pain is usually defined as pain, muscle tension, or stiffness localized below the costal margin and above the inferior gluteal folds, with or without leg pain.

Behavioral and Psychopharmacologic Pain Management, ed. Michael H. Ebert and Robert D. Kerns. Published by Cambridge University Press. © Cambridge University Press 2011.

It is typically classified as being specific or non-specific, acute or chronic. Specific low back pain is defined as symptoms caused by underlying disease process. This can include spinal fractures, cancer, infection, and disc herniation. Non-specific low back pain accounts for the majority of cases with no readily identifiable cause. The point at which acute pain becomes chronic is a subjective matter, with most authorities defining chronic pain as pain that persists 3 months or more after onset as a chronological landmark.

Acute back pain is commonly described as a very sharp pain or a dull ache, usually felt deep in the lower part of the back, and can be more severe in one area, such as the right side, left side, center, or the lower part of the back. Acute pain can be intermittent, but is usually constant, only varying in terms of severity. Acute back pain may be caused by injury or trauma to the back, but just as often has no known cause.

The initial treatment of acute low back pain is short-term and usually successful. The recommended treatment stratagies often employ mild analgesics and muscle relaxants, physical therapy, and prevention practices, these patients typically return to full functionality in a few weeks. Occasionally, these patients will re-injure themselves and have to return for a short course of treatment. Patients with acute pain occurring more than three times in one year or who experience longer-lasting episodes of back pain that significantly interfere with functional activities (e.g., sleeping, sitting, standing, walking, bending, riding in or driving a car) tend to develop a chronic condition.

Chronic back pain is commonly described as deep, aching, dull or burning pain in one area of the back or traveling down the legs. Patients may experience numbness, tingling, burning, or a pins-and-needles type sensation in the legs. Regular daily activities may prove difficult or impossible for the chronic back pain patient. They may find it difficult or unbearable to work, for example, even when the job does not require manual labor. Chronic back pain tends to last a long time, and is not relieved by standard types of medical management. It may result from a previous injury long since healed, or it may have an ongoing cause, such as nerve damage or arthritis.

Spinal anatomy

It is essential to understand normal spinal anatomy in order to aid in locating pathology that may specifically be responsible for a patient's pain. Experimental and clinical studies suggest that low back pain may originate from many spinal structures, including ligaments, facet joints, the vertebral periostium, the paravertebral musculature and fascia, the annulus fibrosis, and spinal nerve roots.

Overview of the spine

This schematic view of a lumbar motion segment demonstrates normal spine anatomy:

- The vertebral body with the interposing intervertebral discs
- The neuroforamen bound by pedicles
- The vertebral body anteriorly
- Laminae and facet joints posteriorly
- Each foramen has an exiting nerve root with its ventral and dorsal rami
- The central canal is comprised mainly of the spinal sac with the intrathecal nerve roots.

Vertebrae

There are 33 vertebrae in the spine and although the vertebrae have slightly different appearances as they range from the cervical spine to the lumbar spine, they all have the same basic structures, and the structures have the same names. Only the first and second cervical vertebrae are structurally different in order to support the skull.

Each vertebra is composed of posterior elements forming a vertebral arch posteriorly and the body anteriorly. The pedicles connect the body to the posterior elements forming the vertebral canal and serve to form a lateral opening in the spinal canal, known as a foramen, through which individual spinal nerves pass.

Discs connect one vertebral body to another to allow motion of the spine and cushion it against heavy loads. Together, the vertebral bodies and discs bear about 80% of the load to the spine. The pedicles are two short cylinders of bone that extend from the vertebral body. Nerve roots branch off the spinal cord and exit to the body between the pedicles of two vertebrae. If the spine becomes unstable, the pedicles may compress the nerve root, causing pain or numbness.

Lamina are two flattened plates of bone that form the walls of the posterior arch. Over time, the lamina may thicken, a process called stenosis. This thickening may compress the spinal cord and/or nerves causing pain or numbness. The articular, transverse, and spinous processes project off the lamina. Ligaments and tendons attach to the processes. Ligaments connect the vertebrae

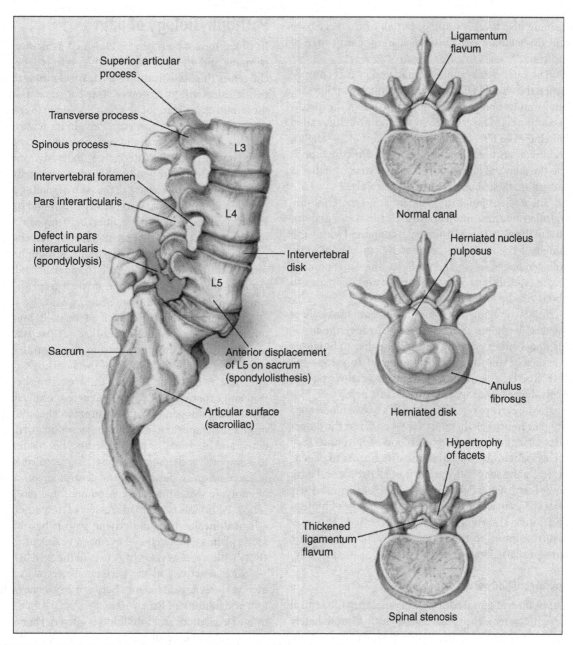

Figure 17.1 Reprinted with permission from *New Engl J Med*. Ref. [5]

to each other and include the anterior and posterior longitudinal ligaments and the ligamentum flavum.

The articular processes join one vertebra to another posteriorly. Movement of the vertebral column is made possible by articulations of several types and is constrained by various ligaments. The orientation of the facet joints dictates the movements possible between two adjacent vertebrae. Minimal rotation is allowed at the lumbar level because of sagitally opposing portions of the joint.

Thoracic facets limit flexion but permit rotation. In the cervical spine, movement in all planes is less restricted.

Intervertebral discs

Intervertebral discs are located between each vertebra from C2–C3 to L5–S1. Combined, they make up one-fourth the height of the spinal column. The discs act as shock absorbers to the loads placed on the spine and allow movement of the spine. Movement at a single disc level is limited, but all of the vertebrae and discs combined allow for a significant range of motion.

The intervertebral disc is made up of two components: the annulus fibrosus and the nucleus pulposus. The annulus fibrosus is the outer portion of the disc. It is composed of layers of collagen and proteins, called lamellae. The fibers of the lamellae slant at 30° angles, and the fibers of each lamella run in a direction opposite the adjacent layers. This creates a structure that is exceptionally strong, yet extremely flexible.

The nucleus pulposus is the inner gel material surrounded by the annulus fibrosus. It makes up about 40% of the disc. This ball-like gel is contained within the lamellae. The nucleus is composed primarily of loose collagen fibers, water, and proteins. The water content of the nucleus is about 90% at birth and decreases to about 70% by the fifth decade of life.

Injury or aging of the annulus fibrosus may allow the nucleus pulposus to be squeezed through the annulus fibers either partially, causing the disc to bulge, or completely, allowing the disc material to escape the disc. The bulging disc or nucleus material may compress the nerves or spinal cord, causing pain.

In the early years of life, the discs have a blood supply that nourishes them. In the second and third decades, discs gradually lose this blood supply, until they are avascular. At this point, the disc begins to degenerate. By the age of 50, over 95% of all people will have some form of disc degeneration. The disc begins to lose water content and shrinks. The spine's range of motion and shock-absorbing ability are decreased. This may result in injury to the nerves and vertebrae, and the aging disc itself may generate pain.

Spinal cord and nerve roots

The brain and spinal cord together make up the central nervous system. The spinal cord is located immediately below the brain stem. It extends through the foramen magnum, a hole at the base of the skull.

The spinal cord functions as a sophisticated network that carries information from the outer elements of the body (skin, muscles, ligaments, joints) through the sensory tracts, to the cerebral cortex. Data are processed there, and new information such as muscle control is sent out through the motor tracts of the spinal cord. The spinal cord ends as the conus medullaris at the L1 vertebral level, where it branches into the cauda equina, a collection of nerves that extend from the conus medullaris to the sacrum.

Pathophysiology of pain

In broad terms, pain can be classified as nociceptive (somatic and visceral), neuropathic, referred, or psychogenic. This classification is useful in planning therapeutic intervention, however clear cut separations of these pain classes cannot be assumed, and in the case of spinal pain frequently overlap. Pain, in its acute form, is necessary for survival and serves an important role in the way an organism interfaces with its environment by signaling real or impending harm. Occasionally, circumstances lead to activity in the pain-signaling pathway that is not beneficial to the organism and has no survival value. Injury to nerve fibers or their projections may cause conditions that are not usually perceived as painful to become excessively painful. Although most injuries do not lead to clinically important and sustained pain; in some cases, even small degrees of insult can precipitate severe and unremitting pain.

In terms of the experience of pain, it must be remembered that noxious stimuli are not just passively conducted from the periphery to the central nervous system as a large number of mechanisms serve to attenuate, magnify, and extend the organism's perception and experience of pain. The current understanding of the pathogenesis of pain suggests that multiple mechanisms appear to mediate the symptoms of nociceptive and neuropathic pain including, but not limited to, temporal and spatial summation, recruitment of inactive neurons, peripheral and central sensitization, phenotypic switching, and central neuronal reorganization. Although a systematic review of the pathophysiological mechanisms underlying pain is beyond the scope of this chapter they have been reviewed extensively within recent years by others in the field [8–12].

Normal activity in the peripheral nervous system involves a reciprocal balance between neuronal excitation and inhibition. Pain arises when the balance shifts toward excitation, and inhibition is altered. Damage to peripheral nerves results in hyperexcitability in the primary afferent nociceptors (*peripheral sensitization*) that leads to hyperexcitability in central neurons (*central sensitization*) and the generation of spontaneous impulses within the axon, as well as the dorsal root ganglion of the peripheral nerves. When the nerve is able to repair itself, the sensitization resolves; however, if the nerve is unable to effect this repair or the insult continues, continued sensitization and altered processes in nociceptors lead to further generation of spontaneous symptoms.

Unresolved injury causes a multitude of changes in gene transcription and activation of various kinases and

Table 17.1 Pathophysiological factors in spinal pain

Mechanical low back or leg pain	Nonmechanical spinal pain	Visceral disease
Lumbar strain, sprain	*Neoplasia*	*Disease of pelvic organs*
Degenerative disc disease	Multiple myeloma	Prostatitis
Herniated disc	Metastatic carcinoma	Endometriosis
Internal disc disruption	Lymphoma and leukemia	Chronic pelvic inflammatory disease
Facet arthropathy	Spinal cord tumors	*Renal disease*
Foraminal stenosis	Retroperitoneal tumors	Nephrolithiasis
Spinal stenosis	Primary vertebral tumors	Pyelonephritis
Spondylolysis	*Infection*	Perinephric abscess
Spondylolisthesis	Osteomyelitis	*Aortic aneurysm*
Sacroiliitis	Septic discitis	*Gastrointestinal disease*
Piriformis syndrome	Paraspinous abscess	Pancreatitis
Osteoporotic compression fracture	Epidural abscess	Cholecystitis
Traumatic fracture	*Inflammatory arthritis*	Penetrating ulcer
Congenital disease	Ankylosing spondylitis	
Severe kyphosis	Psoriatic spondylitis	
Severe scoliosis	Reiter's syndrome	
Transitional vertebrae	*Paget's disease of the bone*	
	Osteochondrosis	

proteins involved in the transmission and amplification of noxious stimuli, including enhanced N-methyl-D-aspartate (NMDA) receptor activity [13, 14]. At the cellular level of the nerve these alterations can lead to the formation of new channels, upregulation of certain receptors and downregulation of others, and altered local or descending inhibition which are some of the biological features that can contribute to hyperexcitability, factors assumed to be a sine qua non for chronic pain [15–17].

It is the altered expression of these channels that results in neurons becoming hyperexcitable and generating ectopic activity, which is thought to lead to the genesis of chronic spontaneous and paroxysmal pain. Beyond this, neuronal hyperexcitability has a wide spectrum of secondary manifestations including, expansion of neuronal receptive fields, change of modality to which neurons respond, recruitment of silent neurons or circuits and a neuronal reorganization in the dorsal horn and within the central nervous system.

It is not entirely unexpected that a genetic component may also contribute to the individual experience of pain and may contribute to the diverse phenotype of individuals with apparently similar lesions, some of whom develop chronic neuropathic pain and many others do not. In the past many genes have been identified that contribute to the development of non-neuropathic pain conditions; however only one gene, thus far – GTP cyclohydrolase 1 (GCH1) – has been implicated specifically in neuropathic pain [18].

It is, therefore, not surprising that given the multiplicity of cellular alterations occurring subsequent to nerve injury, a host of neuroplastic changes take place in which the somatosensory information can be distorted in several ways secondary to the reorganization of all of the structures participating in the transduction, transmission, and translational processing of noxious information.

Spinal pain patterns

The presence of chronic neck or low back pain, whether of peripheral or central origin, continues to present a significant burden to individuals and society by increasing disability, reducing productivity and diminishing the quality of life all with concomitant increases in healthcare resource utilization and costs.

Many clinicians, including primary care physicians, psychologists, physical therapists, and other non-pain specialists, will encounter patients with chronic pain of spinal origin. The clinical spectrum of spinal pain ranges from barely discernible to severely disabling and as previously mentioned is caused by a wide range of disease processes as listed in Table 17.1.

The assessment and differential diagnosis of cervical and lumbar spinal pain syndromes is complex and challenging for the clinician. In patients presenting with chronic spinal pain, the underlying pain mechanism or mechanisms are often difficult to diagnose, and a distinction between nociceptive and neuropathic types of pain is sometimes challenging because conditions such as diabetes mellitus, cancer, and other neurological diseases can produce mixed pain pictures. It is important, of course, that the clinical assessment of a patient with suspected spinal pain should focus on ruling out treatable conditions (e.g., spinal cord compression, neoplasm), confirm a diagnosis or formulate a differential diagnosis and identify clinical features (e.g., anxiety, depression, insomnia, etc.) that might help individualize treatment. Crucial to any pain assessment is the clinician's acknowledgment that the patient is experiencing pain and that the pain is real. This validation of the patient's pain is critical in developing rapport with the patient and establishing a meaningful therapeutic relationship. Without this, any further steps in the care of the pain patient are unproductive, if not meaningless.

Although the differential diagnosis of cervical and lumbar spinal pain is extensive, certain pain patterns emerge which may help to guide the clinician in their diagnostic and classification efforts. Many patients with spinal pain will have pain along the axis of the spine (axial pain), as well as pain extending into one or more extremity (radicular or referred pain), and differentiating axial from radicular pain is critical to guiding therapy. The American College of Physicians and the American Pain Society have recently published clinical guidelines for the diagnosis and treatment of low back pain which recommend that the practitioner attempt to classify patients with low back pain into one of three broad categories: non-specific low back pain, back pain potentially associated with radiculopathy or spinal stenosis, and back pain potentially associated with another spinal cause [19].

History

The first step in the diagnostic evaluation of any patient with spinal pain is the history and physical examination. The pain history should note the pain location, time of onset, intensity, character, associated symptoms, and factors aggravating and relieving the pain, response to past treatments, co-morbid conditions and coping skills. Characteristic features of the pain presentation should be sought and are important in differentiating it from any other source of pain, thereby differentiating nociceptive vs. neuropathic pain. Although it is common for patients with chronic spinal pain to have a "mixed" presentation with signs and symptoms suggestive of both nociceptive and neuropathic pain states. A guide to help in the assessment and evaluation of patients with a suspected neuropathic pain syndrome is presented below (Table 17.2).

Positive symptoms that are typical of neuropathic pain include (1) paresthesias – non-painful, spontaneous sensory phenomena such as "pins and needles" sensation or tingling; (2) dysesthesias – unpleasant spontaneous or evoked sensory phenomena such as burning; (3) hyperesthesia – increased sensitivity to stimuli, often with an unpleasant quality; (4) hyperpathia or hyperalgesia – exaggerated pain response elicited by a normally painful stimulus.

In addition, the effect of pain on quality of life and functional status issues is extremely important. Specific pain measures such as the Neuropathic Pain Scale, Neuropathic Pain Questionnaire, Pain DETECT Questionnaire may be used to quantify the patient's pain as well as its effect on the quality of life. These tools share common features and in general have a similar accuracy rate of up to 80% [20]. These scales are particularly helpful for patients involved in clinical therapeutic trials and may be used to assess the efficacy of treatment regimens. It must be remembered that although these questionnaires aid in the identification of neuropathic pain syndromes and serve as reliable screening tools, they do not replace a detailed medical history and physical examination.

Physical examination

The physical examination should be guided by the patient history. The goal of the physical examination is to characterize the pattern, symmetry and distribution of abnormalities and to determine which modalities are involved (motor, sensory, autonomic). The examination should include a focused general medical examination and neurological assessment.

The general medical examination is an integral part of any diagnostic evaluation. One aspect of the general medical examination to be emphasized is the status of the skin, noting whether changes in skin color (red,

Table 17.2 A guide to the evaluation of patients with chronic spinal pain

History	Deep tendon reflexes
Pain intensity	May be diminished or absent distal to involved nerves
0–10 rating scale (0=no pain, 10 = worst pain imaginable	*Sensory examination*
Rate pain at the initial visit and at each subsequent visit to track treatment response	Light touch, pin prick, vibration and proprioception sense may be diminished or absent distal to involved nerves
Sensory descriptors	Sensory abnormalities may extend beyond normal dermatomal, myotomal and/or sclerotomal boundaries.
Pain qualities: burning, electric, hot, cold, stabbing.	Dynamic allodynia (pain due to cotton lightly moving across the skin)
Unusual sensations: "pin and needles," tingling, itching etc.	Thermal allodynia (burning sensation in response to ice or alcohol on skin)
Temporal variation	Pinprick hyperalgesia (exaggerated pain following light pinprick to skin)
Neuropathic pain often becomes worse at the end of the day, with cold and/or damp weather	Possible presence of Tinel's sign (distally radiating paresthesias upon percussion of damaged or regenerating nerve fibers)
Suspect neoplastic process if the pain has progressively worsened over several months	*Skin examination*
Functional/psychological impact	Alterations in temperature, color, sweating, hair and/or nail growth suggestive of complex regional pain syndrome
The effect of pain on sleep patterns, activities of daily living, work and hobbies	Residual dermatomal scars consistent with previous herpes zoster infection
The effect of pain on mood, social and sexual functioning, suicidal ideation	Characteristic skin changes consistent with diabetes mellitus
Previous treatment modalities	**Special tests**
Neuropathic pain is resistant to NSAIDs and acetaminophen	*CT and MRI scans*
Determine and document adequacy of dose titration for previously trialed drugs (dose reached, duration of treatment, and drug stopped due to adverse effects or lack of efficacy)	Facilitate specific diagnosis (e.g., disc herniations, nerve infiltration/compression by tumor)
Substance abuse history	*Electromyography and nerve conduction studies*
Administer opioid screening tools (COMM or STOP)	May provide objective evidence of nerve injury or dysfunction. Nerve conduction studies evaluate large fiber function, small fiber neuropathy cannot be ruled out if results of NCS are normal
Addiction history may affect decision to prescribe opioids.	*Three-phase nuclear medicine bone scan*
Consider safety of opioids, muscle relaxants and/or hypnotics in the presence of alcohol use	May aid in the diagnosis of complex regional pain syndrome. However, CRPS may be present despite negative study
If substance abuse positive, consider earlier involvement with a psychologist, psychiatrist or addiction specialist	*Clinical biochemistry*
Physical examination	Perform tests to help identify cause of neuropathy; i.e., glucose tolerance test, thyroid function, vitamin B12 levels, CD 4+ T-lymphocyte count
Gross motor examination	
Motor weakness may occur distal to involved nerves	
Attempt to distinguish between true weakness and weakness secondary to pain	

pale, bluish, mottled), rashes, swelling, changes in hair or nail growth, and temperature abnormalities are present or absent. In addition, attention should be paid to a musculoskeletal evaluation including the status of the joints, muscles, and ligaments noting any swelling, laxity, tenderness and limitation of motion are present.

As previously mentioned, patients may present with positive and/or negative sensory symptoms. This means that stimuli such as light touch, pinprick, cold, warm, vibration and two point discrimination may be perceived as either exaggerated or diminished. In patients with positive neuropathic symptoms, there are often correlative signs on the physical examination. Simple bedside tests, such as the use of von Frey filaments, a tuning fork, and pinprick testing are helpful somatosensory tests. Allodynia, for example, may be elicited by lightly stroking the involved area or by testing with a cold instrument. Hyperalgesia or hyperpathia may be elicited during pinprick testing. These examination findings are important, because they are unique to patients with neuropathic pain.

Patients with spinal pain may experience motor symptoms and signs which could also be viewed as negative and/or positive motor signs and symptoms. Negative signs include hypotonia, decreased muscle strength, tremor, dystonia and dyskinesia. Positive signs may include hypertonia, spasm, and exaggerated deep tendon reflexes.

Despite this, it is common for there to be relatively modest demonstrable clinical neurological deficits in patients with significant spinal pain, and in some conditions there may be a completely normal clinical examination. It must be remembered therefore that a lack of significant physical findings does not exclude the diagnosis of spinal pain and should not be dismissed as psychogenic pain or as malingering.

Treatment options

Effective pain management for spine-related pain requires ongoing evaluation, patient education and reassurance. Diagnostic evaluation of treatable underlying conditions (e.g., spinal cord compression, herniated disc, neoplasm) should continue concurrently with ongoing pain management efforts. Patients should be provided with education regarding the natural history of their condition and realistic treatment expectations (e.g., current treatments are not curative and analgesia is rarely complete).

Conventional medical treatment, provided in the primary care setting, is often the first-line therapy

for spine related pain syndromes. This would include treatment modalities such as providing general advice on self-management of non-specific back pain with recommendations to remain active, the application of heat, appropriate body mechanics and exercise regimens. Non-pharmacological treatment options often employed include various combinations of physical therapy, transcutaneous electrical nerve stimulation (TENS), massage, ultrasound, and acupuncture. In addition, the primary care provider may implement the use of pharmacological therapy including the use of acetaminophen, non-steroidal anti-inflammatory drugs (NSAIDs), skeletal muscle relaxants, and opioids when appropriate and necessary. Unfortunately, as much as we would like, no single drug or therapeutic modality works well for all chronic spinal pain states. Given the multiplicity of etiologic causes, diversity of pain mechanisms involved, and individual patient circumstances, treatment regimens must be individualized.

In addition, when considering treatment options for patients with spine-related pain, it must be remembered that behavioral and psychiatric co-morbidities are very common in patients with chronic pain and may be a consequence of delayed diagnosis or inappropriate treatment. In particular depression, anxiety disorders, and sleep disturbances are more common among patients with chronic pain than seen in the general population and may be accompanied or complicated by issues of substance abuse. The use of behavioral and psychopharmacological interventions has proven useful in adding to the armamentarium of therapeutic options available.

Current behavioral and psychopharmacological treatment paradigms

Behavioral treatment options

Contemporary biopsychosocial models of chronic pain differ in important ways from earlier psychological or medical models of pain. Rather than viewing pain as a symptom of some underlying psychological or medical disorder, current biopsychosocial models acknowledge a role for the biologic factors in pain, but also argue that psychosocial variables can influence pain and functioning in all persons, regardless of the source of pain or presence of psychopathology.

Psychological factors such as mood, beliefs about pain and coping style have been found to play an important role in an individual's adjustment to chronic pain. If pain persists over time, a person may avoid performing or engaging in regular activities for fear of further injury or increased pain. This can include activities such as work, social activities, or hobbies. As the individual withdraws and becomes less active, their muscles may become weaker, they may begin to gain or lose weight, and their overall physical conditioning may decline. This can contribute to the belief that one is *disabled*. As pain persists, the person may develop negative beliefs about their experience of pain (e.g., this is never going to get better) or negative thoughts about themselves (e.g., I'm worthless to my family because I can't work). These types of thoughts, along with decreased participation in enjoyable and reinforcing activities, may lead a person to feel depressed and anxious.

One particular psychological treatment approach that has been found to be effective in helping patients to reduce pain, disability and distress is cognitive behavioral therapy (CBT). The major goal of CBT is to replace maladaptive patient coping skills, cognitions, emotions, and behaviors with more adaptive ones. Use of the term CBT varies widely [21] and may be used to denote self-instructions (e.g., distraction, imagery, motivational self-talk), relaxation and/or biofeedback, development of adaptive coping strategies (e.g., minimizing negative or self-defeating thoughts), changing maladaptive beliefs about pain, and goal setting.

Although CBT alone does not address all of the important variables potentially contributing to chronic spinal pain (e.g., pathophysiological factors) it may improve care for patients with psychological co-morbidities. Cognitive behavioral therapy has been found to be effective in patients who had chronic pain from various causes [22]. The addition of even a very brief schedule of CBT to standard care from primary care providers has been shown to reduce pain and anxiety, though such effects may not persist over time [23].

In an early study, Morley *et al.* reported the results of a systematic review and meta-analysis of the existing randomized controlled trials (RCTs) of the efficacy of CBT, and behavioral therapy, for chronic pain in general [24]. Their findings concluded that such treatment is effective for a variety of chronic pain conditions in producing improvement in the important areas of: (1) pain experience; (2) pain behavior and activity level; (3) cognitive coping and appraisal; and (4) social functioning. Similarly, in a recent meta-analysis of 22 individual reported studies of psychological interventions

for the treatment of chronic low back pain noted positive short-term effects on pain interference and positive long-term effects on return to work [25].

In addition, numerous well-conducted studies have demonstrated the therapeutic efficacy of CBT techniques, which are a key component in most multidisciplinary pain management programs. A randomized control trial compared the relative efficacy of lumbar spinal fusion vs. CBT, including exercise, for patients who had low back pain and documented underlying pathophysiology [26]. A total of 64 participants were randomized into one of these two treatment options. At the 1-year follow-up, it was determined that differences between the groups given the lumbar fusion and cognitive intervention and exercise was neither clinically important nor significant. Both groups displayed significant clinical improvement on a wide range of measures. In a more recent RCT comparing the effectiveness of CBT intervention to lumbar fusion in patients with chronic low back pain, who also had a previous surgery for disc herniation, again, no differences in treatment efficacy were found [27].

The biopsychosocial approach to chronic pain management has moved away from the outdated view that monotherapy is the best approach to achieve optimum therapeutic improvement. Multiple factors including the biological, psychological and social must be simultaneously addressed and CBT serves an effective role in dealing with the psychosocial aspects of chronic spinal pain.

Psychopharmacologic treatment options

As previously mentioned there is a substantial overlap of psychiatric diagnoses with chronic pain conditions, and behavioral and psychiatric co-morbidities are very common in patients with chronic pain. In particular depression, anxiety disorders, and sleep disturbances are more common among patients with chronic pain than seen in the general population and the use of psychopharmacological interventions has proven useful, adding to the armamentarium of therapeutic options available.

The most common pharmacologic approach to the management of chronic spinal pain employed in the primary care setting includes the use of NSAIDs, skeletal muscle relaxants, and opioid analgesics. In addition, various psychopharmacologic agents may serve as "adjuvant analgesics" which refer to classes of drugs that can be used for pain relief, although that may not be the primary indications for their use. Many of these agents have multiple mechanisms of action, accounting for their dual effects. The three major classes of psychopharmacologic medications that have been found helpful for treating chronic pain syndromes are antidepressants, anticonvulsants/mood stabilizers, and anxiolytic agents.

Antidepressants

Antidepressants often serve a dual role: treating a mood disorder and independently addressing pain symptoms. One of the earliest form of currently used antidepressants was tricyclic antidepressants (TCAs). These were the drugs of choice for treating depression until the 1980s, when the selective serotonin reuptake inhibitors (SSRIs) were found to possess substantial antidepressant efficacy, and revolutionized the treatment of depression by offering efficacy with greatly reduced side effect profiles. Over the past decade, numerous atypical antidepressants have been developed, including norepinephrine and dopamine reuptake inhibitors (NDRIs), serotonin-norepinephrine reuptake inhibitors (SNRIs), and serotonin-2 antagonist/reuptake inhibitors (SARIs).

When first reported as having analgesic activity, antidepressants were thought to work by relieving the depression component of pain. Although it is well known that relieving depression by any method is likely to decrease pain, some antidepressants appear to have independent analgesic properties of their own. A third mechanism of action is the potentiation or enhancement of opioid analgesia by modulating serotonergic, noradrenergic, and cholinergic effects.

Tricyclic antidepressants

Tricyclic antidepressants have been shown to be safe and effective in the treatment of nociceptive and neuropathic pain. Commonly used agents include amitriptyline, nortriptyline, imipramine, and desipramine. These agents have been studied in double-blind, randomized controlled trials with results suggesting that each of them reduces pain independent of their effect on depression [28]. They are thought to exert their analgesic effect by inhibiting norepinephrine and serotonin reuptake in the central nervous system.

For neuropathic pain conditions, TCAs have been investigated more extensively than SSRIs, SNRIs, and other agents. As noted above, pain relief appears to occur independent of any antidepressant effect [29, 30]. In a systematic review of antidepressants in the treatment of neuropathic pain conditions, 30% of patients given antidepressants had more than 50% pain relief [31, 32]. The number needed to treat (NNT), defined as the number of patients needed to treat with a certain drug to obtain one patients with at least a 50% reduction in pain intensity, has been used to evaluate the pain relieving effects of numerous medications used for chronic pain. The average NNT for TCAs was 2.6 with a range of 2.2 to 3.3 when comparing several different studies involving several different pain conditions [33]. Comparing individual TCAs among each other is difficult, as dosages in some trials were titrated to perceived benefits and side effects, whereas other studies targeted optimal plasma drug concentrations.

Unfortunately, they also effect cholinergic, histaminergic, and adrenergic transmission, resulting in some limiting side effects. These include sedation, orthostasis, cardiac arrhythmia, and urinary retention which may limit their usefulness in certain patient populations, especially the elderly.

Selective serotonin reuptake inhibitors

Since the introduction of fluoxetine (Prozac) in 1987, several other SSRIs have been introduced and have expanded first line therapy for depression. Although SSRIs initially were introduced for use in major depressive disorders, the FDA has approved other indications for these agents, including anxiety disorders, bulimia nervosa, and obsessive compulsive disorder. In addition, SSRIs are often used by clinicians for a variety of other conditions including premenstrual syndrome, chronic fatigue syndrome, and chronic pain management.

The immediate effect of the SSRIs on the central nervous system (CNS) is the blockade of the presynaptic serotonin reuptake pump. Of 19 studies examining the effect of SSRIs on pain, 12 found that SSRIs provide clinically important pain relief [34]. When SSRIs were compared to TCAs, the latter were shown to be superior to analgesics in four out of six trials.

Although SSRIs have fewer side effects than the older antidepressants, they may still cause some undesirable symptoms. Possible CNS effects include headaches, stimulation or sedation, fine tremor, and akathisia. Gastrointestinal effects include nausea, vomiting, anorexia, bloating, and diarrhea. Additionally, other serotonergic drugs should be avoided or used with caution given the possibility of causing serotonergic syndrome. Approximately 10–15% of patients taking an SSRI will experience sexual side effects of decreased libido, impotence, ejaculatory disturbances, and anorgasmia.

Selective serotonin and norepinephrine reuptake inhibitors

The SSRIs and SNRIs are among the newest class of antidepressants, and their ability to reduce pain in various neuropathic syndromes has also been examined. Potential analgesia is suggested by its profile of dual inhibition of serotonin and norepinephrine reuptake that is similar to proven analgesic antidepressants such as imipramine, amitriptyline, and desipramine.

Duloxetine (Cymbalta) is an SNRI that is currently FDA approved for depression and neuropathic pain. Several double-blinded, placebo-controlled RCTs of duloxetine have shown improvement of major depressive disorders and also demonstrated improvement of visual analog scale ratings of physical symptoms associated with depression including reductions in overall pain and back pain [35–37].

Venlafaxine (Effexor)is another SNRI with some evidence of efficacy in the treatment of chronic pain. Several studies evaluated venlafaxine for neuropathic pain conditions. In a comparison of venlafaxine to imipramine, patients with neuropathic pain had improvement of symptoms with either medication compared with placebo, though the NNT for venlafaxine (5.2) was higher than for imipramine (2.7) [38, 39].

The side effect profile of these agents is similar to SSRIs, including nausea, headache, somnolence, dry mouth, dizziness, nervousness, constipation, anxiety, anorexia, blurred vision, and sexual dysfunction.

Serotonin-2 antagonist reuptake inhibitor

Trazadone (Desyrel) is an SARI by virtue of blocking serotonin-2 receptors as well as serotonin reuptake. This agent was first marketed as an antidepressant, but is used primarily for insomnia now, due to its sedating effect. Its usefulness in the treatment of chronic pain is undetermined but given the incidence of insomnia in patients with chronic pain, it may offer at least an adjuvant role.

Norepinephrine dopamine reuptake inhibitors

Other classes of antidepressants have been developed to target specific neurotransmitter interactions at the synaptic level. These classes of antidepressants maximize therapeutic benefits while minimizing side effects. Metabolism of NDRIs, e.g., bupropion

(Wellbutrin) produces hydroxybupropion, an inhibitor of both noradrenergic and dopamine pumps. This agent differs from most other antidepressants in that it has psychostimulant properties. There have been no RCTs of its efficacy in the treatment of chronic pain; however, its stimulating properties offer advantages in treating depression in patients on sedating drugs such as opioids.

Antiepileptic/mood stabilizers

The classic anticonvulsant agents phenytoin and carbamazepine have been used in the treatment of neuropathic pain since the 1960s. Anticonvulsants are thought to inhibit seizures by multiple mechanisms, including functional blockade of voltage-gated sodium channels, functional blockade of voltage-gated calcium channels, direct or indirect enhancement of inhibitory GABAergic neurotransmission, and inhibition of glutamatergic neurotransmission [40]. The result is that they reduce the neuronal hyperexcitability that is fundamental to seizure disorders.

Because neuropathic pain, and perhaps other chronic pain states, is also characterized by neuronal hyperexcitability [41], clinicians and researchers have reasoned that anticonvulsants might alleviate it through similar mechanisms of action. This supposition is supported by a substantial amount of empirical data on the clinical effectiveness of anticonvulsants in neuropathic pain, as well as multiple studies that have been the subject of recent systematic reviews [42, 43].

Unfortunately, the side effect profile of many of the antiepileptics preclude their routine use in the treatment of chronic low back pain with radiculopathy. The clinical usefulness of carbamazepine is limited by significant side effects such as Steven-Johnson syndrome, agraulocytosis, aplastic anemia, and hepatic toxicity. Similarly, phenytoin is infrequently used for chronic pain secondary to adverse reactions and toxicity. One study attempted to evaluate topiramate's role in treating chronic low back pain and had a substantial drop out rate (26%) due to intolerable side effects [44]. Other antiepileptics such as valproic acid, felbamate, and zonigran lack both FDA approval and any meaningful clinical evidence supporting their usage for the treatment of chronic low back pain or neuropathic pain.

Antiepileptic medications with a more favorable side effect profile include gabapentin (Neurontin) and pregabalin (Lyrica) and both are currently used in the treatment of chronic low back pain with and without radiculopathy.

Gabapentin is a α-2-delta subunit voltage-gated calcium-channel antagonist, that has repeatedly demonstrated analgesic efficacy and improvements in mood and sleep in several randomized controlled trials [45, 46]. Similarly, pregabalin, a gabapentin analogue with a similar mechanism, higher calcium-channel affinity and better bioavailability has also been shown to be effective in several RCTs in peripheral neuropathy and post-herpetic neuralgia [46]. Other anticonvulsants, including valproate, and lamotrigine have had equivocal results [46].

The side effect profile of these agents include dizziness, somnolence, peripheral edema, weight gain, ataxia, and vertigo. Although several antiepileptic medications are frequently used in the treatment of chronic low backpain, particularly in the presence of an associated radiculopathy, there is limited high quality evidence directly evaluating their efficacy at the present time.

Anxiolytics

Anxiety disorders may occur in a large percentage of patients with chronic pain. These disorders include panic disorder, generalized anxiety disorder, obsessive compulsive disorder, and post-traumatic stress disorder. These disorders often present with somatic symptoms including chest pain, gastrointestinal disturbances, and neurologic symptoms such as headache, dizziness, syncope, and paresthesias. Treatment of chronic pain that is co-morbid with an anxiety disorder may include anxiolytics as part of the analgesic strategy.

Benzodiazepines depress the CNS at the level of the limbic system, brain stem reticular activating system, and the cortex by binding to and facilitating the action of γ-aminobutyric acid (GABA) as a primary inhibitory neurotransmitter. Although not primary analgesics, benzodiazepines often have a role in the overall analgesic strategy.

In a recent review published in the *Annals of Internal Medicine* [47], for the treatment of acute low back pain, one higher-quality trial found no differences between diazepam and placebo, but another, lower-quality trial found diazepam superior for short-term pain relief and overall improvement. In the treatment of chronic low back pain, pooled results from a lower quality, placebo-controlled trial of diazepam for chronic low back pain found no clinical benefit.

The most common side effects of benzodiazepines are sedation and respiratory depression.

Rapid withdrawal from benzodiazepines can result in rebound insomnia, anxiety, delirium, psychosis, and seizures. Dosages should be discontinued by a gradual taper.

Although the evidence supporting the use of psychopharmacologic adjunctive agents for chronic pain is limited, it appears reasonable to use low dose TCAs in mild to moderately painful radicular syndromes after acetaminophen and NSAIDs have been tried. In younger patients, amitriptyline may be the medication of choice; if side effects become prominent and intolerable, other TCAs such as nortriptyline may be considered.

After those medications have been considered, antiepileptics such as gabapentin can also be used. This medication requires titration of dosing with constant vigilance for side effects. If the above fails, SNRIs and newer generation antiepileptics can be considered. If chosen appropriately, psychopharmacologic adjunctive analgesics can play an important role in the treatment of spinal pain disorders.

Treatment algorithms

Treatments with the lowest risk of adverse effects should be tried first. Studies of chronic pain management suggest that a combination of psychological, pharmacological, and physical therapies, tailored to the needs of the individual patient, may be the best approach [48]. Evidence supporting conservative non-pharmacologic treatments (e.g., physiotherapy, exercise, transcutaneous electrical nerve stimulation, CBT, acupuncture) is limited but growing and given their presumed safety, non-pharmacologic treatments should be considered whenever appropriate. Additionally, early referrals to a pain clinic for nerve blocks or other interventional therapy may be warranted in some cases to facilitate physiotherapy and pain rehabilitation.

Needless to say, spinal pain is best managed with a multidisciplinary approach, however, several different treatments can be initiated in the primary care setting (Table 17.3) and a simplified treatment algorithm is outline below.

Despite the previously noted treatment limitations, it is important to remember that even a 30% pain reduction is clinically important to patients [49]. Other than analgesia, factors to consider when individualizing therapy include tolerability, other benefits (e.g., improved sleep, mood and quality of life), low likelihood of serious adverse events and cost-effectiveness to the patient and the healthcare system.

Table 17.3 Algorithm for the management of chronic spinal pain

Step 1		Pain assessment, history and physical examination, obtain release of information to review previous diagnostic studies and treatment records	
Step 2		Consider non-pharmacologic modalities (physiotherapies, psychological interventions such as cognitive behavioral therapy, bio/neuro-feedback, or early referral for nerve blocks in some cases to facilitate rehabilitation.	
Step 3		Initiate conservative medical management (acetaminophen, NSAIDs, skeletal muscle relaxants, topical analgesics)	
Step 4		Initiate first-line monotherapy (gabapentin or pregabalin *or* tricyclic antidepressant (TCA) or serotonin-norepinephrine reuptake inhibitor (SNRI),	
	Response	*Ineffective or not tolerated*	*Partial treatment response*
Step 5		Switch to alternative first-line drug monotherapy (TCA or SNRI *or* gabapentin or pregabalin)	Consider adding first-line drug (TCA or SNRI *or* gabapentin or pregabalin)
	Response	*Ineffective or not tolerated*	*Partial treatment response*
Step 6		Initiate monotherapy with tramadol or opioid analgesic Consider use of opioid risk screening tool, medication management agreement and informed consent	Consider adding tramadol or opioid analgesic Consider use of opioid risk screening tool, medication management agreement and informed consent
	Response	*Ineffective or not tolerated*	
Step 6		Refer patient to pain specialty clinic for consideration of third-line drugs, interventional treatments and pain rehabilitation programs	

Note. TCA: tricyclic antidepressant; SNRI: serotonin-norepinephrine reuptake inhibitor.

Although little is known about whether the response to one drug predicts the response to another, combining different drugs may result in improved results at lower doses and with fewer side effects. However, if the first oral medication tried is ineffective or not tolerated, one might switch to alternate monotherapy. In the event that all of the first-line oral mono-therapies tried are ineffective or poorly tolerated, we would then recommend initiating monotherapy with tramadol or an opioid analgesic.

Many patients with spinal pain currently receive drug combinations [50], often in the absence of supportive evidence. Nevertheless, clinical experience suggests that poly-pharmacy may be helpful. For example, in a recent RCT, analgesia with a morphine–gabapentin combination was found to be superior to treatment with either drug alone [51]. Therefore, in the event of a partial response to any single drug, one could add an alternate drug. Future trials are needed to evaluate optimal drug combinations and dose ratios as well as safety, compliance, and cost-effectiveness. If none of the above treatments is effective or tolerated, referral to a pain clinic is warranted for consideration of third-line drugs, interventional treatments and pain rehabilitation programs.

Conclusion

Pain syndromes of spinal origin remain a clinical challenge for effective treatment. Any medication used to treat chronic pain syndromes must be weighed for benefits and risks before using. It may take several trials to find an effective therapeutic modality, medication or combination of medications. Patients may need support throughout the process. Effective pain treatment often requires a combination of physical, psychosocial, pharmacologic and non-pharmacologic modalities in order to achieve adequate pain relief. Currently available therapies clearly show varying degrees of clinical efficacy, but it is hoped that future advances in this active field of investigation will further expand the clinicians' armamentarium of treatments for this challenging pain syndrome.

References

1. Hart LG, Deyo RA, Cherkin DC. Physician office visits for low back pain. Frequency, clinical evaluation, and treatment patterns from a U.S. national survey. *Spine* 1995; **20**: 11–19.

2. Hardt J, Jacobsen C, Goldberg J, Nickel R, Buchwald D. Prevalence of chronic pain in a representative sample in the United States. *Pain Med* 2008; **9**: 803–12.

3. Strine TW, Hootman, JM. US national prevalence and correlates of low back and neck pain among adults. *Arthritis Rheum* 2007; **57**: 656–65.

4. Andersson GB. Epidemiological features of chronic low-back pain. *Lancet*, 1999; **354**: 581–5.

5. Deyo RA, Weinstein JN. Low back pain. *N Engl J Med* 2001; **344**: 363–70.

6. Hestbaek L, Leboeuf-Yde C, Manniche C. Low back pain: what is the long-term course? A review of studies of general patient populations. *Eur Spine J* 2003; **12**: 149–65.

7. Deyo RA, Phillips WR. Low back pain. A primary care challenge. *Spine* 1996; **21**: 2826–32.

8. Baron R. Peripheral neuropathic pain: from mechanisms to symptoms. *Clin J Pain* 2000; **16**(2 Suppl): S12–20.

9. Besson JM. The neurobiology of pain. *Lancet* 1999; **353**: 1610–5.

10. Pace MC, Mazzariello L, Passavanti MB, *et al.* Neurobiology of pain. *J Cell Physiol* 2006; **209**: 8–12.

11. Pasero C. Pathophysiology of neuropathic pain. *Pain Manag Nurs*, 2004. **5**(4 Suppl 1): 3–8.

12. Waxman SG. Neurobiology: a channel sets the gain on pain. *Nature* 2006; **444**: 831–2.

13. Wilson JA, Garry EM, Anderson HA, *et al.* NMDA receptor antagonist treatment at the time of nerve injury prevents injury-induced changes in spinal NR1 and NR2B subunit expression and increases the sensitivity of residual pain behaviours to subsequently administered NMDA receptor antagonists. *Pain* 2005; **117**: 421–32.

14. Ultenius C, Linderoth B, Meyerson BA, Wallin J. Spinal NMDA receptor phosphorylation correlates with the presence of neuropathic signs following peripheral nerve injury in the rat. *Neurosci Lett* 2006; **399**: 85–90.

15. Waxman SG, Cummins TR, Dib-Hajj SD, Black JA. Voltage-gated sodium channels and the molecular pathogenesis of pain: a review. *J Rehabil Res Dev* 2000; **37**: 517–28.

16. Matthews EA, Bee LA, Stephens GJ, Dickenson AH. The Cav2.3 calcium channel antagonist SNX-482 reduces dorsal horn neuronal responses in a rat model of chronic neuropathic pain. *Eur J Neurosci* 2007; **25**: 3561–9.

17. Cummins TR, Sheets PL, Waxman SG. The roles of sodium channels in nociception: Implications for mechanisms of pain. *Pain* 2007; **131**: 243–57.

18. Tegeder I, Costigan M, Griffin RS, *et al.* GTP cyclohydrolase and tetrahydrobiopterin regulate pain sensitivity and persistence. *Nat Med* 2006; **12**: 1269–77.

19. Chou R, Qaseem A, Snow V, *et al.* Diagnosis and treatment of low back pain: a joint clinical practice guideline from the American College of Physicians and the American Pain Society. *Ann Intern Med* 2007; **147**: 478–91.

20. Bennett MI, Attal N, Backonja MM, *et al.* Using screening tools to identify neuropathic pain. *Pain* 2007; **127**: 199–203.

21. Gatchel RJ, Okifuji A. Evidence-based scientific data documenting the treatment and cost-effectiveness of comprehensive pain programs for chronic nonmalignant pain. *J Pain* 2006; **7**: 779–93.

22. Morley S, Keefe FJ. Getting a handle on process and change in CBT for chronic pain. *Pain* 2007; **127**: 197–8.

23. Moore JE, Von Korff M, Cherkin D, Saunders K, Lorig K. A randomized trial of a cognitive-behavioral program for enhancing back pain self care in a primary care setting. *Pain* 2000; **88**: 145–53.

24. Morley S, Eccleston C, Williams A. Systematic review and meta-analysis of randomized controlled trials of cognitive behaviour therapy and behaviour therapy for chronic pain in adults, excluding headache. *Pain* 1999; **80**: 1–13.

25. Hoffman BM, Papas RK, Chatkoff DK, Kerns RD. Meta-analysis of psychological interventions for chronic low back pain. *Health Psychol* 2007; **26**: 1–9.

26. Brox JI, Sorensen R, Friis A, *et al.* Randomized clinical trial of lumbar instrumented fusion and cognitive intervention and exercises in patients with chronic low back pain and disc degeneration. *Spine* 2003; **28**: 1913–21.

27. Brox JI, Reikeras O, Nygaard O, *et al.* Lumbar instrumented fusion compared with cognitive intervention and exercises in patients with chronic back pain after previous surgery for disc herniation: a prospective randomized controlled study. *Pain* 2006; **122**: 145–55.

28. Portenoy RK, Rapscak S, Kanner R. Tricyclic antidepressants in chronic pain. *Pain* 1984; **18**: 213–5.

29. Sindrup SH, Otto M, Finnerup NB, Jensen TS. Antidepressants in the treatment of neuropathic pain. *Basic Clin Pharmacol Toxicol* 2005; **96**: 399–409.

30. Finnerup NB, Otto M, McQuay HJ, Jensen TS, Sindrup SH. Algorithm for neuropathic pain treatment: an evidence based proposal. *Pain* 2005; **118**: 289–305.

31. McQuay HJ, Tramer M, Nye B A, *et al.* A systematic review of antidepressants in neuropathic pain. *Pain* 1996; **68**: 217–27.

32. McQuay HJ. Neuropathic pain: evidence matters. *Eur J Pain*, 2002; **6** Suppl A: 11–8.

33. Sindrup SH, Jensen TS. Pharmacologic treatment of pain in polyneuropathy. *Neurology* 2000; **55**: 915–20.

34. Jung AC, Staiger T, Sullivan M. The efficacy of selective serotonin reuptake inhibitors for the management of chronic pain. *J Gen Intern Med* 1997; **12**: 384–9.

35. Mallinckrodt CH, Goldstein DJ, Detke MJ, *et al.* Duloxetine: A new treatment for the emotional and physical symptoms of depression. *Prim Care Companion J Clin Psychiatry* 2003; **5**: 19–28.

36. Goldstein DJ, Lu Y, Detke MJ, *et al.* Effects of duloxetine on painful physical symptoms associated with depression. *Psychosomatics* 2004; **45**: 17–28.

37. Detke MJ, Lu Y, Goldstein DJ, McNamara RK, Demitrack MA. Duloxetine 60 mg once daily dosing versus placebo in the acute treatment of major depression. *J Psychiatr Res* 2002; **36**: 383–90.

38. Tasmuth T, Hartel B, Kalso E. Venlafaxine in neuropathic pain following treatment of breast cancer. *Eur J Pain* 2002; **6**: 17–24.

39. Yucel A, Ozyalcin S, Koknel Talu G, *et al.* The effect of venlafaxine on ongoing and experimentally induced pain in neuropathic pain patients: a double blind, placebo controlled study. *Eur J Pain* 2005; **9**: 407–16.

40. Challapalli, V, Tremont-Lukats, IW, McNicol, ED, Lau, J, Carr, DB. Systemic administration of local anesthetic agents to relieve neuropathic pain. *Cochrane Database Syst Rev* 2005: CD003345.

41. Artus, M, Croft, P, Lewis, M. The use of CAM and conventional treatments among primary care consulters with chronic musculoskeletal pain. *BMC Fam Pract* 2007; **8**: 26.

42. Dworkin, RH, O' Connor, AB, Backonja, M, *et al.* Pharmacologic management of neuropathic pain: evidence-based recommendations. *Pain* 2007; **132**: 237–51.

43. Stacey, BR, Management of peripheral neuropathic pain. *Am J Phys Med Rehabil* 2005; **84**(3 Suppl): S4–16.

44. Khoromi, S, Patsalides, A, Parada, S, *et al.* Topiramate in chronic lumbar radicular pain. *J Pain* 2005; **6**: 829–36.

45. Gilron, I. Gabapentin and pregabalin for chronic neuropathic and early postsurgical pain: current evidence and future directions. *Curr Opin Anaesthesiol* 2007; **20**: 456–72.

46. Finnerup, NB, Otto, M, Jensen, TS, Sindrup, SH. An evidence-based algorithm for the treatment of neuropathic pain. *MedGenMed* 2007; **9**: 36.

47. Chou R, Huffman LH. Medications for acute and chronic low back pain: a review of the evidence for an American Pain Society/American College of Physicians clinical practice guideline. *Ann Intern Med* 2007; **147**: 505–14.

48. Turk DC, Swanson KS, Tunks ER. Psychological approaches in the treatment of chronic pain patients – when pills, scalpels, and needles are not enough. *Can J Psychiatry* 2008; **53**: 213–23.

49. Farrar JT, Young Jr JP, LaMoreaux L, Werth JL, Poole RM. Clinical importance of changes in chronic pain intensity measured on an 11-point numerical pain rating scale. *Pain* 2001. **94**: 149–58.

50. Gilron I, Bailey JM. Trends in opioid use for chronic neuropathic pain: a survey of patients pursuing enrollment in clinical trials. *Can J Anaesth*, 2003; **50**: 42–7.

51. Gilron I, Bailey JM, Tu D, *et al.* Morphine, gabapentin, or their combination for neuropathic pain. *N Engl J Med*, 2005; **352**: 1324–34.

Management of musculoskeletal pain

Akiko Okifuji and Bradford D. Hare

Fibromyalgia syndrome is a chronic, musculoskeletal pain disorder that is characterized by diffuse body pain and heightened hyperalgesia. It is typically associated with a range of functional and psychological disturbances, such as chronic fatigue, non-restorative sleep, cognitive slowness, headaches, functional bowel disorder, paresthesia, stiffness, anxiety, and depression [1]. Fibromyalgia syndrome symptoms are common, with estimated prevalence ranging from 0.7% to 11% [2–6]. The National Arthritis Data Working group has recently estimated that up to 5 million Americans suffer from this condition [7].

History of fibromyalgia syndrome

Fibromyalgia syndrome is not a new illness of the post-modern era. The first published description of FMS appeared in the mid 1800s in Germany. A cluster of FMS-like symptoms were collectively labeled as "Muskelschwiele" (muscle callus), which was considered as exquisite muscle tenderness associated with rheumatism [8]. In the early 1900s, Stockman described patients whose primary complaints consisted of hyperalgesia to pressure and worsening of pain in response to physical activities, and he considered the condition to be "muscular rheumatism" [9]. Around the same time, a more familiar term, "fibrositis" was introduced by an English physician, Gowers, to define the disorder as an inflammatory disorder in the connective tissues [10]. Unfortunately, as we will describe later, this term did not do much to help advance the field. The assumed inflammatory process was never confirmed and the term became a trash can category of chronic pain taxonomy. It took an additional 80 years before the field accepted a more etiologically neutral term and fibromyalgia was introduced, literally meaning pain in the muscles, tendons, and ligaments [11].

Studies of FMS during the first part of the 1900s, as reviewed by Valentine, were mostly small experiments and clinical notes, with mostly inconsistent and conflicting results [12]. A major difficulty stemmed from the absence of demonstrative pathology, either laboratory or imaging based, that could serve as a gold standard to define FMS. Also problematic was the lack of precision in clinically describing the phenomenon. The obtuse applications of various terms to describe FMS resulted in the inclusion of a heterogeneous group of pain phenomena. These problems seriously undermined the scientific understanding of the disorder and development of therapy approaches.

By mid century, the term fibrositis had become more of a wastebasket term that included all sorts of multi-symptom functional complaints. Anyone with pain and fatigue for which no objective confirmation could be obtained was given this diagnosis. In turn, outcomes from treatment approaches that were applied to such a heterogeneous group of patients yielded conflicting results and the lack of consistency in diagnosis prevented any appreciative research advancement. A standardized means to classify the condition was desperately needed.

The first classification criteria were developed by Kraft and his associates [13]. The criteria consisted of a "jump sign" (a behaviorally exaggerated flinching response to pressure), vasomotor instability of affected regions, delayed analgesic response to deep, aching pain, and what they referred as "fibrositic nodules," a ropey consistency of affected muscles. However, the clinical validity of these criteria was never established, and their adaptation was limited. The systematic attempts to delineate relevant factors and consistent use of the same criteria were sorely needed to advance the understanding of the phenomenon.

In 1972, Smythe took an approach to define the syndrome as a disorder of diffuse pain and stiffness,

Behavioral and Psychopharmacologic Pain Management, ed. Michael H. Ebert and Robert D. Kerns. Published by Cambridge University Press. © Cambridge University Press 2011.

Table 18.1 History of fibromyalgia syndrome classification criteria

Smythe 1972[a]. Diagnostic criteria from the clinical studies
Obligatory criteria
1. Subjective aching of 3 months or longer
2. Subjective stiffness of 3 months or longer
3. Local point tenderness
4. Point tenderness in 2 other sites
5. Normal ESR, SGOT, rheumatoid factor, ANF, muscle enzymes and sacroiliac films
Minor criteria
1. Chronic fatigue
2. Emotional distress
3. Poor sleep
4. Morning stiffness
Smythe 1979[b]
History of widespread pain of 3 months or longer
Tenderness at 12 of 14 specified sites
Disturbed sleep with morning fatigue and stiffness
Normal ESR, SGOT, rheumatoid factor, ANF, muscle enzymes and sacroiliac films.
Yunus criteria 1989
Diagnosis of primary fibromyalgia syndrome requires major or minor criteria plus obligatory criteria.
Obligatory criteria
1. Presence of pain or stiffness or both, at 4 or more anatomic sites for 3 months or longer
2. Exclusion of an underlying condition which may be responsible for the overall features of fibromyalgia
Major criteria
Presence of 2 or more of 6 historical variables, plus 4 or more of 14 specified tender points.
Minor criteria
Presence of 3 or more of the 6 historical variables, plus 2 or more tender points

Sources. [a] Ref [14]; [b] Ref. [184].

focusing primarily upon the typical clinical presentations of FMS [14]. In addition to diffuse pain and stiffness, the criteria noted that the symptoms often start following a minor injury and included generalized hyperalgesia, sleep disturbance with morning fatigue and stiffness (see Table 18.1). Additionally, the criteria introduced some exclusion criteria to help distinguish FMS from other rheumatologic conditions.

A decade later, Yunus *et al.* extended the Smythe's criteria into a more elaborate set of diagnostic criteria based upon the comparisons of 63 FMS patients to 32 patients with rheumatoid arthritis and 30 healthy people (see Table 18.1) [15]. These criteria yielded over 90% sensitivity and specificity. Thus, the classification criteria for FMS were rapidly evolving in the 1970s and 1980s. The clinically based classification criteria stimulated a proliferation of FMS research. Unfortunately these studies used criteria inconsistently, and it was difficult to ascertain if the findings from one study would be applicable to others [16].

In order to move towards more systematic, empirically driven criteria to classify FMS, a multicenter study was launched in the late 1980s, involving approximately 300 patients with FMS and 285 control subjects [1]. The essential point of this study was to delineate factors that could, with good sensitivity and specificity, differentiate FMS patients from people with other chronic pain conditions. Of course, trying to determine the eligibility of study patients to define the very disorder those patients were afflicted with presented a problem of circular logic. The multicenter study dealt with this by defining the 300 FMS patients by the "usual" method that each participating clinician had been using [1]. Based upon the results, the American College of Rheumatology (ACR) criteria were suggested; FMS patients should present (1) a history of widespread pain of 3 months or longer, and (2) presence of pain responses to at least 11 of 18 designated tender points (TPs). The locations of the TPs are described in Table 18.2 and drawn in Figure 18.1.

The validity of the ACR criteria, just like the validity of the previously recommended criteria, is difficult to evaluate due to the absence of an absolute "gold standard" for diagnosing FMS, and this leads to the logical cul-de-sac. The diagnosis is further complicated by the fact that FMS frequently co-occurs with other functional disorders that also are characterized by the symptoms commonly associated with FMS, such as fatigue, sleep disorder, and mood disturbance. Furthermore, since these problems are also common in other chronic pain conditions, they did not show enough discriminating power to be included into the ACR classification criteria. But this exclusion of common clinical complaints has made many wonder how valid the ACR criteria really are [17, 18]. It is generally granted that the ACR criteria were developed to improve consistency in defining the study population. Nevertheless, it is disconcerting that many clinicians do not use the ACR

Table 18.2 American College of Rheumatology criteria for classification of FMS

1. Presence of widespread pain for at least 3 months. Pain must be present in all of the body quadrants and axial skeletal area.
2. Presence of pain in at least 11 of 18 tender points on digital palpation with approximately 4 kg force. Tender points are located in 9 bilateral sites as described below:

Occiput: at the suboccipital muscle insertions.

Low cervical: at the anterior aspects of the intertransverse spaces at C5–C7.

Trapezius: at the midpoint of the upper boarder.

Supraspinatus: at origins, above the scapula spine near the medial boarder.

Second rib: at the second costochondral junctions, just lateral to the junctions on upper surfaces.

Lateral epicondyle: at 2 cm distal to the epicondyles.

Gluteal: in upper outer quadrants of buttocks in anterior fold of muscle.

Greater trochanter: posterior to the trochanteric prominence.

Knee: at the medial fat proximal to the joint line.

Adapted from Wolfe et al. 1990.

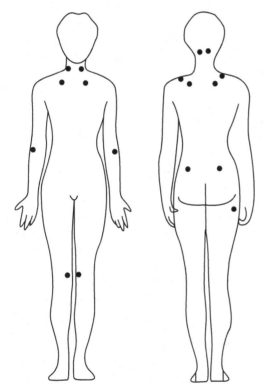

Figure 18.1 American College of Rheumatology designated tender points.

criteria to diagnose FMS [19] and makes one wonder about the external validity of research findings. The concordance between FMS classification by the ACR criteria and clinical diagnosis is only modest (kappa= 0.5) [20]. There are not many disease entities showing such discrepancy in the diagnostic approach between research and clinical practices.

To add to the confusion, the issues of what the TP criterion actually is have not been resolved. There are a large number of individuals who report chronic widespread pain (CWP) who do not qualify as FMS patients because they do not have 11 specific painful tender points; these people too suffer from various functional and affective disorders [18]. It is not clear whether FMS and CWP without TPs are distinct from one another or related in some ways. It is possible that the presence of multiple painful TPs reflects underlying dysfunction of nociception of provoked pain responses. However, the number of painful TPs is only moderately correlated with clinical pain report [21] yet TPs are generally related to the indices of psychological distress [22, 23]. These findings lead us back to the basic unanswered question of what TPs are from the pathophysiological and phenomenological perspectives.

For now, however, the ACR criteria have provided a research tool to identify cases of FMS, and the majority of the published reports on FMS specify their subjects with the ACR criteria, thereby making the integration of knowledge across published reports possible. The significance of the contribution of the ACR criteria to FMS research is apparent. While the clinical diagnosis of FMS still relies largely upon clinical presentations of the symptoms, patients can now at least be identified as ACR-criteria positive or negative.

Cost of FMS

Fibromyalgia syndrome is not lethal or progressive. However, the condition is debilitating and patients with FMS report severely compromised quality of life (QOL). These patients tend to report a lowered sense of physical well-being; indeed, they are concerned about their health [24] and tend to overuse the healthcare resources [25, 26]. When FMS coexists with other chronic illness, such as systemic lupus, FMS adds significantly to the overall disability [27]. When directly assessed, the QOL of FMS patients is significantly poorer than that of patients with other chronic illnesses.

Functional disability

One of the prominent features associated with low QOL in FMS is functional disability. Some have shown that functional disability associated with FMS may be comparative to other chronic illness, such as rheumatoid arthritis [28] and spondyloarthropathy [29]. Others have demonstrated that FMS patients report a greater degree of disability as compared to people with chronic physical problems such as spinal cord injury [30].

Relatively little is known about the factors contributing to the decline in functional ability in FMS patients. Mood disturbance, such as depression and anxiety, is significantly related to self-reported disability [31–33]. Lifestyle of patients may also impact the self-evaluation of their disability. Non-smoking FMS patients report a lower degree of functional disability than FMS patients who are smokers [25]. Obesity in FMS may be related to the sedentary lifestyle, and may also be associated with self-reported disability [34] and actual physical ability in FMS [35]. However, as will be discussed later, subjective disability may not necessarily correspond with objective findings in FMS. Furthermore, despite the general assumption that the illness severity should be the primary determinant of disability, self-reported disability seems fairly independent of disease severity [36].

Exercise intolerance is also frequently noted for FMS patients. At times this creates a clinical challenge when a treatment plan includes activating physical therapy. Research investigating the baseline level of physical conditioning for FMS patients, however, has yielded conflicting results. Some studies showed a below average level of aerobic conditioning in the majority of FMS patients [37], whereas others reported that FMS patients' aerobic capacity did not differ from age-matched healthy individuals, even though FMS patients consistently rated the exercise as more demanding [38]. Research shows much greater consistency with muscle strength; FMS patients exhibit a significantly lower degree of muscle strength and

endurance than do healthy people [39] and chronic myofascial pain patients [40]. Yet, surface electromyographic activity during isokinetic tasks reveals no specific abnormality in the fatigue mechanisms in muscles of FMS patients [41].

Healthcare utilization

Fibromyalgia syndrome is a costly illness. The first multicenter study on the healthcare utilization of FMS patients was conducted in seven healthcare centers [42]. On average, FMS patients had one hospitalization every 3 years and approximately 10 outpatient visits per year. The mean annual cost for outpatient care, medication costs, and hospitalization in 1996 US dollars was $2274. In Canada, FMS patients reported to have had seven physician visits in the 6 months [43]. Another study also estimated seven physician visits per 6 months and seven additional visits to non-physician, alternative therapy visits per 6 months [44]. Medical costs for FMS exceed the costs for osteoarthritis patients, another very common chronic pain [45].

The results from the present study suggest that the healthcare cost for FMS may be rapidly climbing. Based upon the claim data of the Fortune 100 manufacturers, the annual medical, pharmaceutical, and work-loss costs were compared between FMS claimants and randomly selected control claimants [46]. The comparisons revealed that the cost for the FMS claimants were substantially greater ($5945–7776) than that of the control claimants ($2486) per year.

Work disability

Given the persisting symptoms such as fatigue, pain and poor sleep affecting day-to-day functioning of individuals, it should perhaps not be surprising that many FMS patients find it difficult to maintain their productivity at the workplace. It has been estimated that approximately 35% of FMS patients and over 50% of FMS patients with concurrent chronic fatigue syndrome are unable to maintain gainful employment due to their illness [25].

A small study also found that 30% of their patients, mostly in their 40s, had to reduce their work hours and 65% faced a reduction in their family income [28]. Similarly, it has recently been estimated that about a half of FMS patients may eventually lose their jobs due to the hardship associated with the illness [47]. Even for those who maintain the employment, typically working hours are reduced by 25%.

This is not to say that all FMS patients willingly terminate their employment. The results from narrative interviews indicate that FMS patients regard a work role as an important part of their self-image, and the loss of work, therefore, often results in a compromised self-image [48]. The interviews also revealed that the physical aspects of the work environment, such as physical demands of work, requirement for exertion and freedom to move around become critical determinants when they evaluate their ability to stay in the workforce. Moreover, the availability of psychosocial support at work seems essential. Many FMS patients feel that others do not understand their pain and suffering that stems from their "invisible" illness. The lack of acceptance for their frequent medical leaves also seems to adversely impact their sense of well-being at work.

The presence and extent of various co-morbid conditions may also influence their ability to stay being employed. Work-disabled FMS patients, relative to working FMS patients, report greater fatigue, irritability and gastrointestinal discomfort, despite their comparable demographics and pain histories [49].

Compensation issues

The inability to sustain a gainful work status may lead FMS patients to seek disability compensation. The prevalence of financial compensation for FMS patients is hard to determine for several reasons. The decision to award compensation is based not very much on the clinical factors but more on political and economical factors. Thus large regional variations are present and the logic behind such variations is not always easily understood. In addition, the complexity of FMS symptoms makes it very difficult to determine whether a person is receiving the compensation for their pain or psychiatric condition. Thus study results need to be evaluated with these points in mind.

In one small study, 55% of their FMS sample were receiving disability compensation, either temporary or permanent [28]. In the multicenter study, 15% of the study patients were receiving social security disability benefit and an additional 10% were receiving other types of financial compensation for their disability [50].

Some FMS patients report that their symptoms began following an injury. There is some evidence that FMS with injurious onset may be associated with greater symptom severity than FMS with insidious onset [51]. The role of litigation, in terms of the financial incentives worsening symptoms of disability,

has been of considerable interest. However, the self-reported disability was still greater with the injurious onset FMS even after the compensation status was statistically controlled. Similarly, the resolution of litigation for post-accident FMS does not seem to improve FMS symptoms [52].

Pathophysiology

Muscles

Despite the early abnormal biopsy finding in the affected muscles in FMS [53], it is generally agreed upon that the diffuse nature of FMS symptoms points more to a central model than to a peripheral hypothesis of FMS pathophysiology. Research has failed to support any electrodiagnostic evidence of ongoing denervation [54] or increased muscle sympathetic nerve discharge [55] in FMS. By and large, there is no microscopic evidence of definitive pathology in the muscle tissues of FMS patients [56].

However, peripheral abnormality in muscles may still play some, albeit limited, role in FMS. For example, localized hypoxia [38] and metabolic abnormality [57] in the affected areas may be observed in FMS patients. The P-31 magnetic resonance spectroscopic analysis of muscles may show significantly lower levels of ATP and phosphocreatine (PCr) levels in FMS [58]. Below normal levels of ATP and PCr suggest the presence of weakness and fatigability, possibly associated with metabolic dysfunction of the muscle. Conditions that may contribute to the peripheral abnormality include physical deconditioning, abnormalities in phospholipids, focal muscle contraction and ischemia [59].

A concept of "tension myalgia" was introduced under which various musculoskeletal pain disorders (e.g., FMS, myofascial pain) could be described [60]. In this model, abnormal muscle tension due to several possible reasons (e.g., overuse, poor posture, spasm, emotional stress) significantly contributes to the development and maintenance of chronic musculoskeletal pain. The term also implies the presence of persistently elevated muscle tension, leading to the notion that FMS patients may suffer from diffuse and generalized muscle tension. However, FMS patients do not differ from healthy people in the resting levels of surface electromyographic (EMG) values [54, 61] or even show decreased tension levels [62, 63].

Alternatively, pain may result from a phasic increase in muscle tension in response to acute stressors ("stress-tension hyperactivity-pain" model). Note that this model requires that two conditions be met consecutively; first, stress must increase tension and then tension must increase pain. There is some evidence for the first link. Increase in EMG values in response to experimentally induced stress has repeatedly shown in patients with chronic pain disorders such as back pain, temporomandibular pain, and headaches [64]. However, FMS patients seem to show rather heterogeneous psychophysiological patterns in response to stress [63]. Furthermore, there is no reliable evidence that increased tension leads to increased pain, and the validity of this model in the pathophysiology of pain has been questioned. Interestingly, however, FMS patients commonly cite that stress is a major aggravating factor for their pain [65]. The mechanisms underlying this relationship, and whether muscle tension plays a role, are yet to be clarified.

Sleep

The complaint of non-restorative sleep is common in FMS. Experimental studies have shown that FMS-like symptoms develop following repeated deprivation of stage IV sleep [66, 67]. Electrocephalographic (EEG) data showing the presence of alpha wave intrusion during the delta wave sleep has spurred the hypothesis that perhaps FMS is primarily a sleep disorder [68]. However, subsequent research failed to confirm that the alpha intrusion is a universal phenomenon in FMS; approximately a third of FMS patients seem to experience this abnormality [69].

The interruption in Stage IV sleep may also disrupt the production of growth hormone, which is essential for muscle homeostasis and repair. A diminished level of IGF-1, production of which is stimulated by growth hormone, has been observed in many patients in some studies [70] but not all [71].

Psychological disturbance

The lack of specific pathology has led some to speculate that FMS may be a psychological disorder in origin [72, 73]. This premise largely depends on the findings that depression is far more common in FMS than in the general public and that FMS patients report greater emotional distress than healthy people [51, 74]. However, the support for this hypothesis is, at best, weak. Not all FMS patients are depressed [75], nor is depression specific to FMS. Depression is common in other chronic illnesses. Depression rates seem to be comparatively high, about 23–55% in rheumatoid arthritis [76], cancer [77], and systemic lupus erythematosus [78]. Whereas a positive response to dexamethasone suppression test is expected in psychiatrically depressed patients, depression-free FMS patients are negative to the test [79]. Reactivity of the hypothalamic pituitary adrenal (HPA) axis [80] and urinary neopterin response [81] are different in FMS patients from those who are depressed.

As a related, yet alternative concept, FMS has been considered to be a part of the affective spectrum disorder (ASD) [82]. Unlike the psychogenic model, the ASD model does not necessarily suggest a causal relationship between depression and FMS. Instead, the model proposes that there is a family of functional and psychiatric disorders (e.g., irritable bowel syndrome, depression, headaches) that share common pathophysiology. However, the underlying pathology that connects all these different illness entities is not clear at this time. Abnormalities in serotonin have been suggested as a culprit as it seems to be dysregulated in both depression and FMS [83, 84]. Significant family association in both diseases [85–87] suggests the potential involvement of genetic polymorphism that affects the serotonergic system [88]. However, the actual contribution of impaired serotonergic activities to the experience of depression and FMS is still controversial [89, 90]. The ASD model is more heuristic at this point than theoretical or empirically guided.

Abnormal pain modulation

Unremitting pain is a cardinal feature of FMS. Clinically, FMS is associated with greater pain response to digital palpation [91]. Laboratory research has consistently shown lowered pain thresholds to experimentally induced noxious stimuli in FMS patients than healthy individuals regardless of the type of stimulus delivery [92–96]. Fibromyalgia syndrome patients show increased windup (WU) sensitivity (i.e., abnormally heightened temporal summation of pain) and maintain the WU sensitivity [97], suggesting the increased excitability of spinal cord neurons related to central sensitization. Cortical activities reflecting the pain modulation also show consistent patterns of central sensitization. For example, evoked somatosensory response to noxious stimulation in FMS is exaggerated [93, 98]. Regional cerebral blood flow reacts abnormally to pain testing in FMS [99, 100]. In an imaging study, FMS patients show a comparable level of cortical activation with healthy people but at the lower level of noxious stimuli [101], also suggesting the presence of centrally dysregulated pain modulation in FMS.

Central pain dysregulation is the most studied and considered mechanism that may underlie FMS. Readers who are interested in learning details of the studies reviewed here are encouraged to read a recently published review chapter specifically on this topic [102].

Serotonin/catecholamine abnormality

As briefly discussed earlier, the role of the serotonergic abnormality in FMS has gained considerable interest given the widespread influence of serotonin in pain, sleep, and mood. Research is fairly consistent in showing abnormal plasma serotonin [89], transfer ratio of tryptophan [39], CFS concentration [103], and reuptake site density [83].

More recently, there seems to be accumulated evidence that FMS is associated with disturbance in dopaminergic neurotransmission. There is an association with an augmented prolactin response to a buspirone challenge test, suggesting altered sensitivity in dopamine receptors in these patients [104]. A preliminary study based upon tracing L-DOPA uptake with positron emission tomography suggests that FMS may be related to the disrupted presynaptic dopamine activity [105]. The amount of dopamine release in the basal ganglia is correlated to pain reports in response to painful stimulation in healthy people whereas there is no such relationship observed in FMS patients [106].

Our understanding of how exactly these neurotransmitters are involved in FMS is, however, still at the primitive stage. Large individual variations in the neurotransmitter levels can be expected even within a group of FMS patients. Indeed, the correlations of FMS/depression symptoms with the serotonin level were in the opposite direction in one study [89]. Clinical correlates of the neurotransmitter levels are yet to be clarified.

Hypothalamic-pituitary-adrenal dysfunction

Stress commonly exacerbates FMS symptoms; FMS patients seem to have trouble regulating their stress, showing blunted sympathetic responses to various types of stressors [107, 108]. Research has suggested that alteration of the basal pituitary-adrenal function may be present in FMS. Elevated serum cortisol levels in the afternoon [109] and increased daytime plasma or salivary cortisol levels [110, 111] have been shown in FMS patients. There is also an association with dysregulated reactivity of the HPA axis to stress with decreased adrenocorticotropic hormone (ACTH) in response to hypoglycemia [111] and pro-inflammatory stimulation by injecting interleukin (IL)-6 [112]. Post-exercise plasma cortisol was significantly lowered in FMS relative to healthy people [107]. Dysfunction in the HPA axis has a range of adverse consequences in pain and sleep, suggesting that the somatic, cognitive, and emotional symptoms of FMS may be critically influenced by such dysfunction.

Immunological vulnerability

A number of cytokines are implicated in various sickness phenomena including pain, fatigue, sleep disturbance, and depression. In animal studies, exposure to pro-inflammatory cytokines such as IL-1, IL-6, and tumor necrosis factor (TNF)-alpha results in hyperalgesia in rodents [113–115]. Acute exposure to IL-6 in healthy men induces disturbance in slow-wave sleep [116] and impairment in physical task performance (running) [117]. Observations that patients develop FMS-like symptoms after receiving interferon-alpha for chronic hepatitis [118] and IL-2LAK cell therapy for terminal renal cell carcinoma or melanoma [119], have also helped heightened the interest in the role of cytokines in FMS. Increased levels of serum pro-inflammatory cytokines, e.g., IL-2, IL-8, and IL-1ra, are seen in FMS patients compared to healthy people [119, 120, 121] with the greater levels with longer duration of symptoms. Skin biopsies have shown the presence of IL-1 beta, IL-6, and TNF-alpha in up to a third of FMS patients compared to none in healthy people [122].

Treatment

Pharmacological modalities

Anti-inflammatory drugs

Corticosteroids were one of the first classes of medications that investigators tested for FMS, probably because corticosteroids were the common choice of drug for rheumatic and other inflammatory disorders. However, a double-blind, crossover trial of prednisone [123] showed no appreciable treatment benefit. Similarly, double-blind, placebo-controlled trials evaluating the efficacy of non-steroidal anti-inflammatory drugs (NSAIDs) – common over-the-counter analgesics such as ibuprofen and naproxen – have consistently demonstrated no treatment benefit [124, 125]. Thus, even though NSAIDs continue to be commonly used to treat FMS [42], research does not provide any support for the use of anti-inflammatory agents.

Sedatives/hypnotics

Benzodiazepine or non-benzodiazepine hypnotic agents are also commonly used on the basis that improvement of sleep and mood may help FMS symptoms. However, controlled studies showed no benefit [52, 124, 126]. Moreover, the improvement in sleep has not been consistently reported, and there is no evidence of improved mood as a result of using hypnotic drugs. Thus, in general, hypnotics/sedatives appear to be of only limited use in the treatment of FMS. Indeed some consider these as a class of drugs to avoid given the potential complication associated with long-term use [127].

Tricyclic antidepressants

Amitriptyline and cyclobenzaprine are two tricyclic antidepressant (TCA) compounds that show promising effects. Typically, the dosage of amitriptyline is much lower than the therapeutic dose for treating depression. Starting doses of 10 mg/day for amitriptyline or 5 mg at bedtime for cyclobenzaprine are commonly recommended [127]. Research has also shown that a higher dose does not necessarily have improved therapeutic benefit [128]. Meta-analysis evaluating the efficacy of these drugs shows good treatment benefit in treating pain, fatigue, and sleep disturbance associated with FMS [129]. However, the degrees of the efficacy seem to vary greatly across studies as well as patients within a study. It has been estimated that approximately a third of FMS patients respond to this regimen [130]. Nortriptyline, which has a better side effect profile seems to improve some FMS symptoms although to a lesser extent than does amitriptyline [131].

Selective serotonin reuptake inhibitor and serotonin norepinephrine reuptake inhibitor

The introduction of selective serotonin reuptake inhibitor (SSRIs) was received with great enthusiasm since SSRIs are a safer alternative to TCAs that could still address the serotonin dysregulation in FMS. Initially, however, trials testing SSRI for FMS showed only a modest degree of improvement in pain, sleep and mood [125, 132] and somewhat better (but still

modest) results with flexible dose therapy [133]. These studies suffered from high attrition rates and this may have affected the results. Alternatively, the poorer results with SSRIs relative to TCAs with norepinephrine uptake inhibition suggest that the blockade of norepinephrine reuptake has additive benefit in pain control of FMS. Indeed, the combined therapy of fluoxetine and amitriptyline results in superior efficacy compared to use of each drug alone [125]. The results of the trials testing the serotonin norepinephrine reuptake inhibitor also seem to support the contention that the increased availability of both serotonin and norepinephrine may help FMS related pain and disability [134, 135].

Other antidepressants

A randomized controlled trial to evaluate the use of inhibitors of monoamine oxidase (MAO), such as moclobemide for FMS patients who were free of psychopathology showed very limited benefit [136]. Given the potential side effects and drug interactions of MAO inhibitors, their use for FMS does not seem justifiable. Another type of antidepressant drug, mirtazapine (Trade name Remeron), was tested in a 6-week open trial with 29 patients and showed significant improvement in pain, fatigue and sleep in 30% ($n = 10$) patients [137]. This treatment needs to be tested in a larger controlled trial.

Opioid analgesics

The exact prevalence for the use of opioids to treat FMS is not known but typically it does not seem to be very common, at least among those who are referred to a tertiary pain care clinic [138]. This may be sanctionable as evidence supporting the use of opioids for FMS is weak [139]. Experts seem to agree that opioids are not recommended for FMS patients [127].

Anesthetics

There are some reports from pilot, small sample studies that the use of intravenous anesthetic infusion therapy (lidocaine) may be helpful for FMS pain [140, 141]. Similarly, patients with both FMS patients with concurrent myofascial pain syndrome (MPS) may respond well to trigger point injections; a pilot study with 11 patients showed that FMS patients with MPS experienced comparable benefit from the injection with MPS patients without FMS, although FMS patients showed prolonged post-injection soreness [142]. As noted, these studies are not well controlled and replications of the results are needed from prospective, controlled studies with a larger sample size before any conclusions about the value of local anesthetic infusion therapy can be drawn.

Antiepileptic drugs

The antinociceptive effects of antiepileptic drugs (AED), particularly in neuropathic pain, have sparked much interest in using this class of medications for FMS. Several double-blind, placebo-controlled trials suggest that pregablin (Lyrica®) leads to significantly better outcomes in pain, fatigue, and sleep than placebo, although significant response variations exists in terms of therapeutic and adverse effects [143–145]. The most common side effects are dizziness and somnolence, and many patients seem to feel that weight gain and peripheral edema are also a significant issue. The drug gained the FDA approval in 2007. A recent study suggests that a related drug gabapentin (Neurontin®) may also have similar treatment effects [146]. So far, the AED trials only tested the short-term benefit; further studies to evaluate the longer-term effects are needed.

Dopamine agonist

An open trial with a small group of patients for using ropinirole (Requip®), a dopamine agonist, showed some promising results in reducing FMS symptoms [147]. A recent double-blind placebo controlled study tested the efficacy of Pramipexole (Mirapax®), another dopamine agonist that is frequently used to treat Parkinson's disease and restless leg syndrome [148]. After 14 weeks of the therapy, a significantly greater proportion of patients in the treatment group than those in the placebo group reported reduction in pain, fatigue, and disability. While the effects maybe consistent with the hypothesis that a disturbance in the dopaminergic system is involved in FMS, the mechanism by which the dopamine agonists reregulate the disturbance is not understood at this time. Furthermore, the two aforementioned studies are at variance in their side-effect related drop-out rates, making it difficult to understand the tolerability of dopamine agonists. Clearly, this is still preliminary research with some promising pilot results. Further research with long-term follow-ups is needed to establish the efficacy, effectiveness, and safety of this treatment for FMS.

Growth hormone

Since the low level of IGF-1 (which is stimulated by growth hormone) is commonly observed in FMS patients, Bennett and his colleagues [149] conducted a double-blind, placebo-controlled study evaluating the effects of daily growth hormone injections for 9-months in FMS patients with known IGF-1 deficiency. The injections increased the level of IGF, and patients experienced greater improvement 6 months into the treatment than did the placebo group, but not to the point of remission. Unfortunately, this is an expensive protocol. As a related treatment, the use of pyridostigmine was tested in combination with regular exercise, with the assumption that pyridostigmine should improve the growth hormone response to exercise [150]. The therapy improved the IGF level but did not change pain and fatigue. Sleep and anxiety did show significant improvement, making the investigators speculate that it may improve the vagal tone of FMS patients.

Non-pharmacological modalities: physical modalities

Exercise

It has been repeatedly demonstrated that FMS patients are physically deconditioned and this may contribute to the FMS symptoms [151]. It is generally considered that incorporating a fitness program into FMS treatment is desirable. However, the empirical evidence indicates that the efficacy of fitness programs, when used as the sole treatment modality, depend upon the content and intensity of the program. As the results are not always positive, the benefit of any fitness programs should be judged against the specific content of the programs.

Thus far, research seems to point to the direction that fitness programs for FMS patients should impose some exertional efforts. Programs that included submaximal aerobic exercises [152, 153] as well as a combination of cardiovascular and muscle strengthening training [154] have shown significant reduction in clinical pain and hyperalgesic TP responses. Resistance, endurance and strengthening programs can be helpful in improving body strength [155] and may provide pain relief for FMS [156, 157]. Similarly, water-based aerobics seem to be as beneficial as land-based aerobic programs [158], and the therapeutic benefit is reversible if one stops exercising [159]. On the other hand, low-impact exercises seem to have much lesser impact on FMS [160, 161].

General recommendations seem to indicate that high intensity exercise is acceptable for FMS as long as it stays below the pain and fatigue thresholds [162]; however, this often creates a dilemma for clinicians as FMS patients typically show significant exercise intolerance. Another problem is high attrition; over 40% drop-out rates are not uncommon in trials testing exercise for FMS. Relatedly, poor compliance may attenuate the efficacy of exercise. Some have suggested that although the benefit of exercise therapy may not solely depend upon the improved physical capacity per se, compliance to regimen seems critical in achieving and maintaining the treatment gain [153, 163].

Manipulation therapy

Chiropractic therapy is one of the most popular physical modalities for FMS. For example, 40% of FMS patients who were evaluated at a tertiary pain care clinic reported to have undergone chiropractic therapy [51]. However, very little empirical research has been conducted to test the efficacy of chiropractic therapy in general. Thus far, available evidence is not very supportive for treating FMS [164]. Recently, daily connective tissue manipulation, combined with ultrasound therapy for 20 days showed modest improvement in some FMS symptoms [165]. Clearly more research needs to be done in this area, and future studies should include a larger sample size and an attention-control group. The latter is particularly important since patients in the treatment group receive extensive "hands-on" care. Wait-list controls would not be sufficient to rule out a possibility that the observed efficacy may be due to non-specific effects based upon personal interaction between a therapist and patients. A control group receiving therapist contact to control the attentional factor is needed.

Acupuncture

A recent randomized control trial [166] suggests that modest benefit, at least for a relatively short period of time, could be expected by adding acupuncture to medication management and exercise therapy. Another trial, testing the efficacy of electroacupuncture [54] showed that compared to the sham insertion of the needles 2 cm away from the true points, the true treatment resulted in statistically greater improvement. Despite the results, however, many patients remained highly sensitive to pain at the post-treatment.

Light therapy

A series of bright light therapy sessions have been tested for FMS patients with a significant level of seasonal alteration in their symptoms [167]. Since light therapy is commonly applied for seasonal affective disorder, it was examined in this subgroup of FMS patients. However, there was no significant difference in symptom improvement between the treated patients and patients in the placebo control group.

Magnet therapy

Based upon the hypothesized therapeutic effect of a static magnetic field on pain inhibition, the use of magnetic pads for FMS was tested [168]. The results however showed no benefit of the pads; there was no difference in pain 6 months after starting use of the pads between those using the magnetic pads vs. those who used the sham pads.

Non–pharmacological modalities: psychological modalities

Biofeedback

The outcomes of the biofeedback training for treating FMS are equivocal. Some studies [169, 170] yielded promising effects of EMG biofeedback, whereas other studies [170, 171] showed no benefit in improving FMS symptoms. The analysis of EMG biofeedback is somewhat complicated because the training involves several steps. First a patient must learn to readily detect tension, and then he or she must be able to alter that tension state using the learned relaxation skill. The degree to which the efficacy of EMG biofeedback depends upon patients' ability to learn to detect tension and control relaxation response needs to be clarified.

More recently a new wave of biofeedback therapy, heart-rate variability (HRV) feedback, is of great interest. Heart-rate variability is a measure of the changes in the beat-to-beat intervals of heart rate, reflecting how the autonomic nervous system functions. Because heart rate changes as a function of respiration, the feedback is given to modify HRV by consciously manipulating breathing. Despite the general sense of excitement for the HRV biofeedback training, there is only one open trial testing the efficacy of this method [172]. The results showed some improvement in pain, mood and function at the 3-month follow-up.

Hypnosis

The efficacy of hyponotherapy has been evaluated in comparison to a program consisting of massage and relaxation training [173]. Statistically significant improvements in pain, fatigue, sleep, and emotional distress were observed in patients receiving hyponotherapy at the post-treatment and 3-month follow-up. Although the results seem promising, the clinical significance of the changes was not clear. For example, pain levels of 6.0 and 7.1 on a 0–10 scale at post-treatment and follow-up, respectively, in the hypnotherapy group, seem to indicate that considerable levels of pain still were reported by patients following the treatment.

Combined psychological-behavioral techniques

Several investigators have combined different psychological techniques [174–177]. Generally the combination consists of educational lectures and some cognitive and/or behavioral stress management skills. Overall, the interpretation of the results testing the combined psychosocial techniques is not very impressive due to poor methodology (e.g., use of non-parametric analyses, no control group). High drop-out rates are very common in these trials and how different components affect different symptoms of FMS is not clearly delineated. However, the improvement seems to accompany a declining sense of helplessness [177], suggesting that the efficacy of psychologically oriented programs may be best focusing on techniques that can change helplessness.

Multidisciplinary treatments

Given the multifactorial nature of the illness, a growing number of investigators have emphasized the importance of addressing multiple factors associated with FMS [178]. The systematic evaluation of the trials testing various types of multidisciplinary treatment programs for FMS is not easy because the therapy types and parameters of the programs vary greatly. It is also labor and cost intensive to conduct a clinical trial involving multiple treatment options. The systematic reviews suggest that most studies are "poor" quality and it is difficult to interpret the results [179]. On the other hand, the dilemma is that conducting a "high quality" clinical trial of a multidisciplinary treatment often risks it becoming experimentally "sterilized" and removed from reality. When the testing protocols do not mirror what actually goes on in the real world, one faces the irony of pursuing evidence-based medicine that relies upon unrealistic clinical practice.

The majority of multidisciplinary research includes several components: educational, exercise, and psychological therapies that are generally standardized with or without medication management that is generally individually tailored. Typically, the programs that emphasize information provision with less focus on coping skill acquisition [180, 181] result in less success. Programs aiming at the acquisition of coping skills and physical exercises [182, 183] seem to reduce pain, emotional distress, and functional disability. The contrast suggests the importance of putting emphasis on learning, practicing and internalizing new and adaptive coping skills. Intensive rehabilitative programs that included medication management along with physical therapy and psychological modalities [59, 184] also yielded significant improvements in various FMS-related areas including pain, fatigue, mood, and functioning.

It is also interesting to note that these treatment programs all include various treatment components (e.g., physical exercise, psychosocial treatment) that show much more modest results when used as single modalities. Thus, the total effects of a multidisciplinary program seem greater than the sum of all the single therapy components. This suggests that there may be an interactive effect of different treatment components, potentiating the efficacy of each therapeutic component to address various FMS problems.

Case discussions

We would like to present two patients with similar baseline information, both of whom underwent an identical structured therapy program with somewhat different results. The baseline information for these patients is listed in Table 18.3. At the time of the evaluation, both patients were found to be quite deactivated and sedentary. They were intolerant to physical exercise and complained of shortness of breath and sense of racing heart upon very mild exertion. One of the patients (S) used a cane to walk, and complained of unrestorative sleep despite hypersomnia. Patient L also complained of unrestorative sleep with long sleep latency and inability to sustain sleep for longer than 2 hours at a time.

Both patients underwent a 10-week structured rehabilitation program consisting of cognitive behavioral therapy (CBT) and activating physical therapy. The sessions were given weekly in a group format of 4–6 patients. For the first 4 weeks, they received intensive 2-hour CBT per week, aiming at helping them acquire adaptive behavioral and cognitive skills to manage pain and disability. Activating physical therapy started in week 5 in combination with CBT. During weeks 6–9, didactic physical therapy education to help them understand body mechanics, posture, and pacing was included. Physical therapy was 1 hour long, with 20 minutes of stretching (including warm-up and cool-down), 20 minutes of aerobic exercise, and 10 minutes of strengthening. The baseline was determined during

Table 18.3 Background information for two patients

	Patient S	Patient L
Demographic	58-year-old recently widowed female	49-year-old married female
Pain history	8-year history of FMS, insidious and gradual onset	12-year history of FMS, insidious and gradual onset
Treatment history	Physical therapy, chiropractics, ultrasounds, TENS	Physical therapy, medications, chiropractics
Symptomatic complaints	Diffuse pain, joint pain, chronic fatigue, sleep disturbance, irritable bowel syndrome, monthly tension type headaches, depression, feeling unbalanced	Diffuse pain, joint pain, chronic fatigue, sleep disturbance, stress-induced headaches, cold sensitivity, persistent diarrhea, muscle tenderness
Psychiatric diagnosis	Major depressive disorder, characterized with anhedonia, apathy, and lethargy	Dysthymic disorder
Work status	Not working due to pain	Not working due to pain
FMS-related medications	None	Ambien, ibuprofen

FMS: fibromyalgia syndrome; TENS: transcutaneous electrial nerve stimulation.

Table 18.4 Treatment results

	Patient S			Patient L		
	Baseline	Post-treatment	6-month follow-up	Baseline	Post-treatment	6-month follow-up
TP count	18	18	18	12	17	12
TP severity	3.06	2.16	1.61	1.33	2.66	1.50
VAS pain	38	70	18	40	40	30
VAS fatigue	42	70	20	63	68	80
VAS not refreshed in AM	68	64	55	52	72	80
Treadmill distance	0.33	0.25	0.38	0.42	0.6	1.0
Psychiatric diagnosis	MDD	MDD	MDD in Remission	Dysthymia	Dysthymia	Dysthymia

the evaluation and they began their exercise at 70% of their baseline levels to gradually increase the exertion requirement. Daily home exercise plan was developed for each patient and recorded. Table 18.4 shows some symptom and functional parameters across time for these patients.

Patient S showed overall worsening of symptoms (VAS) and function (treadmill walking distance) at the end of the treatment. However, she enjoyed the program and showed excellent compliance with exercise requirements and CBT homework. She rearranged some of the exercise sequences to fit her needs better and continued to apply what she learned in the treatment. At 6 months, she was no longer using the cane, her depression remitted, her sleep and functioning improved, and she was much less symptomatic although her treadmill walking distance did not appear to increase very much from the baseline.

Patient L showed a somewhat different picture. She showed consistent improvement in the distance she walked across time. Although she was compliant with the program requirements and reported a subjective sense of overall improvement at the post-treatment and 6-month follow-up visits, she continued to take Ambien for sleep with no appreciative benefit. She continued to struggle with chronic fatigue and low mood.

These two cases illustrate the complexity of interpreting FMS treatment responses. As reviewed earlier, the combination of exercise and CBT has been shown to be beneficial in clinical trials – that is as a group, patients show better improvement with the combination treatment than those in the control group. In these trials, we rarely focus on individual variations in treatment response. We have two patients here, seemingly presenting similar FMS symptomatology, who showed very different treatment responses. Clearly, the cases show how confusing the treatment results can be. Given that Patient L doubled her walking distance from the baseline to the 6-month follow-up visit, should we consider her a positive responder to the treatment? Patient S showed very little changes in her ability to walk on the treadmill. She actually showed overall worsening at the end of the treatment. However, later on, long after the treatment ended, she showed substantial improvement in all aspects of her FMS and function.

When we treat a multi-symptom disorder with multiple modalities, we often resort to the scientific shot-gun approach, with an assumption that some bullets must hit some symptoms. Clinical trials can tell us what may work as a whole; however, we have very little understanding of how treatment interacts with patients. Take Patient S – how was she able to improve long after completing the program despite her seemingly negative response to treatment initially? The answer may lie somewhere in her personal styles and predispositions. For example, this may reflect her individual needs for gradual adaptation to a healthier and more active lifestyle. Or she may have needed to lift her depression first then started to function better, which resulted in overall improvement in FMS. At this time, we can only speculate.

Patients, although grouped together by common symptoms, are individuals with a variety of personalities, predispositions, learning histories, and environmental circumstances. To understand how these individual characteristics need to be considered in treatment efficacy, we may have to abandon our reductionistic paradigm and start looking into individual causal modeling that takes "person variables" into consideration in the outcome equations. With recent advancement in methodology and statistics, we are better equipped to face this challenge. Only then, we can begin to address the issue of evidence-based, personalized medicine for FMS.

Summary and future directions

Research in the past three decades has greatly enhanced our knowledge on the neurophysiological correlates of FMS. The recurrent theme is the presence of some abnormalities in the neuro-endocrine-immunological system in FMS but no single item explains the entire FMS phenomena. These systems are all an integrated part of human biological entity; thus one system failure is likely to lead to another system failure, creating a complex cascade response set that may not be clearly understood in our current scientific methodology. To further our scientific understanding of FMS, we must work on building a comprehensive and integrative model of the dysregulated systems that contribute to the development and maintenance of FMS. Unfortunately, scientists are often divided into various systems or disciplines, and it is easy for us to become one of those "blind physicians" touching only a small portion of an elephant to describe it. Transdisciplinary efforts are critical for making a major step towards understanding a complex, multi-system pain disorder.

Treatment outcomes, despite a range of protocols, are not convincingly impressive. The quality of the methodology has also dampened the enthusiasm particularly for non-pharmacologic therapies. Even for well-controlled studies, statistical significance that is enlisted as evidence for the efficacy may have questionable clinical significance. For example, if a Drug A showed pain reduction (say 50%) in 25% of the treated patients whereas a placebo drug showed such improvement in 12% of the patients, it still could be statistically significant with a large sample size. From this result, could we conclude that Drug A works for FMS? How would a physician know if a patient sitting in his/her office right at this moment could benefit from this drug?

We clearly have a long way to go before having a significant impact on successful treatment of FMS at the public health level. Advancements in improving outcome research in this field would require us to find better ways to handle the multiple problems associated with FMS. Fibromyalgia outcome variables are far from standardized and this makes it very difficult to integrate the outcome results. To further integrate the clinical reality into FMS treatment outcomes studies, it is important we have better understanding of how these different outcome measures interact with one another. Co-variations of the symptoms across time and across situations do occur in FMS, yet we have very little understanding of them. Clinicians often anecdotally recognize that FMS symptoms do not go away simultaneously, and improvement in one area may be necessary for another symptom to get better. Perhaps some symptoms involve more extensive layers of the neuro-endocrine-immunological systems than others, thereby requiring more extensive treatment for a longer duration. In other words, some outcomes may be "relational", rather than static. Given the complex multi-system nature of the disorder, FMS clinical research will require going over and beyond the traditional approaches and applying innovative and novel conceptual and methodological ventures.

References

1. Wolfe F, Smythe HA, Yunus MB, *et al.* The American College of Rheumatology 1990 Criteria for the Classification of Fibromyalgia. Report of the Multicenter Criteria Committee [see comments]. *Arthritis Rheum* 1990; **33**: 160–72.

2. Forseth KO, Gran JT. The prevalence of fibromyalgia among women aged 20–49 years in Arendal, Norway. *Scand J Rheumatol* 1992; **21**: 74–8.

3. Prescott E, Kjoller M, Jacobsen S, *et al.* Fibromyalgia in the adult Danish population: I. A prevalence study. *Scand J Rheumatol* 1993; **22**: 233–7.

4. Wolfe F, Ross K, Anderson J, Russell IJ, Hebert L. The prevalence and characteristics of fibromyalgia in the general population. *Arthritis Rheum* 1995; **38**: 19–28.

5. Toda K. The prevalence of fibromyalgia in Japanese workers. *Scand J Rheumatol* 2007; **36**: 140–4.

6. Hardt J, Jacobsen C, Goldberg J, Nickel R, Buchwald D. Prevalence of chronic pain in a representative sample in the united states. *Pain Med* 2008; **9**: 803–12.

7. Lawrence RC, Felson DT, Helmick CG, *et al.* Estimates of the prevalence of arthritis and other rheumatic conditions in the United States. Part II. *Arthritis Rheum* 2008; **58**: 26–35.

8. Simons DG. Muscle pain syndromes – Part I. *Am J Phys Med* 1975; **54**: 289–311.

9. Stockman R. The causes, pathology, and treatment of chronic rheumatism. *Edinburgh Med J* 1904; **15**: 107–16.

10. Gowers W. Lumbago: its lessons and analogues. *BMJ* 1904; **1**: 117–21.

11. Yunus M, Masi AT, Calabro JJ, Miller KA, Feigenbaum SL. Primary fibromyalgia (fibrositis): clinical study of 50 patients with matched normal controls. *Semin Arthritis Rheum* 1981; **11**: 151–71.

12. Valentine M. Aetiology of fibrositis: a review. *Ann Rheum Dis* 1947; **6**: 241–50.

13. Kraft GH, Johnson EW, LaBan MM. The fibrositis syndrome. *Arch Phys Med Rehabil* 1968; **49**: 155–62.

14. Smythe H. Nonarticular rheumatism and the fibrositis syndrome. In *Arthritis and Allied Conditions; A textbook of rheumatology* 8th edn [ed. L Hollander]. (Philadelphia, PA: Lea & Febiger, 1972), pp. 874–4.

15. Yunus MB, Masi AT, Aldag JC. Preliminary criteria for primary fibromyalgia syndrome (PFS): multivariate analysis of a consecutive series of PFS, other pain patients, and normal subjects. *Clin Exp Rheumatol* 1989; **7**: 63–9.

16. Raspe H, Croft P. Fibromyalgia. *Baillieres Clin Rheumatol* 1995; **9**: 599–614.

17. Goldenberg DL. Fibromyalgia syndrome a decade later: what have we learned? *Arch Intern Med* 1999; **159**: 777–85.

18. Clauw DJ, Crofford LJ. Chronic widespread pain and fibromyalgia: what we know, and what we need to know. *Best Pract Res Clin Rheumatol* 2003; **17**: 685–701.

19. Fitzcharles MA, Boulos P. Inaccuracy in the diagnosis of fibromyalgia syndrome: analysis of referrals. *Rheumatology (Oxford)* 2003; **42**: 263–7.

20. Katz RS, Wolfe F, Michaud K. Fibromyalgia diagnosis: a comparison of clinical, survey, and American College of Rheumatology criteria. *Arthritis Rheum* 2006; **54**: 169–76.

21. Pamuk ON, Yesil Y, Cakir N. Factors that affect the number of tender points in fibromyalgia and chronic widespread pain patients who did not meet the ACR 1990 criteria for fibromyalgia: are tender points a reflection of neuropathic pain? *Semin Arthritis Rheum* 2006; **36**: 130–4.

22. Wolfe F. The relation between tender points and fibromyalgia symptom variables: evidence that fibromyalgia is not a discrete disorder in the clinic. *Ann Rheum Dis* 1997; **56**: 268–71.

23. McCarberg B, Barkin RL, Wright JA, *et al.* Tender points as predictors of distress and the pharmacologic management of fibromyalgia syndrome. *Am J Ther* 2003; **10**: 176–92.

24. Ejlertsson G, Eden L, Leden I. Predictors of positive health in disability pensioners: a population-based questionnaire study using Positive Odds Ratio. *BMC Public Health* 2002; **2**: 20.

25. Bombardier CH, Buchwald D. Chronic fatigue, chronic fatigue syndrome, and fibromyalgia. Disability and health-care use. *Med Care* 1996; **34**: 924–30.

26. White KP, Speechley M, Harth M, Ostbye T. The London Fibromyalgia Epidemiology Study: direct health care costs of fibromyalgia syndrome in London, Canada. *J Rheumatol* 1999; **26**: 885–9.

27. Middleton GD, McFarlin JE, Lipsky PE. The prevalence and clinical impact of fibromyalgia in systemic lupus

erythematosus [see comments]. *Arthritis Rheum* 1994; **37**: 1181–8.

28. Martinez JE, Ferraz MB, Sato EI, Atra E. Fibromyalgia versus rheumatoid arthritis: a longitudinal comparison of the quality of life. *J Rheumatol* 1995; **22**: 270–4.

29. Heikkila S, Ronni S, Kautiainen HJ, Kauppi MJ. Functional impairment in spondyloarthropathy and fibromyalgia. *J Rheumatol* 2002; **29**: 1415–9.

30. Cardol M, de Jong BA, van den Bos GA, *et al.* Beyond disability: perceived participation in people with a chronic disabling condition. *Clin Rehabil* 2002; **16**: 27–35.

31. Kurtze N, Gundersen KT, Svebak S. Quality of life, functional disability and lifestyle among subgroups of fibromyalgia patients: the significance of anxiety and depression. *Br J Med Psychol* 1999; **72**: 471–84.

32. Sherman JJ, Turk DC, Okifuji A. Prevalence and impact of posttraumatic stress disorder-like symptoms on patients with fibromyalgia syndrome. *Clin J Pain* 2000; **16**: 127–34.

33. White KP, Nielson WR, Harth M, Ostbye T, Speechley M. Chronic widespread musculoskeletal pain with or without fibromyalgia: psychological distress in a representative community adult sample. *J Rheumatol* 2002; **29**: 588–94.

34. Yunus MB, Arslan S, Aldag JC. Relationship between body mass index and fibromyalgia features. *Scand J Rheumatol* 2002; **31**: 27–31.

35. Okifuji A, Bradshaw D, Olso C. Evaluating obesity in fibromyalgia: neuroendocrine biomarkers, symptoms, and functions. *Clin Rheumatol* 2009; **28**: 475–8 .

36. Hawley DJ, Wolfe F, Cathey MA. Pain, functional disability, and psychological status: a 12-month study of severity in fibromyalgia. *J Rheumatol* 1988; **15**: 1551–6.

37. Mannerkorpi K, Burckhardt CS, Bjelle A. Physical performance characteristics of women with fibromyalgia. *Arthritis Care Res* 1994; **7**: 123–9.

38. Bengtsson A, Henriksson KG. The muscle in fibromyalgia – a review of Swedish studies. *J Rheumatol Suppl* 1989; **19**: 144–9.

39. Norregaard J, Bulow PM, Mehlsen J, Danneskiold-Samsoe B. Biochemical changes in relation to a maximal exercise test in patients with fibromyalgia. *Clin Physiol* 1994; **14**: 159–67.

40. Jacobsen S, Holm B. Muscle strength and endurance compared to aerobic capacity in primary fibromyalgia syndrome. *Clin Exp Rheumatol* 1992; **10**: 419–20.

41. Elert JE, Rantapaa-Dahlqvist SB, Henriksson-Larsen K, Lorentzon R, Gerdle BU. Muscle performance, electromyography and fibre type composition in fibromyalgia and work-related myalgia. *Scand J Rheumatol* 1992; **21**: 28–34.

42. Wolfe F, Anderson J, Harkness D, *et al.* Health status and disease severity in fibromyalgia: results of a six-center longitudinal study. *Arthritis Rheum* 1997; **40**: 1571–9.

43. Dobkin PL, De Civita M, Bernatsky S, Kang H, Baron M. Does psychological vulnerability determine health-care utilization in fibromyalgia? *Rheumatology (Oxford)* 2003; **42**: 1324–31.

44. Penrod JR, Bernatsky S, Adam V, *et al.* Health services costs and their determinants in women with fibromyalgia. *J Rheumatol* 2004; **31**: 1391–8.

45. White LA, Birnbaum HG, Kaltenboeck A, *et al.* Employees with fibromyalgia: medical comorbidity, healthcare costs, and work loss. *J Occup Environ Med* 2008; **50**: 13–24.

46. Robinson RL, Birnbaum HG, Morley MA, *et al.* Economic cost and epidemiological characteristics of patients with fibromyalgia claims. *J Rheumatol* 2003; **30**: 1318–25.

47. Assefi NP, Coy TV, Uslan D, Smith WR, Buchwald D. Financial, occupational, and personal consequences of disability in patients with chronic fatigue syndrome and fibromyalgia compared to other fatiguing conditions. *J Rheumatol* 2003; **30**: 804–8.

48. Liedberg GM, Henriksson CM. Factors of importance for work disability in women with fibromyalgia: an interview study. *Arthritis Rheum* 2002; **47**: 266–74.

49. Henriksson C, Liedberg G. Factors of importance for work disability in women with fibromyalgia. *J Rheumatol* 2000; **27**: 1271–6.

50. Wolfe F, Anderson J, Harkness D, *et al.* Work and disability status of persons with fibromyalgia. *J Rheumatol* 1997; **24**: 1171–8.

51. Turk DC, Okifuji A, Sinclair JD, Starz TW. Pain, disability, and physical functioning in subgroups of patients with fibromyalgia. *J Rheumatol* 1996; **23**: 1255–62.

52. Moldofsky H, Wong MT, Lue FA. Litigation, sleep, symptoms and disabilities in postaccident pain (fibromyalgia). *J Rheumatol* 1993; **20**: 1935–40.

53. Bengtsson A, Henriksson KG, Larsson J. Muscle biopsy in primary fibromyalgia. Light-microscopical and histochemical findings. *Scand J Rheumatol* 1986; **15**: 1–6.

54. Durette MR, Rodriquez AA, Agre JC, Silverman JL. Needle electromyographic evaluation of patients with myofascial or fibromyalgic pain. *Am J Phys Med Rehabil* 1991; **70**: 154–6.

55. Elam M, Johansson G, Wallin BG. Do patients with primary fibromyalgia have an altered muscle sympathetic nerve activity? *Pain* 1992; **48**: 371–5.

56. Drewes AM, Andreasen A, Schroder HD, Hogsaa B, Jennum P. Pathology of skeletal muscle in fibromyalgia: a histo-immuno-chemical and ultrastructural study. *Br J Rheumatol* 1993; **32**: 479–83.

57. Sprott H, Rzanny R, Reichenbach JR, Kaiser WA, Hein G, Stein G. 31P magnetic resonance spectroscopy in fibromyalgic muscle. *Rheumatology (Oxford)* 2000; **39**: 1121–5.

58. Park JH, Phothimat P, Oates CT, Hernanz-Schulman M, Olsen NJ. Use of P-31 magnetic resonance spectroscopy to detect metabolic abnormalities in muscles of patients with fibromyalgia. *Arthritis Rheum* 1998; **41**: 406–13.

59. Bennett RM. Fibromyalgia and the disability dilemma. A new era in understanding a complex, multidimensional pain syndrome. *Arthritis Rheum* 1996; **39**: 1627–34.

60. Thompson JM. Tension myalgia as a diagnosis at the Mayo Clinic and its relationship to fibrositis, fibromyalgia, and myofascial pain syndrome. *Mayo Clin Proc* 1990; **65**: 1237–48.

61. Zidar J, Backman E, Bengtsson A, Henriksson KG. Quantitative EMG and muscle tension in painful muscles in fibromyalgia. *Pain* 1990; **40**: 249–54.

62. Bansevicius D, Westgaard RH, Stiles T. EMG activity and pain development in fibromyalgia patients exposed to mental stress of long duration. *Scand J Rheumatol* 2001; **30**: 92–8.

63. Thieme K, Rose U, Pinkpank T, *et al.* Psychophysiological responses in patients with fibromyalgia syndrome. *J Psychosom Res* 2006; **61**: 671–9.

64. Flor H, Turk DC, Birbaumer N. Assessment of stress-related psychophysiological reactions in chronic back pain patients. *J Consult Clin Psychol* 1985; **53**: 354–64.

65. Okifuji A, Turk DC. Stress and psychophysiological dysregulation in patients with fibromyalgia syndrome. *Appl Psychophysiol Biofeedback* 2002; **27**: 129–41.

66. Moldofsky H, Scarisbrick P, England R, Smythe H. Musculosketal symptoms and non-REM sleep disturbance in patients with "fibrositis syndrome" and healthy subjects. *Psychosom Med* 1975; **37**: 341–51.

67. Lentz MJ, Landis CA, Rothermel J, Shaver JL. Effects of selective slow wave sleep disruption on musculoskeletal pain and fatigue in middle aged women. *J Rheumatol* 1999; **26**: 1586–92.

68. Branco J, Atalaia A, Paiva T. Sleep cycles and alpha-delta sleep in fibromyalgia syndrome. *J Rheumatol* 1994; **21**: 1113–7.

69. Carette S, Oakson G, Guimont C, Steriade M. Sleep electroencephalography and the clinical response to amitriptyline in patients with fibromyalgia. *Arthritis Rheum* 1995; **38**: 1211–17.

70. Bennett RM, Cook DM, Clark SR, Burckhardt CS, Campbell SM. Hypothalamic-pituitary-insulin-like growth factor-I axis dysfunction in patients with fibromyalgia. *J Rheumatol* 1997; **24**: 1384–9.

71. Buchwald D, Umali J, Stene M. Insulin-like growth factor-I (somatomedin C) levels in chronic fatigue syndrome and fibromyalgia. *J Rheumatol* 1996; **23**: 739–42.

72. Ercolani M, Trombini G, Chattat R, *et al.* Fibromyalgic syndrome: depression and abnormal illness behavior. Multicenter investigation. *Psychother Psychosom* 1994; **61**: 178–86.

73. Ford CV. Somatization and fashionable diagnoses: illness as a way of life. *Scand J Work Environ Health* 1997; **23**(Suppl 3): 7–16.

74. Krag J, Norregaard J, Larsen JK, Danneskiold-Samsoe B. A blinded, controlled evaluation of anxiety and depressive symptoms in patients with fibromyalgia, as measured by standardized psychometric interview scales. *Acta Psychiatr Scand* 1994; **89**: 370–5.

75. Okifuji A, Turk D, Sherman J. Evaluation of the relationship between depression and fibromyalgia syndrome: why aren't all patients depressed? *J Rheumatol* 2000; **27**: 212–9.

76. Abdel-Nasser A, Abd El-Azim S, Taal E, *et al.* Depression and depressive symptoms in rheumatoid arthritis patients: an analysis of their occurrence and determinants. *Br J Rheumatol* 1998; **37**: 391–7.

77. Aragona M, Muscatello M, Mesiti M. Depressive mood disorders in patients with operable breast cancer. *J Exp Clin Cancer Res* 1997; **16**: 111–8.

78. Gutchinson G, Nehall J, Simeon D. Psychiatric disorders in systemic lupus erythematosus. *West Indian Med J* 1996; **45**: 48–50.

79. Ataoglu S, Ozcetin A, Yildiz O, Ataoglu A. Evaluation of dexamethasone suppression test in fibromyalgia patients with or without depression. *Swiss Med Wkly* 2003; **133**: 241–4.

80. Maes M, Lin A, Bonaccorso S, van Hunsel F, *et al.* Increased 24-hour urinary cortisol excretion in patients with post-traumatic stress disorder and patients with major depression, but not in patients with fibromyalgia. *Acta Psychiatr Scand* 1998; **98**: 328–35.

81. Bonaccorso S, Lin AH, Verkerk R, *et al.* Immune markers in fibromyalgia: comparison with major depressed patients and normal volunteers. *J Affect Disord* 1998; **48**: 75–82.

82. Hudson JI, Pope HG, Jr. Fibromyalgia and psychopathology: is fibromyalgia a form of "affective

spectrum disorder"? *J Rheumatol Suppl* 1989; **19**: 15–22.

83. Russell IJ, Michalek JE, Vipraio GA, *et al*. Platelet 3H-imipramine uptake receptor density and serum serotonin levels in patients with fibromyalgia/fibrositis syndrome [see comments]. *J Rheumatol* 1992; **19**: 104–9.

84. Cowen PJ. Neuroendocrine markers of depression and antidepressant drug action. In *Antidepressants* ed. BE Leonard. (Basel: Birkhauser, 2001).

85. Arnold LM, Hudson JI, Hess EV, *et al*. Family study of fibromyalgia. *Arthritis Rheum* 2004; **50**: 944–52.

86. Arnold LM, Hudson JI, Keck PE, *et al*. Comorbidity of fibromyalgia and psychiatric disorders. *J Clin Psychiatry* 2006; **67**: 1219–25.

87. Bradley LA. Pathophysiologic mechanisms of fibromyalgia and its related disorders. *J Clin Psychiatry* 2008; **69** Suppl 2: 6–13.

88. Buskila D, Sarzi-Puttini P. Biology and therapy of fibromyalgia. Genetic aspects of fibromyalgia syndrome. *Arthritis Res Ther* 2006; **8**: 218.

89. Wolfe F, Russell IJ, Vipraio G, Ross K, Anderson J. Serotonin levels, pain threshold, and fibromyalgia symptoms in the general population. *J Rheumatol* 1997; **24**: 555–9.

90. Cowen PJ. Serotonin and depression: pathophysiological mechanism or marketing myth? *Trends Pharmacol Sci* 2008; **29**: 433–6.

91. Okifuji A, Turk DC, Sinclair JD, Starz TW, Marcus DA. A standardized manual tender point survey. I. Development and determination of a threshold point for the identification of positive tender points in fibromyalgia syndrome. *J Rheumatol* 1997; **24**: 377–83.

92. Arroyo JF, Cohen ML. Abnormal responses to electrocutaneous stimulation in fibromyalgia. *J Rheumatol* 1993; **20**: 1925–31.

93. Gibson SJ, Littlejohn GO, Gorman MM, Helme RD, Granges G. Altered heat pain thresholds and cerebral event-related potentials following painful CO_2 laser stimulation in subjects with fibromyalgia syndrome. *Pain* 1994; **58**: 185–93.

94. Lautenbacher S, Rollman GB, McCain GA. Multi-method assessment of experimental and clinical pain in patients with fibromyalgia. *Pain* 1994; **59**: 45–53.

95. Kosek E, Hansson P. Modulatory influence on somatosensory perception from vibration and heterotopic noxious conditioning stimulation (HNCS) in fibromyalgia patients and healthy subjects. *Pain* 1997; **70**: 41–51.

96. Petzke F, Clauw DJ, Ambrose K, Khine A, Gracely RH. Increased pain sensitivity in fibromyalgia: effects of stimulus type and mode of presentation. *Pain* 2003; **105**: 403–13.

97. Staud R, Price DD, Robinson ME, Mauderli AP, Vierck CJ. Maintenance of windup of second pain requires less frequent stimulation in fibromyalgia patients compared to normal controls. *Pain* 2004; **110**: 689–96.

98. Lorenz J, Grasedyck K, Bromm B. Middle and long latency somatosensory evoked potentials after painful laser stimulation in patients with fibromyalgia syndrome. *Electroencephalogr Clin Neurophysiol* 1996; **100**: 165–8.

99. Bradley LA, McKendree-Smith NL, Alberts KR, *et al*. Use of neuroimaging to understand abnormal pain sensitivity in fibromyalgia. *Curr Rheumatol Rep* 2000; **2**: 141–8.

100. Kwiatek R, Barnden L, Tedman R, *et al*. Regional cerebral blood flow in fibromyalgia: single-photon-emission computed tomography evidence of reduction in the pontine tegmentum and thalami. *Arthritis Rheum* 2000; **43**: 2823–33.

101. Gracely RH, Petzke F, Wolf JM, Clauw DJ. Functional magnetic resonance imaging evidence of augmented pain processing in fibromyalgia. *Arthritis Rheum* 2002; **46**: 1333–43.

102. Gracely RH. Augmented central pain processing in fibromyalgia patients. In *Fundamentals of Musculoskeletal Pain* [eds. T Graven-Nielsen, L Larendt-Nielsen, S Mense]. (Seattle, WA: IASP, 2008), pp. 311–26.

103. Sorensen J, Graven-Nielsen T, Henriksson KG, Bengtsson M, Arendt-Nielsen L. Hyperexcitability in fibromyalgia. *J Rheumatol* 1998; **25**: 152–5.

104. Malt EA, Olafsson S, Aakvaag A, Lund A, Ursin H. Altered dopamine D2 receptor function in fibromyalgia patients: a neuroendocrine study with buspirone in women with fibromyalgia compared to female population based controls. *J Affect Disord* 2003; **75**: 77–82.

105. Wood PB, Patterson JC, 2nd, Sunderland JJ, *et al*. Reduced presynaptic dopamine activity in fibromyalgia syndrome demonstrated with positron emission tomography: a pilot study. *J Pain* 2007; **8**: 51–8.

106. Wood PB, Schweinhardt P, Jaeger E, *et al*. Fibromyalgia patients show an abnormal dopamine response to pain. *Eur J Neurosci* 2007; **25**: 3576–82.

107. van Denderen JC, Boersma JW, Zeinstra P, Hollander AP, van Neerbos BR. Physiological effects of exhaustive physical exercise in primary fibromyalgia syndrome (PFS): is PFS a disorder of neuroendocrine reactivity? *Scand J Rheumatol* 1992; **21**: 35–7.

108. McDermid AJ, Rollman GB, McCain GA. Generalized hypervigilance in fibromyalgia: evidence of perceptual amplification. *Pain* 1996; **66**: 133–44.

109. Crofford LJ, Young EA, Engleberg NC, *et al.* Basal circadian and pulsatile ACTH and cortisol secretion in patients with fibromyalgia and/or chronic fatigue syndrome. *Brain Behav Immun* 2004; **18**: 314–25.

110. Griep EN, Boersma JW, Lentjes EG, *et al.* Function of the hypothalamic-pituitary-adrenal axis in patients with fibromyalgia and low back pain. *J Rheumatol* 1998; **25**: 1374–81.

111. Adler GK, Kinsley BT, Hurwitz S, Mossey CJ, Goldenberg DL. Reduced hypothalamic-pituitary and sympathoadrenal responses to hypoglycemia in women with fibromyalgia syndrome. *Am J Med* 1999; **106**: 534–43.

112. Torpy DJ, Papanicolaou DA, Lotsikas AJ, *et al.* Responses of the sympathetic nervous system and the hypothalamic-pituitary-adrenal axis to interleukin-6: a pilot study in fibromyalgia. *Arthritis Rheum* 2000; **43**: 872–80.

113. Watkins LR, Wiertelak EP, Goehler LE, *et al.* Characterization of cytokine-induced hyperalgesia. *Brain Res* 1994; **654**: 15–26.

114. Oka T, Oka K, Hosoi M, Hori T. Intracerebroventricular injection of interleukin-6 induces thermal hyperalgesia in rats. *Brain Res* 1995; **692**: 123–8.

115. Watkins LR, Goehler LE, Relton J, Brewer MT, Maier SF. Mechanisms of tumor necrosis factor-alpha (TNF-alpha) hyperalgesia. *Brain Res* 1995; **692**: 244–50.

116. Spath-Schwalbe E, Hansen K, Schmidt F, *et al.* Acute effects of recombinant human interleukin-6 on endocrine and central nervous sleep functions in healthy men. *J Clin Endocrinol Metab* 1998; **83**: 1573–9.

117. Robson-Ansley PJ, de Milander L, Collins M, Noakes TD. Acute interleukin-6 administration impairs athletic performance in healthy, trained male runners. *Can J Appl Physiol* 2004; **29**: 411–8.

118. McDonald EM, Mann AH, Thomas HC. Interferons as mediators of psychiatric morbidity. An investigation in a trial of recombinant alpha-interferon in hepatitis-B carriers. *Lancet* 1987; **2**: 1175–8.

119. Wallace DJ, Linker-Israeli M, Hallegua D, *et al.* Cytokines play an aetiopathogenetic role in fibromyalgia: a hypothesis and pilot study. *Rheumatology (Oxford)* 2001; **40**: 743–9.

120. Gur A, Karakoc M, Erdogan S, *et al.* Regional cerebral blood flow and cytokines in young females with fibromyalgia. *Clin Exp Rheumatol* 2002; **20**: 753–60.

121. Bazzichi L, Rossi A, Massimetti G, *et al.* Cytokine patterns in fibromyalgia and their correlation with clinical manifestations. *Clin Exp Rheumatol* 2007; **25**: 225–30.

122. Salemi S, Rethage J, Wollina U, *et al.* Detection of interleukin 1beta (IL-1beta), IL-6, and tumor necrosis factor-alpha in skin of patients with fibromyalgia. *J Rheumatol* 2003; **30**: 146–50.

123. Clark S, Tindall E, Bennett RM. A double blind crossover trial of prednisone versus placebo in the treatment of fibrositis. *J Rheumatol* 1985; **12**: 980–3.

124. Russell IJ, Fletcher EM, Michalek JE, McBroom PC, Hester GG. Treatment of primary fibrositis/fibromyalgia syndrome with ibuprofen and alprazolam. A double-blind, placebo-controlled study. *Arthritis Rheum* 1991; **34**: 552–60.

125. Goldenberg D, Mayskiy M, Mossey C, Ruthazer R, Schmid C. A randomized, double-blind crossover trial of fluoxetine and amitriptyline in the treatment of fibromyalgia. *Arthritis Rheum* 1996; **39**: 1852–9.

126. Drewes AM, Andreasen A, Jennum P, Nielsen KD. Zopiclone in the treatment of sleep abnormalities in fibromyalgia. *Scand J Rheumatol* 1991; **20**: 288–93.

127. Clauw DJ. Pharmacotherapy for patients with fibromyalgia. *J Clin Psychiatry* 2008; **69** Suppl 2: 25–9.

128. Santandrea S, Montrone F, Sarzi Puttini P, Boccassini L, Caruso I. A double-blind crossover study of two cyclobenzaprine regimens in primary fibromyalgia syndrome. *J Int Med Res* 1983; **21**: 74–80.

129. Arnold LM, Keck PE, Jr, Welge JA. Antidepressant treatment of fibromyalgia. A meta-analysis and review. *Psychosomatics* 2000; **41**: 104–13.

130. Carette S, Bell MJ, Reynolds WJ, *et al.* Comparison of amitriptyline, cyclobenzaprine, and placebo in the treatment of fibromyalgia. A randomized, double-blind clinical trial. *Arthritis Rheum* 1994; **37**: 32–40.

131. Heymann RE, Helfenstein M, Feldman D. A double-blind, randomized, controlled study of amitriptyline, nortriptyline and placebo in patients with

fibromyalgia. An analysis of outcome measures. *Clin Exp Rheumatol* 2001; **19**: 697–702.

132. Wolfe F, Cathey MA, Hawley DJ. A double-blind placebo controlled trial of fluoxetine in fibromyalgia. *Scand J Rheumatol* 1994; **23**: 255–9.

133. Arnold LM, Hess EV, Hudson JI, *et al*. A randomized, placebo-controlled, double-blind, flexible-dose study of fluoxetine in the treatment of women with fibromyalgia. *Am J Med* 2002; **112**: 191–7.

134. Arnold LM, Lu Y, Crofford LJ, Wohlreich M, *et al*. A double-blind, multicenter trial comparing duloxetine with placebo in the treatment of fibromyalgia patients with or without major depressive disorder. *Arthritis Rheum* 2004; **50**: 2974–84.

135. Arnold LM, Pritchett YL, D'Souza DN, *et al*. Duloxetine for the treatment of fibromyalgia in women: pooled results from two randomized, placebo-controlled clinical trials. *J Womens Health (Larchmt)* 2007; **16**: 1145–56.

136. Hannonen P, Malminiemi K, Yli-Kerttula U, Isomeri R, Roponen P. A randomized, double-blind, placebo-controlled study of moclobemide and amitriptyline in the treatment of fibromyalgia in females without psychiatric disorder. *Br J Rheumatol* 1998; **37**: 1279–86.

137. Samborski W, Lezanska-Szpera M, Rybakowski JK. Open trial of mirtazapine in patients with fibromyalgia. *Pharmacopsychiatry* 2004; **37**: 168–70.

138. Turk DC, Okifuji A, Starz TW, Sinclair JD. Effects of type of symptom onset on psychological distress and disability in fibromyalgia syndrome patients. *Pain* 1996; **68**: 423–30.

139. Bennett RM, Kamin M, Karim R, Rosenthal N. Tramadol and acetaminophen combination tablets in the treatment of fibromyalgia pain: a double-blind, randomized, placebo-controlled study. *Am J Med* 2003; **114**: 537–45.

140. Posner I. Treatment of fibromyalgia syndrome with intravenous lidocaine: a prospective, randomized pilot study. *J Musculoskel Pain* 1994; **2**: 55–65.

141. Bennett MI, Tai YM. Intravenous lignocaine in the management of primary fibromyalgia syndrome. *Int J Clin Pharmacol Res* 1995; **15**: 115–9.

142. Hong CZ, Hsueh TC. Difference in pain relief after trigger point injections in myofascial pain patients with and without fibromyalgia. *Arch Phys Med Rehabil* 1996; **77**: 1161–6.

143. Crofford LJ, Rowbotham MC, Mease PJ, *et al*. Pregabalin for the treatment of fibromyalgia syndrome: results of a randomized, double-blind, placebo-controlled trial. *Arthritis Rheum* 2005; **52**: 1264–73.

144. Arnold LM, Russell IJ, Diri EW, *et al*. A 14-week, randomized, double-blinded, placebo-controlled monotherapy trial of pregabalin in patients with fibromyalgia. *J Pain* 2008; **9**: 792–805.

145. Crofford LJ, Mease PJ, Simpson SL, *et al*. Fibromyalgia relapse evaluation and efficacy for durability of meaningful relief (FREEDOM): a 6-month, double-blind, placebo-controlled trial with pregabalin. *Pain* 2008; **136**: 419–31.

146. Arnold LM, Goldenberg DL, Stanford SB, Lalonde *et al*. Gabapentin in the treatment of fibromyalgia: a randomized, double-blind, placebo-controlled, multicenter trial. *Arthritis Rheum* 2007; **56**: 1336–44.

147. Holman AJ. Ropinirole, open preliminary observations of a dopamine agonist for refractory fibromyalgia. *J Clin Rheumatol* 2003; **9**: 277–9.

148. Holman AJ, Myers RR. A randomized, double-blind, placebo-controlled trial of pramipexole, a dopamine agonist, in patients with fibromyalgia receiving concomitant medications. *Arthritis Rheum* 2005; **52**: 2495–505.

149. Bennett RM, Clark SC, Walczyk J. A randomized, double-blind, placebo-controlled study of growth hormone in the treatment of fibromyalgia. *Am J Med* 1998; **104**: 227–31.

150. Jones KD, Burckhardt CS, Deodhar AA, *et al*. A six-month randomized controlled trial of exercise and pyridostigmine in the treatment of fibromyalgia. *Arthritis Rheum* 2008; **58**: 612–22.

151. Mengshoel AM, Vollestad NK, Forre O. Pain and fatigue induced by exercise in fibromyalgia patients and sedentary healthy subjects. *Clin Exp Rheumatol* 1995; **13**: 477–82.

152. McCain GA, Bell DA, Mai FM, Halliday PD. A controlled study of the effects of a supervised cardiovascular fitness training program on the manifestations of primary fibromyalgia. *Arthritis Rheum* 1988; **31**: 1135–41.

153. Wigers SH, Stiles TC, Vogel PA. Effects of aerobic exercise versus stress management treatment in fibromyalgia. A 4.5 year prospective study. *Scand J Rheumatol* 1996; **25**: 77–86.

154. Martin L, Nutting A, MacIntosh BR, *et al*. An exercise program in the treatment of fibromyalgia. *J Rheumatol* 1996; **23**: 1050–3.

155. Kingsley JD, Panton LB, Toole T, *et al*. The effects of a 12-week strength-training program on strength and functionality in women with fibromyalgia. *Arch Phys Med Rehabil* 2005; **86**: 1713–21.

156. Figueroa A, Kingsley JD, McMillan V, Panton LB. Resistance exercise training improves heart rate variability in women with fibromyalgia. *Clin Physiol Funct Imaging* 2008; **28**: 49–54.

157. Valkeinen H, Alen M, Hakkinen A, *et al*. Effects of concurrent strength and endurance training on physical fitness and symptoms in postmenopausal women with fibromyalgia: a randomized controlled trial. *Arch Phys Med Rehabil* 2008; **89**: 1660–6.

158. Tomas-Carus P, Gusi N, Hakkinen A, *et al*. Eight months of physical training in warm water improves physical and mental health in women with fibromyalgia: a randomized controlled trial. *J Rehabil Med* 2008; **40**: 248–52.

159. Tomas-Carus P, Hakkinen A, Gusi N, *et al*. Aquatic training and detraining on fitness and quality of life in fibromyalgia. *Med Sci Sports Exerc* 2007; **39**: 1044–50.

160. Mengshoel AM, Komnaes HB, Forre O. The effects of 20 weeks of physical fitness training in female patients with fibromyalgia. *Clin Exp Rheumatol* 1992; **10**: 345–9.

161. Nørregaard J, Lykkegaard J, Mehlgen J, Danneskiold-Samsoe B. Exercise training in treatment of fibromyalgia. *J Musculoskel Pain* 1997; **5**: 71–9.

162. Jones KD, Clark SR. Individualizing the exercise prescription for persons with fibromyalgia. *Rheum Dis Clin North Am* 2002; **28**: 419–36, x–xi.

163. Verstappen F, van Santen-Hoeuftt H, Bolwijn P, van der Linden S, Kuipers H. Effects of a group activity program for fibromyalgia patients on physical fitness and well being. *J Musculoskel Pain* 1997; **5**: 17–28.

164. Blunt KL, Rajwani MH, Guerriero RC. The effectiveness of chiropractic management of fibromyalgia patients: a pilot study. *J Manipulative Physiol Ther* 1997; **20**: 389–99.

165. Citak-Karakay I, Akbayrak T, Demirturk F, Ekici G, Bakar Y. Short and long-term results of connective tissue manipulation and combined ultrasound therapy in patients with fibromyalgia. *J Manipulative Physiol Ther* 2006; **29**: 524–8.

166. Targino RA, Imamura M, Kaziyama HH, *et al*. A randomized controlled trial of acupuncture added to usual treatment for fibromyalgia. *J Rehabil Med* 2008; **40**: 582–8.

167. Pearl SJ, Lue F, MacLean AW, *et al*. The effects of bright light treatment on the symptoms of fibromyalgia. *J Rheumatol* 1996; **23**: 896–902.

168. Alfano AP, Taylor AG, Foresman PA, *et al*. Static magnetic fields for treatment of fibromyalgia: a randomized controlled trial. *J Altern Complement Med* 2001; **7**: 53–64.

169. Ferraccioli G, Ghirelli L, Scita F, *et al*. EMG-biofeedback training in fibromyalgia syndrome. *J Rheumatol* 1987; **14**: 820–5.

170. Drexler AR, Mur EJ, Gunther VC. Efficacy of an EMG-biofeedback therapy in fibromyalgia patients. A comparative study of patients with and without abnormality in (MMPI) psychological scales. *Clin Exp Rheumatol* 2002; **20**: 677–82.

171. van Santen M, Bolwijn P, Verstappen F, *et al*. A randomized clinical trial comparing fitness and biofeedback training versus basic treatment in patients with fibromyalgia. *J Rheumatol* 2002; **29**: 575–81.

172. Hassett AL, Radvanski DC, Vaschillo EG, *et al*. A pilot study of the efficacy of heart rate variability (HRV) biofeedback in patients with fibromyalgia. *Appl Psychophysiol Biofeedback* 2007; **32**: 1–10.

173. Haanen HC, Hoenderdos HT, van Romunde LK, *et al*. Controlled trial of hypnotherapy in the treatment of refractory fibromyalgia. *J Rheumatol* 1991; **18**: 72–5.

174. de Voogd J, Knipping A, de Blécourt A, van Rijswijk M. Treatment of fibromyalgia syndrome with psychomotor therapy and marital counseling. *J Musculoskel Pain* 1993; **1**: 273–81.

175. Kaplan KH, Goldenberg DL, Galvin-Nadeau M. The impact of a meditation-based stress reduction program on fibromyalgia. *Gen Hosp Psychiatry* 1993; **15**: 284–9.

176. Kogstad O, Hintringer F. Patients with fibromyalgia in pain school. *J Musculoskel Pain* 1993; **1**: 261–5.

177. Nicassio PM, Radojevic V, Weisman MH, *et al*. A comparison of behavioral and educational interventions for fibromyalgia. *J Rheumatol* 1997; **24**: 2000–7.

178. Bennett RM. Multidisciplinary group programs to treat fibromyalgia patients. *Rheum Dis Clin North Am* 1996; **22**: 351–67.

179. Karjalainen K, Malmivaara A, van Tulder M, *et al*. Multidisciplinary rehabilitation for fibromyalgia and musculoskeletal pain in working age adults. *Cochrane Database Syst Rev* 2000(2): CD001984.

180. Burckhardt CS, Bjelle A. Education programmes for fibromyalgia patients: description and evaluation. *Baillieres Clin Rheumatol* 1994; **8**: 935–55.

181. Vlaeyen JW, Teeken-Gruben NJ, Goossens ME, *et al*. Cognitive-educational treatment of fibromyalgia: a

randomized clinical trial. I. Clinical effects. *J Rheumatol* 1996; **23**: 1237–45.

182. White KP, Nielson WR. Cognitive behavioral treatment of fibromyalgia syndrome: a followup assessment. *J Rheumatol* 1995; **22**: 717–21.

183. Nielson W, Harth M, Bell D. Out-patient cognitive-behavioral treatment of fibromyalgia: impact on pain response and health status. *Pain Res Manage* 1997; **2**: 145–50.

184. Turk DC, Okifuji A, Sinclair JD, Starz TW. Interdisciplinary treatment for fibromyalgia syndrome: clinical and statistical significance. *Arthritis Care Res* 1998; **11**: 186–95.

185. Smythe H. Nonarticular rheumatism and psychogenic musculoskeletal syndromes. In *Arthritis and Allied Conditions; A textbook of rheumatology* 9th edn. [ed. L Hollander] (Philadelphia, PA: Lea & Febiger, 1979), pp. 881–91.

Management of pain in arthritis

Raphael J. Leo and Thomas J. Romano

Introduction

The negative impact of arthritis on virtually every
aspect of society is so great as to be almost inestima-
ble. In addition to direct costs of care, the indirect
costs resulting from arthritis-related work disability,
absences, and decreased productivity, are monumen-
tal [1–3]. Thus, arthritic conditions not only generate
pain and suffering, but contribute to financial hardship, decreased quality of life, and life dissatisfaction
[4–8]. The resulting social and psychological impact of
arthritic conditions can be staggering.

According to the National Health Interview Survey
[9] over 46 million adults in the USA have some form of
arthritis. Almost half of these adults, i.e., 18.9 million
patients, have limitations in daily activities attributable to the arthritis [10]. Arthritis prevalence increases
with age and is higher among women in every age
group in the USA [11]. Prevalence rates are expected
to rise; by the year 2030 an estimated 67 million adults
in the United States will have diagnosable arthritis [9].
The adverse impact of arthritic conditions is therefore
expected to rise significantly.

Despite these and other problems and challenges
faced by arthritis sufferers, there are now more and
varied treatment options available to them than in
the past. The first portion of this chapter will examine
current diagnostic and treatment approaches to osteoarthritis, rheumatoid arthritis, and systemic lupus erythematosus. The second portion of this chapter will
address psychological and psychopharmacological
treatment approaches, particularly for pain management, in arthritic conditions.

Osteoarthritis

Osteoarthritis (OA) is a musculoskeletal problem that
causes stiffness, loss of mobility, pain, and swelling in
one or more joints. The symptoms are typically due to
inflammation and degeneration in such joint structures
as cartilage, bone, muscles, ligaments, and synovium.
Any joint can be affected by OA but typically weight
bearing joints such as the hips, knees, low back, and
ankles are prone to this disorder. Furthermore injuries
to joints may predispose those parts of the body to early
development of OA such as might be found in relatively
young individuals who have sustained sports injuries,
e.g., from participation in football or basketball. Unlike
systemic inflammatory connective tissue diseases, OA
is not a disorder that is characterized by extra-articular
manifestations, e.g., rheumatoid vasculitis or pleural
pericarditis of systemic lupus erythematosus. That is
not to imply, however, that OA cannot be extremely
painful and does not deserve serious consideration.

Typically, the pathology of OA follows a progression
starting with the loss of cartilage matrix which predisposes the affected joint to further injury. As OA progresses
there tends to be alterations to underlying bone as well as
associated wear and tear on the cartilage with the development of bony outgrowths called osteophytes at the
periphery of the affected joint. Often debris, cartilage
and bone degradation products occupy the joint space,
and eventually more cartilage breakdown occurs when
the synovium or joint lining becomes inflamed due to
the release of inflammatory mediators such as cytokines
and enzymes. Further cartilage damage and reactive
bone formation occurs and eventually, if unchecked, the
affected joint may become totally dysfunctional leading
to significant morbidity and impairment.

Osteoarthritis is the most common joint disorder
not only in the USA but worldwide. Radiographic evidence of OA is present in most people age 65 years or
older and in over 80% of those older than 75 years.
Furthermore, approximately 11% of people older than
64 years have knee OA that is causing pain, and/or
stiffness and/or functional limitations [12]. Knee OA
has been cited frequently as a cause of impairment and

Behavioral and Psychopharmacologic Pain Management, ed. Michael H. Ebert and Robert D. Kerns. Published by
Cambridge University Press. © Cambridge University Press 2011.

disability [13, 14]. There are many reasons for that. The knee is a weight-bearing joint and is often injured by work and/or sporting activities. Many patients often gain weight as they age. Being overweight or obese can be a risk factor in the development and/or exacerbation of knee OA [15–17]. In addition to obesity, age is the most common identifiable risk factor for OA. Certainly genetics may also play a role. Bone abnormalities or inherited traits such as dysplasia or malalignment can subject joints to unusual stresses which could increase the likelihood of the development of OA. There is also slight sex difference, particularly in location of OA independent of age or physical activity. For example, hand OA is more prevalent in women while men are more prone to develop hip OA.

Osteoarthritis is an extremely costly disease. It is the most common cause of disability in the USA. One study measured both direct medical payments and lost productivity and came to the conclusion that the cost to the USA was $86 billion in 1997 [18]. The costs are bound to rise. A subcommittee of the American College of Rheumatology (ACR) estimated that more than 20 million Americans will develop OA [19] as the population ages and as obesity becomes more prevalent.

The diagnosis of OA is usually made after taking a history, doing a physical examination and performing appropriate radiographic and laboratory tests. Typically, a patient with OA will complain of pain on use of a joint associated with gelling and stiffness of the joint. Gelling and stiffness, if present, typically last less than 30 minutes and often patients will say once they start moving the joint they will feel a grinding, clicking, or crunching of the joint in question. Other signs include atrophy of the muscles surrounding the joint and, in the case of OA of weight-bearing joints, an altered gait would often be present. Instability of joints occurs in late stages of OA. X-rays typically show marginal osteophytes, joint space narrowing, some bony sclerosis and cyst formation as well as malalignment [20, 21].

As opposed to rheumatoid arthritis and systemic lupus erythematosus, laboratory investigations are not particularly helpful in the diagnosis of OA, although negative tests will assist with ruling out other disorders. For example, the erythrocyte sedimentation rate (ESR), typically a very sensitive test for systemic inflammation, tends to be normal or only slightly elevated in OA compared to the autoimmune mediated rheumatologic diseases. Moreover, serology tends to be negative or weakly positive. Synovial fluid analysis may be helpful in that results tend to show a relatively non-inflammatory pattern. The typically clear, yellow or straw-colored fluid tends to be slightly viscous and has only a few thousand leukocytes compared to the more intensely inflammatory joint fluid seen in other arthropathies. There has been evidence that suggests that inflammation of the synovial membrane augers poorly as it is often associated with a faster disease progression and ensuing impairment [22]. Furthermore, frequent use of magnetic resonance imaging (MRI) has also been helpful in determining the severity of OA. One study suggested that bone marrow lesions detected by MRI correlated fairly well with higher levels of pain in OA patients. Also those patients with knee OA and such lesions did have more rapidly progressing disease.

The pain experienced by OA sufferers tends to be multi-factorial in its generation and perpetuation. Both peripheral and central mechanisms contribute to the misery experienced by many OA patients. The periphery-linked wear and tear and/or injury cause activation of inflammatory mediators such as interleukin-1 and prostaglandins which can lead to disease progression [23]. In particular, prostaglandin E_2 can contribute to the inflammatory process by sensitizing peripheral nociceptor terminals producing localized pain. This may be due to a direct effect or due to the increase in cyclooxygenase-2 [24, 25]. The central nervous system gets involved after the A-delta fibers and C fibers transmit the nociceptor impulses through the peripheral nerve up to the dorsal root into the dorsal horn of the spinal cord and eventually to the central nervous system. The nociceptive impulses are interpreted via connections between the thalamus and cortex resulting in a conscious awareness of the pain, discussed in Chapter 2.

It is not an uncommon clinical occurrence for joint inflammation to be successfully treated with pharmacologic agents only to have the patient still complaining bitterly of pain. It should be borne in mind that many patients with arthritis have concomitant fibromyalgia [26] and other co-morbidities contributing to global perception of pain. In the absence of co-morbid conditions, it is conceivable that objectively verifiable pathology (e.g., damage seen by X-ray or number of swollen joints) may appear to be at odds with the patients' reported pain level. Such discrepancies suggest that psychological and emotional determinants may be extremely important in the appreciation of subjective pain ratings. Merely addressing the adverse nociceptive stimuli from inflamed joints would be inadequate to help the patient in an optimal way and other interventions may be needed to optimize the ability of the patient to function [27, 28].

Several treatment modalities are available to the patient with OA; several pharmacologic approaches have been reviewed in the ACR sub-committee on osteoarthritis guidelines [29]. First and foremost, the patient must be informed about his condition and how he can actively participate in his treatment. Each patient should be made aware of any aggravating factors peculiar to his situation. For example, the "weekend warrior" who persists in doing strenuous exercise which includes impact loading on the joints must be cautioned that these activities could result in a worsening of his OA. Those exercises and activities causing little impact loading on the joints, e.g., swimming or aqua-aerobics, are preferred. If the patient is over-weight a weight reduction regimen should be initiated.

Other non-pharmacologic treatments include supplementation with chondroitin sulfate 800 mg to 1200 mg daily [30]. Available over-the-counter, chondroitin sulfate is relatively inexpensive and has been shown to be effective in OA [31]. Of interest is that benefits of chondroitin sulfate persist up to 6 months after therapy was discontinued.

The use of medications such as non-steroidal anti-inflammatory drugs (NSAIDs) has been the mainstay of drug therapy for many years. These medications tend to decrease pain, stiffness and swelling, but have never been touted to stop the progression of OA. In fact, there is some evidence that certain NSAIDs may lead to progression of disease [32, 33]. Acetaminophen has also been used successfully to treat the pain associated with mild OA, but this medication may be hepatotoxic and should be used with caution in patients with pre-existing liver disease and those who drink alcohol. Tramadol is a centrally acting analgesic, possessing both weak opioid influences as well as inhibiting the uptake of serotonin and norepinephrine; but lacks anti-inflammatory properties. It is generally well tolerated but in some patients there is an increased risk of seizures.

Patients in whom NSAIDs, acetaminophen and tramadol have proven ineffective may require stronger analgesics such as opioids. Many physicians are reluctant to use opioids for patients who do not have malignancies for a variety of reasons, among which are fear of causing addiction, fears of possible oversight, and concerns about possible diversion. However, these medications can be of great benefit in certain patients and should be prescribed with caution but not withheld unnecessarily.

If pharmacologic and non-pharmacologic treatments for osteoarthritis fall short of the mark other courses of action may be necessary. Intra-articular injection with a corticosteroid and local anesthetic mixture has been used for decades and can be quite effective in providing temporary pain relief in an affected joint [34]. However, there is no proven benefit in terms of the halting of disease progression. Visco-supplementation is an alternative approach for patients who failed the above therapies. There are several products on the market, all of which have been termed "hyaluronans." Because OA patients tend to have a decreased concentration of decreased molecular weight of hyaluronic acids in the joint space those substances no longer provide the necessary shock absorption and lubrication, as they had done in the past. Hyaluronan supplementation has been used to help replenish and restore normal joint function by replacing the hyaluronic acid molecules that have been heretofore degraded and changed. The active ingredient in all of the five available hyaluronans on the market to date have been extracted from chicken combs or made from bacterial cells. All of the products are indicated for knee osteoarthritis but, in principle, they can be used for osteoarthritis of any joint. They have a good safety profile and there is some evidence that preparations can promote normal cartilage growth [35]. Clinical acumen must dictate how and when these agents should be used. In contrast to intra-articular corticosteroid injections hyaluronans do not raise blood sugar and have not been shown to have an adverse affect on cartilage or the surrounding structures.

When all else fails surgery should be considered. Surgery can help relieve pain and improve joint mobility and can enhance the quality of life for many patients who otherwise would not be able to ambulate or perform even the most modest of activities of daily living. Arthroscopic surgery can be used to provide short-term relief in some cases but for the most definitive result conventional surgery may be necessary. There are several operations available, including osteotomy, hip resurfacing, partial joint replacement, and complete joint replacement. Naturally, the latter procedures are major surgical endeavors, and there are significant risks involved including deep venous thrombosis, infection, pulmonary embolism, prosthesis fracture, and dislocation. Post surgery, the patients must participate in an extensive rehabilitation program that must be followed carefully in order to obtain optimal results.

In summary while osteoarthritis is not a systemic inflammatory connective tissue disease and is not associated with extra-articular manifestations, it can cause tremendous pain and disability. Osteoarthritis can be extremely costly in terms of direct costs (i.e. treatment modalities) as well as indirect costs (e.g., lost wages, decreased production, disability). To obtain the best results the clinician must consider all co-morbidities as well as the pharmacologic and non-pharmacologic approaches to treatment.

Rheumatoid arthritis

Rheumatoid arthritis (RA) is a systemic inflammatory connective tissue disease. In addition to multi-joint involvement, typically presenting as a symmetrical polyarthritis, there are several potential extra-articular manifestations of the disorder causing serious internal organ pathology, diminished longevity, and in rare cases, death. In this way it differs from OA.

It has been estimated that approximately 1% of the population of the USA has RA, the majority being women [36]. Although it can occur at any time, it most often presents in the second, third and fourth decades of life [37]. The joints most often affected are the metacarpal-phalangeal joints, the proximal phalangeal joints, knees, ankles, and metatarsal phalangeal joints. In fact, in many patients the first manifestations of RA are in the lower extremities, particularly noticeable since they are weight-bearing joints. In addition to joint pain and inflammation, patients with RA typically have morning stiffness, gelling phenomenon, and fatigue. Over 30% of RA patients have a normochromic, normocytic anemia thought to be mediated by the cytokine, interleukin-6 (IL-6); such anemia is unresponsive to nutritional supplements such as vitamin B-12, folic acid or iron [38]. Rather, only control of the underlying disease will tend to normalize the blood count.

When RA strikes, it typically strikes during a worker's peak years of productivity. In 1996 the cost of treating RA was estimated at being approximately $6 billion. Some of those patients require corrective surgery within 10 years of disease onset [39] adding to the medical and non-medical costs. The direct cost of RA in terms of its impact to society was estimated at being approximately $20 000 per patient per year, more than 60% of which was attributed to lost work productivity [40]. It is interesting to note that even if a patient with RA continues to work but at a diminished capacity, the economic impact of RA has been estimated to be almost three times more than for a patient who is not disabled [41]. Once a patient with RA becomes

disabled it is unusual for him to return to work [42], and often such patients have difficulty even performing household tasks [43]. Therefore, RA severely impacts a patient's physical health, employability, and adaptive functioning.

Since RA is such a devastating disease, it is imperative that an accurate diagnosis is established promptly and effective treatment be initiated as soon as possible to reduce the individual (and societal) burdens of the disorder. The ACR (formerly known as the American Rheumatism Association) published criteria for codifying RA [44]. At least four of the following seven criteria would need to be met for a patient to be classified as having RA: (1) morning stiffness of greater than 1 hour most mornings for at least 6 weeks; (2) arthritis and soft tissue swelling of more than 3 of 14 joints/joint groups present for at least 6 weeks; (3) arthritis in hand joints present for at least 6 weeks; (4) symmetric arthritis present for at least 6 weeks; (5) subcutaneous nodules in specific places; (6) rheumatoid factor at a level above the 95th percentile; (7) radiological changes suggestive of joint erosion. Ultimately, however, the diagnosis is a clinical one. When a patient presents with symmetrical joint pain, morning stiffness, synovitis typically of the proximal small joints of the hands and feet, a diagnosis of RA should be suspected, although other arthritides may be responsible for the above symptoms and should be considered in the differential diagnosis.

Laboratory testing can be helpful. For example, a positive rheumatoid factor (RF), especially a high titer, strongly suggests a diagnosis of RA, although about 30% of patients with RA have a negative RF and RF can be positive in other disorders [45]. This is not surprising since RF is an autoantibody caused by immune dysregulation. More recently, a serum cyclic citrullinated peptide antibody test has been used in order to help the clinician diagnose a patient with RA. This particular blood test is more specific for RA and positive in approximately 80% of RA patients but rarely positive in patients who do not have RA resulting in a specificity of approximately 98% [46]. One benefit of this particular test is that it is often positive in early stages of RA and can often herald disease onset. Other tests can be important such as the ESR which is often elevated in inflammatory conditions, C-reactive protein (CRP), and anti-nuclear antibody (ANA). X-rays and even MRI scanning can be helpful in the diagnosis of RA but typically erosions do not occur until the disease has been established. Of interest is that cardiovascular disease has become the leading cause of death in patients

Table 19.1 FDA-approved biologics employed for rheumatoid arthritis treatment

Agent	Target	Route of Administration	Dosing	Risks
Etanercept (Enbrel[R])[a]	TNF-alpha	SC	every week	Increased risk of infection [f]
Infliximab (Remicade[R])[b]	TNF-alpha	IV	every 6–9 weeks	Infusion reactions; increased risk of infection and malignancy [g]
Adalimumab (Humira[R])[c]	TNF-alpha	SC	every 2 weeks	Increased risk of infection [h]
Anakinra (Kineret[R])	IL-1	SC	every day	Increased risk of infection
Rituximab (Rituxan[R])[d]	CD-20 on B lymphocytes	IV		Infusion reactions; increased risk of infection
Abatacept (Orencia[R])[e]	T lymphocytes	IV	every 2–4 weeks	Infusion reactions; increased risk of infection and malignancy

Sources. [a] Ref. [54, 55]; [b] Ref. [57, 58]; [c] Ref. [60]; [d] Ref. [62]; [e] Ref. [63, 64] [f] Ref. [56]; [g] Ref. [59]; [h] Ref. [59, 61].

TNF-alpha: tumor necrosis factor-alpha; IL-1: interleukin-1; CD-20: cell-surface antigen; SC: subcutaneous; IV: intravenous.

with RA may be related to the elevation of C-reactive protein as well as other acute phase reactants [47]. Within the first year of RA erosions can be identified on X-rays in up to 30% of patients [48]. Within 3 years of diagnosis up to 90% of patients have bone erosions and joint space narrowing noted on plain film X-rays [49]. While X-rays are very helpful, MRI and ultrasonography may detect changes earlier than conventional radiographs [50].

In the past a very popular treatment algorithm for RA was a representative pyramid with initial treatment modalities at the base (e.g., anti-inflammatory medication and physical therapy) rising to the use of slow acting disease modifying agents and eventually to immunosuppressive therapy. It is recognized that RA can rapidly progress leading to significant joint destruction and deformity as well as extra-articular manifestations in the form of lung disease, vasculitis, etc., as such there has been emphasis on early and aggressive treatment. Anti-inflammatory medications, i.e., NSAIDS and corticosteroids, can be useful in alleviating symptoms of RA but do nothing to halt disease progression. Traditional disease modifying anti-rheumatic drugs (DMARDs), used in addition to the anti-inflammatory medications, have been shown to slow radiographic progression in patients with RA

[51]. Including methotrexate, azathioprine, leflumonide, cyclosporin as well as injectable and oral gold salts, combinations of DMARDs have been shown to be more effective in suppressing RA activity than one agent alone [52, 53]. For patients who have failed a combination of anti-inflammatory medications and DMARDs the use of biologics, which target inflammatory mediators such as tumor necrosis factor alpha (TNF-alpha) and interleukin-1 (IL-1), as well as B and T lymphocytes, may be the next logical step in treatment (see Table 19.1). The early use of biologics is indicated once a diagnosis of RA has been established; their use, however, should not be delayed until significant joint deformity or extra-articular pathology has occurred. Unfortunately, side effects associated with the use of biologics include increased risk of serious infections with slightly increased risk of development of malignancy [56, 59, 61, 63]. Other biologic treatments are being developed in an attempt to improve efficacy while decreasing toxicity risks.

The decision to initiate potentially harmful treatment in patients with RA needs to be made with extreme caution. It is important to weigh the risks of treatment against the possibility that undue hesitation, or inadequate treatment, may expose the patient to increased morbidity and even early mortality due to the aggressive and pernicious nature of RA. Furthermore, while pharmacologic therapy is important, the prudent clinician needs to also advise his patient regarding activity modification, stress reduction, and the need for physical therapy, assistive devices, counseling, and other healthcare resources available to patients who suffer from this devastating illness.

Systemic lupus erythematosus

Unlike RA, systemic lupus erythematosus (SLE) has such protean manifestations early in the course of the disease as to confound the clinician. While joint pain and swelling can occur in many patients with SLE, often the patient will initially present with anything from seizures to skin rashes, often different from the typical "butterfly" malar rash, one of the hallmarks of the disease [65]. Constitutional symptoms, e.g., fatigue and pain, abound in SLE [66–68]. Neuropsychiatric symptoms, including depression and psychosis are common features of SLE [69, 70] contributing significantly to dysfunction.

Systemic lupus erythematosus is an autoimmune disease characterized by the production of antibodies directed against components of the nuclei of the patients' cells. It primarily presents in young women although it can affect anyone at any age and at any time. The prevalence of SLE has been estimated at 1 in 2000 Americans but there is variability due to ethnicity, socioeconomic standing, and race [71]. Because it often affects young people, the impact of the disease can be devastating not only in terms of ill-health but also because of its adverse psychological effects due to the negative impact of SLE on appearance and body-image [72, 73].

Because SLE can involve any organ system at the outset and, therefore, mimic other diseases, its true nature may remain hidden for some time and the diagnosis of SLE can be delayed. For example, some patients present with anemia but the anemia may only be part of the picture. The same goes for other problems such as arthritis or pleurisy. Any part of the body can be affected by SLE but most often harms the nervous system, kidneys, blood vessels, lungs, skin, joints, heart and liver. Periods of increased activity (flares) often alternate with periods of disease quiescence. To further challenge the clinician, SLE can potentially be induced by many commonly used medications most notably procainamide, hydralazine, and quinidine [74] medications used to treat cardiac arrythmias and hypertension. Recently, there have been cases of drug-induced SLE occurring in patients receiving biologic agents used to treat RA, such as etanercept [75]. The diagnosis of drug-induced SLE can be made by history, physical exam and laboratory testing [76]; it is reversible upon discontinuation of the offending agent and implementation of symptomatic treatment.

The ACR first established SLE criteria in 1982; these were revised in 1997 [77]. These criteria were not intended to be used to diagnose specific patients but rather for use in clinical trials. Patients must present with four of the following eleven signs and symptoms to be considered to have SLE: malar rash, discoid lesions, photosensitivity, oral ulcers, arthritis, renal disorder, neurologic disorder, serositis, hematologic disorder, positive ANA test, and immunologic disorder with other antibodies being positive. Alternative criteria were published in 1998 [78]. What all of these criteria have in common is an autoimmune condition characterized by inflammation in various body structures associated with abnormal serology, such as a positive ANA test, positive anti-Smith antigen test, or positive anti-double stranded DNA test. Most importantly, the clinician needs to have a high index of suspicion that the patient indeed has systemic lupus in order to consider the diagnosis, then confirm or reject it.

Since SLE can mimic virtually any disease the clinician must always be circumspect in approaching patients who have inflammation, particularly of several different organ systems. It is not uncommon for patients to have unexplained symptoms and, therefore, untreated SLE for many years. The initial complaints can be non specific: fever, malaise, joint pains, myalgias, and fatigue. With the exception of a drug-induced SLE, the cause of this disease is unknown. Triggers for SLE exacerbations include stress, exposure to sunlight (i.e., UV radiation), female hormones, and infections, among others factors.

A good screening test is the ANA test; while a positive ANA is not specific for SLE, a negative ANA effectively excludes the disease. More specific tests for lupus are the anti-Smith antigen test and the anti-double stranded DNA antibody test [79]. Other tests can be used to monitor the course of SLE. For example, the ESR is a very sensitive but extremely non-specific test for inflammation. It often rises with disease flares and falls when the disease goes into remission. Similarly serum complement levels can be useful since low levels of complement suggest consumption and, therefore, depletion by an over stimulated immune system. Low serum complements have often been very useful in predicting and monitoring SLE flares. Naturally tests to monitor end organ function can be useful to assess the SLE patient as well. For example, if kidneys are at risk repeat urinalyses and serum tests for blood urea nitrogen and creatinine can be extremely useful in monitoring the progress of therapy for SLE. Occasionally, renal biopsy may be needed to stage disease level [80]. This is also true for serial white blood cell counts or platelet counts if those cells are the targets of the SLE disease process [81]. It cannot be overemphasized that SLE must be considered in any patient who presents with multi-system problems particularly in women of childbearing age. Systemic lupus erythematosus can present in numerous ways such as patchy hair loss (alopecia), mouth, nasal and vaginal ulcers, joint pain and stiffness, anemia, chest pain, problems such as pericarditis, myocarditis and endocarditis, seizures or psychosis. It is a condition that does not exist in a vacuum; afflicted patients can likewise have other common conditions, e.g., osteoarthritis, fibromyalgia, diabetes, atherosclerotic heart disease.

The bedrock of SLE management is education of the patient so that she better understands the nature of the illness, the treatment options available, and the need for complying with the treatment regimen. Patients should be cautioned about avoiding undue exposure to sunlight and must even use caution when taking potentially photosensitizing medications such as certain antibodies. As previously mentioned, some drugs can induce SLE while others such as estrogen preparations may exacerbate SLE disease activity [82, 83]. As with other chronic diseases, a therapeutic alliance must be forged between patient and doctor in an atmosphere of trust and open communication. Many books and pamphlets are available through the Arthritis Foundation or commercially [84] to facilitate patient education; support groups can also be a good venue whereby patients could learn about SLE and get much-needed psychosocial support.

Pregnancy can be very hazardous for some SLE patients and many medications used to control the disease, such as cyclophosphamide and hydroxychloroquine, are contraindicated in pregnancy. Thus, family planning and safe birth control methods need to be discussed with SLE patients of child-bearing age. Furthermore since SLE and some of the medications used to treat SLE, i.e., immunosuppressives, can lower patients' resistance to infection, the clinician must take symptoms such as fever, cough, sore throat, and dysuria very seriously.

The mainstay of therapy consists of the anti-inflammatory medications, e.g., NSAIDs and corticosteroids. Musculoskeletal symptoms, mild serositis, and low-grade fever due to SLE typically respond to NSAIDs and low-dose oral steroids. Higher doses of steroids such as prednisone or methylprednisolone are often used for SLE flares to rapidly control symptoms. Additionally, DMARDs may be needed to prevent or minimize end-organ damage. One group of DMARDs, the anti-malarial drugs, are particularly useful in controlling musculoskeletal pain and stiffness as well as relieving constitutional symptoms. Such medications should not be abruptly discontinued due to the risk of an SLE flare [85]. The most commonly used antimalarial, hydroxychloroquine, is commonly associated with adverse effects, e.g., gastrointestinal problems and minor skin rashes which can generally be easily managed. Rarely neuropsychiatric side effects include psychosis, seizures, ataxia, so they should not be used in patients with CNS involvement in the lupus disease process. Another side effect, though rare, is retinal toxicity [86]. Screening and follow-up ophthalmologic examinations are necessary in patients taking anti-malarials so that the medication can be tapered and, eventually, discontinued to avoid permanent eye damage.

Another DMARD useful in the treatment of SLE, particularly arthritis, serositis, skin rashes and constitutional signs and symptoms, is methotrexate usually given in once-weekly oral doses. Methotrexate's elimination depends on adequate renal function (i.e. glomerular-filtration and tubular secretion) so it should be used with extreme caution in patients with lupus nephritis. Major organ involvement, particularly, lupus nephritis as well as other serious forms of the disease affecting the central nervous system, vasculature, and blood cells require such aggressive treatment as the use of immunosuppressive therapy. Cyclophosphamide, an alkylating agent, is a very effective drug in managing severe SLE [87, 88]. However, it must be used with caution due to its potential to cause such side effects as leukopenia and hemorrhagic cystitis. Azathioprine, a purine analog, can be used instead of cyclophosphamide and is preferable some cases due to its more favorable toxicity profile, but it is generally considered to be a less effective alternative. Cyclosporine A, a medication often used to suppress the immune system in transplant recipients, has been used to treat both renal [89] and non-renal [90] SLE manifestations. Hormonal therapies have helped some SLE patients. Avoidance of estrogen and the use of male hormones have been effective in many patients. For example, danazol, an attenuated androgen, has been reported to manage lupus thrombocytopenia [91]. Dehydroepiandrosterone (DHEA), an adrenal hormone, has also been used to treat patients with SLE [92]. When faced with a patient with immediately life-threatening lupus problems such as thrombotic thrombocytopenic purpura, pulmonary hemorrhage or vasculitic, plasma exchange (plasmapheresis) may need to be employed [93]. When followed by intravenous cyclophosphamide, plasma exchange has resulted in some long-term SLE remissions [94].

Many SLE patients suffer from chronic pain. Moderate pain can typically be treated with propoxyphene/acetaminophen preparations, hydrocodone/acetominophen preparations, or anti-inflammatory medication such as salicylates or ibuprofen. However, moderate to severe chronic pain may need stronger opioids such as oxycodone, oxymorphone, immediate release preparations as well as long-term preparations containing morphine (e.g., AvinzaR, KadianR), oxycodone (OxycontinR), oxymorphone (Opana ERR) or methadone. A transdermal fentanyl patch may also be needed for chronic persistent pain because of its ability to act over a period of several days. Patients who require steroids frequently may develop complications such as diabetes mellitus, osteoporosis, obesity, fluid retention, and hypertension.

Since the signs and symptoms of SLE and fibromyalgia can overlap it is important to determine which problem is acting up in an SLE patient who complains of increased chest pain, joint pain, muscle pain, fatigue, decreased stamina, and malaise. Many SLE patients also have fibromyalgia [95]. For example if a patient's musculoskeletal pain is increased because of a lupus flare the use of corticosteroids would be very beneficial. However, if the increase in musculoskeletal pain is due to a flare of fibromyalgia, then systemic corticosteroids would not only be ineffective, but would expose the patient to inordinate adverse effects. Diagnosis and treatment of SLE can be challenging. Good treatment is available but the mortality and morbidity from this terrible disease depends on many factors including ethnicity [71, 96].

Psychopharmacologic and psychological aspects of arthritis pain treatment

While osteoarthritis, rheumatoid arthritis, and systemic lupus erythematosus can ravage the body, the profound impact on one's functioning can also damage the psyche and assault the spirit. Allopathic medicine, while very helpful, is only one arm of treatment. Current medical treatments cannot cure RA or OA nor entirely eliminate arthritis-related pain and disability. Chronic pain conditions, such as the varied arthritic syndromes, can best be understood and approached when one considers them from the biopsychosocial perspective (discussed extensively in Chapters 3 and 16). The pain associated with arthritic conditions can adversely affect one's general functioning, produce disability, and reduce one's sense of self-efficacy. Additionally, one's capacity for relationships may be adversely affected, and changes in roles induced by the chronic condition can strain existing relationships. There may be concomitant impairments in economic and social functioning, leading to heightened dependency on others, loss of autonomy, and isolation. Combined, these factors can contribute to the distress associated with having a chronic medical condition lending one toward lowered self-esteem, depression, and anxiety. Focusing exclusively on medical interventions for arthritic conditions can only partially address the impact they have on one's general functioning; and as such, psychological interventions have been invoked to enhance functioning and adaptation to having such chronic illnesses [97].

Conversely, psychological and social factors are likely to have a reciprocal relationship on one's health status. Specifically, disease activity may not be the main predictor of perceived pain and associated dysfunction. In RA, pain is not significantly related to variables such as ESR, grip strength, joint swelling or radiographic changes; but instead appears to be related to psychological variables, e.g., social stress, lack of social support, helplessness, catastrophizing, and ineffective coping strategies [98–100]. In OA, depression is a robust predictor of perceived disability, more than radiographic evidence of degenerative changes [101, 102].

As described in Chapter 6 of this text, there are several psychiatric disorders that can accompany pain conditions. Clinical psychopathologic disorders, e.g., depression, anxiety and personality disorders, have been associated with arthritis [103–105]; increasing disability and functional impairments [106]. Left untreated, depression and other co-morbid psychiatric conditions can exacerbate the multiple complications that already beset patients with arthritic conditions. The presence of co-morbid depression has been linked with increased rates of mortality among RA patients in a 4-year observational study [107]. It is unsurprising, therefore, that patients with arthritis who seek medical treatment are more depressed than those with arthritis who do not seek medical care [108]; unfortunately, co-morbid psychiatric disorders are often unrecognized and undiagnosed among patients with arthritic conditions seeking medical treatment [109].

Management of arthritic conditions ought to be aimed at decreasing pain and suffering, enhancing functioning, and improving quality of life [110]. For example, in a recent multi-site, randomized controlled trial consisting of 1001 patients with arthritis, interventions directed at underlying depression (antidepressants and/or psychotherapeutic measures) resulted in improvements in quality of life, pain intensity, perceived pain associated impairments, and improved health status [111]. In another study, the combination of psychotherapy, specifically CBT, did not add to the therapeutic effectiveness of sertraline therapy in the treatment of depression associated with RA [112], however, no direct comparisons of antidepressants vs. CBT (or other psychotherapy modalities) were conducted to compare their relative effectiveness in improving depression complicating arthritic conditions. Nonetheless, it appears that optimal treatment of arthritic pain, and efforts to optimize functioning, will require multi-modal treatment approaches involving psychiatric and psychological consultation and collaborative treatment.

Psychopharmacologic interventions

Extensive research has been devoted to assessment of the analgesic effects of psychopharmacologic agents, particularly antidepressants. Antidepressants may afford patients additional benefits beyond direct analgesic influences, e.g., by mitigating clinical depressive states that accompany chronic painful conditions. There is a substantial co-occurrence of depression with a variety of chronic pain conditions; it is often associated with increased somatic preoccupation, e.g., pain and associated impairments [113–115]. Depression may result in perpetuation of pain, increasing the number and severity of physical symptoms (referred to as pain scale augmentation), and enhancing subjective assessments of pain-related disability [116–118]. Reduction of co-morbid depression with antidepressant use thus may indirectly reduce pain and perceived disability.

Antidepressants may exert direct pain-mitigating effects by several possible mechanisms, including

influences on central and peripheral pain processing as well as synergistic effects with other medications [119, 120]. Centrally, antidepressants may produce pain relief by influencing norepinephrine (NE) and serotonin (5-HT) neurotransmission of the supraspinal modulatory systems influencing dorsal horn pain transmission mechanisms [121]. Additionally, antidepressants may influence peripheral pain transmission mechanisms, through modulation of peripheral 5-HT receptor activity which interact with inflammatory mediators such as prostaglandin E2 or bradykinin [122]. Lastly, antidepressants also may reduce pain through potentiation of opioid analgesia [120, 123].

The bulk of the evidence pertaining to the use of antidepressants in arthritis pain states has been directed at the utility of tricyclic antidepressants (TCAs); the utility of newer antidepressants in addressing arthritis-related pain were generally uninvestigated. Early trials were limited by the fact that they lacked control group comparators and employed small sample sizes. Subsequently, few controlled studies suggest that antidepressants can be efficacious in reducing the pain associated with arthritic conditions, independent of effects on mood [124–127]. Some studies failed to demonstrate an appreciable analgesic influence from the use of antidepressants [112, 128, 129]. It is noteworthy that treatment with paroxetine (a serotonin selective reuptake inhibitor, SSRI) or amitriptyline (a TCA) have been, among patients with RA, demonstrated to reduce pain, depression and associated disability levels [125]. In this study, the particular advantages of use of either of the two antidepressant agents could not be established. It is unclear if pain relieving effects observed with either amitriptyline or paroxetine in this study were attributable to direct analgesic effects or indirect effects, e.g., mitigating patients' tendencies toward somatic preoccupation and pain scale augmentation or facilitating treatment adherence.

Because of the limited empirical support for the use of antidepressants for their analgesic role in arthritis, antidepressant use has been largely relegated to those persons afflicted with arthritis experiencing co-morbid depressive and/or anxiety disorders. The utility of antidepressant agents in addressing arthritis-related pain and associated co-morbidities have as yet to be fully explored in empirical investigations.

Educational approaches

Arthritis education programs serve to enhance patient awareness about the illness, and the utility of measures such as pharmacological and surgical approaches, exercise and joint protection. Information may be provided in several didactic sessions, or in a home-based self-instructional format. Generally, controlled studies suggest that educational approaches have been demonstrated to foster knowledge, but are limited with regard to improving pain or functional disability [130–133].

In a review of studies utilizing educational interventions among patients with OA or RA, only small effects on pain reduction were observed, i.e., an average of 16% pain reduction was found from pre-treatment pain severity ratings in 15 controlled trials [134]. In addition, a meta-analysis of randomized controlled trials assessing the effectiveness of patient education interventions among patients with RA revealed that such programs resulted in positive effects on physical functioning (disability, number of painful joints), and psychological status (depression and anxiety severity) immediately post-intervention, but the effect sizes were small [135]; however, the influence on pain was not found to be significant. Furthermore, the positive effects of patient education programs were not sustained at follow-up. It is noteworthy that studies included in this review encompassed those invoking "pure" didactic and home-based self informational formats along with those involving combinations of treatment approaches, e.g., cognitive-behavioral arthritis education programs that incorporated didactic instruction with coping strategies training, stress management, and reinforcement of health promoting behaviors. Interestingly, whereas combined information-behavioral programs produced significant effects on the aforementioned outcome measures, information-only programs failed to do so [136].

The ineffectiveness of "pure" arthritis education in producing improvements in pain and disability were thought to be due to the fact that the provision of disease information does not naturally generalize to the development and refinement of disease management skills and behavioral strategies with which to cope with the disease. As such, greater emphasis in recent years has been devoted to the integration of psychological therapies into arthritis management approaches.

One reason studies investigating education programs fail to produce significant effects on pain, or for that matter, sustained improvements in other physical and psychological parameters is that patients included in such investigations often vary with regard to the duration and extensiveness of disease. Hence, questions arise as to whether physical and/or psychological improvements in arthritis may be contingent upon intervening with patients earlier in the course of illness, e.g., soon after diagnosis, as opposed to those with later stages who have been entrenched with established disease [132, 135].

Psychological therapies

Psychological therapies have emerged as relatively non-invasive approaches to the management of arthritic conditions; the rationale for their use is based upon a number of considerations. One is that extensive research has demonstrated the importance of psychological factors in the exacerbation and maintenance of arthritis [100, 137]. Patients prone to experiencing helplessness, or who engage in catastrophizing (expecting the worst) or who devote energy toward regulating one's emotional responses to stress tend to report higher pain levels and psychological distress [138–140]. This assertion does not negate the role of joint biomechanical derangements or other systemic effects of arthritic conditions, but emphasizes that the experiences and behaviors of arthritic patients are influenced by factors in addition to strictly mechanical ones. Secondly, like patients with many chronic disorders, arthritis patients can benefit from approaches that emphasize disease management skills.

Psychological therapies focus on modifying the behavioral, cognitive, and physiological responses to pain [120]. The two psychological techniques that have been advocated most in arthritis include cognitive-behavioral therapy (CBT) and self-regulatory treatment (SRT) interventions. These therapies differ with regard to their approach, perspectives, and goals, briefly described below.

Cognitive-behavioral therapy focuses on belief systems and coping strategies that contribute to problematic behaviors of patients with arthritis [141, 142]. Cognitive restructuring, an interactive process involving the Socratic method, is used to teach patients to identify and modify maladaptive, negatively distorted thoughts that may lead them to avoid activities and to experience negative feelings, such as depression, anxiety, and anger. Patients are encouraged to reappraise irrational, self-defeating thoughts and replace them with more rational alternatives. The presumption is that as a result of cognitive restructuring, patients will demonstrate less avoidance of physical activity, and will experience less physiological arousal and less intense pain. The emphasis of the coping strategies training component of CBT is aimed at assisting patients with developing a repertoire of skills for managing pain as well as problem-solving strategies that may be useful in effectively managing stress in a wide range of situations that might otherwise induce pain. Using homework completed by the patient and issues discussed in sessions, the therapist helps the patient identify and assess the utility of currently employed strategies, and develop alternatives. The approach of CBT has been manualized and can be conducted in an individual or group format [143].

Self-regulatory treatments (SRTs) are intended to teach patients techniques to mitigate the experience of pain by reducing the physiological responses that pain tends to elicit. Utilizing such approaches as biofeedback, relaxation training, guided imagery, and hypnosis, which emphasize the patient's ability to reduce muscle tension, sympathetic arousal, and mental distress (e.g., anxiety), SRTs aim to create an internal state that is incompatible with tension and distress and foster in patients a sense of mastery over their pain experiences.

One problem in evaluating individual psychological therapies is that they are often embedded in broad-based medical and rehabilitation programs that include several other types of treatment. Thus, in many studies there is significant heterogeneity in the definitions and content of treatments employed. For example, SRTs such as relaxation training and guided imagery are often provided in combination with CBT therapies rendering it difficult to determine the independent effect of specific psychological treatments.

A second problem involves methodological approaches in existing clinical research. Varying outcome measures, different sample characteristics, e.g., mild vs. moderately-to-severely disabled individuals; varying use of co-interventions, e.g., medication; and variations in data analysis methods [144], may obscure determination of the differential treatment effects of various psychological therapies. For example, marked heterogeneity in the samples of patients employed in studies might conceal any treatment effects derived from such interventions [145, 146].

Cognitive-behavioral therapy treatment of arthritis

The bulk of the literature on psychotherapy efficacy has focused on CBT treatment. Meta-analyses suggest that patients with arthritis who are exposed to CBT, in comparison to no treatment or to standard treatment, have demonstrated post-treatment improvements in physical (i.e., perceived pain intensity, life interference from pain, health related quality of life), and psychological functioning, i.e., depression severity [147; see also reviews in 132, 135]. However, taken in the aggregate, the effect sizes for impact on pain, perceived disability, coping, depression, and self-efficacy were small, but nonetheless statistically significant [147]. The impact of CBT on analgesic medication requirements has been largely unexamined; although one study suggested that utilization of coping strategies was associated with reductions in analgesic medication use [148]. Additionally, some studies suggest that patients trained in CBT demonstrate less utilization of medical resources, perhaps reflecting the positive influences on coping and emotional stabilization as a result of such interventions [149, 150].

Cognitive-behavioral therapy had little influence on physiological markers of disease, e.g., ESR, CRP, and rheumatoid factors. One double-blind, controlled study demonstrated that a CBT-focused intervention for patients with early stage RA produced short-term improvements in CRP, but not ESR, as compared with patients in standard medical treatment [151]. Although, the effects on CRP were lost at 6-month follow-up, these data suggest that interventions such as CBT may have an impact on the physical morbidity of arthritis. Furthermore, it remains unclear whether there is a direct influence of psychotherapy on inflammatory activity or an indirect influence, i.e., improving treatment adherence in the intensely followed psychotherapy-treated group. On the other hand, CBT had a positive influence on the number of tender, swollen joints, i.e., a clinical index of disease activity, in meta-analysis of randomized controlled trials [147].

The effectiveness of CBT among patients with OA or RA has been related to modification of three core psychological variables [140]. Specifically, CBT effectiveness has been related to improvements in self-efficacy (one's assessment of his/her ability to cope with pain and associated arthritis symptoms), control (enhancing one's sense of mastery over pain), and reducing helplessness (the expectation that outcomes of events will be independent of one's best efforts). Randomized controlled trials suggest that altering the aforementioned variables was linked to improvements in pain severity and psychological dysfunction as well as reductions in perceived disability among patients with OA and RA [152–157].

However, controversy attends the long-term effectiveness of CBT; studies suggest treatment effects are often unsustained at long-term follow-up [135, 146, 147]. Some patients with RA receiving CBT at 12-month follow-up were able to maintain improvements in pain and depression but were unable to maintain improvements in pain behavior [158]. In another study, improvements in coping strategies and self-efficacy were sustained at 15-month follow-up, but management of daily stress and perceived impairment as a result of RA were not [156]. Carson *et al.* [159] found that the provision of maintenance treatment spanning a 12-week period after the initial treatment session failed to demonstrate any additional benefit over conventional CBT treatment without supplemental maintenance sessions. Thus, despite such encouraging influences, the variability in outcomes among patients with arthritic conditions and the maintenance of positive influences of psychological therapies over the course of illness have been questioned.

There are several factors that can undermine the long-term effectiveness of CBT. First, patients with RA and OA experience progressive biomechanical changes in bones and joints. Disease progression may contribute to reduction in the long-term outcome of interventions such as CBT. Second, the temporal stage in the course of illness when CBT was implemented may influence long-term effects. Similar to those who may gain most from educational interventions, patients with early arthritis may yield greater benefits from CBT than those individuals with late-stage disease [147]. In the latter patients, maladaptive patterns of thinking, coping, and behaviors exacerbating pain and disability may become entrenched and may be recalcitrant to psychotherapeutic intervention [160]. Third, patients may fail to complete homework assignments or fail to implement the strategies acquired during therapy, i.e., cognitive structuring and coping skills, at home when they are no longer in session [161]. The effects of CBT training can be enhanced by including spouses/family members in the training [162–164]; thereby increasing the likelihood that implementation of coping strategies will be encouraged at home.

Most of the literature conducted to date assessing the utility of CBT among patients with arthritis has relied on cross-sectional comparisons addressing groups of subjects. Specifically, a group of subjects treated with and instructed in CBT modalities may be compared to groups of control patients, e.g., wait-list controls or those administered conventional medical management. At the conclusion of the intervention period, and perhaps at some follow-up period, the groups are compared with regard to use of coping strategies, pain intensity, and other dependent measures. While efficient for purposes of empirical assessment, aggregate comparisons across groups of participants ignore the point that there is likely to be a great deal of inter-individual variability in terms of responsiveness to CBT, and overlook the fact that the psychological factors influencing arthritis-related pain and associated conditions almost certainly differ from one patient to another. As a result, when a single type of treatment is given to all subjects in a cohort, it may be highly relevant to some of them, but irrelevant to others. There are likely to be subgroups of patients with chronic pain who are reasonably well adjusted and might only derive limited benefits from psychological and psychiatric intervention. By contrast, others with chronic pain identified as having higher levels of distress and dysfunctional cognitive and behavioral characteristics may benefit most from CBT [145, 165–167]. Instead, of a generic approach, treatments may require customizing interventions more closely to the respective patient's needs and circumstances, thereby optimizing treatment benefits [145, 168].

Another pitfall of aggregate comparisons involving patients trained in CBT with other groups of patients is that the presence of coping strategies is treated as a dichotomous variable, i.e., either present or not. In reality, however, such views are short-sighted as coping is a dynamic process, the effects of which unfold over time [169]. One study addressed the patterns of use of coping strategies and the utility of these strategies in intra-individual comparisons of RA patients trained with CBT [170]. Subjects completed daily diaries assessing the types of pain coping strategies invoked, daily mood assessments, joint pain, and assessments of perceived efficacy of the coping strategies employed. Specifically, patients' use of coping strategies was found to be variable from day-to-day depending on that day's perceived pain severity; greater pain severity was associated with more frequent use of several types of coping strategies. Additionally, coping strategies appeared to exert independent influences on emotional distress and pain. Certain coping strategies were more effective in reducing pain (e.g., doing something specific to reduce pain, relaxation, venting emotions to reduce frustration or anxiety) whereas others might be better for enhancing improvements in mood (e.g., diverting attention, seeking emotional support, and venting emotions to reduce frustration or anxiety). Interestingly, there were distinct temporal relationships between the use of coping strategies and resultant improvements in pain or mood. The immediate effects of use of coping strategies led to improvements in mood on the day that such strategies were employed; by contrast, the use of pain coping strategies led to improvements in next-day pain severity ratings. Thus, while pain severity predicted the range and frequency of coping strategies invoked on a particular day, the use of such strategies produced a decline in the pain severity the next day.

Self-regulatory treatment of arthritis

A major problem in determining the effectiveness of SRTs is that they are often provided in combination with CBT therapies. In such cases, it is difficult to ascertain the independent contribution that SRT approaches make.

There are several studies that have attempted to ascertain the potential role of various isolated SRT modalities in arthritic conditions. Two randomized controlled trials demonstrated that guided imagery with relaxation training administered over 12 weeks was able to produce improvements in both self-rated pain severity and quality of life measures among older women with OA as compared with control (standard medical care) participants [171, 172]. Similarly, relaxation training techniques were demonstrated to reduce mental distress (self-rated anxiety and depression) and improved self-rated assessments of well-being among patients with RA as compared with standard medical treatment control participants [173]; relaxation training, however, was unable to produce significant improvements in physiological parameters of RA [173]. In a randomized controlled trial, relaxation training was able to produce enhanced mobility of the upper extremities and muscle function of the lower extremities [174], yet, the positive effects on mobility were unsustained at long-term follow-up (12 months post-treatment). In an uncontrolled trial, multiple SRT approaches, including guided imagery, progressive muscle relaxation, and breathing exercises, were effective in reducing pain and enhancing functioning among children with juvenile rheumatoid arthritis [175]. Lastly, hypnosis was employed in a randomized controlled trial comparing OA patients; comparator groups included a relaxation training group and a standard medical treatment group [176]. In this study, both the hypnosis- and relaxation training-treated groups demonstrated improvements in hip and knee

pain ratings and reduced medication use as compared with subjects in the control group; however, the pain-mitigating effect of hypnosis was appreciated faster in the course of treatment (at approximately 4 weeks) than those of relaxation training conditions (approximately 8 weeks). After continued treatment, the effects of relaxation training and hypnosis conditions did not differ significantly.

Variations in the methodological approaches in existing clinical research, e.g., differences in patient characteristics and disease severity, restrict abilities to conduct meta-analysis pertaining specifically to SRTs or to make definitive statements regarding the treatment effects of various SRT interventions. Systematic analyses of SRT treatment approaches in arthritis may need to assess their utility in randomized controlled trials employing larger sample sizes, and utilizing standard outcome measures thereby facilitating comparisons with investigations employing other treatment modalities.

There is uncertainty regarding the analgesia-related active ingredients of various SRTs. For example, guided imagery, hypnosis, autogenic training, and progressive muscle relaxation share a common relaxation component. Despite modification in application and theoretical orientation, questions arise as to whether it is mere relaxation that accounts for the analgesic efficacy of such approaches. Not all patients are amenable to hypnosis, and in fact, patients differ with regard to their hypnotic suggestibility [120, 177]. Less suggestible patients may be responsive to variant modalities invoking a relaxation response instead. Further research would need to differentiate and clarify the effectiveness of various SRT modalities, and delineate whether certain individual characteristics would predict which patients are likely to benefit from a particular modality (or combination of modalities) than others [176].

Summary

A multidisciplinary approach involving somatic treatments and psychological interventions is advocated for the management of patients with arthritis pain; consultation with psychiatrists, psychologists, and other mental health professionals can facilitate multimodal treatment endeavors. Unfortunately, reimbursement for combined mental health and pain management services provided to patients with arthritis pain is difficult to obtain; as such these services are not likely to be pursued by rheumatologists and primary care physicians consistently. On the other hand, significant reductions in healthcare utilization and associated costs can result from psychopharmacologic and psychological interventions [149, 150, 178].

The utility of psychopharmacologic treatment approaches in the management of patients with arthritis has been largely unexamined. Use of antidepressants can be efficacious in reducing the co-morbidities, e.g., anxiety, depression and to some extent pain, associated with arthritic conditions [111, 124, 126, 127]. Nonetheless, further investigation of the cost effectiveness, tolerability and comparative efficacy of antidepressants, particularly of more recently developed antidepressants, are indicated.

Educational approaches foster knowledge, but may be limited with regard to improving pain or reducing patients' functional disabilities. The provision of disease information does not naturally generalize to the development of behavioral strategies with which to effectively cope with the disease. Further investigations into patient characteristics that predict who will respond best to educational approaches vs. combinations of educational and psychotherapeutic interventions are needed.

The aim of various psychotherapeutic approaches is to modify the emotions, cognitions, and physiological reactivity associated with pain. In the aggregate, there is evidence that psychological interventions (CBT and SRTs) benefit arthritis patients with respect to predominantly self-reported clinical outcomes such as pain relief, improved mood, and subjectively rated functional capacities. It is important to note that these general conclusions obscure several issues that have not been resolved in the studies cited above. One problem in evaluating psychological therapies is that they are often embedded in broad-based intervention programs that include combinations of several types of treatment. As a result, it is difficult to determine the independent effect of the psychological treatments. The literature has been dominated by randomized controlled trials assessing the utility of CBT, demonstrating that it is effective in facilitating psychological adjustment and reducing reported pain levels as compared with standard medical treatment conditions or wait-list control conditions [147]. Less in the way of empirical evidence has been devoted to the utility of SRT interventions in arthritis, even though preliminary investigations appear promising [171–174, 176].

Psychotherapeutic approaches that enhance self-efficacy and perceived control over pain, and reduce maladaptive cognitions, e.g., catastrophizing, appear to reduce arthritis-related pain and associated psychological distress. However, despite encouraging results among patients with arthritis, and in chronic pain conditions in general, variability in patient outcomes and the maintenance of treatment benefits over time is a point of increased concern [136, 142]. Further efforts need to be directed at exploring strategies that preserve positive influences of such interventions over the long term.

Most of the investigations summarized in this chapter have involved patients that were carefully screened to ensure that they met diagnostic criteria and treatment interventions were monitored continuously to ensure quality. The true test of the effectiveness of psychotherapeutic interventions rests with assessment of their utility in general clinical settings in which extraneous variables are uncontrolled, e.g., where patients may have multiple co-morbidities, therapists may be less experienced, and so on [141]. In a related manner, the applicability of psychological therapies among pediatric populations, e.g., afflicted with juvenile RA, and individuals vulnerable to greater disease-related morbidity, e.g., individuals with lower socioeconomic status, have been largely overlooked in existing research. Direct comparisons of the efficacy of various psychotherapeutic modalities as related to pain and resultant disability, along with assessment of the potential utility of various psychotherapeutic measures on physiologic parameters of disease, illness course, and progression warrant further attention. Such efforts may be strengthened by employing the use of observational outcome measures, e.g., overt pain behaviors, quantifiable assessments of functional status, analgesic requirements, sick leave durations, and return to work, may be more meaningful than subjectively rated assessments.

Acknowledgment

The authors thank Wendy Quinton, Ph.D. for her editorial comments and valuable suggestions.

References

1. Li X, Gignac MA, Anis AH. The indirect costs of arthritis resulting from unemployment, reduced performance, and occupational changes while at work. *Med Care* 2006; **44**: 304–10.

2. Newhall-Perry K, Law NJ, Ramos B, *et al.* Direct and indirect costs associated with the onset of seropositive rheumatoid arthritis. Western Consortium of Practicing Rheumatologists. *J Rheumatol* 2000; **27**: 1156–63.

3. Puolakka K, Kautiainen H, Pekuriner M, *et al.*
Monetary value of lost productivity over a five year
follow-up in early rheumatoid arthritis estimated on
the basis of official register data on patients' sickness
absence and gross income: experience from the FIN-
RACo trial. *Ann Rheum Dis* 2006; **65**: 899–904.

4. Abell JE, Hootman JM, Zack MM, Moriarty D,
Helmick CG. Physical activity and health related
quality of life among people with arthritis. *J Epidemiol
Community Health* 2005; **59**: 380–5.

5. Bazzichi L, Maser J, Piccinni A, *et al.* Quality of life in
rheumatoid arthritis impact of disability and lifetime
depressive spectrum symptomatology. *Clin Exp
Rheumatol* 2005; **23**: 783–8.

6. Burman P, Toy GG, Babao S, *et al.* A comparative
evaluation of quality of life and life satisfaction in
patients with psoriatic and rheumatoid arthritis. *Clin
Rheumatol* 2007; **26**: 330–4.

7. Nunez M, Sanchez A, Nunez E, *et al.* Patients
perceptions of health related quality of life in
rheumatoid arthritis and chronic low back pain. *Qual
Life Res* 2006; **15**: 93–102.

8. Ofluoglu D, Berker N, Guven Z, *et al.* Quality of life in
patients with fibromyalgia syndrome and rheumatoid
arthritis. *Clin Rheumatol* 2005; **24**: 490–2.

9. Hootman J, Bolen J, Helmick C, Langmaid G.
Prevalence of doctor-diagnosed arthritis and
arthritis-attributable activity limitation – United
States, 2003–2005. *Morb Mortal Wkly Rep* 2006;
55: 1089–92.

10. Hootman JM, Helmick CG. Projections of U.S.
prevalence of arthritis and associated activity
limitations. *Arthritis Rheum* 2006; **54**: 226–9.

11. Theis KA, Helmick CG, Hootman JM. Arthritis burden
and impact are greater among U.S. women than
men: intervention opportunities. *J Women's Health*
2007; **16**: 441–53.

12. Mjanek NJ, Lane NE. Osteoarthritis: current concepts
in diagnosis and management. *Am Fam Physician* 2000;
61: 1795–1804.

13. Centers for Disease Control and Prevention (CDC).
Prevalence of disabilities and associated health
conditions – United States, 1999. *Morb Mortal Wkly
Rep* 2001; **50**: 120–5.

14. Leveille SG, Fried LP, McMullen W, Guralnik JM.
Advancing the taxonomy of disability in older adults. *J
Gerontol A Biol Sci Med Sci* 2004; **59**: 86–93.

15. Anderson JJ, Felson DT. Factors associated with
osteoarthritis of the knee in the first national Health
and Nutrition Examinaton Survey (HANES I).
Evidence for an association with overweight, race,

and physical demands of work. *Am J Epidemiol* 1988;
128: 179–85.

16. Ettinger WH, Davis MA, Neuhas JM, Mallon KP.
Long-term physical functioning in persons with
knee osteoarthritis from NHANES I: effects of
comorbid medical conditions. *J Clin Epidemiol* 1994;
47: 809–15.

17. Felson DT, Anderson JJ, Naimark A, Walker AM,
Meenan RF. Obesity and knee osteoarthritis. The
Framingham Study. *Ann Intern Med* 1988; **109**: 18–24.

18. Center for Disease Control. Update: direct and indirect
costs of arthritis and other rheumatic conditions-
United States, 1997. *Morb Mortal Wkly Rep* 2004;
53: 388–9.

19. Recommendations for the medical management
of osteoarthritis of the hip and knee: 2000 update.
American College of Rheumatology Subcommittee
on Osteoarthritis Guidelines. *Arthritis Rheum* 2000;
43: 1905–15.

20. Altman R, Asch E, Bloch D, *et al*, Diagnostic and
Therapeutic Criteria Committee of the American
Rheumatism Association. Development of criteria
for the classification and reporting of osteoarthritis.
Classification of osteoarthritis of the knee. *Arthritis
Rheum* 1986; **29**: 1039–49.

21. Altman RD, Hochberg M, Murphy WA, Wolfe F,
Lequesne M. Atlas of individual radiographic features
in osteoarthritis. *Osteoarthritis Cartilage* 1995; **3**(suppl
A): 3–70.

22. Dougados M. Evaluation of disease progression
during nonsteroidal anti-inflammatory drug
treatment: imaging by arthroscopy. *Osteoarthritis
Cartilage* 1999; **7**: 345–7.

23. Felson DT, Chaisson CE, Hill CL, *et al.* The
association of bone marrow lesions with pain in knee
osteoarthritis. *Ann Intern Med* 2001; **134**: 541–9.

24. Dougados M. The role of anti-inflammatory drugs in
the treatment of osteoarthritis: a European viewpoint.
Clin Exp Rheumatol 2001; **19** (Suppl 25): S9–S14.

25. Samad TA, Moore KA, Sapirstein A, *et al.* Interleukin-1
beta-mediated induction of COX-2 in the CNS
contributes to inflammatory pain hypersensitivity.
Nature 2001; **410**: 471–5.

26. Romano TJ. Fibromyalgia syndrome in other
rheumatic conditions. *Lyon Mediterr Med Med Sud Est*
32: 2143–6.

27. Calfas KJ, Kaplan RM, Ingram RE. One-year evaluation
of cognitive-behavioral intervention in osteoarthritis.
Arthritis Care Res 1992; **5**: 202–9.

28. Pariser D, O'Hanlon A. Effects of telephone
intervention on arthritis self-efficacy, depression, pain

and fatigue in older adults with arthritis. *J Geriatr Phys Ther* 2005; **28**: 67–73.

29. American College of Rheumatology Subcommittee on Osteoarthritis Guidelines. Recommendations for the medical management of osteoarthritis of the hip and knee: 2000 update. American College of Rheumatology Subcommittee on Osteoarthritis Guidelines. *Arthritis Rheum* 2000; **43**: 1905–15.

30. Pavelka K, Manopulo R, Bucsi L. Double blind, dose-effect study of oral chondroitin 4&6 sulphate 1200 mg, 800 mg, 200 mg and placebo in the treatment of knee osteoarthritis. *Litera Rheumatologica* 1999; **24**: 21–30.

31. Mazieres B, Combe B, Phan Van A, Tondut J, Grynfeltt M. Chondroitin sulfate in osteoarthritis of the knee: a prospective, double blind, placebo controlled multicenter clinical study. *J Rheumatol* 2001; **28**: 173–81.

32. Huskisson EC, Berry H, Gishen P, Jubb RW, Whitehead J. on behalf of the LINK Study Group. Effects of anti-inflammatory drugs on the progression of osteoarthritis of the knee. *J Rheumatol* 1995; **22**: 1941–6.

33. Reijman M, Bierma-Zeinstra SM, Pols HA, *et al.* Is there an association between the use of different types of nonsteroidal anti-inflammatory drugs and radiologic progression of osteoarthritis? The Rotterdam Study. *Arthritis Rheum* 2005; **52**: 3137–42.

34. Hollander JL, Brown EM, Jessar RA, Brown CY. Hydrocortisone and cortisone injected into arthritic joints: comparative effects of and use of hydrocortisone as a local antiarthritic agent. *J Am Med Assoc* 1951; **147**: 1629–35.

35. Altman RD, Moskowiwtz R. Intraarticular sodium hyaluronate (Hyalgan) in the treatment of patients with osteoarthritis of the knee: a randomized clinical trial. *J Rheumatol* 1998; **25**: 2203–12.

36. Lawrence RC, Helmick CG, Arnett FC, *et al.* Estimates of the prevalence of arthritis and selected musculoskeletal disorders in the United States. *Arthritis Rheum* 1998; **41**: 778–99.

37. Woolf AD, Pfleger B. Burden of major musculoskeletal conditions. *Bull World Health Organ* 2003; **81**: 646–56.

38. Wilson A, Yu HT, Goodnough LT, Nissenson AR. Prevalence and outcomes of anemia in rheumatoid arthritis: a systemic review of the literature. *Am J Med* 2004; **116**(Suppl 7A): 50–7.

39. Kvien TK. Epidemiology and burden of illness of rheumatoid arthritis. *Pharmacoeconomics* 2004; **22**(suppl): 1–12.

40. Yelin E. The costs of rheumatoid arthritis: absolute, incremental, and marginal estimates. *J Rheumatol Suppl.* 1996; **44**: 47–51.

41. Birnbaum HG, Barton M, Greenberg PE, *et al.* Direct and indirect costs of rheumatoid arthritis to an employer. *J Occup Environ Med.* 2000; **42**: 588–96.

42. Sokka T. Work disability in early rheumatoid arthritis. *Clin Exp Rheumatol* 2003; **21**(suppl 31): S71–S74.

43. Reisine ST, Goodenow C, Grady KE. The impact of rheumatoid arthritis on the homemaker. *Soc Sci Med* 1987; **25**: 89–95.

44. Arnett F, Edwardworthy S, Bloch D, *et al.* The American Rheumatism Assocation 1987 revised criteria for the classification of rheumatoid arthritis. *Arthritis Rheum* 1988; **31**: 315–24.

45. Nell VP, Machold KP, Stamm TA, Eberl G *et al.* Autoantibody profiling as early diagnostic and prognostic tool for rheumatoid arthritis. *Ann Rheum Dis* 2005; **64**: 1731–6.

46. Raza K, Breese M, Nightingale P, *et al.* Predictive value of antibodies to cyclic citrullinated peptide in patients with very early inflammatory arthritis. *J. Rheumatol* 2005; **32**: 231–8.

47. Gonzalez-Gay MA, Gonzalez-Juanatey C, Martin J. Rheumatoid arthritis: a disease associated with accelerated atherogenesis. *Semin Arthritis Rheum* 2005; **35**: 8–17.

48. van der Heijde DM, van Leeuwen MA, van Riel PL, van de Putte LB. Radiographic progression on radiographs of hands and feet during the first 3 years of rheumatoid arthritis measured according to Sharp's method (van der Heijde modification). *J Rheumatol* 1995; **22**: 1792–96.

49. Fuchs HA, Kaye JJ, Callahan LF, Nance EP, Pincus T. Evidence of significant radiographic damage in rheumatoid arthritis within the first 2 years of disease. *J Rheumatol* 1989; **16**: 585–91.

50. Tersley L, Torp-Pedersen S, Savnick A, *et al.* Doppler ultrasound and magnetic resonance imaging of synovial inflammation of the hand in rheumatoid arthritis: a comparative study. *Arthritis Rheum* 2003; **48**: 2434–41.

51. Calguneri M, Pay S, Caliskaner Z, *et al.* Combination therapy versus monotherapy for the treatment of patients with rheumatoid arthritis. *Clin Exp Rheumatol* 1999; **17**: 699–704.

52. Boers M, Verhoeven AC, Markusse HM, *et al.* Randomized comparison of combined step-down prednisolone, methotrexate and sulphasalazine with sulphasalazine alone in early rheumatoid arthritis. *Lancet* 1997; **350**: 309–18.

53. Landewe RB, Boers M, Verhoeven AC, *et al.* COBRA combination therapy in patients with early rheumatoid arthritis: long-term structural benefits of a brief intervention. *Arthritis Rheum* 2002; **46**: 347–56.

54. Bathon JM, Martin RW, Fleischmann RM, *et al.* A comparison of entanercept and methotrexate in patients with early rheumatoid arthritis. *N Engl J Med* 2000; **343**: 1586–93.

55. Weinblatt ME, Kremer JM, Bankhurst AD, *et al.* A trial of etanercept, a recombinant tumor necrosis factor receptor: Fc fusion protein, in patients with rheumatoid arthritis receiving methotrexate. *N Engl J Med* 1999; **340**; 253–9.

56. Curtis JR, Patkar N, Xie A, *et al.* Risk of serious bacterial infections among rheumatoid arthritis patients exposed to tumor necrosis factor alpha antagonists. *Arthritis Rheum* 2007; **56**: 1125–33.

57. Lipsky PE, van der Heijde D, St. Clair EW, *et al.* Anti-Tumor Necrosis Factor Trial in Rheumatoid Arthritis with Concomitant Therapy Study Group. Infliximab and methotrexate in the treatment of rheumatoid arthritis. *N Engl J Med* 2000; **343**: 1594–602.

58. Maini R, St. Clair EW, Breedveld F, *et al.* ATTRACT Study Group. Infliximab (chimeric anti-tumor necrosis factor alpha monoclonal antibody) versus placebo in rheumatoid arthritis patients receiving concomitant methotrexate: a randomized phase III trial. *Lancet* 1999; **354**: 1932–9.

59. Bongartz T, Sutton AJ, Sweeting MJ, *et al.* Anti-TNF antibody therapy in rheumatoid arthritis and the risk of serious infections and malignancies: systemic review and meta-analysis of rare harmful effects in randomized controlled trials. *JAMA* 2006; **295**: 2275–85.

60. Weinblatt ME, Keystone EC, Furst DE, *et al.* Adalimunab, a fully human anti-tumor necrosis factor a monoclonal anti-body, for the treatment of rheumatoid arthritis in patients taking concomitant methotrexate: the ARMADA trial. *Arthritis Rheum* 2003; **48**: 35–45.

61. Weinblatt ME, Keystone, EC, Furst DE, *et al.* Long term efficacy and safety of adalimumab plus methotrexate in patients with rheumatoid arthritis: ARMADA 4 year extended study. *Ann Rheum Dis* 2006; **65**: 753–9.

62. Cohen SB, Emery P, Greenwald MW, *et al.* REFLEX Trial Group. Rituximab for rheumatoid arthritis refractory to anti-tumor necrosis factor therapy: results of a multicenter, randomized, double-blind, placebo-controlled, phase III trial evaluating primary efficacy and safety at twenty-four weeks. *Arthritis Rheum* 2006; **54**: 2793–806.

63. Abatacept (Orencia) for rheumatoid arthritis. *Med Lett Drugs Ther* 2006; **28**: 17–18.

64. Genovese MC, Becker JC, Schiff M, *et al.* Abatacept for rheumatoid arthritis refractory to tumor necrosis factor inhibition. *N Engl J Med* 2005; **353**: 1114–23.

65. Sontheimer RD, Gilliam JN. Systemic lupus erythematosus and the skin. In *Systemic Lupus Erythematosus*, 2nd edn., ed. RG Lahita. (New York: Churchill Livingstone, 1992), pp. 657–81.

66. Kozora E, Ellison MC, West S. Depression, fatigue, and pain in systemic lupus erythematosus (SLE) relationship to the American College of Rheumatology SLE neuropsychological battery. *Arthritis Rheum* 2006; **55**: 628–35.

67. Jump Rl, Robinson ME, Armstrong AE, *et al.* Fatigue in systemic lupus erythematosus: contributions of disease activity, pain, depression, and perceived social support. *J Rheumatol* 2005; **32**: 1699–705.

68. Laboni A, Ibanez D, Gladman DD, Urowitz MB, Moldofsky H. Fatigue in systemic lupus erythematosus: contributions of disordered sleep, sleepiness, and depression. *J Rheumatol* 2006; **33**: 2453–7.

69. Kozora E, Arciniegas DB, Zhang L, West S. Neuropsychological patterns in systemic lupus erythematosus patients with depression. *Arthritis Res Ther* 2007; **9**: art. No. R48.

70. Stojanovich L, Zandman-Goddard G, Pavlovich S, Sikanich N. Psychiatric manifestations in systemic lupus erythematosus. *Autoimmun Rev* 2007; **6**: 421–6.

71. Ward MM, Pyun E, Studenski S. Long-term survival in systemic lupus erythematosus. Patient characteristics associated with poorer outcomes. *Arthritis Rheum* 1995; **38**: 274–83.

72. Hale ED, Treharne GJ, Norton Y, *et al.* "Concealing the evidence": the importance of appearance concerns for patients with systemic lupus erythematosus. *Lupus* 2006; **15**: 532–40.

73. Monaghan SM, Sharpe L, Denton F, *et al.* Relationship between appearance and psychological distress in rheumatic disease. *Arthritis Care Res* 2007; **57**: 303–9.

74. Vasoo S. Drug-induced lupus: an update. *Lupus* 2006; **15**: 757–61.

75. Shakoor N, Michalska M, Harris CA, Block JA. Drug-induced systemic lupus erythematosus associated with etanercept therapy. *Lancet* 2002; **259**: 579–80.

76. Rubin RL, Teodorescu M, Beutner EH, Plunkett RW. Complement-fixing properties of anti-nuclear antibodies distinguish drug-induced lupus from systemic lupus erythematosus. *Lupus* 2004; **13**: 249–56.

77. Hochberg MC. Updating the American College of Rheumatology revised criteria for the classification of

systemic lupus erythematosus. *Arthritis Rheum* 1997; **40**: 1725.

78. Hughes GR. Is it lupus? St. Thomas's Hospital "alternative" criteria. *Clin Exp Rheumatol* 1998; **16**: 250–2.

79. Reeves WH, Satoh M, Wang J, Chou CH, Ajmani AK. Antibodies to DNA, DNA-binding proteins and histones. *Rheum Dis Clin North Am* 1994; **20**: 1–28.

80. Gladman DD, Urowitz MB, Cole E, *et al.* Kidney biopsy in SLE. A clinical-morphological evaluation. *Quart J Med* 1989; **73**: 1125–53.

81. Miller MH, Urowitz MB, Gladman DD. The significance of thrombocytopenia in systemic lupus erythematosus. *Arthritis Rheum* 1983; **26**: 1181–6.

82. Julkunen HA. Oral contraceptives in systemic lupus erythematosus: side-effects and influence on the activity of SLE. *Scand J Rheumatol* 1991; **20**: 427–33.

83. Petri M. Exogenous estrogen in systemic lupus erythematosus: oral contraceptives and hormone replacement therapy. *Lupus* 2001; **10**: 222–6.

84. Wallace DJ. *The Lupus Book: A Guide for Patients and their families* (New York: Oxford University Press, 1995).

85. The Canadian Hydroxychloroquine Study Group. A randomized study of the effect of withdrawing hydroxychoroquine sulfate in systemic lupus erythematosus. *N Engl J Med* 1991; **324**: 150–4.

86. Spalton DJ, Verton Roe GM, Hughes GRV. Hydroxychloroquine dosage parameters and retinopathy. *Lupus* 1993; **2**: 355–8.

87. Klippel JH. Is aggressive therapy effective for lupus? *Rheum Dis Clin N Amer* 1993; **19**: 249–61.

88. Neuwelt CM, Lacks S, Kaye BR, Ellman JB, Borenstein DG. Rose of intravenous cyclophosphamide in the treatment of severe neuropsychiatric systemic lupus erythematosus. *Am J Med* 1995; **98**: 32–41.

89. Radhakrishnan J, Kunis Cl, D' Agati V, Appel GB. Cyclosporin treatment of lupus membranous nephropathy. *Clin Nephrol* 1994; **42**: 147–54.

90. Tokuda M, Kurata N, Mizogushi A, *et al.* Effect of low-dose cyclosporin A on systemic lupus erythematosus. *Arthritis Rheum* 1994; **37**: 551–8.

91. West SG, Johnson SC. Danazol for the treatment of refractory autoimmune thrombo cytopenia in systemic lupus erythematosus. *Ann Intern Med* 1988; **108**: 703–6.

92. Chang DM, Lan JL, Lin HY, Luo SF. Dehydroepiandrosterone treatment of women with mild to moderate systemic lupus erythematosus: a multicenter randomized, double-blind, placebo-controlled trial. *Arthritis Rheum* 2002; **46**: 2924–7.

93. Stricker RB, Davis JA, Gershow J, Yamamoto KS, Kiprov DD. Thrombotic thrombocytopenic purpura complicating systemic lupus erythematosus: case report and literature review from the plasmapheresis era. *J Rheumatol* 1992; **19**: 1469–73.

94. Euler HH, Schroeder JO, Harten P, Zeuner RA, Gutschmidt HJ. Treatment-free remission in severe systemic lupus erythematosus following synchronization of plasmapheresis with subsequent pulse cyclophosphamide. *Arthritis Rheum* 1994; **37**: 1784–94.

95. Romano TJ. Coexistence of the fibromyalgia syndrome and systemic lupus erythematosus. *Am J Pain Manage* 1992; **2**: 211–4.

96. Krishnam E, Hubert HB. Ethnicity and mortality from systemic lupus erythematosus in the U.S. *Ann Rheum Dis* 2006; **65**: 1500–5.

97. Morley S, Eccleston C, Williams A. Systematic review and meta-analysis of randomized controlled trials of cognitive-beaviour therapy and behaviour therapy for chronic pain in adults, excluding headache. *Pain* 1999; **80**: 1–13.

98. Hagglund KJ, Haley WE, Reveille JD, Alarcon GS. Predicting individual differences in pain and functional impairment among patients with rheumatoid arthritis. *Arthritis Rheum* 1989; **32**: 851–8.

99. Parker JC, Frank R, Beck N, *et al.* Pain in rheumatoid arthritis: relationship to demographic, medical, and psychological factors. *J Rheumatol* 1988; **15**: 433–7.

100. Young LD. Psychological factors in rheumatoid arthritis. *J Consult Clin Psychol* 1992; **60**: 619–27.

101. Creamer P, Lethbridge-Cejku M, Hochberg MC. Factors associated with functional impairment in symptomatic knee osteoarthritis. *Rheumatology (Oxford)* 2000; **39**: 490–6.

102. Van Baar ME, Dekker J, Lemmens JA, Oostendorp RA, Bijlsma JW. Pain and disability in patients with osteoarthritis of hip or knee. *J Rheumatol* 1998; **25**: 125–33.

103. Covic T, Tyson G, Spencer D, Howe G. Depression in rheumatoid arthritis patients: demographic, clinical, and psychological predictors. *J Psychosom Res* 2006; **60**: 469–76.

104. McWilliams LA, Clara IP, Murphy PDJ, Cox BJ, Sareen J. Associations between arthritis and a broad range of psychiatric disorders: findings from a nationally representative sample. *J Pain* 2008; **9**: 37–44.

105. McWilliams LA, Cox BJ, Enns MW. Mood and anxiety disorders associated with chronic pain: an examination in a nationally representative sample. *Pain* 2003; **106**: 127–33.

106. Katz PP, Yelin EH. Prevalence and correlates of depressive symptoms among persons with rheumatoid arthritis. *J Rheumatol* 1993; **20**: 790–6.

107. Ang DC, Choi H, Kroenke K, Wolfe F. Comorbid depression is an independent risk factor for mortality in patients with rheumatoid arthritis. *J Rheumatol* 2005; **32**: 1013–9.

108. Dexter P, Brandt K. Distribution and predictors of depressive symptoms in osteoarthritis. *J Rheumatol* 1994; **21**: 279–86.

109. Memel DS, Kirwan JR, Sharp DJ, Hehir M. General practitioners miss disability and anxiety as well as depression in their patients with osteoarthritis. *Br J Gen Pract* 2000; **50**: 645–8.

110. Felson DT, Lawrence RC, Hochberg MC, *et al.* Osteoarthritis: new insights. Part 2: treatment approaches. *Ann Intern Med* 2000; **133**: 726–37.

111. Lin EH, Katon W, Von Korff M, *et al.* Effect of improving depression care on pain and functional outcomes among older adults with arthritis. A randomized controlled trial. *JAMA* 2003; **290**: 2428–34.

112. Parker JC, Smarr KL, Slaughter JR, *et al.* Management of depression in rheumatoid arthritis: a combined pharmacologic and cognitive-behavioral approach. *Arthritis Rheum* 2003; **49**: 766–77.

113. Dionne CE, Koepsell TD, von Korff M, *et al.* Predicting long-term functional limitations among back pain patients in primary care settings. *J Clin Epidemiol* 1997; **50**: 31–43.

114. Katon W, Sullivan M, Walker E. Medical symptoms without identified pathology. *Ann Intern Med* 2001; **134**: 917–25.

115. Lamb SE, Guralnik JM, Buchner DM, *et al.* Factors that modify the association between knee pain and mobility limitation in older women. *Ann Rheum Dis* 2000; **59**: 331–37.

116. Burns JW, Johnson BJ, Mahoney N, *et al.* Cognitive and physical capacity process variables predict longterm outcome after treatment of chronic pain. *J Consult Clin Psychology* 1998, **66**: 434–9.

117. Holzberg AD, Robinson ME, Geisser ME, Gremillion HA. The effects of depression and chronic pain on psychosocial and physical functioning. *Clin J Pain* 1996; **12**: 118–25.

118. Murphy H, Dickens C, Creed F, Bernstein R. Depression, illness perception and coping in rheumatoid arthritis. *J Psychosom Res* 1999; **46**: 155–64.

119. Fields HL. Pain modulation. *Prog Brain Res* 2000; **122**: 245–53.

120. Leo RJ. *Clinical Manual of Pain Management in Psychiatry* (Washington, DC. American Psychiatric Publishing, Inc., 2007).

121. Yaksh TL. Central pharmacology of nociceptive transmission, In *Textbook of Pain*, 4th edn. eds. PD Wall and RG Melzack. (Edinburgh: Churchill Livingstone, 1999), pp. 253–308.

122. Abbott FV, Hong Y, Blier P. Persisting sensitization of the behavioural response to formalin-induced injury through activation of serotonin 2A receptors. *Neuroscience* 1997; **77**: 575–84.

123. Schreiber S, Bleich A, Pick CG. Venlafaxine and mirtazapine: different mechanisms of antidepressant action, common opioid-mediated anti nociceptive effects: a possible opioid involvement in severe depression? *J Molecular Neuroscience* 2002; **18**: 143–9.

124. Ash G, Dickens CM, Creed FH, Jayson MI, Tomesnson B. The effects of dothiepin on subjects with rheumatoid arthritis and depression. *Rheumatology (Oxford)* 1999; **38**: 959–67.

125. Bird H, Broggini M. Paroxetine versus amitriptyline for treatment of depression associated with rheumatoid arthritis. *J Rheumatol* 2000; **27**: 2791–7.

126. Fishbain D. Evidence-based data on pain relief with antidepressants. *Ann Med* 2000; **32**: 305–16.

127. Frank RG, Kashani JH, Parker JC, *et al.* Antidepressant analgesia in rheumatoid arthritis. *J Rheumatol* 1988; **15**: 1632–8.

128. Grace EM, Bellamy N, Kassam Y, Buchanan WW. Controlled double-blind randomized trial of amitriptyline in relieving articular pain and tenderness in patients with rheumatoid arthritis. *Curr Med Res Opin* 1985; **9**: 426–9.

129. Sarzi-Puttini P, Cazzola M, Boccassini L, *et al.* A comparison of dothiepin versus placebo in the treatment of pain in rheumatoid arthritis and the association of pain with depression. *J Int Med Res* 1988; **16**: 331–7.

130. Barlow JH, Turner AP, Wright CC. A randomised controlled trial study of the arthritis self-management programme in the UK. *Health Educ Res* 2000; **15**: 665–80.

131. Hammond A. Joint protection behaviour in patients with rheumatoid arthritis following an education program: a pilot study. *Arthritis Care Res* 1994; **7**: 5–9.

132. Hawley DJ. Psycho-educational interventions in the treatment of arthritis. *Baillieres Clinical Rheumatology* 1995; **9**: 803–23.

133. Helliwell PS, O'Hara M, Holdsworth J, *et al.* A 12-month randomized controlled trial of patient education on radiographic changes and quality of life

in early rheumatoid arthritis. *Rheumatology* 1999; **38**: 303–8.

134. Mullen PD, Laville EA, Biddle AK, Lorig K. Efficacy of psychoeducational interventions on pain, depression, and disability in people with arthritis: A meta-analysis. *J Rheumatol* 1987; **14** (Suppl 15): 33–9.

135. Riemsma RP, Taal E, Kirwan JR, Rasker JJ. Systematic review of rheumatoid arthritis patient education. *Arthritis Rheum* 2004; **51**: 1045–59.

136. Keefe FJ, Van Horn Y. Cognitive-behavioral treatment of rheumatoid arthritis pain: maintaining treatment gains. *Arthritis Care Res* 1993; **6**: 213–22.

137. Keefe FJ, Caldwell DS, Queen KT, *et al*. Pain coping strategies in osteoarthritis patients. *J Consult Clin Psychol* 1987; **55**: 208–12.

138. Affleck G, Tennen H, Keefe FJ, *et al*. Everyday life with osteoarthritis or rheumatoid arthritis: independent effects of disease and gender on daily pain, mood, and coping. *Pain* 1999; **83**: 601–9.

139. Keefe FJ, Lefebvre JC, Egert J, *et al*. The relationship of gender to pain, pain behavior, and disability in osteoarthritis patients: the role of catastrophizing. *Pain* 2000; **87**: 325–34.

140. Keefe FJ, Smith SJ, Buffington AL, *et al*. Recent advances and future directions in the biopsychosocial assessment and treatment of arthritis. *J Consult Clin Psychol* 2002; **70**: 640–55.

141. Keefe FJ, Abernethy AP, Campbell LC. Psychological approaches to understanding and treating disease-related pain. *Annu Rev Psychol* 2005; **56**: 601–30.

142. Keefe FJ, Caldwell DS. Cognitive behavioral control of arthritis pain. *Med Clin North Am* 1997; **81**: 277–90.

143. Thorn BE, Kuhajda MC. Group cognitive therapy for chronic pain. *J Clin Psychol* 2006; **62**: 1355–66.

144. Nielson WR, Weir R. Biopsychosocial approaches to the treatment of chronic pain. *Clin J Pain* 2001; **17**(4 suppl): 114–27.

145. Gatchel RJ. A biopsychosocial overview of pretreatment screening of patients with pain. *Clin J Pain* 2001; **17**: 192–9.

146. Mc Cracken LM. Cognitive-behavioral treatment of rheumatoid arthritis: a preliminary review of efficacy and methodology. *Ann Behav Med* 1991; **13**: 57–65.

147. Astin JA, Beckner W, Soeken K, Hochberg MC, Berman B. Psychological interventions for rheumatoid arthritis: A meta-analysis of randomized controlled trials. *Arthritis Rheum* 2002; **47**: 291–302.

148. Gustafsson M, Gaston-Johansson F, Aschenbrenner D, Merboth M. Pain, coping and analgesic medication usage in rheumatoid arthritis patients. *Patient Educ Counsel* 1999; **37**: 33–41.

149. Cronan TA, Hay M, Groessl E, *et al*. The effects of social support and education on health care costs after three years. *Arthritis Care Res* 1998; **11**: 326–34.

150. Young LD, Bradley LA, Turner RA. Decreases in health care resource utilization in patients with rheumatoid arthritis following a cognitive behavioral intervention. *Biofeedback Self Regul* 1995; **20**: 259–68.

151. Sharpe L, Sensky T, Timberlake N, *et al*. A blind, randomized, controlled trial of cognitive-behavioural intervention for patients with recent onset rheumatoid arthritis: preventing psychological and physical morbidity. *Pain* 2001; **89**: 275–83.

152. Keefe FJ, Caldwell DS, Williams DA, *et al*. Pain coping skills training in the management of osteoarthritic knee pain: a comparative study. *Behav Ther* 1990; **21**: 49–62.

153. Keefe FJ, Caldwell DS, Williams DA, *et al*. Pain coping skills training in the management of osteoarthritic knee pain II: follow-up results. *Behav Ther* 1990; **21**: 435–47.

154. Kraaimaat FW, Brons MR, Geenen R, Bijlsma JW. The effect of cognitive behavior therapy in patients with rheumatoid arthritis. *Behav Res Ther* 1995; **33**: 487–95.

155. Leibing E, Pfingsten M, Bartmann U, Rueger U, Schuessler G. Cognitive-behavioral treatment in unselected rheumatoid arthritis outpatients. *Clin J Pain* 1999; **15**: 58–66.

156. Parker JC, Smarr KL, Buckelew SP, *et al*. Effects of stress management on clinical outcomes in rheumatoid arthritis. *Arthritis Rheum* 1995; **38**: 1807–18.

157. Sinclair VG, Wallston KA, Dwyer KA, Blackburn DS, Fuchs H. Effects of a cognitive-behavioural intervention for women with rheumatoid arthritis. *Res Nurs Health* 1998; **21**: 315–26.

158. Bradley LA, Young LD, Anderson KO, *et al*. Effects of psychological therapy on pain behavior of rheumatoid arthritis patients. *Arthritis Rheum* 1987; **30**: 1105–14.

159. Carson JW, Keefe FJ, Affleck G, *et al*. A comparison of conventional pain coping skills training and pain coping skills training with a maintenance training component: a daily diary analysis of short- and long-term treatment effects. *J Pain* 2006; **7**: 615–25.

160. Sinclair VG, Wallston KA. Predictors of improvement in a cognitive-behavioral intervention for women with rheumatoid arthritis. *Ann Behav Med* 2001; **23**: 291–7.

161. Parker JC, Frank R, Beck N, *et al.* Pain management in rheumatoid arthritis: a cognitive-behavioral approach. *Arthritis Rheum* 1988; **31**: 593–601.

162. Keefe FJ, Caldwell DS, Baucom D, *et al.* Spouse-assisted coping skills training in the management of knee pain in osteoarthritis: long-term followup results. *Arthritis Care Res* 1999; **12**: 101–11.

163. Keefe FJ, Caldwell DS, Baucom D, *et al.* Spouse-assisted coping skills training in the management of osteoarthritic knee pain. *Arthritis Care Res* 1996; **9**: 279–91.

164. Radojevic V, Nicassio PM, Weisman MH. Behavioral intervention with and without family support for rheumatoid arthritis. *Behav Ther* 1992; **23**: 13–30.

165. Turk DC. Customizing treatment in chronic pain patients, who, what, and why. *Clin J Pain* 1990; **6**: 255–70.

166. Turk DC, Rudy TE. The robustness of an empirically derived taxonomy of chronic pain patients. *Pain* 1990; **43**: 27–35.

167. Turk DC, Rudy TE. Toward an empirically derived taxonomy of chronic pain patients: integration of psychological assessment data. *J Consult Clin Psychol* 1988; **56**: 233–8.

168. Evers AW, Kraaimaat FW, van Riel PL, de Jong AJL. Tailored cognitive-behavioral therapy in early rheumatoid arthritis for paients at risk: a randomized controlled trial. *Pain* 2002; **100**: 141–53.

169. Lazarus RS, Folkman S. *Stress, Appraisal, and Coping* (New York: Springer, 1984).

170. Keefe FJ, Affleck G, Lefebvre JC, *et al.* Pain coping strategies and coping efficacy in rheumatoid arthritis: a daily process analysis. *Pain* 1997; **69**: 35–42.

171. Baird CL, Sands L. A pilot study of the effectiveness of guided imagery with progressive muscle relaxation to reduce chronic pain and mobility difficulties of osteoarthritis. *Pain Manag Nurs* 2004; **5**: 97–104.

172. Baird CL, Sands LP. Effect of guided imagery with relaxation on health-related quality of life in older women with osteoarthritis. *Res Nurs Health* 2006; **29**: 442–51.

173. Bagheri-Nesami M, Mohseni-Bandpei MA, Shayesteh-Azar M. The effect of Benson relaxation technique on rheumatoid arthritis patients: extended report. *Int J Nurs Pract* 2006; **12**: 214–19.

174. Lundgren S, Stenstrom CH. Muscle relaxation training and quality of life in rheumatoid arthritis. A randomized controlled clinical trial. *Scand J Rheumatol* 1999; **28**: 47–53.

175. Walco G, Varni JW, Bowite NT. Cognitive-behavioral pain management in children with juvenile rheumatoid arthritis. *Pediatrics* 1992; **89**: 1075–9.

176. Gay MC, Philippot P, Luminet O. Differential effectiveness of psychological interventions for reducing osteoarthritis pain: a comparison of Erikson hypnosis and Jacobson relaxation. *Eur J Pain* 2002; **6**: 1–16.

177. Nadon R, Laurence JR, Perry C. Multiple predictors of hypnotic susceptibility. *J Pers Soc Psychol* 1987; **53**: 948–60.

178. Simon GE, von Korff M, Barlow W. Health care costs of primary care patients with recognized depression. *Arch Gen Psychiatry* 1995; **52**: 850–6.

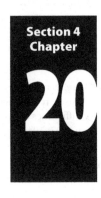

Integrative approaches to the management of painful medical conditions

Management of neuropathic pain

Robert L. Ruff and Suzanne S. Ruff

This chapter provides an overview of neuropathic pain syndromes followed by a discussion of how a health psychologist can contribute to the treatment of neuropathic pain. This chapter does not dwell on medical treatments or surgical interventions for neuropathic pain.

Overview of neuropathic pain

Neuropathic pain, which is also known as neuralgia, refers to pain that results from activation, usually dysfunctional, of the peripheral or central nervous system. Neuralgia results from neurological structural or physiological alteration. In distinction from nociceptive pain, neuropathic pain can exist in the absence of nociceptive input. Neuropathic pain exists without tissue injury directly activating nociceptive receptors in the peripheral nervous system or viscera. Neuropathic pain usually has an electric-like or burning character. It is often perceived in the distribution of a peripheral or cranial nerve or involving a region of the body. Headaches are usually not included in neuropathic pain conditions; however, some headache syndromes, such as migraine and cluster headaches, are not associated with primary activation of nociceptors through tissue injury and can be considered as neuropathic syndromes [1].

Terms often associated with neuropathic pain are allodynia and hyperalgesia. Allodynia is perceived pain that is elicited by innocuous stimuli, such as light touch in a region of the body with allodynia. Hyperalgesia is an intensified perception of pain, so that what should be perceived as low intensity pain is perceived as very intense pain.

Neuropathic pain syndromes

Complex regional pain syndrome (CRPS), is a chronic neuropathic pain condition that is believed to result from dysfunction in the central or peripheral nervous systems that produces pain associated with altered autonomic nervous system function involving a region of the body. Clinical features include changes in the color and temperature of the skin over the affected body region, swelling, intense burning pain, and allodynia. There are two types of CRPS: CRPS type I is triggered by tissue injury with no underlying discernable nerve injury, and was previously referred to as reflex sympathetic dystrophy (RSD), Sudeck's atrophy, reflex neurovascular dystrophy (RND) or algoneurodystrophy; CRPS type II, also referred to as causalgia, has similar features, but symptoms are associated with significant nerve injury. Diagnosis of CRPS is typically made through observation and examination. There is no definitive test for CRPS, but testing of peripheral autonomic nervous system function can be used to document autonomic dysfunction. There is no known cure for either form of CRPS.

Neuropathic pain in the form of CRPS may have been first recognized by Weir Mitchell, an American Union Civil War surgeon, who noticed hyperalgesia and chronic pain in patients who had nerve lesions in the extremities and also some cases where no lesion was observed. Mitchell termed the condition causalgia. As noted above, causalgia in now referred to as CPRS type II.

Other neuropathic syndromes include trigeminal neuralgia (also called Tic Douloureux), atypical trigeminal neuralgia, other pain syndromes associated with cranial or cervical nerves, and post-herpetic neuralgia (caused by shingles or cutaneous herpes zoster). Neuropathic pain can also be pain in the lower or upper extremites such as sciatica (pain associated with nerve root injury and manifesting with pain radiating down a leg), pain radiating into an upper extremity associated with injury to the brachial plexus or cervical/first thoracic nerve root dysfunction.

Behavioral and Psychopharmacologic Pain Management, ed. Michael H. Ebert and Robert D. Kerns. Published by Cambridge University Press. © Cambridge University Press 2011.

Perhaps the most common form of neuropathic pain is pain associated with peripheral nerve injury or degeneration, also know as neuropathy. The most common forms of neuropathy in the Americas are diabetic neuropathy and neuropathy associated with alcohol abuse or alcoholic neuropathy, The nerve injury in degenerative neuropathies such as alcoholic and diabetic neuropathy, can preferentially involve distal small nerve fibers. The pain is often perceived as a burning sensation in the distal extremities associated with allodynia and hyperalgesia. The pain is often most troublesome when the individual is trying to fall asleep.

In trigeminal neuralgia, neuropathic pain is experienced in the distributions of divisions of the trigeminal nerve on one side of the face. The disorder generally causes short episodes or jabs of excruciating pain. The pain can be described in a variety of ways such as "stabbing," "sharp," "like lightning," "burning," and even "pruritic." In the atypical form of trigeminal neuralgia, the pain is perceived as having a continuous or long-lasting component and there may be an aching quality to the persistent pain.

People with trigeminal neuralgia have a phenomena that resembles allodynia, simple stimuli such as eating, making facial expressions, talking, face washing, or other innocuous facial stimulation can trigger an attack of trigeminal neuralgia. The unpredictable nature of this allodynia often results in patients becoming fearful of any facial contact or head movement. The attacks can occur in clusters, or as isolated attacks. In atypical trigeminal neuralgia the pain can be continuous and sustained. Some patients will have facial muscle spasm associated with the pain. Related neuropathic pain syndromes are occipital neuralgia, where pain is perceived in the occiput and neck, and glossopharyngeal neuralgia, where pain is perceived in the throat.

Atypical trigeminal neuralgia is a variant of trigeminal neuralgia. The symptoms can be mistaken for migraine headaches, dental problems such as temporomandibular joint syndrome, musculoskeletal issues, and a somatoform disorder such as hypochondriasis. Atypical trigeminal neuralgia can have a wide range of symptoms and the pain can fluctuate in intensity from mild aching to a crushing or burning sensation. The perceived pain intensity varies among patients and can be as intense as the extreme pain experienced with trigeminal neuralgia. Atypical trigeminal neuralgia pain can be described as heavy, aching, or burning. Sufferers have a constant migraine-like head pain and experience pain in all three trigeminal nerve branches.

They may experience electric shock-like stabs of pain in addition to lasting pain. Unlike typical trigeminal neuralgia, the atypical neuralgia can also cause pain in the scalp and neck. Pain tends to worsen with talking, facial expressions, chewing, and certain environmental triggers such as a cool breeze. Several underlying processes have been associated with atypical trigeminal neuralgia including compression of the trigeminal nerve, dental or sinus infections and physical trauma.

Occipital neuralgia, also called C2 neuralgia, or Arnold's neuralgia is characterized by chronic pain in the upper neck, back of the head, and behind the eyes. The pain can vary in character among patients including stabbing, burning, aching, or electric-like. This syndrome is recognized by its location. However, the pain location can overlap with tension headaches [1].

Post-herpetic neuralgia is a neuropathic pain syndrome that follows a cutaneous outbreak of herpes zoster (aka varicella zoster) or shingles. Shingles is painful. The primary shingles pain is in the distribution of the nerves where there is a vesicular outbreak. The primary herpetic pain resolves as the vesicles (the shingles) resolve. Postherpetic neuralgia refers to neuropathic pain that develops as the skin vesicles are beginning to resolve or shortly after they have resolved. Women are more likely to be affected than men, and those over 50 are at the greatest risk.

The International Headache Society classification for headaches includes several headache syndromes that could be considered as neuropathic pain syndromes including migraine headaches and cluster headaches [1]. The most common form of migraine headaches are migraine without aura, which is also called common migraine. The criteria for common migraine are recurrent episodes of pain lasting for 4 to 72 hours with at least two of the following four characteristics: (1) unilateral, (2) pulsating quality, (3) moderate or severe intensity or (4) aggravated by or causing avoidance of routine physical activity. In addition, migraines have at least one of the following two characteristics: (1) nausea, vomiting or both, or (2) phono- or photophobia or both.

Cluster headaches, also called trigeminal autonomic cephalgia, are a head pain syndrome that overlaps with trigeminal neuralgia in terms of distribution of [1]. The diagnostic criteria require that an individual experience more than five attacks before an individual has a diagnosis of cluster headache. There are two forms of cluster headaches, episodic, and chronic. Episodic cluster headaches consist of severe unilateral orbital, supraorbital, and/or temporal pain that would last 15–180 minutes without treatment. Cluster headaches have at least one of the following criteria on the side of the pain for criteria 1–4: (1) ocular conjunctival injection or lacrimation, (2) nasal congestion or rhinnorrhea, (3) forehead, eyelid or facial edema, (4) miosis or ptosis, or (5) a sense of agitation or restlessness. Episodic cluster headaches have an attack frequency of every other day to eight times a day with periods of remission of at least 1 month. Chronic cluster headaches occur for more than a year with periods of remission of less than 1 month. Paroxysmal hemicrania is a related pain syndrome in which the attacks are of shorter duration, typically 2–30 minutes. Paroxysmal hemicrania is more common in women and is extremely responsive to indomethacin to the extent that response to indomethacin is considered by some to be a characteristic of the syndrome.

Pathophysiology of neuropathic pain

The way that nervous tissue responds to injury may potentiate the development of neuropathic pain. Following trauma to a nerve fiber, a short onset of afferent impulses, termed "injury discharge," occurs. While lasting only minutes, the injury discharge has been linked to the onset of neuropathic pain [2, 3]. After an axon is severed, the distal axon segment degenerates and is absorbed by neuroglia (Schwann cells in the peripheral nervous system and oligodendroglia in the central nervous system [CNS]). The proximal axon segment fuses, retracts, and enlarges to form a "retraction bulb." The nucleus of the damaged axon undergoes chromatolysis in preparation for axon regeneration. Neuroglia in the region of the distal stump of the nerve and a series of chemical markers in the basal lamina secreted by neuroglia help stimulate regeneration of the distal axon and guide regeneration toward the original target. However, neuroglia that proliferate in the region of axonal injury can form a glial scar that blocks axons from reconnecting with their proper targets. The regenerating axon must make connections with the appropriate receptors for effective regeneration. If the axon does not properly reconnect, aberrant reinnervation may occur. If the progress of the regenerating axon is stopped by damaged tissue or scar tissue, the axon may generate a collection of neurofibrils to form a mass known as a neuroma [2, 3]. The electrical properties of the neuroma are invariably abnormal with the neuroma producing spontaneous electrical activity that is propagated to the cell body.

Trauma to neurons in the CNS causes a proliferation of glial cells that produce a glial scar. The glial scar can block new axonal formation and impair the reestablishment of correct CNS connections. In addition, damaged nerve terminals at the site of CNS injury may swell. The swelling combined with glial proliferation can inhibit the proper reconnection of axon terminals with the proper target cell bodies. Additionally, damaged neurons may become inexcitable if they are severely damaged or develop abnormal excitability in response to altered membrane integrity and altered expression of excitable ionic channel and receptors for neurotransmitters. When a group of neurons lose their function or begin to malfunction, abnormal signals sent to the brain may be translated as painful signals [2, 3].

There are several factors that can contribute to the genesis of neuropathic pain: (1) Alteration in the number, distribution or gating properties of the ion channels involved in generating and suppressing neural action potentials; (2) Changes in the structure of neurons that enable abnormal linking of neurons which facilitates the firing of networks of neurons; (3) Abnormal electrical linkage of cells that result in the ephaptic electrical connection between cells that are normally not electrically coupled; (4) A critical part of central pain processing is a pain regulatory network that includes neurons expressing neurotransmitters that are endogenous opioids such as met- and leu-enkephalin. The pain modulatory system is essential for somatic sensory focusing and endogenous modulation of the perceived intensity of pain. Malfunction of the pain regulatory system disrupts the normal processes that regulate perceived pain intensity. With respect to neuropathic pain, impairment of the pain regulatory function can increase the intensity of neuropathic pain as well as potentiating the genesis of neuropathic pain.

An example of how altered expression of ionic channels can contribute to neuropathic pain is that after peripheral nerve injury altered regulation of voltage gated sodium channel expression results in hyperexcitability of injured primary spinal sensory neurons in dorsal root ganglia (DRG) [4]. Specifically, there is upregulated expression of Nav1.3 mRNA and channel protein in DRG neurons of adult rats after several types of peripheral nerve injury including axotomy [5, 6] and chronic constriction injury [7]. The gating properties of the Nav1.3 channels permits neuronal firing at higher than normal frequencies with lower thresholds for activation [8, 9]. The incorporation of Nav1.3 channels leads to hyperexcitability of sensory nerve fibers. The pathologically high firing rate of the altered neurons is likely misinterpreted by the CNS as pain.

Central nervous system hyperexcitability occurs in response to some forms of CNS injury and contributes to the genesis of neuropathic pain after such injury. Hyperexcitability of dorsal horn neurons is well documented after experimental spinal cord injury and is associated with allodynia and hyperalgesia [10]. The processes responsible for neuronal hyperexcitability are being uncovered. A factor that contributes to hyperexcitability is increased microglia-neuron signaling by prostaglandin E2, associated with an increase in the expression of Nav1.3, resulting in increased excitability of pain-processing cells in the dorsal horn region of the spinal cord and likely in the comparable region of the brainstem, the spinal nucleus of cranial nerve V, which is involved with processing of facial pain information [11].

Diagnosis

Diagnosis of neuropathic pain syndromes involves recognizing specific syndromes and sometimes locating the damaged elements of the peripheral or central nervous system by identifying missing or altered sensory or motor function. A variety of diagnostic procedures can help to establish a diagnosis. The tests that may be needed can include EMG and/or nerve conduction tests, tests of autonomic nervous system function such as sweating and quantitative assessment of skin temperature, and detailed quantitative sensory testing. A full discussion of the diagnostic testing used to diagnose different neuropathic syndromes is beyond the scope of this paragraph. A detailed discussion of different surgical treatments for neuropathic pain is also beyond the scope of this chapter.

Since pain is subjective to the patient, it is important to use a pain assessment scale, such as the McGill Pain Questionnaire [12]. Qualifying the severity of the pain is helpful in diagnosis and in evaluating the effectiveness of the treatment. However, for chronic pain it is equally important to evaluate how effectively an intervention increases an individual's level of activity and extent of community interaction.

Pharmacological treatments for neuropathic pain

The primary medications for treating neuropathic pain are listed in Table 20.1. Because neuropathic pain is often associated with hyperexcitability of components of the central or peripheral nervous system and disruption of the normal pain modulation system, medical treatments for neuropathic pain incorporate agents that can combat membrane hyperexcitability such as specific anticonvulsant medications and agents that enhance the pain modulation system such as agents that enhance the action of the neurotransmitter serotonin [2, 3, 12–14].

The use of opioid medications for neuropathic pain has been controversial. However, when other medications, including combinations of agents listed in Table 20.1, are not able to produce an acceptable level of pain control and function, then opioid medications can be considered. Long-acting opioids are associated with better outcome measures: increased comfort, increased functioning, and less tolerance. Short-acting opioids may be considered for activity-related pain, to enable a patient to fall asleep or in other special circumstances. When long-term use of opioids is planned, the patient and pain treatment team should enter into a pain agreement [15]. The agreement is an education tool. Its language should be respectful and clearly articulate the responsibilities of the patient and the treatment team. Specific education of the patient is needed when using opioid medication so that the patient appreciates the side effects of the medication and that it will likely only reduce pain by about 30%. Tolerance and dependence are physiological sequelae of long-term use of opioid medication; they are not to be confused with addiction.

Gate control theory was a seminal event in pain management [16]. The medical model alone did not explain the range of clinical presentations of patients with similar types of underlying neuropathology causing pain. The biopsychosocial model is now widely accepted and provides a more robust understanding of a patient's experience of and reaction to pain, particularly chronic pain. Three systems are involved in processing pain signals: sensory-discriminative, cognitive-evaluative, and affective-motivational. While the first is the purview of the medical model, the cognitive and affective may best be addressed by a health psychologist. Cognitive factors include a patient's beliefs about their pain, their appraisal of their pain and their expectancy about how their chronic pain will affect their ability to function in the future. These cognitive factors are potential areas of intervention for the health psychologist. A patient's perception of the validity of the diagnosis and uncertainty about the prognosis

Table 20.1 Pharmacological treatment for neuropathic pain

Medication class	Uses	Dosing	Side effects	Comments
TCA				
Nortriptyline Desipramine Doxepin Amitriptyline	All classes of neuropathic pain	25 mg at bedtime increase by 25 mg weekly 150 mg usual max 100 mg max with cardiac disease Check levels Avoid amitriptyline with risk for arrhythmia	Sedation, dry mouth, weight gain, constipation, urinary retention, blurred vision	Nortriptyline and desipramine preferred agents, amitriptyline effective and has strong empirical support, but greater likelihood of side effects
SSNRI	All classes		Nausea	Both agents may improve depression Do not use with tramadol Avoid rapid cessation Avoid duloxetine with renal or liver disease, alcohol abuse
Duloxetine		30 mg daily increase by 30 mg weekly to 60 mg twice a day		
Venlafaxine		37.5 mg daily increase by 37.5 to 75 mg weekly to 225 mg daily		
Anticonvulsant	All classes			
Gabapentin		100 mg three times a day, increase weekly by 100 mg to reach 300 mg three times a day	Sedation, light-headedness and peripheral edema	Slower dosing increase reduces side effects. Monitor renal and hepatic function.
Pregabalin	Pregabalin indicated for neuropathy	Can be given twice or three times a day – 75 mg every 12 h or 50 mg every 8 h daily, increase daily dose by 150 mg weekly to 600 mg daily dose	Sedation comes with rapid dose increase	Carbamazepine is an older effective agent that is less likely to be tolerated due to side effects of sedation and light headedness. It can be useful for trigeminal and other cranial neuralgias
Topirimate	Topirimate indicated for migraine, but can be used for other neuropathic pain syndromes	25 mg daily increase by 25 mg weekly to 50–100 mg every 12 h		
Carbamazepine		Start at 100 mg daily increase slowly by 100 to 200 mg per week to a final daily dose of 800 mg in 2 to 4 doses		
Opioids				
Methadone	Use when all conservative measures have failed to make the patient more functional.	Time-based dosing Can start at 2.5 mg daily may give every 6 h, use as low a dose as possible	Constipation, sedation, cognitive clouding	Must anticipate constipation Methadone has been associated with cardiac QT prolongation Oxycontine has a higher potential for abuse

Table 20.1 *(Cont.)*

Medication class	Uses	Dosing	Side effects	Comments
Sustained action morphine		Start at 15 mg every 12 hours, titrate to effectiveness		Prolonged use will lead to tolerance and dependency, which should not be confused with addiction If long term – use an opioid agreement
Fentanyl patch		25 mcg applied every 3 days – higher doses can be used as needed		
Tramadol	Short acting analgesic that can be used to treat pain preventing sleep, activity relate pain or other pain flares	Start at 50 mg daily or every 12 h, may increase the dosing as needed to 400 mg per day	Nausea, emesis, drowsiness, light headedness Lowers seizure threshold	Avoid with history of substance abuse or suicidal behavior history Impaired motor function particularly at onset can impair driving – do not operate heavy machinery Use with SSNRI, SSRI or TCA agents can trigger serotonin syndrome
Topical lidocaine and potentially other topical anesthetics	Best for pain associated with peripheral neuropathy	Can be applied as a gel or via patch. Apply patch to area 12 h on and off for 12 h. Can use an occlusive dressing for lidocaine gel	Should not have systemic interactions, but will impair peripheral sensation	Can be used alone or as applied before using capsaiscin Lidocaine patches are costly
Topical capsaicin	Peripheral neuropathy, but not post-herpetic neuralgia	Strengths 0.025%, 0.075%, over the counter 0.010% and 0.035%. Apply up to 4 times a day	Burning sensation	Can apply lidocaine first to block burning. Do not apply to mucosa, eyes or other sensitive areas. Wear gloves or use applicator

TCA: tricyclic antidepressant; SSNRI: selective serotonin and norepinephrine reuptake inhibitor; SSRI: selective serotonin reuptake inhibitor.

can have an impact on a patient's motivation to move beyond a purely medical model. The psychologist needs to appreciate how a patient appraises their own ability to control their pain and the patient's perception of the extent of their own skills to adapt to pain. Affective factors include anxiety, fear, anger, and depression. Pain is by definition an emotional experience, yet the affective factors are sometimes ignored by both patients and clinicians. Emotional factors can have a direct impact on chronic pain. For example, muscle tensing and sympathetic arousal can increase pain. Emotional aspects of pain can also alter pain perception. Neuropathic pain will respond to psychological interventions that are widely used for other types of chronic pain. Yet, psychological interventions are often overshadowed by pharmacological treatment, surgical interventions and other procedures in the treatment of non-radicular neuropathic pain.

Defining the role

Patients can be concerned that seeing a psychologist means that the pain is being relegated to the category of being psychosomatic. It is important to assure the patient that the psychologist is acting as a member of a care team and that medical treatment will not halt. The initial interaction between the psychologist and the patient should validate the patient's pain. At the initial contact it is important to begin educating the patient on three aspects of their condition: (1) that the pain is an established condition that will not be immediately and permanently corrected; (2) the patient needs to understand their pain diagnosis and its prognosis; and (3) that by working with members of the care team including psychologists, physicians and therapists that the patient can become more functional. The order of discussion will depend upon the patient's needs and receptivity. How the patient describes their pain may suggest the initial tenor of the interaction. If the patient describes their pain primarily with distress terms (e.g., agonizing, excruciating, horrible, unbearable) then the patient may need to vent before they will hear and retain information. Unfortunately, health psychologists are often involved in pain management after the patient has undergone extensive and often multiple, detailed medical assessments. The focus on the testing and evaluation is important in establishing a diagnosis, but can create a belief that if an additional stone is overturned that a cure will suddenly become apparent. It may be useful to suggest to the individual that a full diagnostic evaluation has been conducted and that attention needs to be given to improving treatment.

The health psychologist should encourage the patient to keep a pain diary. The diary should log activities and amount of time spent at work or out of the home as well as when pain occurred and its perceived intensity. The diary serves several purposes. The diary enables the pain intervention team to monitor the course of pain to help determine if interventions are beneficial. The diary may help to identify factors that are triggering or worsening pain that the patient was not aware of. The diary can be used to monitor activity levels and to see how interventions are having an impact on activity levels.

The patient needs to understand that effective treatment interventions need to be applied long term. Therefore, it is important to establish that the pain condition is long standing and that the goal is to increase the patient's function as an indication of the effectiveness of pain treatment. After seeing multiple practitioners, patients often have formed incorrect perceptions of what their pain condition is and how it will affect them. For example, an individual with radicular back pain may believe that their spinal cord is being damaged and that if the pain does not stop that they will become paralyzed. Therefore, it is important to review what the patient believes their condition/diagnosis is and the implications/prognosis of their condition. Care needs to be taken to be sure that the patient actually understands their diagnosis and prognosis and that they are not simply parroting medical terms that they do not understand. The patient needs to appreciate that medication and surgical/anesthesia interventions are not the only way to treat pain. For chronic pain, interventions may no longer be effective and the side effects of medications may limit their long-term utility. The patient needs to become actively involved in physical/occupational therapy and other treatments that can provide the patient with ways of increasing their functionality and reducing their pain. The non-surgical and non-pharmacological treatment approaches can empower the patient to have an active role in their treatment.

Medication counseling

Patients will often benefit from discussion of the appropriate use of medications and their role in treating chronic neuropathic pain. The following points may be useful in directing a discussion about pain medication: (1) medication alone may reduce but will usually not eliminate neuropathic pain; (2) medication needs to be taken in a manner that will prevent pain rather than solely to treat pain flare ups; (3) the primary outcome in treating chronic neuropathic pain is to increase function; (4) non-surgical and non-pharmacological interventions such as therapy can reduce the overall reliance on medication; and (5) opioids are not well suited to the long-term management of non-terminal pain.

While medications can be an important component in managing neuropathic pain, patients need to have realistic expectations of the benefits of medication. Medication can reduce, but will usually not eliminate pain. The benefits of pain medication to increase functionality can be enhanced through therapy and behavioral modification. In addition, long-term use of medication can be associated with side effects and tolerance to the effects of the medications. Patients need to recognize that many types of pain medication work best if the patient maintains constant medication levels rather than to use the medication only for flares of pain. Patients need to appreciate the importance of taking pain medication on a time-dependent around the clock fashion. When a patient with neuropathic pain sees a health psychologist, they may have been taking opioid medication for a long time. Such patients may feel threatened by the initial suggestion to stop the opioid medication. In order to establish an effective therapeutic relationship, it is prudent not to begin by modifying the opioid treatment. Rather, the initial interventions should be directed at education. After other treatment, management strategies are in place, an opioid wean may be started. Education about what to expect in a wean is also very important.

Monitoring activity

Patients who have neuropathic pain that is worsened by movements can develop an aversion to activity, kinesiophobia [17]. Low activity levels may lead to impaired joint function, which can lead to joint pain. In addition, reduced activity can lead to obesity, which can further interfere with the patient's activity level. Patients with neuropathic pain due to radiculopathy, neuropathy, and CRPS need to understand that appropriately supervised activity will not worsen their underlying pathology. These patients need to have therapy initially aimed at regaining normal ranges of motion. Activity needs to be increased gradually as the patient tolerates. It may be beneficial to adjust pain medication schedules so that patients receive pain medications 30–60 minutes prior to therapy to facilitate a patient's participation in therapy.

Patients need to learn how to manage their activity levels. A common mistake is to do too much on days with less pain ("good days") and to do too little on days with more severe pain ("bad days"). Health psychologists need to counsel patients on pacing their activity to enable the patients to have more consistent activity levels, which will facilitate community reintegration and return to work. Teaching patients how to modulate their activity levels and the importance of doing such will enable patients to gain control over their pain, which can reduce their fear of activity.

Pacing is a very important concept to teach patients with chronic pain. In reviewing pain diaries, a psychologist can help patients determine what activities aggravate pain. They can learn to time those activities and intersperse non-aggravating activities so that they conserve energy, do not aggravate their pain, and are more productive in the long run.

Role of sleep in pain

The health psychologist needs to pay careful attention to the patient's sleep hygiene. Neuropathic pain is often associated with impaired sleep [18–20]. Clearly, pain can impair sleep. However, impaired sleep can also alter pain perception, which can heighten the perceived pain severity. Sleep deprivation can trigger neuropathic pain [21]. In a recent study of neuropathic head pain caused by combat head trauma, patients with impaired sleep reported more severe pain [22]. Consequently, addressing sleep impairment is an important component of treating neuropathic pain. There are several tools that can be employed to assess an individual's sleep hygiene [23]. The Epworth Sleepiness Scale is an easy to administer questionnaire to assess daytime sleepiness and is a good indicator of the quality of night-time sleep [24].

The health psychologist should provide sleep hygiene counseling. As appropriate, sleep hygiene counseling should include the following instructions: (1) adapt a fixed bedtime routine; (2) avoid activities that may trigger pain prior to sleep; (3) avoid agitating video or audio programs/movies within 6 hours of bedtime; (4) stop watching television 1 hour before bedtime and engage in calming activities such as reading or engaging in intimacy with your partner; (5) sleep only when sleepy, engage in a boring activity if not sleepy at bedtime; (6) avoid caffeinated beverages such as coffee, sodas and "power drinks" and avoid nicotine and alcohol within 6 hours of bedtime; (6) avoid sleeping during the day; (7) engage in exercise during the day, but not within 4 hours of bedtime; (8) take a hot bath or shower about an hour before bedtime; and if obesity is not an issue (9) take a light snack before bedtime.

Avoiding naps during the day is an important point to press. It is often helpful to help patients distinguish between tiredness and sleepiness – a physical and a mental state, respectively. One must recover from physical tiredness, but sleepiness is under volitional control. If sleepiness occurs during the day, a patient can have a list of things to do when sleepy to avoid napping, thus improving sleep during the night.

The function of a pain group

The health psychologist should strongly consider establishing a pain group. There are basically two types of pain groups: psycho-educational and process.

Patients are at different stages of acceptance as well as education of their pain conditions. Groups offer an opportunity for all patients to learn – whether they are able to actually make behavioral changes at the time they attend group. A "stages of change" model is often useful to evaluate an individual's readiness to make changes [25–29]. This model has been used to understand how people move from being unreceptive to change to being able to change and to prevent return to prior behavior patterns. The five stages of change are: (1) precontemplative – the patient does not agree that he needs to change; (2) contemplative – the patient is willing to consider change; (3) preparation – the patient is thinking about how to change, but has not begun to change; (4) action – the patient is changing; (5) maintenance and relapse prevention – the patient incorporates behavioral changes over a long-term basis. Patients may need to travel through the stages of change several times before the change becomes truly established behavior patterns. Individual sessions can be used to help each patient advance through their stages of change and to reinforce a patient's positive actions.

It is often most helpful to start with a psycho-educational group. Topics can include information about pain in general, developing realistic expectations about how much medical treatments/medications can help, how they can manage some of their pain, and how to become more functional. Pacing, assertive communication – both in medical appointments and with friends and family – and effective coping skills are core components of pain management groups. A logical segue to process groups would include groups on relaxation training. Diaphramatic breathing techniques should be a first step in this group (or series of classes). A physiological rationale for the use of this technique might win over any skeptics in the group.

A process group allows patients to learn that others have experienced the same frustrations, isolation, changes in self-perception, depression/anxieties and express themselves openly. At times, this may be the first time patients are among others with chronic pain. It is helpful to have family sessions as well. Care should be taken to learn how the group wishes to incorporate family sessions. It would be unwise to open the group to non-patients if that negates the opportunity for free expression.

The psychologist should try to end the group on a positive note. It may be helpful to ask each patient for a success at the end of the group, encouraging those who have difficulties with this exercise.

As the group members develop supportive interactions, both older members and newer members will start to voice their concerns and to determine if their concerns are validated or refuted by the other group members. Patients can also learn coping strategies from other members of the group. It is important that the health psychologist direct, but not control the group so that individuals are able to freely express themselves. In forming the groups, the psychologist should consider trying to have patients with similar conditions in the same group so that they are addressing similar issues. It is probably wise to exclude patients with psychosis or prominent thought disorders as such individuals may be disruptive to a pain group.

Positive psychology

The role of positive psychology [30–33] has expanded in the health psychology setting. Positive psychology can be used in pain management once a patient starts to feel some relief and control over the pain. Positive psychology focuses on character strengths that enable a person to become resilient during periods of physical or emotional stress [31]. Having chronic pain leads to a state of deconditioning and debility that can put a patient into a negative frame of mind. The health psychologist can help the patient shift the way that the patient thinks about pain.

Shifting the focus of the patient towards pain is within the purview of cognitive behavioral therapy [34]. Cognitive-behavioral therapy shifts the patient's focus on pain from negative to a more neutral stance. Positive psychology can be used to shift a patient's thoughts from neutral to positive [32, 33]. Rather than asking for pain ratings the psychologist can ask the patient for a comfort rating (we use a 0–10 scale where 0 is extreme discomfort and 10 is fully comfortable and functioning in all areas – family, social, vocational).

Another useful step is to have patients keep a gratitude journal at night [30]. This focuses their attention on what is going well in their lives. Positive emotions can empower patients, provide them with emotional resiliency and heightens their abilities to combat stress and distress [31].

Helping a patient to identify and utilize their strengths can enable them to have more control over their pain. A useful exercise is to have the patient take the VIA Signature Strengths Questionnaire (www.authentichappiness.sas.upenn.edu/Default.aspx or www.authentichappiness.org) to learn their character strengths. The patient can print out the results of the questionnaire and bring them to an individual appointment to review with the psychologist [32]. The authentic happiness website contains other tests such as a gratitude questionnaire.

Conclusion

Neuropathic pain is common and often misunderstood. The health psychologist is an important member of the pain treatment team who can educate the patient about the pain, thereby demystifying the condition. In addition, the health psychologist can help the patient recognize what behavioral changes they need to make to be as functional as possible with their pain and to guide patients through the paths of change.

Acknowledgment

Supported by the Rehabilitation Research Service of the Department of Veterans Affairs.

References

1. Headache Classification Subcommittee of the International Headache Society. The International Classification of Headache Disorders, 2nd edition. *Cephalgia* 2004; **24** (Suppl 1): 9–160.

2. Dworkin RH, Backonja M, Rowbotham MC, Allen RR, Argoff CR. Advances in neuropathic pain – diagnosis, mechanisms, and treatment recommendations. *Arch Neurol* 2003; **60**: 1524–34.

3. Jensen TS. An improved understanding of neuropathic pain. *Eur J Pain* 2002; **6**: 3–11.

4. Waxman SG, Dib–Hajj SD, Cummins TR, Black JA. Sodium channels and pain. *Proc Natl Acad Sci USA* 1999; **96**: 7635–9.

5. Black JA, Cummins TR, Plumpton C, *et al.* Upregulation of a silent sodium channel after peripheral, but not central, nerve injury in DRG neurons. *J Neurophysiol* 1999; **82**: 2776–85.

6. Black JA, Liu S, Tanaka M, Cummins TR, Waxman SG. Changes in the expression of tetrodotoxin-sensitive sodium channels within dorsal root ganglia neurons in inflammatory pain. *Pain* 2004; **108**: 237–47.

7. Dib-Hajj SD, Fjell J, Cummins TR, *et al.* Plasticity of sodium channel expression in DRG neurons in the chronic constriction injury model of neuropathic pain. *Pain* 1999; **83**: 691–700.

8. Cummins TR, Waxman SG. Downregulation of tetrodotoxinresistant sodium currents and upregulation of a rapidly repriming tetrodotoxin-sensitive sodium current in small spinal sensory neurons following nerve injury. *J Neurosci* 1997; **17**: 3503–14.

9. Waxman SG, Hains BC. Fire and phantoms after spinal cord injury: Na+ channels and central pain. *Trends Neurosci* 2006; **29**: 207–15.

10. Hains BC, Waxman SG. Activated microglia contribute to the maintenance of chronic pain after spinal cord injury. *J Neurosci* 2006; **26**: 4308–17.

11. Zhao P, Waxman SG, Hains BC. Extracellular signal-regulated kinase-regulated microglia-neuron signaling by prostaglandin e2 contributes to pain after spinal cord injury. *J Neurosci* 2007; **27**: 2357–68.

12. Gilron I, Watson CPN, Cahill CM, Moulin DE. Neuropathic pain: a practical guide for the clinician. *Canad Med Assoc J* 2006; **175**: 265–75.

13. Dworkin RH, O'Connor AB, Backonja M, *et al.* Pharmacologic management of neuropathic pain: evidence-based recommendations. *Pain* 2007; **132**: 237–51.

14. Moulin DE, Clark AJ, Gilron I, *et al.* Pharmacological management of chronic neuropathic pain – consensus statement and guidelines from the Canadian Pain Society. *Pain Res Manag* 2007; **12**: 13–21.

15. Hariharan J, Lamb GC, Neuner JM. Long-term opioid contract use for chronic pain management in primary care practice. A five year experience. *J Gen Intern Med* 2007; **22**: 485–90.

16. Melzack R, Casey KL. Sensory, motivational and central control determinants of pain: a new conceptional model. In *The Skin Senses*, ed. D Kenshalo (Springfield, IL: Thomas, 1968), pp. 423–43.

17. Strine TW, Hootman JM, Chapman DP, Okoro CA, Balluz L. Health-related quality of life, health risk behaviors, and disability among adults with pain-related activity difficulty. *Am J Public Health* 2005; **95**: 2042–8.

18. Dick BD, Rashiq S. Disruption of attention and working memory traces in individuals with chronic pain. *Anesth Analg* 2007; **104**: 1223–9.

19. Hans G, Masquelier E, De Cock P. The diagnosis and management of neuropathic pain in daily practice in Belgium: an observational study. *BMC Public Health* 2007; **7**: 170–82.

20. Zelman DC, Brandenburg NA, Gore M. Sleep impairment in patients with painful diabetic peripheral neuropathy. *Clin J Pain* 2006; **22**: 681–5.

21. Smith MT, Edwards RR, McCann UD, Haythornthwaite JA. The effects of sleep deprivation on pain inhibition and spontaneous pain in women. *Sleep* 2007; **30**: 495–505.

22. Ruff RL, Ruff SS, Wang X-F. Headaches among veterans of operations Iraqi Freedom and Enduring Freedom with mild traumatic brain injury associated with exposures to explosions. *J Rehabil Res Dev* 2008; **45**: 941–53.

23. Mastin DF, Bryson J, Corwyn R. Assessment of sleep hygiene using the Sleep Hygiene Index. *J Behav Med* 2006; **29**: 223–7.

24. Johns MW. Sensitivity and specificity of the multiple sleep latency test (MSLT), the maintenance of wakefulness test and the Epworth sleepiness scale: failure of the MSLT as a gold standard. *J Sleep Res* 2000; **9**: 5–11.

25. Kerns RD, Habib S. A critical review of the pain readiness to change model. *J Pain* 2004; **5**: 357–67.

26. Kerns RD, Rosenberg R. Predicting responses to self-management treatments for chronic pain: application of the pain stages of change model. *Pain* 2000; **84**: 49–55.

27. Kerns RD, Rosenberg R, Jamison RN, Caudill MA, Haythornthwaite J. Readiness to adopt a self-management approach to chronic pain: the Pain Stages of Change Questionnaire (PSOCQ). *Pain* 1997; **72**: 227–34.

28. Prochaska JO, DiClemente CC, Norcross JC. In search of how people change. *Am Psychol* 1992; **47**: 1102–4.

29. Prochaska JO, Velicer WF, Rossi JS, *et al.* Stages of change and decisional balance for 12 problem behaviors. *Health Psychol* 1994; **13**: 39–46.

30. Emmons RA, McCullough ME. Counting blessings versus burdens: an experiment investigation of gratitude and well-being in daily life. *J Personality Social Psychol* 2003; **84**: 377–89.

31. Fredrickson B. The role of positive emotions in positive psychology. *Am Psychol* 2001; **56**: 218–26.

32. Peterson C, Seligman MEP. *Character Strengths and Virtues: A classification and handbook* (New York: Oxford University Press, 2004).

33. Seligman MEP, Csikszentmihaly M. Positive psychology: an introduction. *Am Psychol* 2000; **55**: 5–14.

34. Turk DC, Winter F. *The Pain Survival Guide. How to Reclaim Your Life* (Washington, DC: American Psychological Association, 2006).

Management of headache pain

Donald B. Penzien, Morris Maizels and Jeanetta C. Rains

Introduction

Recurrent or chronic benign headache disorders, such as migraine, tension-type, and cluster headache, are amongst the most common painful conditions encountered in medical practice and are the focus of this chapter. Headache impacts a large percentage of the population and poses substantial economic burden as well as personal suffering and disability. A careful headache history following established headache diagnostic nosology generally discriminates such benign headaches from other pathologic conditions. Behavioral risk factors for headache are increasingly recognized as potentially important variables in the progression of headache from episodic to chronic. Headaches are comorbid with a number of psychiatric, pain, and medical disorders, and the coprevalence increases in cases of more frequent and severe headaches. Headache may present in the context of chronic pain as the primary pain disorder, or more commonly, in association with another chronic pain problem. While headache itself is a ubiquitous symptom, the patient with chronic, daily, and refractory headache presents a unique challenge both in diagnosis and treatment. A wide range of acute and prophylactic pharmacologic treatments are available for treatment of headache. There are also effective non-pharmacologic treatments for migraine and tension-type headache that may be administered in combination with medication or as monotherapy. Psychological and behavioral strategies may also be employed to improve adherence with pharmacologic measures or address co-morbid psychiatric disorders.

Epidemiology and impact of headache

Headache is the most common pain-related complaint and the seventh leading ailment seen in medical practice,

accounting for 18 million physician visits a year [1], with migraine and tension-type headache accounting for the majority of headache presentations. Although physician consultations for headache in the USA have increased in the past 15 years, headache remains substantially underdiagnosed and undertreated [2]. A recent review of population studies estimated worldwide current prevalences were 47% for headache, 10% for migraine, 38% for tension-type headache, and 3% for chronic daily headache, with lifetime prevalences somewhat higher (66% for headache, 14% for migraine, and 46% for tension-type headache) [3].

Females exhibit a higher prevalence of migraine than males (18% vs. 6% of the population, respectively) at all ages, with peak prevalence between 25 and 55 years of age [3]. Although episodic tension-type headache is only slightly more prevalent among women than men (42% vs. 36%; prevalence ratio = 1.16), chronic tension-type headache is substantially more prevalent among women (2.8% vs. 1.4%; prevalence ratio = 2.0) [1]. Like migraine, the prevalence of tension-type headache also varies by age, peaking in the third and fourth decades of life.

Annual direct medical costs for migraine care have been estimated to exceed $1 billion annually – a figure, however, far less than the costs of productivity losses due to migraine at an estimated $13 billion [4]. Both tension-type headache and migraine are associated with chronic or recurrent episodes of impairment, and migraineurs in particular are frequently disabled during their acute headaches. In a recent study, 90% of migraineurs reported functional impairment with their headaches and 53% exhibited severe impairment requiring bed rest, nearly a third had missed at least one day of work or school in the past 3 months, and 51% reported productivity was reduced by at least half due to headache [2].

Relative to migraine, less is known about the psychosocial impact of tension-type headache. A recent epidemiologic study indicated that 8.3% of episodic

Behavioral and Psychopharmacologic Pain Management, ed. Michael H. Ebert and Robert D. Kerns. Published by Cambridge University Press. © Cambridge University Press 2011.

tension-type headache sufferers missed workdays due to headache (average 9 days per year), and 43.6% reported reduced effectiveness in the work, home and school [1]. Among chronic tension-type headache sufferers, 11.8% missed workdays (average 20 days per year) and 46.5% reported reduced productivity due to headache.

Co-morbidities also play an important role in the presentation of migraine and other primary headache disorders. A recent epidemiologic survey of 5700 adults in the USA revealed that 83% of migraineurs and 79% of persons with other severe types of headache had some form of co-morbidity [5]. Compared with headache-free subjects, migraineurs were at significantly increased risk for psychiatric disorders (odds ratio [OR] 3.1), other pain conditions (OR 3.3), and physical diseases (OR 2.1), with similar ORs for non-migraine headache patients. Migraineurs also experienced role disability on 25.2% of the last 30 days compared with 9.7% of the days for persons without headache, with co-morbid conditions explaining 65% of the role disability associated with migraine.

Headache classification

Primary headache disorders – those without an underlying cause – may be categorized as those lasting longer than 4 hours and those lasting less than 4 hours. Cluster headache is the best known example of severe headache lasting less than four hours. This chapter will focus on the longer-lasting, primary headache disorders.

The most common long-lasting headaches are migraine and tension-type headache. Both of these primary headache disorders may be classified as episodic (i.e., with headache-free intervals) or chronic (occurring on a daily or near-daily basis). Migraine and tension-type headache most typically begin as episodic disorders, and with time, may evolve or transform into a daily headache syndrome.

Formal diagnostic criteria have been established, such as the International Classification of Headache Disorders-2 (ICHD-2) for primary and secondary headache disorders [6]. Table 21.1 lists the main diagnostic considerations in the patient with chronic, daily, and refractory headache. Approximately 5% of adults experience chronic daily headache: about half of these chronic migraine and half tension-type headache (with medication overuse a factor in both). Although far less common, it is important to consider unusual causes of daily headache in the patient who presents with a refractory headache disorder.

Table 21.1 Differential diagnosis of chronic daily headache syndromes (lasting longer than 4 hours)

Chronic migraine
Chronic tension-type headache
Medication-overuse headache
New daily persistent headache
Hemicrania continua
Idiopathic intracranial hypertension
Spontaneous intracranial hypotension

Table 21.2 International Headache Society diagnostic criteria for episodic migraine

Migraine without aura

A. At least five attacks fulfilling criteria B-D

B. Headache attacks lasting 4–72 hours (untreated or unsuccessfully treated)

C. Headache has at least two of the following characteristics:
1. Unilateral location
2. Pulsating quality
3. Moderate or severe pain intensity
4. Aggravation by or causing avoidance of routine physical activity (e.g., walking or climbing stairs)

D. During headache at least one of the following:
1. Nausea and/or vomiting
2. Photophobia and phonophobia

E. Not attributed to another disorder

Table 21.2 lists the ICHD-2 diagnostic criteria for episodic migraine. Chronic migraine is variably defined as 8–15 days/month of migraine headache; typically, patients experience milder headaches on a daily or near-daily basis. Chronic migraine is further discussed below. Tension-type headache is essentially a headache that lacks migraine features.

New daily persistent headache is a headache that essentially starts "out of the blue" and persists. By definition, it is not due to an underlying disorder, although onset may occur in relation to an infection or viral illness. New daily persistent headache may spontaneously remit over time, but otherwise it is often poorly responsive to usual therapies.

Hemicrania continua is a rare but important cause of refractory daily headache. Headache is constant, in a fixed unilateral location, and more severe episodes of pain may be associated with autonomic phenomena, such as ipsilateral tearing or rhinitis. Hemicrania continua is uniquely responsive to indomethacin, and in fact relief of headache with an adequate trial of indomethacin (up to 75 mg three times per day) is a diagnostic criterion for the disorder [6].

High and low pressure headache syndromes should be considered in the differential diagnosis of any patient with refractory chronic daily headache. Idiopathic intracranial hypertension (IIH), also known as pseudotumor cerebri, most commonly occurs in obese young women, and may occur in association with certain medications. Spontaneous intracranial hypotension (SIH) is due to a spontaneous dural leak, sometimes presenting after very minor trauma. Although initially the headache has postural features, suggesting a dural puncture headache, with time the postural component may disappear, leaving a daily headache with non-specific features. Although both IIH and SIH may have characteristic MRI findings, they require lumbar puncture to confirm that opening pressures are abnormal. Idiopathic intracranial hypertension and SIH are two syndromes which may be missed despite imaging with CT or MRI.

Chronic migraine

Migraine as an episodic disorder can transform over time into chronic daily headache. The transformation or progression of migraine from episodic to chronic and daily is a widely recognized phenomenon supported by an emerging body of evidence [7]. Citing research reporting brain abnormalities in migraineurs (e.g., brain infarction and white matter lesions, iron deposits in periaqueductal gray correlating with headache duration, central sensitization), Bigal and Lipton [8] have suggested migraine may in some cases be conceptualized as a chronic progressive disorder. Since migraine is known to progress in selected patients but does not progress in all or even most patients, they suggest migraine is best conceptualized as a chronic disorder with episodic manifestations which is progressive in some patients.

The conceptualization of migraine as a progressive disorder highlights the value of identifying potentially modifiable risk factors associated with onset and progression, risk factor modification (primary prevention), and early intervention to limit progression (secondary prevention). Although some implicated risk factors for migraine chronification are not modifiable (e.g., age, low socioeconomic status, head injury), other risk factors have key behavioral components that can be recognized and modified (e.g., analgesic

overuse, depression, stressful life events, sleep variables, obesity [9]). Thus screening and behavioral risk-reduction (i.e., behavioral self-management) strategies theoretically could prevent chronification.

Although many headache patients do not suffer from a co-morbid psychological disorder, epidemiological research consistently confirms the co-morbidity of headache with mood, anxiety, and substance abuse disorders (see Table 21.3 [10]). Headache patients (particularly those with migraine and chronic tension-type headache) are approximately 2–5 times more likely to suffer from a depressive or anxiety disorder than are individuals without headache disorders [10–12]. Up to one-third of migraineurs will meet criteria for major depression at one point in their lifetime and more than half will meet criteria for an anxiety disorder, with panic disorder and phobias being particularly prevalent. As referenced above, a growing body of literature has implicated psychiatric co-morbidity as a risk factor for chronification of migraine, and many patients with chronic forms of migraine and tension-type headache endorse higher levels of depression and anxiety than do their non-headache counterparts [13, 14]. Co-morbid depression and anxiety also are associated with poorer long-term headache outcomes and satisfaction with treatment [15, 16], considerably higher medical costs and healthcare utilization [17], and increased headache-related disability [16].

Medication overuse headache

A unique and important cause of chronic daily headache is medication overuse headache (MOH), previously also known as drug rebound headache. It is a refractory daily headache, maintained by daily or frequent use of symptomatic medications, which ultimately improves after discontinuation of those medications [6, 18].

The ICHD criteria specify 10–15 days/month of use as comprising medication overuse, depending on the medication involved (10 days for opiates and butalbital compounds, 15 days for most others). Pragmatically, the use of symptomatic medications more than 3 days/week on an ongoing basis is likely to represent medication overuse. Medication overuse has been described for all symptomatic medications used to treat headache, including simple analgesics (aspirin, acetaminophen, non-steroidal anti-inflammatories), compound analgesics (especially those containing caffeine), and triptans. Caffeinated beverages also are a potential cause of MOH. Medications especially problematic for

Table 21.3 Lifetime prevalence of migraine and psychiatric disorders

Diagnosis	Migraine	Control	Odds ratio[a]
Major depression	34%	10%	4.5
Dysthymia	9%	2%	4.4
Bipolar II	4%	1%	5.1
Manic episode	5%	1%	5.4
Panic disorder	11%	2%	6.6
Anxiety (GAD)	10%	2%	5.7
Obsessive-compulsive disorder	9%	2%	5.1
Phobia	40%	21%	2.6
Illicit drug use	20%	10%	2.2
Nicotine dependence	33%	18%	2.2

[a] Odds ratios adjusted for gender.
GAD: generalized anxiety disorder.

Table 21.4 Common treatment strategies for medication overuse headache

1. Patient education
2. Withdraw all symptomatic medications including caffeine
3. Transition regimen (no evidence supports one regimen over another)
A. steroid burst (e.g., dexamethasone 4 mg bid x 3 days, 4 mg qd x 3 days)
B. daily long-acting non-steroidal anti-inflammatory (NSAID) (e.g., meloxicam)
C. daily long-acting triptan (naratriptan or frovatriptan) or daily self-injection of dihydroergotamine bid
D. "rescue" regimens
   1) dihydroergotamine 1mg IM bid (+/- ketorolac 60 mg IM) (may be given as self-injection)
   2) valproic acid (1000 mg IV)
   3) neuroleptics
   4) antihistamines
4. Maximize standard prophylactic regimens

MOH, in addition to caffeine-containing compounds, are opiates and butalbital compounds.

Common strategies for treatment of MOH are listed in Table 21.4. The treatment begins with patient education. Lack of understanding of MOH (both by physician and patient) may result in incomplete and unsuccessful withdrawal regimens, resulting in the patient resuming the previous offending agents. It is critical that the patient be informed that: (1) 80% of patients with MOH respond to detoxification with return to a pattern of episodic headache; (2) patients who do not withdraw from symptomatic medication do not respond to additional pharmacologic or behavioral treatments; and (3) patients typically experience headache exacerbation in the first week of withdrawal. Successful treatment of MOH requires complete withdrawal of all symptomatic medications and implementation of appropriate prophylaxis. Typically, a "transition regimen" is used to minimize the headache exacerbation which occurs in the first week following medication withdrawal. Numerous withdrawal and transition regimens have been described, although none studied in a rigorous scientific manner. Zed and colleagues [19] found essentially no difference in outcome between gradual vs. abrupt withdrawal of overused medications, no difference between use of transition medications as compared to no transition medications, and no difference among the various transition medications (non-steroidal anti-inflammatories, triptans, etc.).

Pharmacologic treatment of chronic migraine

The main categories of migraine preventive therapies are antihypertensive, antidepressant, and antiepileptic medications [20]. In research trials, a headache preventive is considered effective if 50% of patients respond with at least a 50% decrease in headache attacks. However, overall, headache preventives by themselves are associated with a modest improvement in headache control [20]. Pharmacotherapy combined with behavioral headache therapy has been shown to be more effective than either therapy alone (cf. Holroyd *et al.* [21]).

General principles of headache preventive therapies

Preventive therapies are recommended when headaches are: daily; require use of symptomatic medications more than 2 days/week; frequent enough to interfere with usual activities, or are poorly relieved with acute therapies, even if infrequent [20]. Headache preventives typically require at least 4 weeks for efficacy, and an adequate medication trial may require up to 3 months. No preventive medication has been shown to be more efficacious than another, so the choice of preventive is often based on tolerability.

Beta blockers (propranolol and others) are effective for migraine prevention, but are less commonly used for daily headache syndromes. Physiologically, their efficacy may be based on their effect on contingent negative variation, a marker of cortical hypersensitivity.

Similar to findings in chronic pain treatment studies, antidepressants with mixed noradrenergic and serotonergic properties are effective as headache preventives. Tricyclic antidepressants (especially amitriptyline and nortriptyline) are the most frequently prescribed headache preventives, and may improve sleep and reduce muscle spasm. Typical doses of tricyclics for headache prevention range from 10–75 mg, and efficacy is not necessarily dose-related. Limiting side effects include sedation and weight gain, while anticholinergic side effects (dry mouth and constipation) are common but usually tolerated. Venlafaxine, a serotonergic noradrenergic reuptake inhibitor (SNRI) has been widely used instead of tricyclics, because it does not typically cause weight gain – efficacy has been reported in open-label but not double-blind studies. Several studies of serotonin specific reuptake inhibitors (SSRIs) have found little efficacy as headache preventives.

Several antiepileptic drugs are effective for headache prevention, specifically valproate, gabapentin, and topiramate. Of these three, only gabapentin has been found also to be useful for chronic pain, suggesting that the mechanisms of action for headache prevention and chronic pain differ. Side effect profiles again influence the choice of medication. Valproate

use is specifically discouraged in women of childbearing age because of teratogenicity (although use of any headache preventive in pregnancy is usually discouraged, and should be based on a risk-benefit discussion). Both valproate and gabapentin commonly cause weight gain, and topiramate is the only antiepiletic headache preventive that is not associated with weight gain. However, cognitive side effects of topiramate frequently limit its use.

Verapamil and other calcium channel blockers have been cited as effective headache preventives, but clinically their efficacy appears to be small.

Natural supplements that have at least some evidence of efficacy include vitamin B2 (100–200 mg, twice daily), magnesium (300 mg, twice daily), coenzyme Q10 (150 mg, twice daily) and butterbur root (75 mg, twice daily).

Headache preventives of different classes are often combined, although there have been no randomized trials of combined therapies.

The refractory (chronic migraine) headache

Recently, the first formal criteria for refractory migraine were proposed (see Table 21.5) [22]. Hallmarks of the refractory migraine criteria include ongoing significant interference with functioning or quality of life and failure of adequately administered medication treatment regimens (both preventive and abortive). In a review published in tandem with these proposed criteria, Dodick [23] suggested failure of behavioral treatments be added as a criterion because of the strong evidence in support of such therapies (see italics in Table 21.5). If headache remains refractory to appropriate therapy (including treatment of medication overuse headache), a trial of repetitive intramuscular (outpatient) or intravenous (inpatient) dihydroergotamine is indicated. The intravenous protocol, first described by Raskin in 1986 has been reported to be effective in over 90% of patients with refractory headache [24].

Interventional therapies of headache

Although in widespread use, several randomized double-blinded studies of botulinum toxin have consistently failed to show efficacy for episodic or chronic migraine, and a guideline from the American Academy of Neurology stated that it probably is ineffective for episodic migraine or chronic tension-type headache [25]. Occipital nerve stimulators have

Table 21.5 Proposed criteria for definition of refractory chronic migraine, with an additional proposed criterion in italics

Criteria	Definition
Primary diagnosis	A. ICHD-II migraine or chronic migraine
Refractory	B. Headache causes significant interference with function or quality of life despite modification of triggers, lifestyle factors, and adequate trials of acute and preventive medications.
	1. Failed adequate trials of preventive medicines from at least two of following: beta blockers, anticonvulsants, tricyclics, calcium channel blockers.
	2. Failed adequate trials of abortive medicines, to include triptans and non-triptan medicines.
	3. *Failed adequate trial of behavioral therapies, to include relaxation and/or cognitive behavioral therapy.*
Adequate trial	At least 2 months at optimum or maximal-tolerated dose
Modifier	With or without medication overuse

Source. Modified from Schulman *et al.* [22], with an additional proposed criterion in italics.

recently been introduced as a therapeutic option for patients with severe headache refractory to aggressive therapies [26]. The experience with this modality is limited, and it appears to offer best efficacy for patients with unilateral headache syndromes, such as cluster headache, hemicrania continua, and fixed unilateral chronic migraine. Problems with lead migration and battery failure remain technological challenges. Acupuncture is commonly used and widely available modality that appears to have efficacy for headache prevention, although the difficulty of including sham acupuncture leads to difficulty in demonstated efficacy.

Treatment of chronic migraine contrasted with treatment of chronic pain

Epidemiologic studies have demonstrated that patients with migraine or frequent headaches are at increased risk of co-occurring non-headache pain compared to those without headache, with the best current evidence data related to musculoskeletal pain or arthritis [27]. Moreover, there is evidence to indicate that the presence of multiple pain conditions is a negative prognostic factor for pain recovery [27]. Several antidepressants and antiepileptic drugs are useful both as headache preventives and for chronic pain disorders, but important differences exist, suggesting overlapping but distinct neuroanatomic pathways may underlie the two disorders (see Table 21.6).

Headache patients with co-morbid chronic pain disorders

Managing headache patients who present with other co-morbid chronic pain problems can prove challenging. Co-morbid chronic pain disorders that commonly influence headache management are fibromyalgia, chronic neck pain, and chronic low back pain. Fibromyalgia has been found to be present in 35.6% of patients with chronic daily migraine [28]. Headaches were more often incapacitating in patients with fibromyalgia, and there was a higher prevalence of depression, anxiety, and insomnia in patients with the co-morbidity. Conversely, chronic headaches were present in 76% of treatment-seeking fibromyalgia patients [29]. Both antidepressants and antiepileptic drugs are commonly used to treat both of these conditions, although their effect on fibromyalgia is typically modest.

Aside from fibromyalgia, the prevalence of chronic headache was four times higher in a population with musculoskeletal symptoms, with neck pain in particular associated with headache [30]. Although definitions of cervicogenic headache differ, it is generally defined as a unilateral headache of the cervical and occipital region, triggered or exacerbated by neck movement with objective findings of abnormal cervical movement or tenderness [31]. Selective nerve blocks of upper cervical facets have been reported to be diagnostic and therapeutic [32], although epidural blocks are not considered effective. The use of occipital nerve blocks is

Table 21.6 Antidepressants and antiepileptics used for headache prophylaxis and chronic pain

	Migraine	Neuropathic pain	Non-neuropathic pain
Antidepressants			
Tricyclic antidepressants	A	A	B
Selective serotonin reuptake inhibitors	-	-	-
Serotonin-norepinephrine reuptake inhibitors			
– venlafaxine	C	?	?
– duloxetine	?	A (FDA*)	A (FDA)
Bupropion	?	A	?
Antiepileptics			
Valproate	A (FDA)	-	-
Gabapentin	A	A (FDA)	-/?
Topiramate	A (FDA)	-	-
Pregabalin	?	A (FDA)	A (FDA)

Levels of evidence: A (strong evidence); B (moderate evidence); C (evidence from open-label trials or consensus). - : little or no evidence for efficacy, or weak efficacy; ?: efficacy uncertain or not studied. ªFDA: FDA-approved.

widely promoted, although scientific evidence of the efficacy of this procedure is lacking [33].

Headache patients with co-morbid chronic pain disorders and opiates

A particularly challenging problem is the headache patient with a co-morbid chronic pain problem that is being treated with opiates. No aspect of management distinguishes chronic pain from headache more than the use of opioids. Opioid therapy is a mainstay of the treatment of chronic pain disorders. Long-acting opioids (LAOs) are often promoted, although the benefit of LAOs has been questioned [34]. For migraine, however, the use of opioids is discouraged, as it may render the migraineur less responsive to triptan therapy, and frequent use is associated with MOH.

The use of daily opiates in the patient with refractory chronic daily headache is controversial. In the largest and longest observational study of LAOs for patients with refractory chronic daily headache, 76% of patients failed to benefit or dropped out of therapy over a 3-year period. Of the 24% who were considered good responders (>50% improvement in an index of severe headache activity), many remained disabled to the extent that physician's assessment of improvement did not support the patient's assessment of benefit [35]. However, other authors have reported more favorable

Table 21.7 Suggestions for the treatment of patients with refractory chronic daily headache and a co-morbid chronic pain problem requiring opiates

Identify the primary headache diagnosis.

Maximize non-pharmacological (behavioral) therapies.

Treat medication overuse of non-narcotics (e.g., butalbital, caffeine compounds).

Consider withdrawal of opiates to establish a new baseline for headache and chronic pain.

If opiates are necessary, consider long-acting opiates.

Consider interventional therapies.

Monitor headache and chronic pain activity concomitantly.

Establish goals for and monitor function and disabilities specific to chronic daily headache and chronic pain.

shorter-term outcomes, with up to 70% of patients who demonstrated benefit in the first 2 months maintaining benefit over 1 year [36]. Patients often responded at low doses (methadone 7.5–30 mg daily), and relapsed to chronic daily headache (CDH) if opiates were discontinued. Neither of the latter reports, however, addresses the patient with refractory CDH with a co-morbid chronic pain problem known to respond to opiates. There are no observational studies or treatment guidelines for this population, of which we are aware. We suggest guidelines for the patient for the

Table 21.8 Why headache treatments fail

Diagnosis is incomplete or incorrect.
- incorrect primary headache diagnosis
- migraine headache diagnosed as sinus or tension headache
- cluster headache diagnosed as migraine headache
- hemicrania continua
- secondary disorders unrecognized
- high and low pressure headache syndromes
- chronic sinusitis or other sinus etiologies
- cervical disorders

Exacerbating factors have been missed
- medication overuse
- hormonal factors
- dietary factors
- lifestyle factors
- occupational/environmental factors

Inadequate pharmacotherapy
- acute therapy
- lack of migraine-specific therapy
- delay of treatment during an attack
- failure to use combined therapy (triptan + anti-inflammatory or anti-emetic)
- preventive therapy
- failure to titrate to therapeutic dose for adequate period of time
- hesitance to use rational polypharmacy
- patient non-compliance

Inadequate non-pharmacologic therapy
- relaxation therapy and cognitive-behavioral therapy
- myofascial therapies

Other factors: co-morbid disorders
- other chronic pain disorders
- psychiatric disorders

Source. Adapted from Ref. [37].

headache patient requiring use of opiates for another pain disorder (see Table 21.7).

Why headache treatments fail

Lipton and colleagues [37], in an excellent review, have categorized the reasons why headache treatments fail (see Table 21.8). It is our opinion that aside from medication overuse headache, the most common reasons for failure of headache therapies are inadequate attention to lifestyle and biopsychosocial factors. Holroyd and colleagues have shown that pharmacotherapy alone is associated with only 38% improvement in headache, while the combination of pharmacotherapy and cognitive/relaxation therapies are associated with 64% improvement [21]. The following section addresses biobehavioral care of headache.

Behavioral management of headache

As primary headaches are *psycho*-physiological disorders (i.e., a physical disorder subject to psychosocial influences and environmental stressors), they are amenable to the application of behavioral treatment strategies that can be implemented to augment or in lieu of pharmacologic headache treatment.

Several behavioral headache interventions enjoy strong empirical support and thus they have become standard components for head pain management in many headache treatment centers and pain practices. The widely implemented behavioral treatments target a patient's headache-related physiological responses (relaxation skills training, biofeedback) or headache-related behaviors, emotions, and cognitions (cognitive-behavioral therapy, stress-management training). Physiologic self-control regulation training, education regarding stress/headache relationships, and active problem solving are common foci of these standard behavioral headache treatments.

Behavioral interventions can be appropriately administered to headache patients with a broad variety of headache characteristics, medical and psychiatric conditions, and medical treatment contraindications. Nearly all headache patients could benefit from behavioral interventions that include identification and modification of trigger factors, pacing, and basic cognitive and relaxation therapy skills. Patients with the following characteristics may be particularly well suited for behavioral headache therapy: poor tolerance of drug treatments; medical contraindications for drug treatment; inadequate response to drug treatments; a preference for non-drug interventions; pregnancy, planned pregnancy, or nursing; a history of frequent or excessive use of analgesic or other acute medications; and significant life stress/deficient stress-coping skills [38]. Many headache patients possess a number of these attributes, and in our judgment, a patient possessing even one merits consideration for behavioral headache self-management training.

Table 21.9 Headache precipitants or "triggers"

Lack of food: fasting, insufficient food, delayed meals

Specific foods: aged cheese, alcohol, chocolate, nuts, etc

Sleep: excessive sleep or oversleeping, insufficient sleep, abrupt changes in sleep schedule

Ovarian hormones: menstruation, oral contraceptives, pregnancy, menopause

Environment: heat, cold, lights, noise, perfume, smoke, odors, fumes

Exercise

Allergy/smoking

Weather

Stress: during stress, after stress (i.e., "let-down headache")

Caffeine

Behavioral self-management of headache trigger factors

Failure to address triggering or exacerbating factors is cited as one of the most common reasons for the failure of headache treatment [37]. General population studies indicate stress, sleep difficulties (e.g., irregular sleep/wake schedule, non-refreshing sleep, insufficient sleep), and dietary factors (e.g., skipping meals, alcohol, specific trigger foods) are among the most frequently identified triggers for migraine and tension-type headache [39]. There is, in fact, an important behavioral component to nearly all of the identified headache triggers (see Table 21.9). Thus, identification of headache triggers provides valuable opportunities for behavioral intervention and headache self-management.

In behavioral headache self-management training, patients prospectively monitor potential headache triggers to identify individual variables that can help them take actions to prevent or manage their headaches [40]. Once associations between usual precipitants and headache episodes are identified, patients develop (after initial instruction from a therapist) appropriate responses to avoid, modify, or learn strategies to cope more effectively with triggers. The behavioral self-management training is a core construct for each of the standard behavioral headache treatments.

Standard behavioral headache treatments

Standard behavioral interventions can be broadly categorized as relaxation training, biofeedback training, cognitive-behavioral therapy and/or stress-management training), or some combination of these approaches [41].

Relaxation training

Relaxation skills enable headache sufferers to modify their own headache-related physiological responses and decrease sympathetic arousal. Protocols for headache often include progressive muscle relaxation training, autogenic training involving self-instructions (such as warmth and heaviness) to promote a state of deep relaxation; and meditative or passive relaxation. Within-session training generally is facilitated by materials and instructions for home practice. Over time, training abbreviates and integrates relaxation skills into everyday responses until relaxation is achieved through simple recall and eventually becomes an automated response. Relaxation techniques are often used in combination with biofeedback and stress-management.

Biofeedback training

Biofeedback training employs technologies to monitor physiological processes that are usually considered either involuntary or outside of conscious awareness (e.g., muscle tension, pulse, blood pressure, peripheral blood flow). Information about the physiological process is converted and amplified into a signal (visual or auditory) and then *fed back* to the individual. Patients can then learn strategies to enhance control over the response. The two most common forms of biofeedback for headache have been thermal biofeedback or "hand warming" for migraine and electromyographic (EMG) biofeedback for tension-type headache. Training often is facilitated by instructing patients in relaxation exercises and home practice. The biofeedback device is gradually eliminated as self-regulation skills are consolidated.

Cognitive-behavioral therapy

Cognitive-behavioral therapy (CBT) combines two psychological treatment approaches: cognitive therapy and behavior therapy. It essentially modifies overt behavior by altering thoughts, interpretations of events, assumptions, and usual behavioral responses to events or stressors. Applied to headache, such interventions alert patients to the role of thought processes in stress responses and the relationships between stress, coping, and headaches. Patients are assisted in identifying the psychological or behavioral factors that trigger or aggravate their headaches, and taught to employ more effective strategies for coping with headache-related stress. Often, treatment is administered in conjunction with relaxation or biofeedback training for headache.

The evidence for behavioral management of headache

The first empirical study evaluating a behavioral headache intervention for recurrent headache was published in 1969; 30 years later, reviewers identified over 300 studies evaluating behavioral treatments for migraine [42]. The overwhelming majority of clinical trials have yielded positive outcomes leading a large number of professional practice organizations to endorse use of behavioral headache treatments alongside pharmacologic treatments for primary headache.

An important evidence-based guideline for migraine management was produced by the US Headache Treatment Guideline Consortium, whose membership included the American Academy of Family Physicians, American Academy of Neurology, American Headache Society, American College of Emergency Physicians, American College of Physicians, American Osteopathic Association, and the National Headache Foundation [20, 38]. Focused on management of migraine by the primary care practitioner, the guideline is available online in its entirety (www.aan.com). The Consortium's principal recommendations pertaining to behavioral interventions for migraine include:

(a) relaxation training, thermal biofeedback combined with relaxation training, EMG biofeedback, and cognitive-behavioral therapy may be considered as treatment options for prevention of migraine;

(b) behavioral therapy may be combined with preventive drug therapy to achieve added clinical improvement for migraine.

Efficacy of behavioral headache management

Migraine

With support from the Agency for Healthcare Research and Quality (AHRQ), Goslin and colleagues [42] produced a comprehensive meta-analysis of the behavioral literature. They employed conservative study inclusion criteria to examine six treatment conditions plus a wait-list control condition. The behavioral interventions yielded 32–49% improvement in migraine from pre- to post-treatment as compared

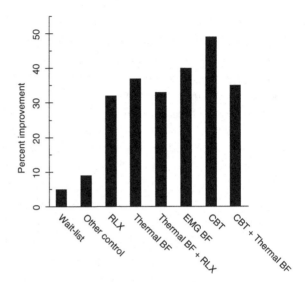

Figure 21.1 Meta-analysis of behavioral treatments for migraine RLX: Relaxation training; BF: Biofeedback training; EMG: Electromyographic; CBT: Cognitive behavioral therapy. Source. Ref. [42].

to 5% reduction for controls (Figure 21.1). Effect size estimates revealed relaxation training, thermal biofeedback combined with relaxation training, EMG biofeedback training, and cognitive-behavioral therapy all were significantly more effective than the control condition.

Few studies have directly assessed the comparative efficacy of behavioral vs. drug therapies for migraine. However, meta-analytic comparisons yield similar levels of improvement in migraine with propranolol (a beta-blocker FDA-approved for migraine prophylaxis; 32 trials), flunarizine (a calcium channel blocker widely used in Canada and Europe for migraine prophylaxis; 31 trials), and combined relaxation and biofeedback training (35 trials) [43, 44]. The average patient receiving propranolol, flunarizine, or behavioral interventions showed greater than a 50% improvement in migraine, whereas patients receiving pill placebos showed only a 12% improvement. Thus, while the two treatment modalities are likely to offer differing advantages and disadvantages within particular subgroups of patients, the best of the prophylactic medications and behavioral therapies appear to be similarly viable for migraine management.

Tension-type headache

Employing methodology closely paralleling the Goslin *et al.* migraine review [42], McCrory and colleagues produced a meta-analysis of behavioral treatments for

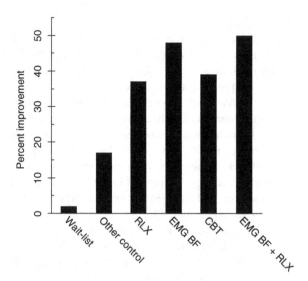

Figure 21.2 Meta-analysis of behavioral treatments for tension-type headache
RLX: Relaxation training; BF: Biofeedback training;
EMG: Electromyographic; CBT: Cognitive behavioral therapy.
Source. Ref. [45].

tension-type headache that examined four treatment and two control conditions (wait-list control, other controls) [45]. The behavioral interventions yielded on average 37–50% headache reduction from pre- to post-treatment vs. 2% reduction for no-treatment, and 9% for other controls (Figure 21.2). The effect size estimates revealed that all of the behavioral interventions were significantly more effective than the control conditions.

The study by Holroyd and colleagues [21] provides the best available comparison of behavioral and pharmacologic treatment for tension-type headache. Over 200 patients were randomly assigned to one of four conditions: (1) tricyclic antidepressant medication; (2) stress-management training; (3) combined antidepressant and stress-management; or (4) medication placebo. Compared to placebo, medication and behavioral therapy each produced larger reductions in headache activity, analgesic medication use, and headache-related disability, but the medication condition yielded more rapid improvements in headache activity. Moreover, a higher proportion of patients receiving the combined therapy experienced a clinically meaningful headache reduction (64% of patients) compared to antidepressant medication (38%) or stress management training (35%). Thus, whereas each treatment strategy is modestly effective when used singly, improved outcomes were achieved with a combined approach.

Maintenance of treatment gains

Considerable evidence indicates that among patients initially responsive to therapy, the effects of behavioral treatments endure well over time, with the longest follow-up occurring 7 years post-treatment [46]. For example, Blanchard and colleagues [47] found that 78% of tension-type sufferers and 91% of migraineurs remained significantly improved 5 years after completing behavioral treatment.

Behavioral treatment formats

Behavioral treatment for headache can be effectively administered in a variety of formats and settings.

Clinic-based treatment

Standard clinic-based treatments typically involve 6 to 12 weekly sessions that last 45–60 minutes for individual treatment and 60–120 minutes for group treatment. This format had the advantage of maximizing patients' time with, and attention from, a healthcare provider time, but it also is the most costly to deliver with respect to clinician time as well as patient travel.

Limited contact treatment

The limited therapist contact treatments have adapted therapy components from the standard clinic-based behavioral treatments to generate interventions that typically involve only three- to four- monthly clinic sessions. Clinic visits introduce headache management skills and address problems encountered in acquiring or using these skills, and patients are provided treatment manuals and audio recordings that guide the learning and refinement of skills to be practiced at home, with clinician assistance via phone calls. Meta-analyses have demonstrated the utility of the minimal-contact treatment approach, indicating that for many patients such treatments can be as effective as those delivered in a clinic setting [48].

Non-professionally administered treatment

The self-management literature has emphasized use of groups led by trained non-professional leaders who suffer from a chronic disorder. Well-established certification programs have been established for lay leaders, and detailed guides for conducting lay-led but professionally supervised self-management groups for chronic disorders such as arthritis, asthma, diabetes, and chronic back pain have been produced (e.g., http://patienteducation.stanford.edu). Recently, lay-led migraine education or self-management groups have demonstrated potential for yielding at least modest benefit with respect to improved headache outcomes, reduced healthcare utilization, and enhanced patient self-efficacy [49, 50].

No professional contact treatment

No contact treatment refers to programs that are designed to enable individuals to acquire and successfully use behavioral headache self-management skills without clinic visits or face-to-face instruction from a clinician. Learning at home or at the workplace, community library, or other setting may be supervised by a behavioral clinician via the telephone or via the Internet. Alternately, the need for supervision by a "live" behavioral clinician might be eliminated altogether.

Few studies have yet evaluated strictly self-help programs, and those reported have suffered from high attrition rates. For example, Kohlenberg and Kahn [51] reported a substantial 62% headache reduction with their self-help book vs. only 14% with information control, but their dropout rate exceeded 60%. A principal shortcoming for static self-help interventions may be their lack of corrective feedback and motivational assistance that is often needed during the several weeks required to develop and integrate behavioral headache self-management skills into daily routines. Noteworthy efforts are underway to develop headache treatments that take advantage of the Internet and other media that have demonstrated considerable promise. The use of electronic media and communications technologies allows interventions to be interactive and suitably tailored to individual patients' needs, which is likely to help overcome the limitations of static self-help approaches [52, 53].

Although these new formats for administering behavioral treatment will not be suitable for all patients, they offer promising cost-effective alternatives to clinic-based behavioral treatment.

Co-morbid mood and anxiety disorders

Epidemiologic studies indicate that mood and anxiety disorders frequently are co-morbid with migraine [11, 12]. Although population data are limited for tension-type headache, mood and anxiety disorders appear co-morbid with chronic (but not episodic) tension-type headache [54]. Probably because of selection factors, mood and anxiety disorders are reported at higher rates in clinical samples than in population samples, with the highest rates reported in specialty headache centers. Mood and anxiety disorders also have been reported more frequently among chronic than episodic migraine or tension-type headache sufferers and in the presence of medication overuse [54, 55]. Personality disorders have been less frequently examined in the empirical headache literature than affective and anxiety disorders, but they clearly can markedly complicate headache management [56, 57].

It is important to identify and manage mood and anxiety disorders among patients presenting for headache treatment because they further impair the daily functioning and quality-of-life of individuals already burdened with a headache disorder [16, 58]. Moreover, when present, psychiatric co-morbidity often complicates headache management and portends a poorer prognosis for headache treatment [59, 60]. The reader is referred to the detailed review by Maizels *et al.* for a discussion of screening for psychopathology among headache patients [61]. Integrated cognitive-behavioral therapy for headaches as well as psychological symptoms offers a logically consistent approach to the management of headaches and co-morbid mood or anxiety disorders [10, 62].

Behavioral facilitation of medication compliance

Nonadherence with medical regimens represents a substantial challenge in medicine and is particularly relevant to headache since symptoms may worsen in the context of medication overuse. Adherence to long-term medication therapy for various chronic illnesses averages only about 50% [63, 64], and reported adherence rates among headache sufferers have been similarly poor [65]. Only one-half to two-thirds of headache patients are adherent to their prophylactic medication regimens, and only one-quarter used their medications as prescribed after 1 year.

Risk factors for non-compliance have not been objectively assessed among headache sufferers, but the literature of various chronic conditions probably can be extrapolated to headache (e.g., adherence with medication regimens decreases with the frequency and complexity of the dosing regimen, with multiple medications, and with increasing side effects and cost).

Table 21.10 Adherence enhancing strategies

Education about headache and treatment
  Prophylactic vs. acute, abortive, consequences of overuse

Involve patient in decision-making and plan
  Collaborative alliance, negotiated rather than dictate, discussion of barriers (e.g., cost, side effects)

Simplify treatment regimen
  Minimize number of medications, minimize number of daily dosings

Provide written medication/treatment plan
  Detailed and "negotiated" treatment plan

Provider communication/rapport skills
  Environment, active listening, empathy, adjust language to patient, cultural sensitivity

Assess and treat co-morbid depression, anxiety

Assess and track compliance
  Medication reminder systems and cueing

Although very limited, available evidence suggests that behavioral compliance-enhancing interventions for migraine hold considerable promise [66]. A variety of behavioral compliance enhancing strategies well suited for headache management are presented in Table 21.10.

Conclusion

Headache, particularly migraine and tension-type headache, are the most common pain conditions encountered in medical practice. Headache shares commonalities with other chronic pain disorders discussed in this volume with respect to diagnostic tools, treatment armamentarium, and the importance of managing psychiatric co-morbidities. Interestingly, it is now recognized that headache patients often present with multiple pain problems such as fibromyalgia and other musculoskeletal pains. Headache patients present with some unique treatment challenges, and direct application of standard chronic pain treatment strategies generally does not provide for optimal care. Arguably the most important difference between management of headache vs. other chronic pain conditions may involve medication overuse headache; the analgesic and abortive medications that can be efficacious for acute management of headache may over time complicate the headache picture – transforming headache from episodic to chronic and daily pain, and rendering the headache sufferer unresponsive to traditional treatments.

Fortunately, as described in this chapter, effective pharmacological and non-pharmacologic treatments for headache are available. Randomized controlled trials indicate that the average headache sufferer may expect to experience approximately a 50% improvement in headache with either prophylactic medication or behavioral treatment. However, it is also well recognized that treatment failures are not uncommon. Medication overuse, inadequate medication trials, and non-adherence undermine treatment effectiveness. A substantial number of headache sufferers also present with psychiatric complications, and the presence of psychological symptoms generally portends a poorer outcome for headache management.

There is emerging evidence that multidisciplinary or combined pharmacologic plus behavioral treatment may improve outcomes in standard care and likely is necessary in the management of complicated and refractory cases. While few patients historically have had access to behavioral treatments, a number of abbreviated behavioral treatments have recently been presented. Self-management strategies addressing behavioral modification for headache triggers and medication adherence lend themselves to medical practice and would facilitate traditional medical care. Modifications of standard behavioral treatments and broader implementation of self-management principals into primary care and neurology practice settings where most headache patients receive treatment is needed to fully realize the impact of behavioral management with headache.

References

1. Schwartz BS, Stewart WF, Simon D, Lipton RB. Epidemiology of tension-type headache. *JAMA* 1998; **279**: 381–3.

2. Lipton RB, Stewart WF, Diamond S, Diamond ML, Reed M. Prevalence and burden of migraine in the United States: Data from the American Migraine Study II. *Headache* 2001; **41**: 646–57.

3. Lipton RB, Bigal ME, Hamelsky S, Scher A. Headache: epidemiology and impact. In *Wolff's Headache and Other Head Pain,* 8th edn., eds. SD Silberstein, RB Lipton and DW Dodick (New York: Oxford University Press, 2008), pp. 45–62.

4. Hu XH, Markson LE, Lipton RB, Stewart WF, Berger ML. Burden of migraine in the United States: Disability and economic costs. *Arch Intern Med* 1999; **159**: 813–8.

5. Saunders K, Merikangas K, Low NC, Von Korff M, Kessler RC. Impact of comorbidity on headache-related disability. *Neurology* 2008; **70**: 538–47.

6. Olesen J, Headache Classification Subcommittee of the International Headache Society. The International Classification of Headache Disorders: 2nd edn. *Cephalalgia* 2004; **24**(Suppl 1): 1–160.

7. Penzien DB, Rains JC, Lipton RB. Introduction to the special series on the chronification of headache: Mechanisms, risk factors, and behavioral strategies aimed at primary and secondary prevention of chronic headache. *Headache* 2008; **48**: 5–6.

8. Bigal ME, Lipton RB. Modifiable risk factors for migraine progression. *Headache* 2006; **46**: 1334–43.

9. Scher AI, Midgette L, Lipton RB. Risk factors for headache chronification. *Headache* 2008; **48**: 16–25.

10. Lake AE III, Rains JC, Penzien DB, Lipchik GL. Headache and psychiatric comorbidity: Historical context, clinical implications, and research relevance. *Headache* 2005; **45**: 493–506.

11. Hamelsky SW, Lipton RB. Psychiatric comorbidity of migraine. *Headache*, 2006; **46**: 1327–33.

12. Penzien DB, Peatfield RC, Lipchik GL. Headache in patients with co-morbid psychiatric disease. In *The Headaches,* 3rd edn., eds. J Olesen, P Goadsby, N Ramadan, P Tfelt-Hansn, and KMA Welch, (Philadelphia: Lippincott, Williams, Wilkins, 2006), pp. 1117–24.

13. Karakurum B, Soylu O, Karataş M, *et al.* Personality, depression, and anxiety as risk factors for chronic migraine. *Intern J Neurosci* 2004; **114**: 1391–9.

14. Zwart JA, Dyb G, Hagen K, *et al.* Depression and anxiety disorders associated with headache frequency. The Nord-Trøndelag Health Study. *Eur J Neurol* 2003; **10**: 147–52.

15. Guidetti V, Galli F, Fabrizi P, *et al.* Headache and psychiatric comorbidity: Clinical aspects and outcome in an 8-year follow-up study. *Cephalalgia* 1998; **18**: 455–62.

16. Lantéri-Minet M, Radat F, Chautart MH, Lucas C. Anxiety and depression associated with migraine: Influence on migraine subjects' disability and quality of life, and acute migraine management. *Pain* 2005; **118**: 319–26.

17. Pesa J, Lage MJ. The medical costs of migraine and comorbid anxiety and depression. *Headache* 2004; **44**: 562–70.

18. Silberstein S., Olesen J., Bousser MG., *et al.* The International Classification of Headache Disorders, 2nd edn. (ICHD-II)-revision of criteria for 8.2 Medication-overuse headache. *Cephalalgia* 2005; **25**: 460–5.

19. Zed PJ, Loewen PS, Robinson G. Medication-induced headache: Overview and systematic review of therapeutic approaches. *Ann Pharmacother* 1999; **33**: 61–72.

20. Silberstein SD. Practice parameter: Evidence-based guidelines for migraine headache (an evidence-based review): Report of the Quality Standards Subcommittee of the American Academy of Neurology. *Neurology* 2000; **55**: 754–62.

21. Holroyd KA, O'Donnell FJ, Stensland, *et al.* Management of chronic tension-type headache with tricyclic antidepressant medication, stress management therapy, and their combination: A randomized controlled trial. *JAMA* 2001; **285**: 2208–15.

22. Schulman EA, Lake AE III, Goadsby PJ, *et al.* Defining refractory migraine and refractory chronic migraine: Proposed criteria from the refractory headache special interest section of the American Headache Society. *Headache* 2008; **48**: 778–82.

23. Dodick DW. Reflections and speculations on refractory migraine: Why do some patients fail to improve with currently available therapies? *Headache* 2008; **48**: 828–37.

24. Silberstein SD, Schulman EA, Hopkins MM. Repetitive intravenous DHE in the treatment of refractory headache. *Headache* 1990; **30**: 334–9.

25. Naumann M, So Y, Argoff CE, *et al.* Assessment: Botulinum toxin for the treatment of autonomic nervous disorders and pain (an evidence-based review). Report of the Therapeutics and Technology Assessment Subcommittee of the American Academy of Neurology. *Neurology* 2008; **70**: 1707–14.

26. Schwedt TJ, Dodick DW, Hentz J, Trentman TL, Zimmerman RS. Occipital nerve stimulation for chronic headache – long-term safety and efficacy. *Cephalalgia* 2007; **27**: 153–7.

27. Scher AI, Stewart WF, Lipton RB. The comorbidity of headache with other pain syndromes. *Headache* 2006; **46**: 1416–23.

28. Peres MFP, Young WB, Kaup AO, Zukerman E, Silberstein SD. Fibromyalgia is common in patients with transformed migraine. *Neurology* 2001; **57**: 1326–8.

29. Marcus DA, Bernstein C, Rudy TE. Fibromyalgia and headache: An epidemiological study supporting migraine as part of the fibromyalgia syndrome. *Clin Rheumatol* 2005; **24**: 595–601.

30. Hagen K, Einarsen C, Zwart J-A, Svebak S, Bovim G. The co-occurrence of headache and musculoskeletal symptoms amongst 51050 adults in Norway. *Eur J Neurol* 2002; **9**: 527–33.

31. Biondi DM. Cervicogenic headache: Diagnostic evaluation and treatment strategies. *Curr Pain Headache Rep* 2001; **5**: 361–8.

32. Fredriksen TA. Cervicogenic headache: Invasive procedures. *Cephalalgia* 2008; **28** Suppl 1: 39–40.

33. Ashkenazi A, Levin M. Greater occipital nerve block for migraine and other headaches: Is it useful? *Curr Pain Headache Rep*, 2007; **11**: 231–5.

34. Chou R, Clark E, Helfand M. Comparative efficacy and safety of long-acting oral opioids for chronic non-cancer pain. A systematic review. *J Pain Symptom Manage* 2003; **26**: 1026–48.

35. Saper JR, Lake AE III, Hamel RL, *et al.* Daily scheduled opioids for intractable head pain: Long-term observations of a treatment program. *Neurology* 2004; **62**: 1687–94.

36. Rothrock JF. Treatment-refractory migraine: The case for opioid therapy. *Headache* 2008; **48**: 850–4.

37. Lipton RB, Silberstein SD, Saper JR, Bigal ME, Goadsby PJ. Why headache treatment fails. *Neurology* 2003; **60**: 1064–70.

38. Campbell JK, Penzien DB, Wall EM. *Evidence-based guidelines for migraine headache in the primary care setting: Behavioral and physical treatments*; 2000. www.aan.com/professionals/practice/pdfs/gl0089.pdf [accessed June 2010].

39. Kelman L. The triggers or precipitants of the acute migraine attack. *Cephalalgia* 2007; **27**: 394–402.

40. Penzien DB, Rains JC, Lipchik GL, Creer TL. Behavioral interventions for tension-type headache: overview of current therapies and recommendation for a self-management model for chronic headache. *Curr Pain Headache Rep* 2004; **8**: 489–99.

41. Rains JC, Penzien DB, McCrory DC, Gray RN. Behavioral headache treatment: History, review of the empirical literature, and methodological critique. *Headache* 2005; **45**(Suppl): S91–108.

42. Goslin RE, Gray RN, McCrory DC, Penzien D, Rains J, Hasselblad V. *Behavioral and physical treatments for migraine headache*. Technical review 2.2. February 1999. Prepared for the Agency for Health Care Policy and Research under Contract No. 290-94-2025.

43. Davis MK, Holroyd KA, Penzien DB. Flunarizine and propranolol: Comparative effectiveness in the treatment of migraine headaches. *Headache* 1999; **39**: 349.

44. Holroyd KA, Penzien DB. Pharmacological vs. nonpharmacological prophylaxis of recurrent migraine headache: A meta-analytic review of clinical trials. *Pain* 1990; **42**: 1–13.

45. McCrory DC, Penzien DB, Hasselblad V, Gray RN. *Evidence report: Behavioral and physical treatments for tension-type and cervicogenic headache.* (Des Moines, IA: Foundation for Chiropractic Education and Research, Product No. 2085, 2001).

46. Blanchard EB. Psychological treatment of benign headache disorders. *J Consult Clin Psychol* 1992; **60**, 537–51.

47. Blanchard EB, Appelbaum KA, Guarnieri P, Morrill B, Dentinger MP. Five year prospective follow-up on the treatment of chronic headache with biofeedback and/or relaxation. *Headache* 1987; **27**: 580–3.

48. Haddock CK, Rowan AB, Andrasik F, *et al.* Home-based behavioral treatments for chronic benign headache: A meta-analysis of controlled trials. *Cephalalgia* 1997; **17**: 113–8.

49. Mérelle SY, Sorbi MJ, van Doornen LJ, Passchier J. Lay trainers with migraine for a home-based behavioral training: A 6-month follow-up study. *Headache* 2008; **48**: 1311–25.

50. Rothrock JF, Parada VA, Sims C, *et al.* The impact of intensive patient education on clinical outcome in a clinic-based migraine population. *Headache* 2006; **46**: 726–31.

51. Kohlenberg RJ, Kahn T. Self-help treatment for migraine headaches: A controlled outcome study. *Headache* 1981; **21**: 196–200.

52. Devineni T, Blanchard EB. A randomized controlled trial of an Internet-based treatment for chronic headache. *Behav Res Ther* 2005; **43**: 277–92.

53. Hicks C, von Baeyer C, McGrath P. Online psychological treatment for pediatric recurrent pain: A randomized evaluation. *J Pediatr Psychol* 2006; **31**: 1–13.

54. Heckman BD, Holroyd KA. Tension-type headache and psychiatric comorbidity. *Curr Pain Headache Rep* 2006; **10**: 439–47.

55. Juang K, Wang S, Fuh J. Comorbidity of depressive and anxiety disorders in chronic daily headache and its subtypes. *Headache* 2000; **40**: 818–23.

56. Saper JR., Lake AE. III. Borderline personality disorder and the chronic headache patient: Review and management recommendations. *Headache* 2002; **42**: 663–74.

57. Saper JR. "Are you talking to me?" Confronting behavioral disturbances in patients with headache. *Headache* 2006; **46**(Suppl.3): S151–S156.

58. Baskin SM, Lipchik GL, Smitherman TA. Mood and anxiety disorders in chronic headache. *Headache* 2006; **46**(suppl 3), S76–87.

59. Puca F, Genco S, Prudenzano MP, *et al.* Psychiatric comorbidity and psychosocial stress in patients with

tension-type headache from headache centers in Italy. The Italian Collaborative Group for the Study of Psychopathological Factors in Primary Headaches. *Cephalalgia* 1999; **19**: 159–64.

60. Lake AE III. Behavioral and nonpharmacologic treatments of headache. *Med Clin North Am* 2001; **85**: 1055–75.

61. Maizels M, Smitherman TA, Penzien DB. A review of screening tools for psychiatric comorbidity in headache patients. *Headache* 2006; **46**(suppl 3): S98–S109.

62. Lipchik GL, Smitherman TA, Penzien DB, Holroyd KA. Basic principles and techniques of behavioral therapy for comorbid psychiatric disorders in headache patients. *Headache* 2006; **6**(suppl 3): S119–32.

63. Gottlieb H. Medication nonadherence: Finding solutions to a costly medical problem. *Drug Benefit Trends* 2000; **12**: 57–62.

64. Dunbar-Jacob J, Mortimer-Stephens MK. Treatment adherence in chronic disease. *J Clin Epidemiol* 2001; **54** Suppl 1: S57–60.

65. Rains JC, Lipchik GL, Penzien DB. Behavioral facilitation of medical treatment for headache – part I: Review of headache treatment compliance. *Headache* 2006; **46**: 1387–94.

66. Rains JC, Penzien DB, Lipchik GL. Behavioral facilitation of medical treatment for headache – part II: Theoretical models and behavioral strategies for improving adherence. *Headache* 2006; **46**: 1395–403.

Section 4
Chapter

22

Integrative approaches to the management of painful medical conditions

Management of pain in palliative medicine

Victor T. Chang, Brooke Myers-Sorger, Lawrence J. Weinberger, Mark E. Jones and Ellyn Poltrock Stein

Introduction

Palliative medicine addresses the care of patients with a terminal illness, where the expected lifespan is usually in the range of 6 months or less. The field has its roots in oncology and the development of hospice care, and the 6-month expected survival in the USA is defined by the Medicare Hospice Benefit. The scope of palliative medicine has expanded to include patients with advanced stages of other illnesses, such as congestive heart failure, chronic obstructive pulmonary disease, cirrhosis, HIV infection, end stage renal disease, and dementia. Palliative medicine is now delivered in settings other than home hospice, including acute care hospitals, intensive care units, and nursing homes. Managing the pain of patients at the end of life presents its own distinct challenges in assessment and management. These challenges arise from the scale of physical and psychological issues faced by the patient and caregivers, as well as the limited amount of time available. The issues that often have to be simultaneously addressed by psychologists include assessing concurrent pain management, mood disorders, cognition, psychological tasks specific to palliative care, and coping by the patient and family. While recent advances have increased the number of medical interventions for pain in palliative care, psychological approaches remain an important aspect of pain management. Assessment and interventions for pain have been studied mostly in the oncology setting, and these will be the main focus of this chapter. Interested readers are referred to additional texts for further details [1].

Prevalence of pain in palliative medicine populations

Pain is highly prevalent in different palliative medicine settings and is usually associated with other symptoms,

despite the diversity of illnesses and treatment settings denoted by the term "palliative care unit."

The fact that patients with advanced cancer often experience pain is well known. A survey of medical hematology/oncology veterans highlighted the fact that patients with advanced cancer can experience pain from other chronic medical conditions (e.g., arthritis, low back pain), complications of pain medications (e.g., constipation), and painful side effects of treatments for cancer [2].

The SUPPORT study found that in patients with metastatic colon cancer, the prevalence of pain increased from 30% at 6 months prior to death to 45% in the last 3 days, with similar findings for patients with advanced non-small cell lung cancer [3]. Pain was also highly prevalent in other terminal conditions, including 40% of patients with congestive heart failure [4], 20–30% of patients with chronic obstructive pulmonary disease [5], and 40% of patients with end stage liver disease [6].

In a study of hemodialysis patients, 50% had pain. Causes included musculoskeletal disease (63%), dialysis procedures (13.6%), neuropathic pain (12.6%), and peripheral vascular disease (9.7%) [7]. In a multicenter study of deaths of 131 dialysis patients, 42% of the patients available for follow-up were in pain in the last 24 hours of life, and 5% were in severe pain [8]. In a recent multisite survey of AIDS patients receiving palliative care, pain was reported by 65% of the respondents [9].

In other surveys comparing terminally ill patients with cancer and non-cancer diagnoses, symptom distress scores were similar for both groups of patients [10]. In a review, pain, fatigue, breathlessness, depression and nausea all had a high prevalence in five different disease states–cancer, HIV, heart failure, chronic obstructive pulmonary disease, and renal disease [11].

Behavioral and Psychopharmacologic Pain Management, ed. Michael H. Ebert and Robert D. Kerns. Published by Cambridge University Press. © Cambridge University Press 2011.

Prevalence of pain by treatment setting

Recent reviews of hospice patients suggest that pain remains highly prevalent in palliative care settings [12, 13] and hospices [14, 15], and pain is often accompanied by symptoms of lack of energy, dry mouth, and shortness of breath.

Another increasingly important site for palliative care is nursing homes. In a national data set, over 70% of nursing home patients experienced pain, and 50% reported daily pain. Pain intensity was rated as mild for 13%, moderate for 57% and horrible for 30% [16].

Despite growing awareness and implementation of palliative care in medical settings, many patients with terminal, irreversible illnesses eventually die in intensive care units (ICUs). In one study 60% of all hospital deaths in the USA occur in ICUs [17]. This is not surprising considering that ICUs are intended to treat the most acutely ill patients. However, many of the aggressive interventions applied in ICU settings are inappropriate for patients who are actively dying, and they may actually contribute to increased pain and suffering at the end of life [18].

Issues in pain assessment

The data clearly demonstrate that multiple physical symptoms occur in patients with a variety of palliative diseases. Therefore, a focus on the regular monitoring of pain alone is limited. Future improvements in clinical care should focus on measuring multiple symptoms using very simple tools, developing an understanding of which dimensions of pain are most important in palliative medicine, improving pain assessment in the cognitively impaired patient, and delineating the sources of pain in non-cancer palliative care patients [19].

Psychological assessment of the palliative care patient

To understand pain in the palliative care patient, it is important to have a sense of the patient. The first section of this chapter addresses particular issues faced by these patients.

Psychological tasks of the palliative care patient

The psychological tasks in this phase of life include coping with grief, the construction of a meaningful narrative through life review [20], achieving closure (resolution of ongoing conflicts and neuroses), letting go, and saying goodbyes. The patient deals with issues of existential meaninglessness, and balances the paradox of trying to remain connected while at the same time letting go. Within this larger structure are more mundane tasks, such as dealing with medical complications of the illness, preparation of advance directives and wills, etc. [21, 22].

Approach to psychological assessment

A framework for psychological assessment includes developmental issues, the meaning and impact of the illness, coping style, impact of the illness on the self, relationships, stressors, and spiritual resources. Of particular relevance are the issues of fear, anxiety, grief, meaning, hope, loss, loneliness, and the effect of the dying process on relationships, as well as how these are managed in patients with psychiatric conditions [23]. Within the context of dying, all of these factors are often amplified and can become overwhelming to both patients and their loved ones.

Because of the unique aspects of the psychology of the palliative care patient, we will describe some of these features and how they interact with pain assessment. Much of this data comes from studies of cancer patients, but is likely to be relevant to patients with other end stage illnesses. An understanding of these issues will guide the assessment of both the patient and pain experienced by the patient.

Mood disorders in palliative care patients

Even experienced clinicians may be surprised when some patients do not have a depressive reaction. It is a common occurrence to have a patient respond to a question about their mood or a formal questionnaire as reflecting insensitivity or limited empathy from the clinician: "Of course, I'm depressed, I feel sick, have no energy, and I'm dying." In such instances, a role for education is evident. Patients find it reassuring to know that while they feel awful, this does not necessarily represent a true depressive disorder, but rather is an acknowledgement of their deteriorating physical condition.

The large majority of patients seen by psychologists in palliative care experience some form of mood disorder in the form of an adjustment disorder, anxiety, or a depressive disorder. Co-morbidity is common. In the Canadian National Palliative Care Survey, for patients who were diagnosed with an anxiety or depressive disorder, one half met the criteria for a second disorder. Patients who complained of pain were significantly more likely to have an anxiety or depressive disorder. Similar results were found for patients with other physical symptoms [24]. Conversely, patients with a depressive disorder are more likely to report pain and other symptoms [25].

Affective distress, whether an adjustment disorder or a major depression, often complicates interpretations of physical pain, as well as potential limitations in functional capacity. This highlights the need to obtain a detailed account of the patient's history, in terms of both physical and mental illness and personality characteristics including ascribed roles. Although such a conclusion about the importance of a thorough history may seem obvious, an understanding of the impact of the illness upon the patient's trajectory in life is regarded as essential for managing those individuals with unduly persistent or complex pain disorders.

Achieving a reliable bedside assessment of depressive reactions among patients with terminal illness is very difficult. The gold standard remains a structured interview by a mental healthcare professional, but this is not always practical because of limited availability of trained personnel and the limited stamina of many palliative care patients. Much attention has been focused instead on the development and testing of short instruments to screen for depression. Existing survey instruments that include physical symptoms traditionally identified as symptoms of depression (sadness, low energy, sleep disturbances), mimicking the vegetative symptoms inherent in advanced disease (e.g., diminished appetite or weight loss, and sleep disturbance), often generate false positives. Asking the subjective experience and expectations of patients is regarded as a more reliable indicator of mood states than their somatic reactions, with feelings of hopelessness, worthlessness, and guilt suggestive of major depression.

Currently, there are efforts to establish screening tools for anxiety and depression tailored specifically to palliative care patients that attempt to distinguish the existential features of death (i.e., profound sense of loss of social, spiritual, and personal meaning) from the physical symptoms associated with a disease process [26, 27]. This may prevent characterizing the "normal" emotional distress arising from the complications of severe physical illness as pathological. When pain has been aggressively treated, but the patient still reports significant pain, it is important for palliative care specialists (especially mental health professionals) to assess what other factors may be contributing to the patient's pain. It will be important to distinguish between mood-related factors, anxiety, issues related to patient's fears about his condition, fears of dying, feelings related to loss of functional status, and related issues. Psychosocial factors that affect pain will be discussed further below.

Major depression

The incidence of "depression" in patients with cancer consistently is high, with prevalence rates ranging from 15 to 30% in patients with advanced cancer [28]. In a pain and symptom control clinic, 72% of respondents were symptomatic, and 19% had severe symptoms [29]. One reason for the wide variation is the disparate definitions of depression, which range from generalized distress (anxiety and sadness) to criterion-validated major depressive disorder. An important role for consultation-liaison psychologists and psychiatrists is to determine whether an individual is manifesting an adjustment reaction, i.e., a reasonable sense of sadness attributable to dealing with a potentially devastating illness, or a major depressive disorder.

Risk factors include pre-existing affective disorders and those individuals who experience a marked disruption in self-image and social role. Patients with end stage illnesses often experience multiple losses. For example, individuals who define themselves in terms of their jobs and suddenly cannot put in 10–12 hour days can experience a serious emotional void. Disruption in inherent assumptions about the course of one's life, such as "if you work hard you will succeed and enjoy professional success and a fulfilling retirement" can lead to much anxiety and anger. Alternately, interference with relations with significant others, especially when there are dependent parties, can induce intense dysphoria. The inability to maintain financial obligations or oversight responsibilities for children, elderly parents, or disabled siblings often results in anxiety and guilt. One patient experienced repeated episodes of intense pain that coincided with worrying about who would be present to oversee meals for his disabled adult sister who resided in a nursing home as she would eat reliably only when he accompanied her. The demarcation between major depressive disorder and adjustment disorder can sometimes be difficult to discern in the immediate aftermath of an exacerbation of illness. Follow-up may be necessary as an adjustment disorder is, by definition, time limited.

The relationship between pain and depression is important to clarify in patients who are undergoing evaluation for depression. Earlier studies showed a correlation between the severity of pain and distress in cancer patients and hospice patients [30]. More recent surveys with newer instruments have not been able to replicate these findings [31]. The relationship between cancer pain and depression remains problematic on a purely epidemiologic basis because both cancer and depression are associated with aging [32]. However, longitudinal studies of geriatric cancer patients show that more severe symptoms precede the development of depression [33, 34], and intervention studies show that both distress and pain are relieved by treatment of pain [35, 36]. Clinically, patients with severe pain are irritable, withdrawn, and inactive, and a diagnosis of depression should not be made until the pain has been addressed and treated.

Pain, depression and functional status

Pain, depression, and functional status have a complex relationship which is slowly being disentangled. Functional status is linked to the patient's sense of independence and well-being. There is a consistent negative correlation between mood and level of functional capacity [37, 38]. Restrictions in physical activities such as standing, dressing, and eating can induce feelings of sadness because of loss of autonomy, and/or curtailment of recreational interests. The patient may interpret diminishing functional capacity as an indication of the advancement of the illness, which can be perceived as demoralizing. This, in turn, can increase pain. As one patient remarked, "On days I can't button my shirt, the pain is worse." Thus, perception of functional status exerts a central influence upon patients' psychological functioning and, for a substantial percentage of individuals, is the underpinning for their dysphoric affective reactions. Exploration of these issues may help the patient cope with pain. A major goal of palliative medicine is to help patients maintain function, which may depend on pain management.

Closely related is the concept of functional trajectories over time. The majority of studies suggest the following model: disease progression leads to increased pain and other symptoms (e.g., fatigue), physical debilitation, and decreased functional activities (e.g., instrumental activities of daily living and socialization), with associated psychological ramifications. Although many patients and their caregivers expect that it will be a nosedive, trajectories of functional status may vary by disease and can be better described as gradual changes over time, or as a series of plateaus punctuated by occasional crises [39]. Within the last weeks and months of life of cancer patients, generalized psychological distress becomes even more prominent as patients manifest a decline in their overall physical condition and specific physical symptoms become more severe [10,

40]. Thus, in a palliative care population, deterioration in mood may be a marker for impending death. At this point, psychological factors such as existential distress may surpass physical pain in precipitating mood disturbances. Analgesic relief of pain is paramount at this stage, with psychological interventions directed towards providing emotional support and kindness.

Interestingly, it is likely that there are other individuals who may experience depression as a primary symptom which, in turn, hampers their functional status. While the linkage between pain, depression, and outcomes has been established, there is an emerging consensus that the relationship between depression and functional outcomes may be bi-directional in nature [41, 42]. Pending additional longitudinal research, it is paramount that clinicians remain sensitive to and are aware of the relationship between pain, depression, and functional ability to allow for appropriate psychosocial interventions.

Desire for hastened death

The expression of a desire for hastened death requires careful evaluation. These are not uncommon in palliative care patients. Such a request should not be automatically considered a request for euthanasia, or as active suicidal ideation, but as a marker for intense distress which requires further exploration. In-depth assessment reveals a variety of reasons for desire for hastened death, and no two patients are alike [43]. In one study of 106 patients on a palliative care unit, 26% reported a high desire and 41% reported moderate desire. In multivariate analyses controlling for age, gender, and performance status, risk factors for desire for hastened death included pain, lack of appetite, and sadness [44], highlighting the role of pain assessment when seeing these patients. It is important to remember that the desire for hastened death may fluctuate over time in response to clinical developments, and the request may be withdrawn at a later time. In a survey of Dutch physicians of patients who had recently made a request for hastened death, the perception of unbearable suffering, pointless suffering, loss of dignity, and general health problems were associated with patients who did not change their mind, whereas patients with more mental health problems were more likely to change their mind, possibly because of a more labile mental status. Pain and depression were not associated with requests to change the request in this sample [45]. Similar findings on the importance of meaninglessness and pointless suffering were reported for patients with advanced HIV disease [46].

Anxiety and stress disorders

The prevalence of anxiety disorders ranges from 6 to 8% in patients with advanced cancer and up to 15% in patients with terminal illness [28]. Pain generates fear. Neural pain pathways connect to structures in the limbic system such as the amygdala, and can be seen in functional MRI studies [47, 48]. In one survey of patients in a palliative care unit where the Hospital and Anxiety Depression Scale (HADS) was used as a measure of distress, both pain interference (with walking ability, normal work, relations with others), and average pain severity were significantly associated with the anxiety component of the HADS scale [49].

Catastrophizing

The importance of catastrophizing was highlighted in a study of patients with metastatic breast cancer. Higher levels of catastrophizing were associated with greater levels of emotional distress, suggesting that catastrophizing mediates maladaptive responses to pain [50]. In a literature review of coping styles and cancer pain, the presence of catastrophizing was associated with increased pain intensity in three of four studies [51].

Fear of pain during the dying process

Perhaps the most universal and essentially human factor to consider is fear and anxiety about the process of dying itself. Pain is often feared by those who experience serious illness. Indeed, pain consistently is rated as the most distressing aspect of an advanced or terminal illness [52]. Individuals identify being free from symptoms and pain as inherently defining a "good death," while a "bad death" involves prolonged suffering, as well as inadequate analgesia and uncontrolled symptoms [53].

Anxiety of this type is often characterized by intrusive thoughts about unmanaged breakthrough pain or extreme dyspnea. Such fears can often be substantially relieved by appropriate reassurance from trusted providers. Patients are sometimes uncomfortable voicing these concerns, and it is incumbent upon clinicians to encourage frank and open discussion wherein patients can explore their fears in a safe environment. Psychologists often are more comfortable in addressing these matters and should take the initiative if they sense this may be an unspoken issue.

Fears about inadequate analgesia or symptom control can also be assuaged via good communication and clear decision-making with the treatment team [52]. By participating in treatment decisions that anticipate the progression of their illness, the patients become empowered. Their concerns about poor decisions being made in the midst of a crisis or without their consent (e.g., resuscitation or use of powerful opiates) are often alleviated by appropriate preparation.

Patients with post-traumatic stress disorder

The role of enduring attitudes upon pain is well illustrated by studies of individuals with post-traumatic stress disorder (PTSD). Individuals who have been subjected to, and have persistent recollections about, a life-threatening event, such as a serious accident or combat, report more intense pain and affective distress than pain patients without histories of trauma or PTSD. Emotional reactions such as anger and depression are more prominent. In addition, individuals generally manifest higher rates of disability and interference with life activities. A poorer prognosis in response to physical interventions for non-malignant pain has also been reported. Similarly, enduring a life-threatening circumstance prior to the onset of cancer can amplify dysphoric reactions during the course of the illness [54].

Of interest, first-hand experience with a stressor is not essential to induce such elevated depressive reactions. Children of Holocaust (concentration camp) survivors who developed cancer displayed an increased prevalence of depression and agitation [55]. This suggests the possibility that profoundly pessimistic attitudes experienced by victims of extreme trauma (e.g., perceptions of perceived randomness of fate, unavailability of support, or hopelessness) have been conveyed to and adopted by their children, and are reactivated when the children experience their own life-threatening illnesses. Thus, when asking about family history of illness, inquiry about past injuries or parents' adaptation to severe stressors might generate warnings about maladaptive attitudes toward serious illness.

Among clinicians who work in the Veterans' Affairs medical system, anecdotal experiences suggest that there are likely to be psychological ramifications beyond those experienced by the civilian population. In a recent article addressing the potential effects of combat PTSD in a palliative care population, Feldman and Periyakoil [56] suggest that trauma may have a complex influence on dealing with terminal illness and the dying process. The threat to life inherent in terminal illness may mimic an original trauma experienced in the battlefield, exacerbating previous symptoms that may have been controlled. Thus, it is helpful to ask direct questions about military experiences, as well as about other extraordinary life circumstances, including those of immediate family.

Adjustment disorders

Although anxiety and depression are important syndromes in patients with advanced disease states, differentiating those individuals who experience adjustment reactions associated with the consequences of their physical illness from those who experience a profound interruption in world-view and self-efficacy may be critical in recognizing psychopathology and offering appropriate and effective interventions. Much recent work has been devoted to characterizing adjustment disorders in patients with life threatening illnesses. The prevalence of adjustment disorders ranges from 14 to 35% of patients with advanced cancer and from 11 to 16% of patients with terminal illness [28]. These syndromes are summarized below.

Distress

The term distress is a blanket term intended to include psychological, social, and spiritual domains of experience without the stigma patients attach to terms such as depression. Others have used distress to indicate emotional distress (anxiety and depression), existential distress (see below) or other kinds of reactions to the situation at hand. The National Comprehensive Cancer Network has piloted screening for distress with guidelines for management [57]. A recent literature review found a strong relationship between chronic cancer pain and the presence of distress, though the magnitude of the relationship was found to be moderate [51].

Demoralization

A situation characterized by failure to cope that leads to feelings of impotence, isolation, despair, and damaged self-esteem, forms the basis of demoralization, which is thought to represent a common ground between anxiety and depression [58]. For palliative care patients, the sense of breakdown in coping can arise in a variety of ways. A patient may feel trapped in a deteriorating physical body, useless, and helpless. Unrelieved pain or other symptoms can precipitate a sense of demoralization. The patient's hopes and assumptions about life and its meaning may be pervasively disrupted, damaging the individual's general sense of well-being, meaning and purpose, and engendering a sense of helplessness.

The construct of demoralization has been further refined to represent a failure of both problem-focused (problem solving, action oriented) and emotion-focused (flight, cognitive reframing) coping. Such restrictions in world-view lead to a weakening

of self-esteem, and in turn, shame and isolation develop. Hopelessness arises when the patient is demoralized and feels that no help is available. This results in meaninglessness and existential despair. Therapies that restore control over the problems at hand, (e.g., providing better pain and symptom control), or provide a meaning and purpose (e.g., supportive psychotherapy), are central to dealing with demoralization [59]. Currently, there is no DSM code for demoralization.

In a factor analysis of dysphoric symptoms in patients with cancer or motor neuron disease, demoralization was distinguished from depression by the absence of anhedonia in demoralization. Patients in the demoralization cluster tended to express hopelessness, pessimism, discouragement, and helplessness. Additionally, measures of demoralization correlated inversely with measures of cohesive support, whereas depression was associated with severe physical illness, lack of interest, and inability to enjoy activities [60]. The prevalence of demoralization was reported to be 30% and depression 16% in a sample of medical outpatients in two non-overlapping groups [61]. Demoralization should be considered in patients with distress from severe pain or other significant psychosocial aspects of their situation. Appreciating the concept of demoralization helps elucidate the significance of studies that have examined the relationship between pain and depression.

In summary, the degree of demoralization one experiences is likely to affect perception of and coping with physical pain. Identifying which individuals experience a sense of bleakness about their disease process and helping them identify achievable goals within the confines of their physical limitations may ameliorate their demoralization. This, in turn, may yield improvements in depressive symptoms and subjective reporting of pain.

Preparatory grief

Originally termed anticipatory grief, preparatory grief is the sense of loss evoked by previous losses and the losses to come. In the study by Clarke et al. [60] mentioned above, three clusters for dysphoric symptoms were identified – demoralization, depression, and grief. Some items for pain were found in the depression and the grief clusters but most of the pain items did not cluster with any of the three groups. All three groupings scored highly on the usual measures for depression. This suggests that one of the reasons for a higher prevalence rate of depression in surveys of patients at the end of life may be due to the conflation of preparatory grief and demoralization as depression, as these entities have overlapping symptoms and also may coexist. Periyakoil describes the grief process as involving profound sadness, which can manifest on a temporary basis as somatic symptoms, social withdrawal, and fleeting suicidality [27]. Preparatory grief can be distinguished from depression that is more consistent with an affective and/or character-based disorder. Variation in mood is also to be expected. In contrast, depressed patients have a consistent flat affect. They experience persistent hopelessness, helplessness, worthlessness, excessive guilt, anhedonia, and dysphoria, as well as continuous thoughts about death and suicide [27]. Thus, distinguishing the nature of symptoms reported by patients is an essential feature in establishing a reliable diagnosis and treatment interventions.

Existential distress

Existential distress refers to despair induced by a sense of meaninglessness: "What's the point of living like this?" Unresolved existential distress may precipitate requests for hastened death and may result from, and manifest as, intractable pain. The closest counterpart to existential distress in palliative medicine is the term spiritual pain. This term denotes distress that results from a rupture and disconnection that separates individuals from that aspect of their deepest selves that gives meaning, hope, and purpose [62]. Spiritual pain can be impacted by issues such as family and work, aspects of the self that form the basis of one's identity. Therapeutic efforts are directed towards relieving fear and emphasizing how the individual can maintain a connection of those aspects that have been long treasured.

Suffering

Suffering is a holistic concept, which can be defined as a loss of integrity [63]. A related viewpoint defines suffering as the perception of threat to the self, which is engendered when there is a discrepancy between the usual and the actual self. Pain, by interfering with the patient's functioning, leads to a discrepancy and causes suffering [64]. According to a modern definition, suffering is an aversive emotional experience characterized by the perception of personal distress caused by adverse factors that undermine quality of life [65].

In one multisite survey of 381 patients with advanced cancer in palliative care units conducted with semistructured interviews, 25% of patients considered themselves to be suffering at a moderate to severe level. Correlates of suffering were malaise, pain, depression, and weakness; pain was mentioned most frequently in the qualitative interviews. Of the 20 participants with severe-to-extreme pain, 14 (70.0%) indicated that they were suffering significantly compared to 13 (11.5%) of 113 patients with no pain. More than half of the patients with moderate to severe suffering met criteria for a depressive or anxiety disorder [66]. It is possible to treat the illness or the pain, yet increase individuals' suffering by not focusing in on the human experience of the illness and its meaning (e.g., lack of control over symptoms, hope concerning prognosis, perceptions of others) [59].

Other psychological issues

Hope

Hope is an important and poignant concept for patients, caregivers, and healthcare professionals. Many patients can acknowledge the reality of their illness and its consequences and remain hopeful (e.g., they believe that life still has value and/or pleasure and/or meaning despite the severity of their illness). If one thinks of hope as the presence of a meaningful goal, then hope can be redirected towards plans for better pain and symptom control, and realization of shorter-term plans and goals [67].

Cognitive disorders

A significant number of patients will have impaired cognition due to their underlying illness, medications, delirium, or dementia. Cognitive assessment serves a number of purposes – evaluating the patient's pain report, evaluating capacity to make decisions, and determining effective psychotherapeutic treatment modalities, as a patient with impaired cognition will be unable to participate meaningfully in psychotherapy. The assessment and management of pain in these patients remains an active area of investigation [68].

Patients may themselves complain of impaired cognition. One series of 29 patients with cancer pain complained of difficulties in remembering (54%), concentration (46%), and sedation (37%). However, routine screening tests of cognition and sedation, such as the Mini-Mental Status score and the OAA/Sedation scores were not able to detect any abnormalities [69].

It should be noted that standard psychological instruments for cognitive function were developed for evaluating demented patients, and they have been insensitive for detecting the types of cognitive complaints voiced by cancer patients. If one uses Piagetian tasks of judgment as a criterion, the error rate increased significantly in patients who had to spend a good part of the day resting; these patients performed at a level similar to children less than 10 years old [70]. Degree of physical debilitation associated with a terminal illness, rather than age, has been shown to seriously impede higher-order cognitive functions [71].

The role of underlying illnesses and medications should also be considered in patients with impaired cognition. Metabolic abnormalities that result from organ failure, brain metastases, sepsis, and medications may contribute to cognitive impairment. Opioids and benzodiazepines tend to receive more attention by clinicians as a possible cause of delirium.

Delirium

Delirium interferes with the ability of the patient to communicate and remain connected to his environment, and represents the loss of the person to his family and friends. Delirium in the patient is stressful for family and caregivers, and education and patient sedation may be necessary to reduce family distress [72].

The prevalence of delirium has been estimated in hospitalized patients with advanced cancer to range from 28% to 42%, and as high as 88% before death. Although delirium is defined as a reversible state, it may persist in more than half of patients, and no reversible cause may be found [73]. Delirium can affect patient ratings of pain. In 99 patients who underwent hematopoietic stem cell transplantation, a procedure associated with predictable mucositis and related pain, and were followed prospectively, as the number of delirious episodes increased, the severity of pain ratings also increased [74]. Clinical cases have been reported where the presence of unrecognized delirium confounded pain assessment as the patient's ratings of persistent severe pain lead to rapid escalation of pain medications [75].

Demented patients

To assign a magnitude or rating of pain, the patient must be able to interpret a sensation as unpleasant, remember and compare a sensation with other pains, correlate the sensation with a number or descriptor, and then give a verbal response. The ability to respond to a verbal pain assessment is generally associated with level of cognitive impairment [76].

Elderly patients with mild impairment are able to answer questions about pain with visual and hearing aids. Persons with Mini-Mental State Examination scores below 15 are significantly impaired in their ability to complete and comprehend self-report pain rating scales, although some studies show that persons with even moderate impairment (i.e., Mini-Mental State Examination scores as low as 8) are able to respond consistently to verbal pain assessment measures [77].

In patients with moderate-to-severe impairment and verbal assessment difficulties, behavioral observation-based pain assessment scales are the subject of intense research activity. Common behaviors associated with pain in persons with dementia include facial expressions; verbalizations/vocalizations; body movements; changes in interpersonal interactions; changes in activity patterns; or mental status changes [78]. The reader is referred to reviews and websites for a more complete description of pain rating scales built around these behavioral ratings [79]. As these behaviors are not unique to pain, but may be responses to a variety of distressing stimuli, further clinical evaluation is required. In addition to physical examination, this may take the form of an empirical trial of a mild analgesic, such as acetaminophen.

Denial

Clinicians expect patients to have a full understanding and be in accord with treatment plans, yet are often later surprised when patients ask "naïve" questions, express markedly unrealistic expectations or even state they were never apprised of any of the details about their condition. Other clinicians, e.g., nurses, psychologists, often hear about patients' dissatisfaction with their physician's communication despite clear evidence that the physician has indeed imparted such relevant information. Alternately, despite patients' explicit acknowledgement of the "facts" of their condition, compliance with interventions can be erratic which negatively affects symptom presentation and disease progression.

Denial has both adaptive and maladaptive features in patients with end stage disease. On one hand, it provides a defense against the fear of impending death. Conversely, denial can be maladaptive when it results in non-compliance with medical treatments or refusal to acknowledge and/or make decisions relating to end of life issues. A management strategy starts with discussing the patient's desired management approach to his/her illness and short-term life goals. Often, incongruities between the patient's expectations and limitations imposed by the disease state will evoke clues about the patient's underlying fears that lead to such cognitive distortions. Usually these distortions are related to anticipation of intense loss, which can then be addressed through supportive therapy.

One patient who was diagnosed with advanced lung cancer would not acknowledge the grave nature of his condition for nearly 1 year, though he continued to pursue the recommended treatments. His emotional reactions were disparate with his actions. When a doctor stated explicitly that he would "definitely die soon," this patient "couldn't deny what was happening to me," though he admitted that his physicians had been clear about his prognosis for many months. He subsequently expressed hopelessness and a desire to "give up on everything." He believed that "things were better when I was in denial." In therapy sessions with a psychologist, the patient discussed what his life had been like prior to the cancer diagnosis, his ensuing fears, and wishes for the immediate future. The patient was able to focus on "things I still want to do" for himself and for his family. His denial or blunted affective reaction worked to help him "keep living, even though they were telling me I was dying." Yet when faced with the imminence of his death, his denial was no longer an effective defense against anxiety. Explicitly shifting the focus from a vague and indefinite end towards satisfying immediate goals helped ameliorate his anxiety.

Social and situational factors

The availability of supportive friends and caregivers acts as a buffer to the stresses and demands caused by illness. Uncontrolled pain may cause the patient to isolate himself from friends and family, which in turn, may result in the patient withdrawing from support networks causing the patient to become socially isolated. There is an emerging literature that suggests that social factors may have an effect upon pain, by reducing overall stress [80] or by increasing overall satisfaction with quality of life [81]. Patients experience higher levels of pain when they are less engaged in social activities or have a restricted or unstable social network [51]. Presumably the stressors associated with limited community support, financial resources and social status impede a sense of purpose and hamper the ability to determine one's course of healthcare. Family strife over medical treatment and place of death is common at the end of life [82], which can aggravate

pain, and emphasizes the importance of a comprehensive assessment.

An emerging body of work on caregivers is yielding new insights into how the social environment can affect the assessment and management of pain. Understanding caregivers' reaction is crucial in pain assessment because caregivers often become proxy raters, and much psychological counseling may be needed to be devoted to the caregiver and to the communication between the patient, caregiver, and healthcare team about pain. Additionally, it would be helpful to review and discuss how caregivers dispense medications. Caregivers of patients with a history of substance use have been reluctant to administer pain medications for fear of rekindling the older problem of substance use.

Watching a loved one in pain is extremely distressing for caregivers. In one descriptive study, spouses of patients described feeling a sense of helplessness and fear when the patient was in severe pain, and a sense of normalcy and hopefulness when the patient was not in severe pain. Pain control, emotional support, and education are vital in managing these reactions [83]. One study found that caregivers of cancer patients with pain had higher scores for anxiety, depression, and caregiver strain compared to caregivers of patients who did not have cancer pain [84]. These reactions by caregivers are more severe when the patient catastrophizes about pain [85]. Another study demonstrated that spouses' reactions to rheumatoid arthritis patients' pain affected the patient's tendency to catastrophize [86]. One can envision stabilizing or destabilizing cycles of pain depending on how the patient and spouse react to the pain and to each other.

Recent studies in home hospice settings have shown that ratings of pain severity are similar between the patient and caregiver [87]. However, perceptions of caregivers can also reflect the biases and experiences of the caregiver [88, 89]. These assessments are important to determine because many times, patients are unable to give their own assessments, and the caregiver becomes the proxy rater. Caregiver assessments may lead to conflicts with healthcare professionals. Any change in the patient's affect, vocalizations, and movements is likely to be ascribed to pain by the caregiver.

Example: A patient dying from pancreatic cancer was unresponsive, but had occasional groping movements of his arms, causing his caregivers concern about his comfort. He had been on haloperidol and was started on benztropine for presumed akathisia, with cessation of his arm movements.

Caregivers' participation in pain management

One study of 75 dyads in Australia found that caregivers were heavily involved in administering medications and learning about pain management and had more difficulty talking with their relatives than with doctors about pain management [90]. Patients' quality of life is directly affected by how well their spouses or caretakers adapt to the patients' illness. In a study of 63 caregivers and patients, caregivers who rated high on measures of self-efficacy reported less caregiver strain and a more positive mood, and the patients of these caregivers reported improved physical well being, but there was no correlation with patient reports of usual pain or worst pain [91].

An approach to pain

Psychological approaches to pain management are handicapped if pain is severe and uncontrolled. This is especially true in patients with end stage cancer where pain usually results from severe anatomic abnormalities caused by tumor masses. Psychological consultations are often requested for patients with pain where the pain is not responding to treatment, or is associated with a mood disorder. An early step in the consultation response should be to review the assessment and management to date from the chart or in discussion with referring services. Such situations are real opportunities to combine pharmacological and psychological approaches to pain management. We briefly review the medical assessment and management of pain, especially for cancer patients.

The assessment of pain includes:

1. Taking a thorough pain history. Basic elements include patient ratings of pain severity (worst, least, average) over a 24-hour period, site of pain, aggravating, and relieving factors. For patients unable to rate pain with numbers, Likert descriptors (a little bit, somewhat, quite a bit, very much) can convey information about pain severity. Important additional information includes the amount and duration of pain relief with current interventions, the presence of central nervous system side effects from analgesics, and the effect of pain on function and mood. These questions often will lead to an exploration of feelings of hopelessness, fear, isolation, and sadness related to pain, and the meaning of pain to the patient. Knowledge of pain severity ratings will be important in forming judgments about whether possible depressive mood disorders or anxiety disorders are really a manifestation of poorly controlled pain. Patients usually have more than one site of pain, each with its own set of associated features.

The patient's experiences and perceptions of pain treatments should be explored. The amount of relief and side effects attributed to pain treatments, and attitudes about specific pain medications (e.g., "Morphine kills people."), will affect compliance. How patients and their caregivers talk about pain with healthcare providers and each other may also be important.

2. Assessing for important psychosocial issues. The presence of other distressing symptoms and aspects of the psychosocial history which may be overlooked on a medical or surgical service. Additional questions can address past pain experiences that affected the patient's family or caregivers, other deaths directly or indirectly related to the patient's circle of associates, and areas of tension or conflict between the patient, caregivers, and health professionals.

3. Physical examination and relevant imaging studies. This includes a visual inspection, and if possible, gentle palpation of the affected area. It is helpful to have the patient point to the site of pain, as misunderstandings may arise from casual use of anatomical terms by patients. A neurological sensory exam for the presence of allodynia, hyperesthesia will be helpful in identifying a neuropathic pain syndrome. Imaging studies may be painful, but they can be helpful in elucidating an anatomical basis for the pain complaint. Knowledge of the history and physical findings are important when reviewing imaging studies with the radiologists. Some patients with advanced illnesses or who are at home will be unable to have imaging studies done.

4. Assignment of a pain diagnosis. This may or may not be possible, depending on the amount of information available, but will guide recommendations for pain management. Chronic pain syndromes have been classified by the International Association for the Study of Pain [92]. Cancer pain syndromes have been well summarized in textbooks of palliative medicine and review articles [93, 94]. In one large survey of patients with cancer pain, broad categories of pain diagnoses include nociceptive pain (35%),

neuropathic pain (8%), mixed pain syndromes (36%), and breakthrough pain (65%) [95]. Breakthrough pain, often related to bone or nerve involvement by cancer, may be particularly troublesome and difficult to manage.

5. Assessing how effective medical and other interventions have been in providing relief. This includes patient ratings of both the magnitude of pain relief, as well as the duration of pain relief. Ideally, all of the pain should be relieved all of the time with no side effects. In practice, a good amount (50–80%) of relief can be achieved for most of the time. A clinically significant difference is 2 points on the 0–10 scale, or a shift in Likert severity categories, such as from severe to moderate. Even if pain severity does not change, improvements in ability to function are encouraging to the patient and caregivers. During this assessment, be sure to attend to variables such as dosing, timing of medication delivery, and the patient's compliance with medications and regimens. In patients with regional pain syndromes, radiation therapy, and interventional anesthetic approaches ("blocks") may be appropriate.

6. Assessing side effects from pain management, or general disease management to date. Central nervous system side effects are feared by patients and their families:"I don't want to become a zombie." These side effects include sedation (reversible with stimulants), delirium, visual hallucinations, myoclonus, and delirium. When present, the patient should be switched to another opioid. The incidence of these side effects was estimated to range from 6–20% in a series of patients treated for cancer pain [36]. Constipation remains an important side effect. A social side effect is stigma from taking opioids and fears of addiction, and these have to be openly acknowledged and discussed with patients and their caregivers.

Psychological aspects of pain assessment

Dimensions of pain

The overall construct for palliative medicine is maintaining and optimizing quality of life in patients with incurable diseases. Quality of life is defined by the World Health Organization as having domains of physical, social, family, and emotional well-being. Additional domains of existential and spiritual well-being have been incorporated into new instruments for measuring quality of life. A number of terms related to pain are used in palliative medicine. These include the terms spiritual pain – the issue of meaninglessness at the end of life, social pain – disruption of relationships, psychological pain – pain associated with losses, and total pain – the combination of these experiences. Cecily Saunders, the founder of modern palliative medicine, emphasized that pain at the end-of-life has an all-encompassing quality, which goes beyond the physical, and enters into psychological and even metaphysical realms.

Meaning of pain

Beliefs about the meaning of pain play a role in pain perception, especially in patients with cancer. Individuals who attribute their cancer pain to progressive illness, as opposed to a source unrelated to their cancer, suffer more intense pain [96] and experience more interference in daily activities and pleasure [97]. Thus, attribution of the source of pain is critical. The level of detailed knowledge about the specific disease process will affect individual's interpretation of physical sensations and in turn, ameliorate or exacerbate their experience of pain and psychological distress. Psychologists will need to confer with their medical colleagues about the patient's findings and diagnoses. Furthermore, despite recent emphasis on pain treatment, delivery of pain medications can be problematic in practice.

Religious backgrounds may also be important in understanding the meaning of pain. In some traditions, pain at the end of life may be construed as a punishment or expiation of sins committed earlier in life. Other traditions may exalt pain at the end of life, as a fulfillment of a religious ideal, such as the death of Christ [98]. In a similar vein, patients with tobacco-related cancers often feely guilty about having "brought the cancer upon themselves" and feel they deserve to be in pain.

The effects of pain

The presence of uncontrolled pain can aggravate the psychological tasks by increasing fear, exhausting the patient's limited coping resources and attention, and increasing loneliness through social withdrawal.

Coping processes: coping, self-efficacy, and perceived stress

Patients' coping styles are a guidepost to the level of participation they will assume in the management of their illness. Gleaning information during early clinical interactions about the patient's desire for information, attribution of etiology, and attitudes about illness will often provide clues about potential obstacles during the course of care. Self-efficacy (SE) is the term most commonly used to conceptualize the foundation for improvement in pain and adaptive functioning following psychological interventions. Self-efficacy represents an individual's expectation that he/she has the resources (e.g., skills, knowledge, endurance) to accomplish a desired objective and overcome obstacles that might otherwise hamper the endeavor. Another important factor is "perceived stress," a concept that captures patients' interpretations about the limitations imposed by their illness. These subjective assessments address the implications of a patient's physical state, limitations in physical functioning and social relations. Individuals will vary in the degree to which their assessments are regarded as valid (objective), or unrealistic. The latter can involve bimodal inaccuracies, as patients may be deemed unduly favorable (naïve, optimistic, or "in denial"), or unfavorable (pessimistic, hopeless, despairing). Thus, perceived stress can be regarded as the converse of self-efficacy, although perceived stress incorporates additional social and environmental factors and is more broad than self-efficacy. Perceived stress is also determined by long-standing attitudes and personal experiences that can be modified through interventions such as cognitive-behavioral therapy and interpersonal psychotherapies.

Intervention and treatment

The underlying premise for pharmacological, psychological, and behavioral approaches to pain is the biopsychosocial model of pain, with adaptations for special features in patients with terminal illness [99]. We will discuss general strategies for intervention, citing both therapeutic techniques and their application to patients varying in level of psychological distress. Patients with adjustment reactions or those individuals with limited social or financial resources will respond to supportive interventions that emphasize caring and instruction to better manage specific symptoms; this can range from psychoeducational programming to skill training courses. Individuals with

more pronounced psychopathology will require more effort in understanding their world-view, which may entail comprehensive evaluations of their social circumstances, intensive engagement with the therapist, and perhaps a focus upon more existential or spiritual issues to achieve a sense of purpose throughout the final stages of their illness.

Pharmacological pain management

Patient selection for pharmacological management

When embarking on a pharmacological approach to pain management, the quintessential question here is: Who is the person in pain? What are his/her traits/temperament? How do personality characteristics interact to produce reactions to pain? And how does this, in turn, affect how they view their pain, how they deal with their treatment, how they deal with their pain medications (e.g., how they ask, if they ask, when/how much they ask). With these and similar questions, the story will emerge and guide the healthcare professional to treatments more likely to be helpful for the patient. Consider the patient's perspective on pain and pain medications. These may include the following commonly encountered statements:

> Why bother?
> They would offer it to me if they thought it would help.
> I'll become addicted to it.
> I don't need anyone to help.
> Give me enough to keep me out so I don't have to deal with this.
> Is it important to be awake? (Address patient's views on alertness and his/her ability to interact/communicate with others.)
> Do the medications result in more distress (e.g., constipation)? (Assessing the side effects of the medications, and understanding what the patient is willing to tolerate.)
> Does the patient worry about becoming addicted? (what is this about, being in control, being a "good patient", being independent, etc.)

Does the patient have trouble asking for what s/he need from others or from authority figures? (e.g., will they tell you they are in pain or ask for a PRN or will they feel as though they are a bother.)

Pharmacologic modalities for pain treatment

Mainstays of biomedical interventions for cancer pain are pharmacological. Additional modalities include radiation therapy, and anesthesiologic procedures for regional pain syndromes.

Pain medications are prescribed based upon the severity and type of pain. The World Health Organization ladder recommends non-steroidal analgesics for mild pain (e.g., pain severity 1–4), low dose opioids or opioid combination products such as oxycodone/acetaminophen preparations for moderate pain (e.g., pain severity 5–6), and opioids for severe pain (e.g., pain severity 7–10). Pain medications should be scheduled around the clock, with additional doses, often called rescue doses, available on request for additional pain flares.

Nonsteroidal anti-inflammatory drugs (NSAIDs) interfere with prostaglandin pathways that are important in nociception. These drugs are often prescribed for patients with bone pain and joint pain syndromes, and are available in oral and parenteral formulations. These drugs have a ceiling effect for efficacy, and their side effects include gastrointestinal irritation and bleeding, and renal insufficiency.

Opioid combination products where a second medication, usually a NSAID, is combined with an opioid, are widely available. These medications show a synergistic analgesic effect. Another medication, tramadol, is used for mild to moderate pain but is structurally different from opioids.

The opioids available in the United States include morphine, hydromorphone, oxycodone, oxymorphone, meperidine, levodromoran, methadone, and fentanyl. Collectively, opioids are available in oral, mucosal, parenteral, transdermal, rectal, and buccal formulations. Morphine is considered the standard opioid, and the usual recommended initial dose for a patient with severe pain is 30 mg by mouth or 10 mg parenterally. The opioids are all effective, but differ in side effects for an individual patient. Conversions of opioids from one to another or by different routes are often necessary in palliative medicine patients, and tables to assist in these conversions are available in most textbooks of palliative medicine.

Adjuvant medications refer to medications that have an analgesic effect that was discovered serendipitously. We now know that, in general, they affect other signaling pathways that modulate nociception, or stabilize the membrane and prevent nerve firing. Families of these agents include the tricyclic antidepressants, the serotonin specific reuptake inhibitors (SSRIs), serotonin norepinephrine reuptake inhibitors (SNRIs), anticonvulsants, and local anesthetics.

Steroids (e.g., dexamethasone) are used for patients with pain from epidural cord compression and other forms of tumor-related nerve edema. Capsaicin, the active substance in peppers, has been used topically for pain syndromes such as post-herpetic neuralgia.

Readers are referred to palliative medicine textbooks and excellent reviews [100] for more details (also see Table 22.1).

Psychological and behavioral approaches to pain

Emotion-based interventions

Emotional expressive therapy is based upon the concept that the ability to process and express emotions related to stressful events may ameliorate the perception of pain. Patients, especially patients at the end of life, have stories to tell and therein lies the idea of using storytelling in a therapeutic manner [101]. In emotional disclosure, subjects write or talk about thoughts and feelings related to stressful events. Studies on the effectiveness of emotional disclosure in pain control have yielded mixed results. On an individual basis, a single blind randomized controlled trial in Colombia showed that cancer patients with cancer pain assigned to write narrative essays and who wrote essays with high emotional content had lower pain scores than patients who wrote essays with low emotional content, and also when compared to controls [102].

Support groups encourage the expression of emotions and information exchange among group members. Please see the section on supportive-expressive groups for a more detailed discussion.

Existential/meaning-focused interventions

One task of psychotherapy is restoration of meaning [103]. Short-term interventions targeting the personal meaning of illness can supplement more objective or quantifiable stressors (e.g., economic impact, fatigue) and thereby modify emotional distress that accompanies, and can even exacerbate, physiological sources of pain. This is particularly relevant for those patients who report debilitating levels of pain despite high doses of analgesics or whose reports of pain are disproportionate with physical findings. Such individuals may be regarded as manifesting attitudes of hopelessness and despair even as one rechecks biomedical evaluations for sources of pain. It is important to note that such reactions may not be synonymous with major depression, but rather represent an extreme form of an adjustment reaction with a pervasive sense of uncontrollability, which has been deemed to represent "demoralization." Supportive psychosocial interventions derived from existential therapy perspectives are being developed

Table 22.1 Common pharmacological agents

Class	Indications	Agents	Side effects
Opioids	somatic pain	morphine hydromorphone methadone oxycodone oxymorphone	sedation delirium visual hallucinations nausea decreased memory decreased libido
Adjuvant medications			
NSAIDs	musculoskeletal	delirium renal failure	bone pain
Antidepressants			
Tricyclic agents		amitriptyline nortriptyline imipramine	dry mouth delirium
Quarternary SSRI SNRI		mirtazapine citalopram duloxetine venlafaxine	
Anticonvulsants	neuropathic pain (stabbing, intermittent pain) peripheral neuropathy		
		gabapentin, pregabalin carbazepine, oxcarbazepine levatiracetam phenytoin	
Steroids	epidural disease	prednisone dexamethasone	labile mood delirium anxiety
Stimulants	sedation from opioids short term treatment for depression	methylphenidate	anxiety, psychosis
Sympathetic antagonists	complex regional pain syndrome	clonidine	orthostatic symptoms
Anesthetics	neuropathic pain (sodium channel)		
		transdermal lidocaine	
		topiramate	
		tocainide	
	neuropathic pain (vanilloid receptor family)		
		capsaicin	

to target such pervasive dysphoric reactions [104]. Any improvement in a general sense of hope can lead to an implementation of targeted cognitive-behavioral interventions to behavioral functioning or social interactions.

Meaning-centered group psychotherapy is based on Frankl's logotherapy and utilizes didactics, discussion, and experiential exercises that focus on particular themes related to meaning and advanced cancer. It is designed to help patients with advanced cancer to develop, sustain, or enhance a sense of meaning, peace, and purpose in their lives. It provides a supportive community among patients who are suffering with similar day-to-day issues, as well as deeper existential issues, and it facilitates a greater understanding of plausible meaning sources assisting patients to discover sources of meaning in their life prior to and after diagnosis [104]. It aims to increase an individual's sense of meaning, and thus, positively impact his/her quality of life and coping style, although outcome studies have yet to demonstrate the benefits of this mode of psychotherapy. Pain, in particular, is not targeted. By increasing a patient's sense of meaning and self-efficacy, patients' perception of pain may improve.

Another approach frequently used in palliative medicine is life review. The patient's life experiences and his/her achievements are recounted and celebrated, and they seek to provide context and meaning for his current status [20]. The life summary can be recorded and presented to the patient and family as part of the patient's legacy. Interested readers are referred to a review [105].

Established religious traditions may be important for the patient and assist in providing a framework of meaning. Consultations with clergy members can be invaluable in helping patients connect their spiritual values with management of their medical condition.

Educational approaches

Education of patients can reduce pain. In a randomized controlled trial, the knowledge of patients with painful bone metastases about cancer pain management was assessed with a questionnaire and 20% of those who received directed education showed improvement in their knowledge scores compared to 0.5% for those who received usual care [106]. In another randomized controlled trial, hospitalized cancer patients with moderate to severe pain who received a structured pain education had less pain severity and better coping responses to pain [107].

Support groups can be another vehicle for education. These groups are usually highly structured (lectures given by healthcare professionals) and time-limited (5–10 weekly or monthly sessions) with psychoeducational components included. They are often directed at improving coping with illness as well as quality of life.

Cognitive-behavioral therapy

Cognitive behavioral therapy (CBT) presumes that patients monitor their symptoms, and these perceptions modulate behavior. In patients with severe symptoms, the goals of CBT are to alter maladaptive behaviors, alter ongoing images and feelings of the self that interfere with functioning, and alteration of cognitive schema that lead to ineffective functioning [108]. The impact of such interventions is exerted through the impact upon psychological style (e.g., self-efficacy, locus of control), which in turn changes individuals' perception of their pain, and improvement in the broad constellation of affective distress and functional activity. The desired result is to promote well behaviors and improved coping abilities.

Skills taught include relaxation techniques, breathing exercises, attentional training such as distraction, and imagery. Patient selection requires patients who are not overly skeptical, and who have enough mental capacity to participate in cognitive exercises. These techniques work best in patients with mild to moderate pain. Patients are often interested in learning and trying these techniques because of their non-pharmacologic nature and sense of control afforded.

Cognitive-behavioral therapy interventions have been effective in specific symptoms associated with cancer treatment, such as chemotherapy-induced nausea and vomiting [109]. Studies of CBT in patients with cancer pain are few. In one study, patients with cancer pain that required opioids were randomized to distraction, relaxation, and positive mood reinforcement audiotapes. The patients on the distraction and relaxation arms experienced pain relief but it did not last after the session [110].

A meta-analysis of randomized clinical trials of CBT for patients with breast cancer found this therapy to be effective for both distress and pain. This effect had not been detected in previous reviews of more heterogeneous groups of cancer patients [111].

Hypnosis

Reports on series of patients treated with hypnosis for pain management in advanced cancer date to the 1950s and earlier [112, 113] and have steadily appeared since then. Two relevant randomized controlled trials have been reported. In the first, patients with metastatic breast carcinoma in the treatment arm were taught a self-hypnosis exercise to "filter the hurt out of the pain" and to focus on an alternate sensation. Over a 1-year period, pain slopes increased for the control arm but not the treatment arm. There were parallel increases in perceptions of suffering and mood disorder in the control arm [96]. In the second, bone marrow transplant patients were randomized to hypnotic interventions, cognitive behavioral coping skills training, therapist contact, and usual care; the patients who underwent hypnotic interventions had less mucositis pain [114]. Hypnosis has been combined with other approaches, such as existential psychotherapy [115]. A meta-analysis concluded that further research is needed on hypnosis in palliative care for symptom control as the majority of studies in this review reported small sample sizes, variability in techniques utilized, and weak articulation of outcome measures [116].

Psychotherapy

Psychotherapy at its core is the art of restoring hope and meaning [102]. Given that the future of a dying person is inherently bleak, hope takes on new forms, as the therapist joins with the person's experience and allows him or herself to enter the dying person's world. At the center of all therapeutic interventions (across all theoretical orientations and disorders) is the relationship maintained between therapist and patient. Given the level of vulnerability of the dying patient, this concept is central to interventions addressing issues at the end of life. The level of intervention is likely to depend upon the level of intimacy established between the two (when did the relationship begin, during the last days of life vs. at time of diagnosis) as well as the patient's ability to engage in the work (e.g., limits resulting from cognitive impairment and physical discomfort). The therapeutic posture is active and empathetic, and less remote than is customarily seen in psychotherapy.

The extent to which different modes of psychotherapy are effective, in general, and serve to ameliorate pain, in particular, with a palliative care population is largely unknown. The theory is that pain is sustained through unresolved components of existential distress (ambivalence, meaninglessness, death anxiety, unfulfilled goals, and unresolved grief) and that by working through these issues, the pain will become more responsive to medications and other conventional treatments [115].

Generally, because the time is more limited (sometimes only hours or days), less emphasis is placed on developing insights, and more attention is given to maladaptive coping behaviors. Perhaps in part because of this time pressure, patients are capable of significant growth as they tackle the issues they face. Unlike hypnosis, some degree of pain control is required for patients to be able to concentrate and participate in psychotherapy. Psychotherapists who embark on this type of work should also be prepared to examine their own views of death, and be prepared to grieve when the patient dies [21].

Individual. The goal of individual therapy with the terminally ill is to provide support and assistance in adapting to and understanding the illness. It is necessary that patients be physically comfortable enough and cognitively clear enough to participate and this may not allow for group participation. A variety of orientations provide this framework including supportive, insight-oriented, and existential psychotherapies. Therapists may choose to work within one framework or move within and among them as indicated by patient's presentation.

Supportive psychotherapy. This treatment allows for patients to be provided with support, knowledge and skills. The therapist is likely to emphasize past strengths, support successful coping strategies, and teach new coping skills (including relaxation and other CBT techniques, as well as assertiveness and communication skills). The therapist listens and often allows for the comfort to converse open and honestly, allowing for discussion of whatever the patient desires (e.g., death and dying, suffering, life review). Furthermore a supportive psychotherapy relationship provides continuity and stability within the healthcare system.

Insight-oriented psychotherapy. This modality of treatment is intended to promote self-understanding and the development of a new means of coping with a broad range of emotional experience. Insight-oriented therapy is likely to be indicated for those with significant psychological distress or interpersonal issues who are motivated to explore their feelings and themselves. In addition, as those with advanced illness experience their suffering and the reality of their impending death, issues concerning earlier life challenges may come to the forefront and need to be addressed and explored.

Existential psychotherapy. Existential psychotherapy is intended to assist patients to better cope with their diagnosis, adjust to living with their illness, and live more fully with the time they have left. Palliative care patients are confronted with their own mortality, and as a result, they are often troubled by fears of dying, concerns about dying alone, and spiritual questions about meaning and purpose. Existential psychotherapy encourages patients to identify, explore, and address anxieties about death, isolation, and a desire to find meaning. This therapeutic intervention is more present-focused, and it seeks to facilitate self-awareness and acceptance by allowing patients to acknowledge and discuss the difficult questions that arise when patients are faced with the reality of their death.

Group therapy. Supportive-expressive group psychotherapy (SEGT) can best be described as an amalgam of several models of group work (including supportive, existential, cognitive behavioral, interpersonal and psychoeducational interventions) developed to more appropriately serve the needs of those with advanced cancer. The goals of SEGT are multiple, and center on building and strengthening bonds, expressing emotions, detoxifying death and dying, redefining life's priorities, and improving coping. There is a major emphasis on relationships both within the group as well as with outside family, friends, and medical staff. Groups are run by co-facilitators and meet weekly for 90 minutes. Treatment is long-term, often lasting a year or longer. Differences between SEGT and psychotherapy groups lie in their long-term nature, a larger size, and relaxation of boundaries with the promotion of 'out-of-session' contact. Finding psychotherapists with knowledge of modern oncology is difficult. The therapists' task is to draw out and facilitate expression of emotional pain in a group setting. Therapists work with group members about medical therapies, the price of relationships (connectedness vs. separation), and preparation for death. Only half of eligible patients want to participate [117].

Recently, three large randomized controlled trials have been performed to test the hypothesis that SEGT can increase survival in patients with metastatic breast cancer. None showed a difference in survival. The Canadian study intervention arm treated pain with self-hypnosis and relaxation at the end of each meeting, and discussions of fear of opioids when the topic of pain arose. Patients in the intervention arm who had high baseline levels of pain improved, whereas pain did not improve in the control arm [118]. The Australian study showed significant reduction in the incidence of depressive disorders, helplessness/hopelessness, and improved social functioning in the SEGT arm but the report did not provide information about pain [119]. The American study did not report in detail about symptom distress [120].

Coping responses

Self-Efficacy centered approaches

Several studies have shown that individuals with higher innate levels of SE report lower levels of pain and show less restriction in functioning due to pain. Similarly, interventions designed to enhance direct coping and SE reveal modest improvement in patient satisfaction, improvement in pain levels, and partner satisfaction/emotional well-being. In a related vein, individuals who believe that they exert a high level of influence over their environment experience less pain and greater satisfaction than persons who believe that events are the result of outside forces (unmediated events, fate, and influence of others). Challenging patients' implicit beliefs about the negative aspects of their illness and especially a lack of control over their fate often yields benefits. However, in the context of severe pain disorders such as those associated with advanced cancer, ultimately such improvement in attitude is relatively modest in magnitude and duration in the course of disease management.

Interventions for caregivers

Psychoeducational interventions that increase caretakers' understanding of the course of severe illness and provide tangible ways to manage symptoms can improve the atmosphere of hopelessness in a household and in turn, impact quality of life. Thus, human contact, love, support, as well as the expectation that there will be someone available in times of crisis may serve to buffer the psychological effects of physical pain. If caregiver SE is associated with patient pain outcomes, then pain outcomes might be improved by interventions for caregiver self efficacy. Two randomized control trials have recently been reported. In one, patients and their caregivers at the end of life were randomized to usual care compared to three 1-hour educational sessions delivered by a nurse practitioner on the management of cancer pain and other symptoms. Caregivers in the intervention arm reported increased SE and less caregiver strain than those in the control group. Patient pain scores were the same in both arms [121]. In another randomized trial, caregivers of patients entering hospice care were randomized to standard care, standard care and three supportive visits, standard care with visits and education about coping skills. Caregivers in the coping skills arm had improvement in caregiver quality of life, caregiver burden, and patients reported a decreased symptom burden [122].

Special situations

Patients with refractory pain

Psychologists may be called to see the patient whose pain does not seem to be responding to analgesic measures. In approaching these situations, the first steps should include reassessing the pain evaluation and diagnosis with the medical team. The patient should then be asked about his compliance with taking pain medications, as compliance was determined to be an issue for patients with rates of 85% in one study [83]. Reasons for not taking analgesics and preferring to live with moderate to severe pain may include fear of addiction, opiate stigma, fear of side effects, dislike of medications, and as an expression of denial of the illness [123]. In this context, the administration of morphine, but not other opioids, may be seen by patients as an acknowledgment of death rather than an analgesic [124]. The morphine drip has become part of the lay conception of the medical death ritual, and is sometimes ordered by physicians for dying patients even when there is no complaint of pain. The next step is then to assess for psychological aspects of pain, such as suffering or existential distress that is being reported by the patient as pain. Patients, and their physicians, may not realize that patients may lump different pain syndromes into one, where one of the pain syndromes is indeed disease related, and what is reported as pain may also result from character idiosyncrasies or unresolved psychological issues [125].

Pain crisis

The pain crisis refers to situations with cancer patients where a source of pain becomes overwhelming for the patient and leads to hospitalization and other measures for pain control. Psychologists may be consulted as patients and their caregivers frequently experience severe emotional distress at this juncture in the patient's illness [126].

Conclusion

For the vast majority of patients in palliative medicine, pain is a valid symptom of the disease process and not inherently indicative of psychopathology. However, psychological symptoms and ways of being affect the perception and experience of pain. Our increasing understanding of psychological disorders and how they interact with pain assessment and management will lead to more sensitive and tailored psychological assessments of patients. The evidence base is improving for psychological and behavioral interventions to improve pain control in this group of vulnerable patients, and it is paramount that more research be done to better inform clinicians how and when to appropriately intervene. Research utilizing measures of despair, hopelessness,

demoralization, existential distress, spirituality, and other related constructs, while assessing functional activity and magnitude of subjective pain, will allow for a deeper understanding of the nuances in suffering at the end of life, and improve prospects for a "good death".

Acknowledgments

Drs Myres-Sorger, Jones, and Stein were supported in part by the VA Palliative Care Fellowship Program of the VA Bronx and New Jersey. Dr. Chang was supported in part by VA HSRD IIR 2-103.

References

1. Chochinov HM, Breitbart W. *Handbook of Psychiatry in Palliative Medicine* (New York: Oxford University Press, Inc, 2003).

2. Chang VT, Hwang SS, Feuerman M, Kasimis B. Symptom and quality of life survey of medical oncology patients at a Veterans Affair Medical Center. A role for symptom assessment. *Cancer* 2000; **88**: 1175–83.

3. McCarthy EP, Phillips RS, Zhong Z, Drews RE, Lynn J. Dying with cancer: patients' function, symptoms, and care preferences as death approaches. *J Am Geriatr Soc* 2000; **48**: S110–S121.

4. Levenson JW, McCarthy EP, Lynn J, Davis RB, Phillips RS. The last six months of life for patients with congestive heart failure. *J Am Geriatr Soc* 2000; **48**: S101–S109.

5. Lynn J, Ely EW, Zhong Z, McNiff KL, *et al.* Living and dying with chronic obstructive pulmonary disease. *J Am Geriatr Soc* 2000; **48**: S91–S100.

6. Roth K, Lynn J, Zhong Z, Borum M, Dawson NV. Dying with end stage liver disease with cirrhosis: insights from SUPPORT. *J Am Geriatr Soc* 2000; **48**: S122–S130.

7. Davison SN. Pain in hemodialysis patients: prevalence, etiology, severity, and management. *Am J Kidney Dis* 2003; **42**: 1239–47.

8. Cohen LM, Germain M, Poppel DM, Woods A, Kjellstrand CM. Dialysis discontinuation and withdrawal of dialysis. *Am J Kidney Dis* 2000; **36**: 140–4

9. Karus D, Raveis VH, Alexander C, *et al.* Patient reports of symptoms and their treatment at three palliative care projects servicing individuals with HIV/AIDS. *J Pain Symptom Manage* 2005; **30**: 408–17.

10. Tranmer JE, Heyland D, Dudgeon D, *et al.* Measuring the symptom experience of seriously ill cancer and non cancer hospitalized patients near the end of life with the Memorial Symptom Assessment Scale. *J Pain Symptom Manage* 2003; **25**: 420–9.

11. Solano JP, Gomes B, Higginson IJ. A comparison of symptom prevalence in far advanced cancer, AIDS, heart disease, chronic obstructive pulmonary disease and renal disease. *J Pain Symptom Manage* 2006; **31**: 58–69.

12. Walsh D, Donnelly S, Rybicki L. The symptoms of advanced cancer: relationship to age, gender, and performance status in 1000 patients. *Supp Care Cancer* 2000; **8**: 175–9.

13. Potter J, Hami F, Bryan T, Quigley C. Symptoms in 400 patients referred to palliative care services: prevalence and patterns. *Palliat Med* 2003; **17**: 310–14.

14. Kutner JS, Kassner CT, Nowels DE. Symptom burden at the end of life: hospice providers' perceptions. *J Pain Symptom Manage* 2001; **21**: 473–80.

15. McMillan SC, Small BJ. Symptom distress and quality of life in patients with cancer newly admitted to hospice home care. *Oncol Nurs Forum* 2002; **29**: 1421–8.

16. Buchanan RJ, Choi M, Wang S, Huang C. Analyses of nursing home residents in hospice care using the Minimum Data Set. *Palliat Med* 2002; **16**: 465–80.

17. Angus DC, Barnato AE, Linde-Zwirble W. Use of intensive care at the end of life in the United States: An epidemiologic study. *Critical Care Med* 2004; **32**: 638–43.

18. Marik PE. Management of patients with metastatic malignancy in the intensive care unit. *Am J Hosp Pall Med* 2007; **23**: 479–82.

19. Kirkova J, Davis MP, Walsh D, et al. Cancer symptom assessment instruments: a systematic review. *J Clin Oncol* 2006; **24**: 1459–73.

20. Butler RN. The life review: an interpretation of reminiscence in the aged. *Psychiatry* 1963; **26**: 65–76.

21. Cohen ST, Block S. Issues in psychotherapy with terminally ill patients. *Pall Supp Care* 2004; **2**: 181–9.

22. Rodin G, Zimmermann C. Psychoanalytic reflections on mortality: a reconsideration *J Am Acad Psychoanal Dynam Psych* 2008; **36**: 181–96.

23. Block SD. Psychological issues in end-of-life care. *J Palliat Med* 2006; **9**: 751–72.

24. Wilson KG, Chochinov HM, Skirko MG, et al. Depression and anxiety disorders in palliative cancer care. *J Pain Symptom Manage* 2007 Winter; **33**: 118–29.

25. Lloyd-Williams M, Dennis M, Taylor F. A prospective study to determine the association between physical symptoms and depression in patients with advanced cancer. *Palliat Med* 2004; **18**: 558–63.

26. Kissane DW, Wein S, Love A, et al. The Demoralization Scale: a report of its development and preliminary validation *J Palliat Care* 2004 Winter; **20**: 269–76.

27. Periyakoil VS, Kraemer HC, Noda A, et al. The development and initial validation of the Terminally Ill Grief or Depression Scale (TIGDS). *Int J Methods Psychiatr Res* 2005; **14**: 202–12.

28. Miovic M, Block S. Psychiatric disorders in advanced cancer. *Cancer* 2007; **110**: 1665–76.

29. Sela RA. Screening for depression in palliative cancer patients attending a pain and symptom control clinic. *Pall Supp Care* 2007; **5**: 207–17.

30. Kane RL, Berstein L, Wales J, Rothenberg R. Hospice effectiveness in controlling pain. *JAMA* 1985; **253**: 2683–6.

31. Teunissen SCCM, de Graeff A, Voest EE, de Haes JC. Are anxiety and depressed mood related to physical symptom burden? A study in hospitalized advanced cancer patients. *Palliat Med* 2007; **21**: 341–6.

32. Gagliese L, Gauthier L, Rodin G. Cancer pain and depression: a systematic review of age-related patterns. *Pain Res Manage* 2007; **12**: 205–11.

33. Kurtz ME, Kurtz JC, Stomell M, Given CW, Given B. Predictors of depressive symptomatology of geriatric patients with lung cancer – a longitudinal analysis. *Psychooncology* 2002; **11**: 12–22.

34. Kurtz ME, Kurtz JC, Stomell M, Given CW, Given B. Predictors of depressive symptomatology of geriatric patients with colorectal cancer: a longitudinal view. *Support Care Cancer* 2002; **10**: 494–501.

35. Kane RL. Who should be in control? *Rep Natl Forum Hosp Health Aff* 1985; 151–9.

36. Chang VT, Hwang SS, Kasimis B. Longitudinal documentation of cancer pain management outcomes: a pilot study at a VA medical center. *J Pain Symptom Manage* 2002; **24**: 494–505.

37. Akechi T, Okuyama T, Sugawara Y, Nakano T, Shima Y, Uchitomi Y. Major depression, adjustment disorders, and post-traumatic stress disorder in terminally ill cancer patients: associated and predictive factors. *J Clin Oncol* 2004; **22**: 1957–65.

38. Hopwood P, Stephens RJ. Depression in patients with lung cancer: prevalence and risk factors derived from quality-of-life data. *J Clin Oncol* 2000; **18**: 893–903.

39. Lunney JR, Lynn J, Foley DJ, Lipson S, Guralnik JM. Patterns of functional decline at the end of life. *JAMA* 2003; **289**: 2387–92.

40. Hwang SS, Chang VT, Fairclough DL, Cogswell J, Kasimis B. Longitudinal quality of life in advanced cancer patients: pilot study results from a VA medical cancer center. *J Pain Symptom Manage* 2003; **25**: 225–35.

41. Ormel J. Synchrony of change in depression and disability: what next? *Arch Gen Psychiatry* 2000; **57**: 381–2.

42. Evans C, Charney DS, Lewis L, et al. Mood disorders in the medically ill: scientific review and recommendations. *Biol Psychiatry* 2005; **58**: 175–89.

43. Coyle N, Sculco L. Expressed desire for hastened death in seven patients living with advanced cancer. A phenomenologic inquiry. *Oncol Nurs Forum* 2004; **31**: 699–706.

44. Mystakidou K, Parpa E, Katsouda E, Galanos A, Vlahos L. The role of physical and psychological symptoms in desire for death: a study of terminally ill cancer patients. *Psychooncology* 2006; **15**: 355–60.

45. Marcoux I, Onwuteaka-Philipsen B, Jansen-Van der Weide MC, Van der Wal G. Withdrawing an explicit request for euthanasia or physician-assisted suicide: a retrospective study on the influence of mental health status and other patient characteristics. *Psychol Med* 2005; **35**: 1265–74.

46. Rosenfeld B, Breitbart W, Gibson C, Kramer M. Desire for hastened death among patients with advanced AIDS. *Psychosomatics* 2006; **47**: 504–12.

47. Casey KL. Forebrain mechanisms of nociception and pain: analysis through imaging. *Proc Natl Acad Sci USA* 1999; **96**: 7668–74.

48. Price DD. Psychological and neural dimensions of the affective dimension of pain. *Science* 2000; **288**: 1769–72.

49. Mystakidou K, Tsilika E, Parpa E, Katsouda E, Galanos A, Vlahos L. Psychological distress of patients with advanced cancer. Influence and contribution of pain severity and pain interference. *Cancer Nurs* 2006; **29**: 400–5.

50. Bishop SR, Warr D. Coping, catastrophizing and chronic pain in breast cancer. *J Behav Med* 2003; **26**: 265–81.

51. Zaza C, Baine N. Cancer pain and psychosocial factors: a critical review of the literature. *J Pain Symptom Manage* 2002; **24**: 526–42.

52. Steinhauser KE, Christakis NA, Clipp EC, *et al.* Factors considered important at the end of life by patients, family, physicians, and other care providers. *JAMA* 2000; **284**: 2476–82.

53. Vig EK, Pearlman RA. Good and bad dying from the perspective of terminally ill men. *Arch Intern Med* 2004; **164**: 977–81.

54. Smith MY, Egert J, Winkel G, Jacobson J. The impact of PTSD on pain experience in persons with HIV/AIDS. *Pain* 2002; **98**: 9–17.

55. Baider L, Peretz T, Hadani PE, *et al.* Transmission of response to trauma? Second-generation Holocaust survivors' reaction to cancer. *Am J Psychiatry* 2000; **157**: 904–10.

56. Feldman DB, Periyakoil VS. Posttraumatic stress disorder at the end of life. *J Palliat Med* 2006; **9**: 213–8.

57. Murillo M, Holland JC. Clinical practice guidelines for the management of psychosocial distress at the end of life. *Pall Supp Care* 2004; **2**: 65–77.

58. Frank JD. Psychotherapy, the restoration of morale. *Am J Psych* 1974; **131**: 271–4.

59. Clarke DM, Kissane DW. Demoralization: its phenomenology and importance. *Aust N Z J Psychiatry* 2002; **36**: 733–42.

60. Clarke DM, Kissane DW, Trauer T, Smith GC. Demoralization, anhedonia, and grief in patients with severe physical illness. *World Psychiatry* 2005; **4**: 96–105.

61. Mangelli L, Fava GA, Grandi S, *et al.* Assessing demoralization and depression in the setting of medical disease *J Clin Psychiatry* 2005; **66**: 391–4.

62. Kearny M, Mount B. Spiritual care of the dying patient. In *Handbook of Psychiatry in Palliative Medicine*, eds. HM Chochinov, and W Breitbart (New York: Oxford University Press, 2000), pp. 357–73.

63. Cassell EJ. The nature of suffering and the goals of medicine. *N Engl J Med* 1982; **396**: 639–45.

64. Chapman CR, Gavrin J. Suffering: the contributions of persistent pain. *Lancet* 1999; **353**: 2233–7.

65. Cherny NI, Coyle N, Foley KM. Suffering in the advanced cancer patient: a definition and taxonomy. *J Palliat Care* 1994; **10**: 57–70.

66. Wilson KG, Chochinov HM, McPherson CJ, *et al.* Suffering with advanced cancer. *J Clin Oncol* 2007; **25**: 1691–7.

67. Clayton JM, Hancock K, Parker S, *et al.* Sustaining hope when communicating with terminally ill patients and their families: a systematic review. *Psychooncology* 2008; **17**: 641–59.

68. Buffum MD, Hutt E, Chang VT, Craine MH, Snow AL. Cognitive impairment and pain management: review of issues and challenges. *J Rehabil Res Dev* 2007; **44**: 315–30.

69. Klepstad P, Hilton P, Moen J, *et al.* Self reports are not related to objective assessments of cognitive function and sedation with cancer pain admitted to a palliative care unit. *Pall Med* 2002; **16**: 513–9.

70. Cassell EJ, Leon AC, Kaufman SG. Preliminary evidence of impaired thinking in sick patients. *Ann Intern Med* 2001; **134**: 1120–3.

71. Sorger BM, Rosenfeld B, Pessin H, Timm AK, Cimino J. Decision-making capacity in elderly, terminally ill patients with cancer. *Behav Sci Law* 2007; **25**: 393–404.

72. Morita T, Akechi T, Ikenaga M, *et al.* Terminal delirium: recommendations from bereaved families' experiences. *J Pain Symptom Manage* 2007; **34**: 579–89.

73. Lawlor PG, Gagnon B, Mancini IL, *et al.* Occurrence, causes, and outcome of delirium in patients with advanced cancer. A prospective study. *Arch Intern Med* 2000; **160**: 786–94.

74. Fann JR, Alfano CM, Burlington BE, *et al.* Clinical presentation of delirium in patients undergoing hematopoietic stem cell transplantation. Delirium and distress symptoms and time course. *Cancer* 2005; **103**: 810–20.

75. Coyle N, Breitbart W, Weaver S, Portenoy R. Delirium as a contributing factor to "crescendo" pain: three case reports. *J Pain Symptom Manage* 1994; **9**: 44–7.

76. American Geriatric Society Panel on Persistent Pain in Older Persons. The management of persistent pain in older persons. *J Am Geriatric Soc* 2002; **50** Suppl 6: S205–S224.

77. Weiner DK. Assessing persistent pain in older adults: practicalities and pitfalls. *Analgesia* 1999; **4**: 377–95.

78. Feldt KS, Warne MA, Ryden MB. Examining pain in aggressive cognitively impaired older adults. *J Gerontol Nurs* 1998; **24**: 14–22.

79. Herr K, Bjoro K, Decker S. Tools for assessment of pain in nonverbal older adults with dementia: a state of the science review. *J Pain Symptom Manage* 2006; **31**: 170–92.

80. Koopman C, Hermanson K, Diamond S, Angell K, Spiegel D. Social support, life stress, pain and emotional adjustment to advanced breast cancer. *Psycho-Oncology* 1998; **7**: 101–11.

81. Bowling A, Barber J, Morris R, Ebrahim S. Do perceptions of neighbourhood environment influence health? Baseline findings from a British survey of aging. *J Epidemiol Community Health* 2006; **60**: 476–83.

82. Zhang, AY, Siminoff, LA. The role of the family in treatment decision making by patients with cancer. *Oncol Nurs Forum* 2003; **30**: 1022–8.

83. Mehta A, Ezer H. My love is hurting: the meaning spouses attribute to their loved ones' pain during palliative care. *J Pall Care* 2003 Summer; **19**: 87–94.

84. Miaskowski C, Kragness L, Dibble S, Wallhagen M. Differences in mood states, health status, and caregiver strain between family caregivers of oncology outpatients with and without cancer-related pain. *J Pain Symptom Manage* 1997; **13**: 138–47.

85. Keefe FJ, Lipkus I, Lefebvre JC, *et al.* The social context of gastrointestinal cancer pain: a preliminary study examining the relation of patient pain catastrophizing to patient perceptions of social support and caregiver stress and negative responses. *Pain* 2003; **103**: 151–6.

86. Holtzman S, DeLongis A. One day at a time: the impact of daily satisfaction with spouse responses on pain, negative affect and catastrophizing among individuals with rheumatoid arthritis. *Pain* 2007; **131**: 202–13.

87. Kutner JS, Bryant LL, Beaty BL, Fairclough DL. Symptom distress and quality-of-life assessment at the end of life: the role of proxy response. *J Pain Symptom Manage* 2006; **32**: 300–10.

88. Kurtz ME, Kurtz JC, Given CW, Given B. Concordance of cancer patient and caregiver symptom reports. *Cancer Pract* 1996; **4**: 185–90.

89. Redinbaugh EM, Baum A, DeMoss C, Fello M, Arnold R. Factors associated with the accuracy of family caregiver estimates of patient pain. *J Pain Symptom Manage* 2002; **23**: 31–8.

90. Yates P, Aranda S, Edwards H, *et al.* Family caregivers' experiences and involvement with cancer pain management. *J Pall Care* 2004 Winter; **20**: 4, 287–96.

91. Keefe FJ, Ahles TA, Porter LS, *et al.* The self-efficacy of family caregivers for helping cancer patients manage pain at end-of-life. *Pain* 2003; **103**: 157–62.

92. International Association for the Study of Pain Task Force on Taxonomy. *Classification of Chronic Pain*, 2nd edn., eds. H Mersky, and N Bogduk. (Seattle: IASP Press, 1994).

93. Caraceni A, Portenoy RK. An international survey of cancer pain characteristics and syndromes. IASP Task Force on Cancer Pain. *Pain* 1999; **82**: 263–74.

94. Foley KM. Acute and chronic cancer pain syndromes. In *Oxford Textbook of Palliative Medicine*, 3rd edn, eds. D Doyle, G Hanks, NI Cherny, and K Calman. (New York: Oxford University Press, 2004), pp. 298–316.

95. Zech DFJ, Grond S, Lynch J, Hertel D, Lehmann KA. Validation of World Health Organization Guidelines for cancer pain relief. A prospective study. *Pain* 1995; **63**: 65–76.

96. Spiegel D, Bloom JR. Group therapy and hypnosis reduce metastatic breast carcinoma pain. *Psychosom Med* 1983; **45**: 333–9.

97. Daut RL, Cleeland CS. The prevalence and severity of pain in cancer. *Cancer* 1982; **50**: 1913–18.

98. Curlin FA, Roach CJ, Gorawar-Bhat R, Lantos JD, Chin MH. When patients choose faith over medicine. Physician perspectives on religiously related conflict in the medical encounter. *Arch Intern Med* 2005; **165**: 88–91.

99. Sutton LM, Porter LS, Keefe FJ. Cancer pain at the end of life: a biopsychosocial perspective. *Pain* 2002; **99**: 5–10.

100. Cleary J. The pharmacologic management of cancer pain. *J Pall Med* 2007; **10**: 1369–94.

101. Carr DB, Loeser JD, Morris DB. (eds.). Narrative, pain, and suffering. *Progress in Pain Research and Management* (Volume **34**. Seattle: IASP Press, 2005).

102. Cepeda MS, Chapman CR, Miranda N, *et al.* Emotional disclosure through patient narrative may

improve pain and well-being: results of a randomized controlled trial in patients with cancer pain. *J Pain Symptom Manage* 2008; **35**: 623–31.

103. Frank JD. Psychotherapy – the transformation of meanings. *J Roy Soc Med* 1986; **79**: 341–6.

104. Breitbart W, Gibson C, Poppito SR, Berg A. Psychotherapeutic interventions at the end of life: a focus on meaning and spirituality. *Can J Psychiatry* 2004; **49**: 366–72.

105. LeMay K, Wilson KG. Treatment of existential distress in life threatening illness: a review of manualized interventions. *Clin Psychol Rev* 2008; **28**: 472–93.

106. Kim JE, Dodd M, West C, *et al*. The PRO-SELF pain control program improves patients' knowledge of cancer pain management. *Oncol Nurs Forum* 2004; **31**: 1137–43.

107. Lai YH, Guo SL, Keefe FJ, *et al*. Effects of brief pain education on hospitalized cancer patients with moderate to severe pain. *Support Care Cancer* 2004; **12**: 645–52.

108. Turk DC, Feldman CS. A cognitive-behavioral approach to symptom management in palliative care: augmenting somatic interventions. In *Handbook of Psychiatry in Palliative Medicine*, eds. HM Chochinov, and W Breitbart, (New York: Oxford University Press, Inc., 2000), pp. 223–41.

109. Given C, Given B, Rahbar M, *et al*. Effect of cognitive behavioral intervention on reducing symptom severity during chemotherapy. *J Clin Oncol* 2004; **22**: 507–516.

110. Anderson KO, Cohen MZ, Mendoza TR, *et al*. Brief cognitive-behavioral audiotape interventions for cancer related pain. Immediate but not long-term effectiveness. *Cancer* 2006; **107**: 207–14.

111. Tatrow K, Montgomery GH. Cognitive behavioral therapy techniques for distress and pain in breast cancer patients: a meta-analysis. *J Behav Med* 2006; **29**: 17–27.

112. Erickson M. Hypnosis in painful terminal illness. *J Ark Med Soc* 1959; **56**: 67–71.

113. Sacerdote P. Theory and practice of pain control in malignancy and other protracted or recurring painful illnesses. *Int J Clin Exp Hypno* 1970; **18**: 160–80.

114. Syrjala KL, Cummings C, Donaldson GW. Hypnosis or cognitive behavioral training for the reduction of pain and nausea during cancer treatment: a controlled clinical trial. *Pain* 1992; **48**: 137–46.

115. Iglesias A. Hypnosis and existential psychotherapy with end-stage terminally ill patients. *Am J Clin Hypn* 2004; **46**: 201–13.

116. Rajasekaran M, Edmonds PM, Higginson IL. Systematic review of hypnotherapy for treating symptoms in terminally ill cancer patients. *Palliat Med* 2005; **19**: 418–26.

117. Kissane DW, Grabsch B, Clarke DM, *et al*. Supportive-expressive group therapy: the transformation of existential ambivalence into creative living while enhancing adherence to anti-cancer therapies. *Psycho Oncology* 2004a; **13**: 755–68.

118. Goodwin PJ, Leszcz M, Ennis M, *et al*. The effect of group psychosocial support on survival in metastatic breast cancer. *N Engl J Med* 2001; **345**: 1719–26.

119. Kissane DW, Grabsch B, Clarke DM, *et al*. Supportive-expressive group therapy for women with metastatic breast cancer: survival and psychosocial outcome from a randomized controlled trial. *Psycho Oncology* 2007; **16**: 277–86.

120. Spiegel D, Butler LD, Giese-Davis J, *et al*. Effects of supportive-expressive group therapy on survival of patients with metastatic breast cancer. A randomized prospective trial. *Cancer* 2007; **110**: 1130–8.

121. Keefe FJ, Ahles TA, Sutton L, *et al*. Partner-guided cancer pain management at the End of Life: a preliminary study. *J Pain Symptom Manage* 2005; **29**: 263–72.

122. McMillan SC, Small BJ, Weitzner M, *et al*. Impact of coping skills intervention with family caregivers of hospice patients with cancer. A randomized clinical trial. *Cancer* 2005; **106**: 214–22.

123. Weiss SC, Emanuel LL, Fairclough DL, Emanuel EJ. Understanding the experience of pain in terminally ill patients. *Lancet* 2001; **357**: 1311–5.

124. Reid CM, Gooberman-Hill R, Hanks GW. Opioid analgesics for cancer pain: symptom control for the living or comfort for the dying? A qualitative study to investigate the factors influencing the decision to accept morphine for pain caused by cancer. *Ann Oncol* 2008; **19**: 44–8.

125. Strasser F, Walker P, Bruera E. Palliative pain management: when both pain and suffering hurt. *J Pall Care Summer* 2005; **21**: 69–79.

126. Moryl N, Coyle N, Foley KM. Managing an acute pain crisis in a patient with advanced cancer: "this is as much of a crisis as a code". *JAMA* 2008; **299**: 1457–67.

Section 4
Chapter

23

Integrative approaches to the management of painful
medical conditions

Pain-associated disability syndrome in children and adolescents

Gerard A. Banez

Chronic pain in children and adolescents is common, with a prevalence of at least 15%. A significant subset of these patients experiences a downward spiral of increasing functional disability. They do not attend school, interact with peers, and/or participate in sports, extracurricular activities, and other personal/family activities. Though advances have been made on pharmacological and psychologically based treatments, unidisciplinary and symptom-focused strategies may not lead to an acceptable resolution. For severely affected patients, an interdisciplinary rehabilitation approach provides an understandable and useful model of care. The purpose of this chapter is to present an overview of biopsychosocial rehabilitation of children and adolescents with chronic pain and associated functional impairment. First, an introduction to pediatric chronic pain and its treatment will be presented. Second, pain-associated disability syndrome (PADS) will be described. Third, an interdisciplinary rehabilitation approach for children and adolescents with PADS will be discussed. Fourth, the Cleveland Clinic Pediatric Pain Rehabilitation Program will be presented as an example of an interdisciplinary pain rehabilitation program for pediatric PADS. In the final section of the chapter, common clinical challenges will be discussed.

Pediatric chronic pain and its treatment

Chronic pain in children and adolescents is common with prevalence rates ranging between 15% [1] and 32% [2]. In an epidemiological study of almost 750 school-recruited children and adolescents in Germany, Roth Iseigkeit [3] reported that more than 80% had pain during the previous 3 months. One-third of her sample had pain for more than 6 months and one-third reported pain more than once weekly. In a study of 5424 children

and adolescents, Perquin *et al.* reported that 54% had a significant pain episode in the last 3 months and 26% had chronic or recurrent pain [4]. One-third of those who reported chronic pain had severe disabling pain.

The most common pediatric chronic pain condition is headache followed by recurrent abdominal pain (RAP) and musculoskeletal pain [4]. Headache prevalence at age 7 years ranges from 37% to 51.5% and from 7 to 15 years, 57% to 82% [5–7]. Population-based studies suggest that RAP is experienced by 10% to 15% of school-age children [8, 9] and almost 20% of middle school and high school students [10]. Population studies indicate that chronic or recurrent musculoskeletal pain is also common in school-age children with back pain being the most frequent (20%), followed by limb pain (16%) and fibromyalgia (6%) [11–15]. Approximately 5–8% of new referrals to North American pediatric rheumatology centers have a diagnosis of idiopathic musculoskeletal pain syndromes, a small percentage of which are complex regional pain syndrome (CRPS)/reflex sympathetic dystrophy (RSD) [13, 16, 17].

Medical and physical treatments

The existing but limited literature on medical and physical treatments suggests that these treatments may be helpful to some children and adolescents with chronic pain, but are not effective for all patients. A variety of medications are used, including tricyclic antidepressants (TCAs), selective serotonin reuptake inhibitors (SSRIs), beta blockers, anticonvulsants, muscle relaxants, and over-the-counter analgesics such as acetaminophen and ibuprofen. Their use is often based on data extrapolated from adults [18]. In children with migraine there is some evidence in support of acetaminophen, ibuprofen, and sumatriptan nasal spray during attacks [7]. Evidence for efficacy of treatment of RAP in children has been found in therapies that use famotidine, pizotifen, and

Behavioral and Psychopharmacologic Pain Management, ed. Michael H. Ebert and Robert D. Kerns. Published by Cambridge University Press. © Cambridge University Press 2011.

peppermint oil enteric-coated capsules [19]. For musculoskeletal pain such as fibromyalgia and CRPS/RSD, various medications including amitriptyline and gabapentin are used, but empirical support is limited. Overall, existing data suggest that pharmacotherapy may reduce the frequency and severity of chronic pain, but it rarely leads to eradication or elimination of pain and may be associated with adverse side effects.

Psychosocial treatments

Similarly, psychosocial treatments, particularly relaxation and cognitive-behavioral therapy, can be helpful in reducing the severity and frequency of chronic pain, but are not effective for all patients. When effective, these treatments impact pain perceptions and behaviors, alter environmental and behavioral triggers, but do not typically eliminate pain. A systematic review and subset meta-analysis of published randomized controlled trials of psychological therapies for children and adolescents with chronic pain identified 18 papers that met the criteria for inclusion in the review [20]. The majority of these papers reported brief behavioral and cognitive behavioral interventions (e.g., contingency management training for parents, instruction to the child on progressive muscle relaxation, diaphragmatic breathing, cognitive coping) for children with headache, and many were conducted in community (i.e. school) settings. Meta-analysis was applicable for 12 headache trials and one trial of RAP using the Pain Index. The odds-ratio for a 50% reduction in pain was 9.62 and the number needed to treat was 2.32, indicating that the psychological treatments examined are effective in reducing the pain of headache. These findings are consistent with Holden et al., who concluded that relaxation/self-hypnosis is a well established and efficacious treatment for recurrent headache and thermal biofeedback is a probably efficacious treatment [21]. Cognitive-behavioral interventions have also been found to be effective in the treatment of RAP, with five randomized trials reporting statistically significant improvements in pain [19, 22, 23]. Though treatment studies using cognitive behavioral interventions for adults with fibromyalgia have shown effectiveness (e.g., reducing patients' ratings of pain, tender point measures, functional disability), psychological treatments have not been adequately tested in children with fibromyalgia [24].

Pain-associated disability syndrome

The term pain-associated disability syndrome (PADS) was coined to describe chronic pain patients with severe problems in functioning regardless of location or etiology of pain. Children and adolescents with PADS have chronic pain, do not attend school, do not interact with peers, increasingly withdraw from sports and other extracurricular activities, and become less involved with family and home duties. A focus on PADS rather than chronic pain facilitates a shift from an acute disease focus to rehabilitation. It is clinically useful in that it precludes the dualistic and outdated view of pain as physical or psychological. The PADS emphasis addresses not so much the cause of the pain as the related functional impairment [25]. The focus is on management of pain and reduction of associated suffering.

Bursch defined PADS as "a downward spiral of increasing pain-associated disability, lasting at least 3 months, for which symptom-focused strategies have not led to an acceptable resolution" [26]. She noted that the initial pain may be caused by an illness or injury, a developmental challenge, or psychosocial stressor. Bursch acknowledged that it is often not possible to identify the trigger, and she noted that the time frame for the development of PADS varies widely from patient to patient [26]. In the only study to employ Bursch's criteria, Hyman et al. reported on children with visceral, or gastrointestinal (GI), PADS [27]. Participants were 40 children (18 male) who ranged in age from 7 to 21 years and manifested GI symptoms severe enough to prevent school attendance or eating for 2 months. Hyman and colleagues found that these children shared a number of associated factors including learning disabilities, unrealistic goals as well as a perfectionist, high-achieving orientation; early pain experiences, a passive or dependent coping style; marital problems in the home; and chronic illness in a parent. All the children in their study had at least two of these associated factors, and a majority had four or more factors. Possible triggering events for their symptoms included: acute febrile illness ($n = 20$), school change ($n = 11$), trauma ($n = 2$), death of a loved one ($n = 2$), and sexual abuse ($n = 2$). Psychiatric co-morbidity was present in a majority of the children.

Interdisciplinary pain rehabilitation

When treating children and adolescents with PADS, a rehabilitation model of care provides an understandable and useful alternative to the acute pain model, which is focused on eradication of pain. In a rehabilitation model, pain is accepted as a symptom that may or may not be eliminated. The focus of care is on independent functioning (rather than pain), improved coping, and increased self-efficacy. Increased functioning, improved coping skills, and better self-efficacy are viewed as signs of progress. For patients who have shown little response to unidisciplinary and symptom-focused strategies, this approach may be particularly helpful. With adults, interdisciplinary pain rehabilitation programs have been shown to be clinically effective and cost effective [28, 29]. Relative to other widely used medical treatments, adult pain rehabilitation programs provide better outcomes in areas such as functional activities, medication use, and healthcare utilization.

Theoretical influences and an evolving model

Biopsychosocial model of chronic pain

One theoretical influence on our rehabilitation approach to children with PADS is the biospsychosocial model of the etiology and course of chronic pain [30]. This model presumes that a child's condition is a function of multiple interacting determinants, including early life factors (e.g., genetic predisposition, environmental factors), physiological factors, psychosocial factors (e.g., life stress, psychosocial state, coping, social support), and interactions between physiological and psychological factors. According to this model, a child with pain but with no psychosocial problems

as well as good coping skills and social support will have a better outcome than the child with pain as well as coexisting emotional difficulties, high life stress, and limited support. The child's clinical outcome (e.g., daily function, quality of life) will, in turn, affect the severity of the disorder.

Psychosocial model of the development of sick role behavior

A second theoretical influence is the conceptual model developed by Walker to describe the role of psychosocial factors in the course of recurrent abdominal pain (RAP) in middle childhood [31]. This model proposes the psychosocial mechanisms that lead some children with RAP to develop sick role behavior (e.g., frequent somatic complaints, activity restrictions, dependence on caretakers) while others do not, and is relevant to multiple chronic pain conditions in children (see Figure 23.1). According to this model, the amount of activity restriction associated with pain and the extent to which this restriction is perceived, as rewarding or aversive, play significant roles in determining whether or not pain results in functional disability. That is, if missed school days are perceived as rewarding by the child with pain who struggles academically and has no friends at school, they may contribute to more impairment. The child with pain who excels academically, is socially engaged, and views missed school days negatively will attempt to attend school despite pain.

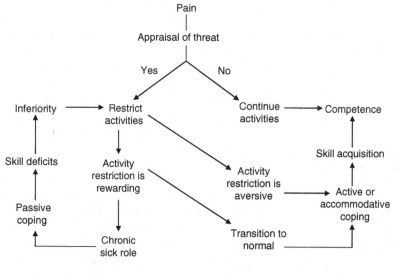

Figure 23.1 Psychosocial model of the development of sick role behavior (using information from Ref. [31]).

Acceptance and change model

A third important influence is the acceptance and change model conceptualized by Hayes et al. [32]. The acceptance/change model emphasizes acceptance of and/or willingness to experience pain/distress rather than trying to control or reduce symptoms. This model is helpful because the traditional focus on controlling pain/distress is only useful when it can be achieved. This focus is problematic when it is not successful, and controlling chronic pain is not always possible. A focus on controlling pain can lead to unwanted side effects, move patients away from things they deem important, and/or lead to sick role behavior and functional disability. The acceptance/change model provides an alternative focus which is consistent with the rehabilitation approach's emphasis on improved functioning with or without pain. Its focus is on reducing the distressing and disabling influences of pain as they concern important areas in patients' lives [33]. The model encourages a shift in perspective, from a symptom-reduction approach to valued living in the presence of pain and distress [34].

Indirect support for the acceptance/change model can be found in research suggesting that pain in itself does not explain functional disability. That is, the amount of impairment that some children exhibit is not directly correlated with the severity of their pain condition. For example, in a study of 104 patients with chronic back pain, Crombez et al. found that pain-related fear predicted poor behavioral performance and was more associated with disability than pain itself [35]. Direct support for an acceptance/change model is found in the research of McCracken [36], who found that acceptance of pain was associated with less pain, disability, depression, and anxiety as well as return to work. McCracken et al. [33] reported that acceptance, in comparison with coping, accounts for more variance in functioning, and Viane et al. found that acceptance reliably predicts mental well-being [37].

Acceptance and commitment therapy

Acceptance and commitment therapy (ACT) is a psychological therapy based on the acceptance/change model [32]. In ACT, acceptance of what cannot be changed (i.e., pain, fear of anticipated pain) is promoted as a means to recognize the things that can. Patients in ACT are provided assistance with identifying and achieving personal values and encouraged to pursue valued living despite pain (e.g., "playing soccer and being part of the team even though I'm in pain").

Pain-related avoidance behavior is considered the cause of disability [34] and, for that reason, exposure to previously avoided personal experiences, like pain or fear, is an important component of ACT. To help children cope with these experiences, they are instructed in learning to notice pain/distress in a non-judgmental, non-elaborative, and non-controlling way (i.e., "my thoughts are just my thoughts"). Once they are able to shift their perspective from symptom reduction to valued living, increased functioning becomes possible.

Wicksell et al. treated 14 consecutive patients between 13 and 20 years old with chronic debilitating pain [38]. Patients were provided with individual sessions of ACT (M = 14.4) and parent sessions (M = 2.4) aimed at improving functioning by increasing the ability to act in line with personal values in the presence of negative thoughts, emotions, or bodily sensations. Improvements in functional ability, school attendance, catastrophizing, and pain (e.g., intensity and interference) were found post-treatment and at 3- and 6-month follow-ups. In a study of 15 adolescents with functional abdominal pain, Greco et al. provided 12 to 14 individual and 2 to 5 parent sessions to promote life quality and decrease functional disability [39]. At the conclusion of treatment, they found significant improvements in quality of life, functioning, and symptom reduction.

Evolving model of chronic pain and functional disability

As influenced by these conceptual models, our evolving conceptualization of chronic pain and functional disability proposes that pain results from an illness, life event, or psychosocial stress that taxes the vulnerable child [26]. In the child who develops PADS, the pain and related symptoms lead to activity restriction that is reinforcing, e.g., missed school days are perceived as rewarding [31]. Over time, sick role behavior develops, and the secondary effects of pain, such as moving children away from things they deem important, contribute to increasing functional disability. To effectively treat, clinicians must identify and interrupt the cycle of decreased functioning, inactivate the fear that improvement is impossible, and reduce the vulnerabilities, physical and psychological, to somatic and behavioral symptoms. A biopsychosocial rehabilitation plan that addresses specific contributors is needed (e.g., parent guidance to encourage normal activity, cognitive approaches to foster hopefulness, physical therapy for strength and endurance, pain coping skills training). In addition to improved coping, acceptance of chronic pain and a commitment to valued living despite pain may be critical. A child's unwillingness to have pain, as illustrated in a failure to engage in valued activities to avoid negative experiences, such as fear of pain, failures, disappointments [34], can be a major obstacle to progress.

Existing literature on pain rehabilitation programs for children and adolescents with PADS

To date, several studies have examined the utility of a rehabilitation approach to children and adolescents with chronic pain and functional disability. In a prospective follow-up, Sherry and colleagues concluded that intense exercise therapy is effective in initially treating childhood CRPS and is associated with a low rate of long-term symptoms or dysfunction [40]. Participants were 103 children (87 girls; mean age = 13.0 years) with CRPS. Forty-nine participants were followed for more than 2 years (mean = 5 years 3 months). Most received a daily program of 4 hours of aerobic, functionally directed exercises, 1–2 hours of hydrotherapy, and desensitization. The mean duration of exercise therapy was 14 days, but in the last 2 years of the research had decreased to 6 days. Ninety-five children (92%) initially became symptom-free. Of those followed for more than 2 years, 43 (88%) were symptom-free, 5 (10%) were fully functional but had some continued pain, and 1 (2%) had functional limitations.

Lee *et al.* conducted a prospective, randomized, single-blind trial of physical therapy and cognitive-behavioral treatment for children and adolescents with CRPS [41]. Children 8 to 17 years of age (*n* = 28) were randomly assigned to one of two groups: (1) physical therapy once per week for 6 weeks or (2) physical therapy three times per week for 6 weeks. Both groups received six sessions of cognitive-behavioral treatment. Assessments of pain and function were repeated at two follow-up time periods. All five measures of pain and function improved significantly in both groups after treatment, with sustained benefit evident in the majority of patients at long-term follow-up. Most children with CRPS showed reduced pain and improved function with the non-invasive treatment approach, with long-term functional outcomes also very good.

In another program integrating intense physical and occupational therapy with cognitive-behavioral therapy, Eccleston and colleagues concluded that their interdisciplinary treatment was a promising approach to the management of a variety of chronic musculoskeletal and other idiopathic pain syndromes, pain related distress, and disability [18]. Fifty-seven adolescents (mean age = 14.28 years) with chronic pain and 57 accompanying adults underwent a three-week residential program of physical and occupational activity, cognitive therapy, and education. Post-treatment adolescents reported significant improvements for self report of disability, physical function, and sit to stand. At 3 months post-treatment adolescents maintained physical improvements and reduced anxiety, disability, and somatic treatment. Following treatment, adults reported significant improvement in their report of adolescent disability, adult anxiety, depression, and parental illness. At 3 months, 64% improved school attendance, and 40% had returned to full-time education.

Cleveland Clinic Pediatric Pain Rehabilitation Program

The Cleveland Clinic Pediatric Pain Rehabilitation Program was designed to assist children and adolescents with chronic pain that interferes with their normal activities. The primary goals of the program are: (1) to help children manage their pain effectively and (2) to restore daily activity. The program differs from previously evaluated programs in that it consists of inpatient and day hospital components. As well, it blends pediatric subspecialty care, behavioral health, and rehabilitation therapies in an individualized but coordinated manner.

In the first 2 weeks of the program, children are admitted to our inpatient rehabilitation unit where their treatment is often delivered apart from their parents. Our view is that the inpatient setting maximizes potential for successful control of the environment and for the interdisciplinary structure to adhere to a common treatment philosophy [42]. Separation of children and parents serves to interrupt maladaptive interactions that are maintaining or worsening pain behaviors and facilitates acquisition of new and more healthy behavioral habits. In their final week, children participate as outpatients and return home with their parents at the end of each day. They continue the activities of the prior weeks but have more opportunities to apply their new skills in real-world situations. Throughout the program, parents and other family members are provided with assistance helping their children return to normal functioning. An important objective of the final week is successful re-entry into home, school, and other community settings.

Children and adolescents referred to our program have shown little to no improvement with past outpatient services (medical, psychological, rehabilitative) of appropriate length, frequency, and/or intensity and have been referred specifically for intensive interdisciplinary pain rehabilitation. Their progress is gradual, with increases in day-to-day activity serving as a better initial indicator of improvement than reductions in pain frequency and severity.

Pediatric subspecialty care

Prior to admission, children being considered for the program are typically seen by the appropriate medical subspecialist (e.g., patient with headaches is evaluated by a pediatric neurologist) to determine program appropriateness. In addition to chronic pain and disability, the necessity of an intensive interdisciplinary pain rehabilitation program needs to be established. Exhaustion of appropriate outpatient resources is a primary consideration. After admission, subspecialists provide consultation as needed. They are involved in planning and supervising medication regimens and offer consultation on daily care as needed. If their evaluations suggest the need, other specialty consultations are requested. Our preference, however, is to complete all subspecialty medical evaluation prior to admission. Pre-admission completion of these evaluations is important because they take time away from the rehabilitation program. Moreover, until evaluation is complete, some patients and parents continue to worry about missed diagnoses and have difficulties committing to the program.

Behavioral health care

Psychological or behavioral health services are a critical component of our program. These services are designed to support patients as they participate in their rehabilitation therapies, enhance pain management skills and resources, and facilitate improved emotional adjustment and familial functioning. Patients in our program participate in individual and/or family therapy three to five times/week. Acceptance of pain and commitment to living with pain are major areas of focus. They also participate in our Mind-Body Skills Training group with other pain rehabilitation patients. This group provides training in evidence-

Figure 23.2 Golden rules of chronic pain

All pain is real
Improvement is first measured by increased functioning
Don't ask your child if she is in pain
Exercise is good for sleep and for chronic pain
Sleep is good
Reduce anxiety
A long-term problem requires a long-term solution

Source. Ref. [43].

based pain management strategies (e.g., progressive muscle relaxation, diaphragmatic breathing, cognitive self-statements) as well as exposure to complementary/alternative techniques, such as aromatherapy and acupressure. Our behavioral health services are not intended to be primary mental health services. As important mental health issues arise, these are brought to the attention of the patient and family, and appropriate follow-up resources are recommended.

Each patient in the program also has a written Individualized Functional Plan (IFP) that identifies specific behavioral treatment goals (see Figure 23.2). These goals are generated by the patient in coordination with program staff and are revised on a weekly basis. On a daily basis at the end of each hour, patients are rated on their effort at goal attainment by staff and by themselves. The objective of the IFP is to promote increased health and wellness. Individual and group incentives are used to increase commitment to this objective.

Rehabilitation therapies

Children in the program are involved in intensive physical and occupational therapies on a daily basis. These therapies are important because the long periods of inactivity often associated with chronic pain can lead to short, overused muscles. Patients' muscles can be weak and atrophied, promoting overuse of agonists and shortening of antagonists. It is not uncommon for our patients to exhibit problems with sitting and standing posture. Because regular exercise has been shown to reduce stress, anxiety, and depression and is predictive of a continued active lifestyle through adulthood, the importance of establishing good exercise habits is stressed. Increased activity and relaxation also help our children learn to understand their bodies better.

Each patient participates in individual physical therapy (PT) and occupational therapy (OT) sessions on a daily basis. These sessions focus on sensory destimulation, postural alignment/body awareness, and durable medical equipment (DME) assessment, such as orthotics, arch supports, shoes, and appropriate clothing. As indicated, kinesiotaping and/or other types of taping are used. During the program, each patient is given ongoing evening exercises to perform independent of their therapy sessions. Prior to discharge, an individualized home exercise program (HEP), including endurance and strengthening activities, is developed. Individualized pictures and directions are provided. As much as possible, age-appropriate peer activities, as opposed to formal exercises, are encouraged.

In addition to their individual rehabilitation therapies, all patients participate in morning exercise and aquatic therapy groups. The morning exercise group is scheduled as the first activity of each day as we have found that the earlier our patients initiate physical activity, the better. Physical, occupational, and recreation therapists collaborate on the aquatic therapy program, which is conducted in pool heated to 92° F. Among the areas targeted in these group therapies are: stretching, strengthening, endurance, relaxation, and team building.

Leisure education and recreation therapy

Leisure education and recreation therapy are provided to enable children to gain a broader understanding of where, why, how, and with whom they can pursue their leisure interests and experiences. These services play an important role in facilitating a return to age-appropriate activities. Therapeutic activities are designed to help our patients unlearn maladaptive leisure skills and learn more functional responses (i.e., develop different types of leisure behaviors that allow for greater flexibility in meeting recreational interests). Through these activities, they develop leisure awareness and activity skills, learn to use leisure resources, and improve social interaction skills during recreational activities.

Parent/family education

Parent/family education plays a critical role in our rehabilitation approach and is provided individually as well as in group sessions. Emphasis is placed on the physical and psychological aspects of pain, disability, and their treatment. Zeltzer's "Golden Rules of Chronic Pain" are used as a starting point and framework for helping parents help their children handle their pain successfully (see Table 23.1) [43]. Guidelines for managing pain

behaviors are presented, with attention to the importance of encouraging normal activity and discouraging pain behaviors [44]. As discharge nears, parents and family members are provided assistance in facilitating a successful transition to home and preventing regression upon discharge.

School re-entry process

Missed school days are a common problem for children with chronic pain and, for many, represent the most significant domain of functional impairment. Some, like Bursch [26], have written that it is common to discover previously undiagnosed learning and communication disorders in children thought to be high functioning before the onset of their pain. Ho and colleagues, however, reported that children and adolescents attending a tertiary-care interdisciplinary pain service ($n = 57$, ages 8–18) scored higher in general intelligence, verbal ability, non-verbal reasoning, word reading, and math reasoning than the general population [45]. The level of academic achievement for most of their participants was consistent with their intellectual ability. They concluded that their data do not indicate overall cognitive impairment or a single atypical achievement pattern and recommended looking beyond cognitive and achievement scores (e.g., stressfulness of intra-individual weaknesses, incongruity between actual achievement and perceived potential) to explore the links between school functioning and chronic pain in children. They also hypothesized that school programs that are flexible enough to allow normalized peer interactions yet accommodate for fluctuations in pain and functioning (e.g., reduced course load, self-paced curriculum, or a combination of school attendance and home-based learning) are best suited for children and adolescents with chronic pain.

To help children in our program keep pace during their time away from school and to facilitate their re-entry into the classroom environment, all patients receive classroom services throughout the 3-week program. They are asked to bring work and assignments from their home schools, and a teacher from the Cleveland Metropolitan School District provides individualized assistance. On the final week of each patient's program, a school re-entry meeting is held. This meeting is attended by the patient, family, and program staff, with home school staff participating by way of conference call. During this meeting, program staff provide the school with information about the child's diagnosis, functioning, and the importance

Name_____   Dates_____

Individualized Functioning Plan – Week 1

Goal (Rated 0- 2*)		Tues.	Wed.	Th.	Fri.	Sat.	Sun. (Parent Rating)
Morning Care							
Nursing Goal 1: Follow Meal/Drinking Recommendations	AM						
	PM						
Nursing Goal 2: Interact w/ others Respectfully	AM						
	PM						
Nursing Goal 3: Minimize pain talk	AM						
	PM						
Individual Goal 1:	Ex. Group					AM	AM
	M-B-S						
	Pool						
	OT						
	PT					PM	PM
	RT						
	PSYC						
	School						
Individual Goal 2:	Ex. Group					AM	AM
	M-B-S						
	Pool						
	OT						
	PT					PM	PM
	RT						
	PSYC						
	School						
Individual Goal 3:	Ex. Group					AM	AM
	M-B-S						
	Pool						
	OT						
	PT					PM	PM
	RT						
	PSYC						
	School						
School Goal: Homework Completion							
Total Points Earned							

* Goals are rated based on effort as a 0 (needs improvement), 1 (getting there), or 2 (doing well).

Table 23.1 Individualized functioning plan – Week 1.

of focusing on the child's abilities and activities, not on pain. Findings such as those of Logan and Curran underscore the importance of this type of meeting [46]. In their study of school personnel's understanding of adolescent chronic pain problems, they found that school personnel cited many challenges to working with adolescents in pain, including high absence rates, wide individual variation in presentation of symptoms and impairment, the need to balance accommodations with school policies, attending to the needs of other students, and dealing with parents. They also identified needs for more information about chronic pain problems and more guidance from healthcare professionals regarding how to manage pain symptoms and pain-related behaviors in the school setting. This study reveals that school personnel struggle when they encounter chronic pain problems in the school setting and feel inadequately educated about how to work effectively with students with chronic pain. The school re-entry meeting improves collaboration between our program and each patient's school and is designed to address the challenges that school personnel identify in working with children with chronic pain.

Preliminary outcomes assessment

Preliminary evaluation of the initial twelve adolescents (mean age = 16.1 years) treated in our 3-week, combined inpatient and day hospital program suggests that the program is accomplishing its goals, particularly in the area of improved functioning. Primary diagnoses included headache ($n = 5$), complex regional pain syndrome ($n = 4$), fibromyalgia ($n = 1$), and back pain ($n = 2$). Mean chronicity of pain was 2.6 years. Our initial results show a 36% improvement in pain severity and a 50% improvement in physical functioning at posttreatment. We have also found a 46% improvement in social functioning and a 50% improvement in pain-specific anxiety at 1-month follow-up. These preliminary data suggest that our interdisciplinary rehabilitation approach can be effective in helping adolescents return to normal activity despite pain. Longer-term, more comprehensive assessment of a larger group of adolescents is ongoing and will be important for better evaluating program effectiveness.

Common clinical challenges

One common clinical challenge is dispelling the belief that medications/surgery are the only helpful treatment strategies for pain. Many patients, parents, and their providers adopt a traditional biomedical approach to pain. The biomedical approach emphasizes accurate diagnosis of the cause(s) of pain as a means of identifying effective treatments. This approach promotes a search for the cure, with elimination or eradication of pain as the primary treatment goal. Those who adhere to this approach are typically not open or fully committed to behavioral approaches or rehabilitation therapies. They do not see the role of non-medical treatments and more easily dismiss them when they do not immediately make pain go away.

A related clinical challenge is the patient and/or family's inability to understand how psychosocial stressors/problems can exacerbate pain. Many patients and families view chronic pain as strictly physical in nature. They do not recognize or acknowledge the psychosocial aspects of pain. Attempts to introduce or address psychosocial contributors are viewed as suggestions that the pain is not real and/or is psychological in nature. Introduction of psychosocial contributors can be upsetting and is often met defensively. In our program, all pain is seen as real pain. The existence or reported severity of pain is not questioned. We emphasize, however, that all pain has a physical component and all pain has a psychological component. In terms of the latter, we know that, at a minimum, life stressors, mood, and emotions impact perceptions of pain and the ways in which children cope with their pain. Though for some, the psychological component can be greater (e.g., clinically significant depressive or anxiety-related symptoms), initial presentation of the psychological aspects in this manner is usually well-accepted and defuses concerns that pain validity is being questioned.

Inability to accept pain and commit to valued living despite pain represents a major obstacle to improvement in a rehabilitation approach. Some patients and families cannot envision a return to normal life in the presence of pain. Their preference is to restrict activity until the pain is eliminated. When the pain is gone, the child will return to normal activity. Until then, they argue that the child cannot do more or he/she will make matters worse. Some are unable to see the point of trying to do things if the pain has not lessened. By putting functioning first, the rehabilitation approach challenges common approaches to pain. For acute pain, bed rest and activity restrictions are often recommended. With chronic pain, a return to valued living despite pain represents a means to improvement. As children return to desired activity, they become less preoccupied with their pain, moods and emotions improve, and strength and conditioning increase in ways that promote even more activity. In our experience, as activity increases and lifestyles normalize, the effects of pain lessen. This approach, however, is counterintuitive for many and can be difficult to accept.

Some patients and families are afraid of additional harm that may result from pushing 'too hard.' They fear that pushing may cause more damage or injury and worsen the underlying cause or condition for the pain [25]. In part, their fear is rooted in the biomedical model and our understanding of acute pain, not chronic pain. As noted, treatments of acute pain, which typically resolves in a reasonable amount of time, may involve rest and restrictions. Educational approaches about the development and maintenance of chronic pain and associated functional disability are important ways of countering these misperceptions. In a related way, efforts to address patient and family stress about pain-related difficulties are critical. Seeing their children in pain is typically rated as one of the most stressful events parents can face. Inability to tolerate their children's pain can lead parents to respond to pain behaviors in ways that are not helpful and may serve to maintain pain-related behaviors.

A final challenge is overcoming a home and family culture of sick role behavior and functional disability. Children with PADS may have parents or other family members who also have chronic pain, somatic complaints, and/or functional disability. Walker and Greene reported that anxiety, depression, and somatization were greater in mothers of children with RAP than mothers of well children [47]. Wasserman *et al.* found a higher incidence of current and prior painful gastrointestinal disorders among family members of children with RAP than among family members of well children [48]. In addition, children with recurrent unexplained pain, compared to children with recurrent explained pain, have been found to identify more models of pain or illness behavior in their environment [49]. In this study, children with recurrent unexplained pain identified more positive consequences of pain behavior while children with explained pain identified more negative consequences. Clearly, the presence of family members with chronic pain and associated disability complicates the process of treating PADS. Familial modeling and support of maladaptive pain behaviors may diminish the child's motivation to learn how to manage chronic pain. In such cases, intensive family therapy focused on the functions served by the pain and the processes maintaining it may be warranted.

Case illustration

GBS is a 17-year-old male who presented with an at least 5-year history of severe abdominal pain. His pain was intense enough to cause a significant number of missed school days. He missed 3 months of school in eighth grade, and he was home schooled in nineth grade. He tried returning to school in tenth grade but missed so many days that he had to enroll in an independent study program to increase his credits. He continued in this program in eleventh grade but was rarely able to attend the one day of school required a week. According to his parents, he had attended about 6 months of school over the past 3 years.

GBS reported severe periumbilical pain that began in the morning. He reported that his pain was constant and noted that nothing helped him feel better. He often stayed in bed for 3 hours before getting up at noon. His mother would call from work to wake him and came home to make his lunch. He spent about 8 hours a day on the computer playing games or interacting with friends. He rarely went out and spent most of his time alone.

GBS used to have problems sleeping until trazadone was started by a psychiatrist. At the time of referral, he was sleeping well. He had problems with nausea but rarely vomited. He did not have constipation, flatulence, bloating, or diarrhea. He had been thoroughly evaluated by two pediatric gastroenterologists, with no specific physical or organic cause found.

GBS was born 1 week prematurely and discharged to home. One week later, his mother was instructed to stop breast-feeding because he had galactosemia. He had feeding problems as an infant, projectile vomited his feeds, and was on Nutramigen until the age of 2 years. His vomiting continued until 6th grade. He had an episode of high heart rate during this time period, but 24 hour Holter monitor was normal. He had a history of migraine headaches as well, but had not had a migraine since starting amitriptyline 2 months earlier.

At age 14, GBS developed Type II diabetes and was started on medication. He had not completed diabetes education and did not check his blood sugar. According to his parents, he was in too much pain to attend his education sessions. He had also seen psychiatrists and psychologists for depression and anxiety but missed many appointments due to his pain. According to parents, he had missed about 75% of his medical appointments because of pain.

Referral diagnoses included irritable bowel syndrome, myofascial headaches with a reported history of past migraines, generalized anxiety disorder with increased anxiety sensitivity, and major depressive disorder with suicidal ideation but no intent. When asked to rate his pain over the past few days, he rated his pain as a "7" on a scale of "0" [no pain] to "10" [maximum]. On the Bath Adolescent Pain Questionnaire (BAPQ), his Physical Functioning score = 11, and his Pain Specific Anxiety score = 12. Of note was the distress and helplessness his parents presented, reporting that their entire family life seemed to revolve around his pain. Parents were frustrated because he did not appear to be doing anything to help himself.

GBS was admitted to the Cleveland Clinic Pediatric Pain Rehabilitation Program for a combined inpatient/day hospital program. His pain and disability were conceptualized from a biopsychosocial perspective, with early life factors such as a predisposition to gastrointestinal difficulties, physiological factors (e.g., dysfunctional pain processing), and psychological factors (e.g., depression, anxiety) presumed to interact and impact his condition. His sense of hopelessness, limited coping resources, and activity restriction had led to significant sick role behavior. Parents' attempts to assist appeared to be inadvertently reinforcing and maintaining his difficulties. He had spiraled into a hole that neither he nor his family believed they could help him escape.

Treatment consisted of individual and/or family psychological therapy three to four times/week, participation in a pain management training group, physical therapy and occupational therapy on a daily basis, pool therapy, leisure education and recreation therapy, and a school program. Over the course of his stay, consultations with a psychiatrist (use of escitalopram for anxiety and addition of melatonin for sleep) and biofeedback therapist (blood volume pulse, surface electromyographic, and respiration biofeedback for relaxation training) were requested, and diabetic education was offered. Treatment goals included a more positive mental attitude, enhanced coping skills, increased strength and endurance, and a return to age-appropriate activities.

GBS was initially slow to warm to the program and slightly resistant. He and his parents were preoccupied with identifying the cause of his pain and shared a sense of hopelessness related to past treatment failures. He participated in therapies, however, because of his desire for a return to normal functioning and past interest in physical exercise. As he began to notice improvements in sleep, strength, and endurance, abdominal pain became less of a problem. He became more accepting of his pain and committed to leading his life despite pain. He began to understand and accept the importance of a rehabilitation approach. By the third week, he appeared to truly embrace the approach and was making good lifestyle changes. He rarely, if ever, complained about abdominal pain and functioned very normally, including sleep. He continued to report benefits from physical and occupational therapies. Over the course of treatment, his parents received individual and group parent education, with an emphasis on promoting normal activity. They learned how to disengage from maladaptive interactions with him and developed strategies to help him help himself. Of particular importance was training in a familial problem-solving approach that they utilized to develop a school re-entry plan that met his academic, social, and physical health needs.

At the time of discharge, parents commented on the changes GBS had made while in the program. He was positive, hopeful, and future-oriented in a way they had not seen in the past. Physically and psychologically, they noted multiple gains. His pain severity rating at discharge was a "4," which represented a 42% improvement over admission. His BAPQ Physical Functioning score = 6 and Pain Specific Anxiety score = 5 at discharge, representing 46% and 58% improvements, respectively.

Summary

Children and adolescents with PADS are among the most physically complex and psychologically challenging patients to treat. For those who have not responded to unidisciplinary and symptom-focused treatments, an interdisciplinary rehabilitation approach, which is focused on independent functioning, may be warranted. The child's acceptance of chronic pain and a commitment to valued living despite pain can be central to progress. The few existing studies examining the rehabilitation approach to children with PADS are most encouraging, demonstrating benefit in both pain and function. Future investigations will be important for determining which patients respond best to the rehabilitation approach, what combinations of services are most beneficial, and the mechanisms that underlie the improvements that result from these programs.

References

1. Goodman JE, McGrath PJ. The epidemiology of pain in children and adolescents: A review. *Pain* 1991; **46**: 247–64.

2. El-Metwally A, Salminen JJ, Auvinen A, Kautiainen H, Mikkelsson M. Prognosis of non-specific musculoskeletal pain in preadolescents: A prospective 4-year follow-up study till adolescence. *Pain* 2004; **110**: 550–9.

3. Roth-Isigkeit A, Thyen U, Stöven H, Schwarzenberger J, Schmucker P. Pain among children and

adolescents: Restrictions in daily living and triggering factors. *Pediatrics* 2005; **115**: e152–62.

4. Perquin CW, Hazebroek-Kampscheur AAJM, Hunfeld JAM, *et al.* Pain in children and adolescents: A common experience. *Pain* 2000; **87**: 51–8.

5. Lipton RB. Diagnosis and epidemiology of pediatric migraine. *Curr Opin Neurol* 1997; **10**: 231–6.

6. Lipton RB, Maytal J, Winner P. Epidemiology and classification of headache. In *Headache in Children and Adolescents,* eds. P Winner and AD Rothner. (Hamilton-London: BC Decker, 2001), pp. 1–19.

7. Rothner AD. Headaches in children and adolescents. *Semin Pediatr Neurol* 1991; **8**: 2–6.

8. Apley J. *The Child with Abdominal Pains*, 2nd edn. (London: Blackwell, 1925).

9. Apley J, Naish N. Recurrent abdominal pain: A field survey of 1,000 school children. *Arch Dis Childhood* 1958; **33**: 165–70.

10. Hyams JS, Burke G, Davis PM, Rzepsaki B, Andrulonis PA. Abdominal pain and irritable bowel syndrome in adolescents: A community-based study. *J Pediatrics* 1996; **129**: 220–6.

11. Abu-Arafeh I, Russell G. Recurrent limb pain in schoolchildren. *Arch Dis Child*, 74 1996; 336–9.

12. Buskila D, Press J, Gedalia A, *et al.* Assessment of nonarticular tenderness and prevalence of fibromyalgia in children. *J Rheumatol* 1993; **20**: 368–70.

13. Maillard SM, Davies K, Khubchandani R, Woo PM, Murray KJ. Reflex sympathetic dystrophy: A multidisciplinary approach. *Arthritis Rheum* 2004; **51**: 284–90.

14. Oster J. Recurrent abdominal pain, headache and limb pains in children and adolescents. *Pediatrics* 1972; **50**: 429–36.

15. Payne WK III, Ogilvie JW. Back pain in children and adolescents. *Pediatr Clin North Am* 1996; **43**: 899–917.

16. Bowyer S, Roettcher P, Pediatric Rheumatology Database Research Group. Pediatric rheumatology clinic populations in the United States: Results of a 3 year survey. *J Rheumatol* 1996; **23**: 1968–74.

17. Malleson PN, Fung MY, Rosenberg AM. The incidence of pediatric rheumatic diseases: Results from the Canadian Pediatric Rheumatology Association Disease Registry. *J Rheumatol* 1996; **23**: 1981–7.

18. Eccleston C, Malleson PN, Clinch J, Connell H, Sourbut C. Chronic pain in adolescents: Evaluation of inter-disciplinary cognitive-behaviour therapy (CBT). *Arch Dis Child* 2003; **88**: 881–5.

19. Weydert JA, Ball TM, Davis MF. Systematic review of treatments for recurrent abdominal pain. *Pediatrics* 2003; **111**: e1–e11.

20. Eccleston C, Morley S, Williams A, Yorke L, Mastroyannopoulou K. Systematic review of randomized controlled trials of psychological therapy for chronic pain in children and adolescents, with a subset meta-analysis of pain relief. *Pain* 2002; **99**: 157–65.

21. Holden EW, Deichmann MM, Levy JD. Empirically-supported treatments in pediatric psychology: Recurrent pediatric headache. *J Pediatr Psychol* 1999; **24**: 91–109.

22. Huertas-Ceballos A, Logan S, Bennett C, Macarthur C. Psychosocial interventions for recurrent abdominal pain (RAP) and irritable bowel syndrome (IBS) in childhood. *Cochrane Database Syst Rev* 2008; **23**: CD003014.

23. Janicke DM, Finney JW. Empirically supported treatments in pediatric psychology: Recurrent abdominal pain. *J Pediatr Psychol* 1999; **24**: 115–27.

24. Kashikar-Zuck S, Graham TB, Huenefeld MD, Powers SW. A review of biobehavioral research in juvenile primary fibromyalgia syndrome. *Arthritis Care Res* 2000; 13: 388–97.

25. Harding V, Williams C de C. Extending physiotherapy skills using a psychological approach: Cognitive-behavioural management of chronic pain. *Physiotherapy* 1995; **81**: 681–8.

26. Bursch B. Pain-associated disability syndrome. In *Pediatric Functional Gastrointestinal Disorders,* ed. P Hyman. (New York: Academy Professional Information Services, 1999), pp. 8.1–8.14.

27. Hymam PE, Bursch, B, Sood M, *et al.* Visceral pain-associated disability syndrome: a dexcriptive analysis. *J Ped Gast Nutr* 2002; **35**: 663–8.

28. Gatchel RJ, Okifuji A. Evidence-based scientific data documenting the treatment and cost-effectiveness of comprehensive pain programs for chronic malignant pain. *J Pain* 2006; **7**: 779–93.

29. Turk DC. Clinical effectiveness and cost-effectiveness of treatments for patients with chronic pain. *Clin J Pain* 2002; **18**: 355–65.

30. Engel GL. The need for a new medical model: A challenge for biomedicine. *Science* 1977; **196**: 129–36.

31. Walker LS. The evolution of research on recurrent abdominal pain: History, assumptions, and a conceptual model. In *Chronic and Recurrent Pain in Children and Adolescents,* eds. PJ McGrath and GA Finley. (Seattle: International Association for the Study of Pain, 1999), pp. 141–72.

32. Hayes SC, Strosahl KD, Wilson KG. *Acceptance and Commitment Therapy: An experiential approach to behavior change.* (New York: Guilford Press, 1999).

33. McCracken LM, Vowles KE, Eccleston C. Acceptance-based treatment for persons with complex, long standing chronic pain: A preliminary analysis of treatment outcome in comparison to a waiting phase. *Behav Res Ther* 2004; **43**: 1335–46.

34. Wicksell RK. Value-based exposure and acceptance in the treatment of pediatric chronic pain: From symptom reduction to valued living. *Pediatric Pain Letter* 2007; **9**: 13–20.

35. Crombez G, Vlaeyen JW, Heuts PH, Lysens R. Pain-related fear is more disabling than pain itself: Evidence on the role of pain-related fear in chronic back pain disability. *Pain* 1999; **80**: 329–39.

36. McCracken LM. Learning to live with the pain: Acceptance of pain predicts adjustment in persons with chronic pain. *Pain* 1998; **74**: 21–7.

37. Viane I, Crombez G, Eccleston C, *et al.* Acceptance of pain is an independent predictor of mental well-being in patients with chronic pain: Empirical evidence and reappraisal. *Pain* 2003; **106**: 65–72.

38. Wicksell RK, Melin L, Olsson G. Exposure and acceptance in the rehabilitation of adolescents with idiopathic chronic pain – a pilot study. *Eur J Pain* 2007; **11**: 267–74.

39. Greco LA, Blomquist KK, Acrea S, Moulton D. Acceptance and commitment therapy for adolescents with functional abdominal pain: Results of a polit investigation. Manuscript submitted for pbulicaton 2008.

40. Sherry DD, Wallace CA, Kelley C, Kidder M, Sapp L. Short- and long-term outcomes of children with complex regional pain syndrome type 1 treated with exercise therapy. *Clin J Pain* 1999; **15**: 218–23.

41. Lee BH, Scharff L, Sethna NF, *et al.* Physical therapy and cognitive-behavioral treatment for complex regional pain syndromes. *J Pediatr* 2002; **141**: 135–40.

42. Calvert P, Jureidini J. Restrained rehabilitation: an approach to children and adolescents with unexplained signs and symptoms. *Arch Dis Child* 2003; **88**: 399–402.

43. Zeltzer LK, Schlank CB. *Conquering Your Child's Pain: A pediatrician's guide for reclaiming a normal childhood.* (New York: HarperCollins, 2005).

44. Masek BJ, Russo DC, Varni JW. Behavioral approaches to the management of chronic pain in children. *Pediatr Clin North Am* 1984; **31**: 1113–31.

45. Ho GH, Bennett SM, Cox D, Poole G. Brief report: Cognitive functioning and academic achievement in children and adolescents with chronic pain. *J Pediatr Psychol* 2009; **34**: 311–6.

46. Logan DE, Curran JA. Adolescent chronic pain problems in the school setting: Exploring the experiences and beliefs of selected school personnel through focus group methodology. *J Adolesc Health* 2005; **37**: 281–5.

47. Walker LS, Green JW. Children with recurrent abdominal pain and their parents: More somatic complaints, anxiety, and depression than other parent groups. *J Pediatr Psychol* 1989; **12**: 224–31.

48. Wasserman AL, Whitington PF, Rivara FP. Psychogenic basis for abdominal pain in children and adolescents. *J Am Acad Child Adolesc Psychiatry* 1988; **27**: 179–84.

49. Osborne RB, Hatcher JW, Richtsmeier AJ. The role of social modeling in unexplained pediatric pain. *J Pediatr Psychol* 1989; **14**: 43–61.

Management of pain in geriatric patients

Stephen Thielke and M. Carrington Reid

During their third year medicine-surgery clerkships, medical students were observed to become less idealistic about two groups of patients: the elderly and people with chronic pain [1]. Working with elderly patients in pain may thus not only challenge the skills of clinicians, but also frustrate their ideals and expectations about their work. We begin with this observation to suggest that improving pain treatment in older adults is not simply a matter of prescribing the right treatment for the disease and the patient, but also of addressing the psychological barriers that clinicians and patients both face in their attempts to deal with pain.

We will argue that the primary difficulty with treating pain in older adults is not the lack of evidence-based treatments, since many exist, but rather the beliefs, expectations, and patterns of behaviors around chronic pain that impair use of potentially effective treatments. In other chronic medical conditions such as hypertension, congestive heart failure, and diabetes, the gap between available treatments and their real-world use is substantial, and adherence to treatment regimens is often low [2]. But the treatment of chronic pain among older adults entails even more complicating issues, such as beliefs about whether pain symptoms are a normal part of aging, whether they should be treated, and whether the treatments are dangerous. Our discussion will focus less on the evidence for specific treatments, and more on how patients use them, what they think of them, and how providers can promote their effective use. We propose that these patient-level and service-related factors are more important for improving the health of older adults with pain than are comparisons of efficacy from controlled studies.

We do not attempt to present a comprehensive approach to the older patient in pain. A number of excellent and updated general reviews of pain in aging exist, many of which include extensive evidence-based recommendations (see Table 24.1). These reviews confirm that chronic pain is a highly prevalent, costly, and often disabling disorder in later life. Prevalence studies indicate that as many as 40% to 50% of older adults report the presence of a chronic pain disorder. The deleterious consequences of inadequately treated pain are far-reaching and include impaired quality of life, sleep, immune function, physical functioning, as well as impairment in activities of daily living (ADLs). Indeed, among older women, pain is the most commonly reported cause of ADL impairment. Interested readers are encouraged to review these publications along with other relevant resources which are included in Table 24.1. In this chapter, we seek to keep a patient-centered rather than disease-centered focus, and to address the most important perspectives on pain in aging that may be new to readers. We introduce this chapter by discussing common myths about aging and pain. We then review research on current treatments that older adults currently use for pain, synthesize the literature about beliefs that patients express about pain and pain treatments, and discuss patients' treatment preferences. Finally, we examine barriers that interfere with more effective pain treatment, and make recommendations for how clinicians can improve treatment of pain in older adults.

Myths of pain and aging

Patients and clinicians have a variety of preconceptions about pain and aging. Unfortunately, most are never scrutinized. For instance, in focus groups of older patients with osteoarthritis, many patients perceived pain as a part of normal aging that required acceptance, not treatment, and their physicians seemed complicit in that. One respondent stated about her pain: "My doctor tells me all the time, 'You're just getting older'"; another remarked, "So I showed my family doctor [where I hurt] and she said it's going to get worse you know. Get used to it." [3]. Some of the key beliefs about pain and aging

---

Behavioral and Psychopharmacologic Pain Management, ed. Michael H. Ebert and Robert D. Kerns. Published by Cambridge University Press. © Cambridge University Press 2011.

commonly expressed are: that pain is a part of getting older; that pain worsens as people get older; that older adults get used to pain; and that patients seek medical treatment as the main way of dealing with pain. These beliefs have more than academic importance, because the values that patients and providers hold about pain and its treatments, and their expectations about these, determine health service use, clinical decisions, and self-management. Examining these preconceptions empirically shows that few of them are true, and suggests further that they stem from oversimplified, stereotyped, and anachronistic notions.

Myth number 1: Pain is a part of getting older

The apparently high prevalence of pain complaints among older adults often leads to the conclusion that normal aging causes pain. Up to two-thirds of older Americans have been found to report persistent pain [4], and as many as 83% of older adults report pain that interferes with daily activities and quality of life [5]. Older age predicts more likely onset of and failure to recover from persistent pain among primary care patients [6]. Many providers approach pain as if it were inevitable as patients get older, advising patients to "get used to it" [3]. These observations, as well as many stereotypes of older adults complaining increasingly of pain, seem to demonstrate that pain is to be expected as people age.

This conclusion is, on further examination, specious in several ways. While the prevalence of chronic pain complaints may be high in older populations, it is not consistently higher with advancing age. A Centers for Disease Control survey conducted from 1999 to 2002 found that any sort of pain persisting for more than 24 hours in the month prior to the interview was reported by 29% of 45–64 year-olds but only 21% of those 65 years and older [7]. A meta-analysis of differences in pain perception with advancing age found that the highest prevalence of chronic pain occurred at about age 65, after which there was a slight decline with advancing age, even beyond age 85 [8]. Other research about the epidemiology of pain across the lifespan have found that the frequency of chronic pain either declines with age [9], or demonstrates no strong association with age [10]. Clinically, many types of pain complaints occur less commonly with advancing age, such as headache, abdominal pain, and chest pain [11], and population-based studies show a lower prevalence of low back, neck, and face pain, as well as migraine or severe headache, among older compared to younger adults [7].

These studies illustrate that pain is not an inevitable consequence of aging, and that for many types of pain and in many circumstances older adults report less chronic pain than their younger counterparts. The evidence refutes preconceptions that most of the pain associated with advanced age is inevitable. While certain types of pain, especially osteoarthritis, increase in prevalence, there is little evidence that the symptoms of pain in general become more common with age.

Myth number 2: Pain worsens as people get older

Both patients and clinicians often express the expectation that pain is more intense and intractable among older compared to younger adults. This belief is encapsulated in the patient's description of the doctor saying that "it's going to get worse you know" [3]. Studies examining the beliefs of patients about aging and pain have confirmed this theme. For instance, older (over 70 years) compared with younger patients were more likely to believe that people should expect to live with pain as they get older [12]. More than one-quarter of patients with osteoarthritis expressed the belief that this disease always gets worse with increasing age [13]. Patients of all ages expressed the belief that aging is associated with greater susceptibility to and suffering from pain [14].

Research on the experience of pain in older adults generates a much more complex picture. First, different individuals experience pain and its sequelae quite differently. Assessments of patients using standardized multiaxial pain measures have indicated that there are at least three primary clusters of pain and pain-related symptoms: about one-quarter with less intense pain, less frequent depression, and less sleep disruption, about one-third with more pain and more functional disability, and the remainder with a combination of characteristics [15]. More general research on symptomatology with advancing age shows that there is enormous heterogeneity in how older adults report and are affected by similar medical complaints [16]. Second, longitudinal studies examining the course of chronic pain complaints corroborate this heterogeneity and disprove any consistent worsening with age. In a cohort of adults with hip and knee osteoarthritis, pain and disability generally worsened over 7 years, but 35% of those initially reporting hip pain and 29% of those initially reporting knee pain improved [17]. Likewise, pain and functional status in knee and hip osteoarthritis has been found to deteriorate slowly, with little change after 3 years of follow-up, and many patients showed improvement [18]. Third, the factors found to be protective against decline in pain-related functioning are telling. Among patients with knee osteoarthritis, these factors include higher levels of joint strength, mental health, self-efficacy, social support, and activity [19]. This finding clearly contradicts the purely biological paradigm in which pain is posited to worsen progressively as a factor of years lived. There is even some evidence that older adults cope better with pain than do their younger counterparts: compared with younger people in pain, older people in pain had higher total quality of life scores, were more satisfied with their material comforts and social life, and reported better mood [20].

Despite the absence of clear age-related trends, there is strong evidence that pain is associated with significant impairments in physical functioning and mental health throughout aging. Persistent hip or knee pain has been found to result in significant declines in physical functioning, as measured by the SF-36 [21, 22]. Increasing number of months of activity-restricting back pain has been shown to be a strong and independent predictor of worsening lower extremity strength [23]. There is a strong direct association between depression and degree of pain severity among older (age 70 and over) but not younger patients [24]. Depression is very strongly associated with pain in older adults, as indicated by numerous lines of research: older adults with chronic pain are far more likely to be depressed than those without pain [25]; significantly more adults with osteorathritis pain have major or minor depression compared to those without it [26]; osteoarthritis pain is strongly associated with depression symptoms and poor perceived health [27], and the strongest predictor of depression in an osteoarthritis cohort was perceived pain [28]. These effects seem also to carry over into treatments applied for pain: more days of activity limitation and poor mental health were strongly associated with a decreased odds of analgesic or antiinflammatory use [29]. Chronic pain may thus not worsen with advancing age, but continues to negatively impact older individuals' functioning, mental health, and use of treatments.

Myth number 3: Older adults get used to living with pain

Physicians who advise older patients living with pain to "get used to it" tacitly suggest that this technique might work, and that older people can acclimate to the experience of pain. There is some evidence that nociception changes with advancing age [30], which might be interpreted to suggest that older adults suffer less for the same amount of tissue pathology. The findings described above about how older adults may cope with pain better than younger adults do [20] could imply that pain has less of an effect on the elderly. Patients may talk as if they had indeed gotten used to living with pain, or that their pain tolerance had increased over time [31].

While the degree of suffering or distress that pain causes in different groups is impossible to measure objectively, some evidence about the effects of pain on the health of aging adults can be inferred from empirical studies. If older adults became used to living with pain, or if pain became a normal part of aging, one would expect that the associated deleterious consequences would become mitigated with age. We will present research about the association of pain with two such associated outcomes, depression and insomnia, and conclude that pain continues to exert a powerful negative effect on individuals throughout the aging process.

There is no simple framework that explains the causal relationship between depression and pain with advancing age, although the association is very strong. For instance, it is not well established whether depression causes pain, pain causes depression, or there is a bidirectional effect. As described above, degree of pain is more strongly associated with depression in older than younger adults [24], which challenges the preconception that older adults might show less mental health effects from pain. In age-related pain conditions, pain negatively impacts depression and increases health service utilization [26, 32]. Among older adults with pain, depression, or both, those with depression combined with pain were more likely to show new functional limitations and to have higher total healthcare expenditures, with no decrease in this association with age [33]. Among elderly nursing home residents, many of whom have significant functional impairments, pain is strongly associated with depression [34]. The negative effects of pain on depression treatment have been described in a variety of older adult populations, and increased pain seems to reduce the likelihood that depression will improve with treatment [35–37]. These data strongly argue against the expectation that older adults can or do get used to living with pain, and indicate that pain exerts persistent powerful negative effects on older adults' mental health.

Sleep is another domain in which pain continues to be associated with negative health effects. Among

older adults with pain, sleep disruption is highly prevalent: 31% reported problems with sleep onset, 81%
with sleep maintenance, and 51% with early morning
awakenings [38]. Pain-related sleep difficulties were
also associated with poorer self-rated health, poorer
physical functioning, and depressive symptoms. In a
national sample of adults, 24.8% of those with arthritis described insomnia, roughly twice the prevalence
among those without arthritis, and pain was a strong
predictor of insomnia [39]. There is thus no evidence
that older adults get used to pain's effects on sleep.

While this research suggests that people do not
acclimate to pain with advancing age, there is some
evidence that older adults complain less about pain
than their younger counterparts. Older adults are often
reticent about pain, or reluctant to label a sensation as
painful [40]. Other research has found that older adults
minimize and underreport pain [41–43]. Older adults
with pain commonly express stoical beliefs about pain,
such as that it is better endured than treated [3, 31]. This
difference in expression may promote the myth of how
older adults get used to living with pain, since in complaining less they appear hardened to it. This research
shows no clear age-related differences in nociception
or the sequelae of pain, but rather suggests consistent
negative effects of pain across all ages, with a more stoical attitude among many older adults.

Myth number 4: Older adults seek medical treatment as the primary way of dealing with pain

From one perspective, medical treatments for pain
could be seen as a success. Healthcare professionals,
including allopathic, complementary, and alternative
providers, perceive their treatments to be first-line, primary mechanisms to relieve pain. They conceptualize
pain as a medical problem, recommend treatments to
patients that are considered evidence-based, and generally believe in the efficacy of their recommendations.
In controlled studies, there are in fact many treatments
for chronic pain that are superior to placebo [44].
Among older adults with chronic pain, 91% described
at least one effective strategy for reducing pain, and the
most common strategy (reported by 59%) was analgesic use [45]. One might thus expect that older adults
in pain were likely to receive medical treatments, especially medications, from their providers, and that these
treatments provided effective pain control. Yet a closer

examination of health services data regarding chronic
pain in older adults shows that this expectation about
the treatment of pain in medical settings is inaccurate
and overly optimistic. We find instead that most medical treatments for pain are suboptimal.

While pain is a common complaint and is assessed
as a "fifth vital sign" across clinical settings, providers
report frustration about interpreting and acting on
reports of pain, even expressing that they were subject
to the "tyranny of pain treatment." As one primary care
provider described:

> The problem is we are told over and over again [to treat pain]. I
> think it leads to some frustration that almost makes me not want
> to ask the question, "Are you in pain?" I'm like, Oh my god, I can't
> deal with it. If this patient has nine out of ten pain, you know the
> medical assistant asks the patient, Do you have pain? [The patient
> responds] Yes, I have nine out of ten pain. And then I'm supposed
> to ask the patient and write in my note how I dealt with the pain.
> And I don't have an answer. (AP Spitz, pers. comm.).

Another provider complained that the Joint Commission on Accreditation of Healthcare (JCAHO)-
mandated stipulation that physicians deal with all pain
above a score of five is impossible to satisfy. Nurses in
home care who communicate patients' pain to physicians describe receiving responses such as "What do
you want me to do with this?" or "I've tried everything
and failed – I can't help you" (Reid, personal communication). The nurses thus felt impotent and fearful about
asking patients about pain because it both did not lead
to any action and also frustrated the physicians. General
internists have expressed particular dissatisfaction about
prescribing opioid analgesics to older adults [46].

Research on patient perspectives discloses this
same theme. Patients describe how their providers
are less-than-eager to hear about pain symptoms, suggested by such advice as "get used to it". Representative
samples of older adults asked about their pain describe
low degrees and quality of medical treatment for it. In
a community sample in Finland, only about 35–40% of
those suffering joint or back pain that impaired daily
functioning had been prescribed an analgesic medication for regular use, and the researchers conclude that
"Pain is markedly undertreated in community-dwelling
older people" [47]. In a large study of older adults with
depression, only half of those who reported pain that
interfered with daily activities reported using a medication for it [48]. Opioid medications have been found
to be used less often for the same indications in older
compared with younger patients with chronic pain
[49]. Among older adults in nursing homes, one study

found that less than half of residents with predictably recurrent pain were prescribed scheduled medications [50], and another found that one-quarter of those with persistent pain were not receiving any analgesic [51]. Using all older adults with pain as the denominator, it appears that many or even the majority of patients with pain are not receiving any medical treatment for it.

Such research does not elucidate the processes underlying care provision for pain in aging adults. It is possible that older adults do not receive medical treatments because they do report pain at the time of a visit, or have side effects from medications, even though providers are applying evidence-based treatments. Yet other studies examining the quality of medical care provided to older patients suggest that chronic pain management is inadequate. Pain programs are less likely to include older adults than their younger counterparts with similar pain problems [52]. Among vulnerable older adults with pain, fewer than 40% reported having been screened for pain by their medical provider over a 2-year period [53]. The same study also showed that while treatment was offered to 86% of those patients identified with pain, follow-up occurred in only 66%. Fewer than two-thirds of patients prescribed opioids reported being offered a bowel regimen, and only 10% of patients prescribed non-steroidal anti-inflammatory drugs (NSAIDs) had appropriate attention paid to potential gastrointestinal toxicity. This research suggests that care for chronic pain in older vulnerable patients is inadequate across many domains: screening, clinical evaluation, follow-up, and attention to potential toxicities. Another study looking at quality indicators around measures of effective care and measures of medication safety for chronic pain in older adults found that both were suboptimal [54]. More subjectively, patients often report that their physicians do not endeavor to understand their concerns about pain treatment. As a study of a cohort with osteoarthritis concludes, "The lack of a patient-centered approach to care leads professionals to ignore key symptoms and issues for individuals, and to a preoccupation with pharmaceutical interventions, rather than treatment options that their patients prefer" [55].

An important mismatch between patient and provider perspectives occurs around the effectiveness of medical treatments. Providers frequently believe that they can offer strong and effective treatments, usually in the form of medications. Yet among older adults living in retirement facilities who reported persistent pain, the most helpful strategy was not medications or

prescribed treatments but prayer. Medications (opioids, NSAIDs, and acetaminophen) were rated as only moderately effective [56]. In another group, although use of analgesic medications was high (reported by 59%), 60% of participants described their pain as still "quite a bit" or "extremely" bothersome [45]. Among older veterans, few medical strategies for pain control were rated as effective [57]. Despite the enthusiasm about and evidence for many medical treatments for pain, the overall service provision for chronic pain in older adults seems inadequate, pain is often not treated, and when it is treated the outcomes are only marginally successful. It may be surprising to clinicians, who are used to equating more adherence with better health, that individuals in pain who described less adherence to pain medications and made fewer visits to the doctor reported better quality of life [58]. While this certainly does not prove that taking medications or seeking medical care impairs quality of life, and while there is considerable selection bias around the use of healthcare for pain, such findings challenge providers' expectations that their prescriptions, when followed, lead to improved patient outcomes.

The next sections, which examine how older adults attempt to treat their pain and what they believe about and prefer in pain treatments, illustrate that many of the approaches used and preferred by patients are not recommended or prescribed by providers, and that patients have very different beliefs about pain than do providers. Medical providers have little grounds for perceiving their treatments as either particularly effective or successful in helping the bulk of older adults who live with pain.

How do older adults treat their pain?

There has been extensive research about treatments used for chronic pain among older adults, most of which challenges the preconceptions described above. The most general finding, that appears throughout qualitative and epidemiological research, is that older adults apply many non-medical and medical strategies for coping with pain, and treat pain as different from their other chronic medical conditions. A telling example of this theme has been uncovered in a cohort of patients aging with osteoarthritis: while most patients took analgesics, they took them at lower doses and less often than recommended, and adhered to analgesics differently than to medications for other chronic conditions [27].

Only 26% took the medications at the full dose recommended, but 94% reported taking at least one herbal remedy or vitamin for their arthritis. Some patients even reported taking their analgesic as prescribed until the time they learned that it was an analgesic, at which point they decreased the dose and limited their use of it. The behaviors and beliefs described by participants reveal how oversimplified a purely medical focus on choosing "the right drug at the right dose" is. In examining the current approaches older adults use to cope with pain, we will address in the following sections both the material treatments (such as activities or medications), as well as the cognitive approaches (such as stoicism or ignoring pain) that have been identified.

Surveys of older adults with persistent pain disclose that they use a mixture of both medical and nonmedical treatments. Among adults aged 65 years and older living in retirement facilities with persistent pain, the most frequently employed treatments included acetaminophen, regular exercise, prayer, and heat and cold. As strategies for controlling pain these treatments were characterized by participants as only moderately helpful at best [56]. Older veterans with chronic pain described a variety of common coping strategies: analgesic medications (78%), exercise (35%), cognitive methods (37%), religious activities (21%), and activity restrictions (20%) [57]. Community-dwelling older adults, when asked to describe their coping mechanisms, reported using exercise, heat and cold, and medications, with medications considered a treatment of last resort [59]. There are likely important cultural differences in the use of oral medications as a treatment for pain: among older adults residing in Hong Kong who reported chronic pain, the majority used non-prescription interventions, most commonly topical analgesics with massage, while only one in five took an oral agent [60]. The majority of participants (58%) perceived non-pharmacologic interventions as very effective, which also differs from the findings among American adults. The application of physical modalities has been found to be generally low in the USA: in a cross-sectional survey of older adults receiving longitudinal care in a geriatric ambulatory care practice, only 16% used exercise and 4% used relaxation to deal with chronic pain, although most were interested in learning about or trying these approaches [61].

The cognitive strategies that older adults apply to deal with pain demonstrate that, even though there is a great deal of heterogeneity and plasticity in how older adults cope with pain [62], there are a number of commonly used approaches. Older adults with chronic pain reported coping with pain most frequently through task persistence (ignoring pain and continuing an activity despite pain), pacing (taking breaks, going slower, and breaking tasks into manageable components), and coping self-statements (purposefully thinking positive thoughts about the pain problem) [63, 64]. The use of guarding (restricting the use or movement of a body part) was found to be a strong predictor of disability. Among community-dwelling older adults, the two most common themes for coping with pain were ignoring the pain and distraction [59]. Interviews with older adults with pain who received home care defined two groups based on their response to pain, the "competent and proud / confident and serene", and the "misunderstood and disappointed / resigned and sad" [65]. Across both groups the most common behavioral strategies used were taking medication, rest, distracting activities, and talking about pain. Respondents reported that they chose strategies by balancing advantages of the activities against the disadvantages these caused for their daily living. Certain pain coping strategies have been found to be strongly associated with self-efficacy and better outcomes, including task persistence, exercise/stretching, coping self-statements, and activity pacing [66].

This research shows that while older adults use a variety of material and cognitive approaches for coping with pain, there appears to be no optimal or preferred strategy, and most of the strategies are described as only moderately beneficial. Medication use is common, but may be less common than non-medical approaches such as herbal supplements or vitamins, but the evidence about this in large populations is limited. Physical modalities seem to be used by a minority of older persons with pain. Older adults reported various ways of coping psychologically with pain, some of which may predict better outcomes. Our review highlights that, within the heterogeneity of treatments and tactics, older adults actively work to manage pain on their own, often without involving their medical providers.

Beliefs about pain and pain treatments

The real-world approaches for coping with chronic pain differ considerably from those that are based on efficacy studies [67]. In order to understand this mismatch, it is important to examine the beliefs that older adults and their providers hold about pain and pain treatments. Beliefs are very important in patients' readiness and capacity to self-manage pain [68], and in how providers approach patients with pain. Although most of this research has focused on patients, important differences in patient and provider beliefs about pain and pain treatment have also been identified, as described below.

Patients often express beliefs about pain that may surprise providers. In a survey of older adults, about one-quarter expressed the belief that nothing could be done with osteoarthritis, and many were fatalistic about the cause and course of the disease and nihilistic about its treatment [69]. In-depth qualitative interviews with older patients with osteoarthritis have demonstrated how perceptions and attitudes about pain and pain medications play an integral role in how older adults approach pain [31]. Many patients reported a high pain tolerance despite experiencing pain-related functional limitations and sleep disturbance, as revealed in comments such as, "I can stand more pain than most people." Pain was seen to be a regular part of life during the aging process: "that's how you know you're alive … you ache." Most of the participants considered medications to be dangerous and dose changes unacceptable: "I don't fool around with my medications. I know a few people who have … bless them … they are not around any longer." Fear of addiction was a major concern for some participants, and some saw using medications as a sign of weakness: "I used to take [painkillers] more often. I think I was a little softer then… I don't take them unless I am really upset about my pain." These patients were quite reluctant to use medications, and generally limited their use.

The contrasts between patients' beliefs and expectations compared to those of primary care providers have been explored in more detail [70]. First, providers focused mainly on biomedical causes of pain, while patients focused on the subjective experience of pain. Second, patients expected straightforward communication about their pain, but often did not receive it during medical appointments. They found it very important to receive a physical exam regardless of the pain complaint, an expectation that was not shared by providers. Third, patients stressed the importance of being trusted by their providers, noting that previous providers had frequently dismissed them as malingerers. In the rubric of trust, patients considered referral for tests as a sign that their problems were taken seriously by providers. Fourth, while patients reported that

education about pain was important, they felt that it was generally impractical, vague, or unclear, and providers felt that there was insufficient time to educate patients. Another study found that older patients with chronic pain and their healthcare providers often had opposing attitudes and goals: providers were focused on diagnosis and treatments, while patients sought to be understood as individuals and to address quality of life, and struggled to have their pain concerns legitimized [71].

Research in primary care settings has confirmed this disconnect between patients and providers. In one recent study, patients, primary care providers, and nurses were surveyed about their expectations about and barriers to providing better management of osteoarthritis [72]. In another study, patients with arthritis were interviewed about their experience of the illness and the care they received for it [73]. In both investigations, patients were found to be worried largely about disability and worsening of their disease, while primary care providers focused mostly on diagnosis. Patients sought to learn about non-pharmacologic and non-traditional health management topics, but providers found it difficult to provide this information. Patients sought lifestyle changes to improve their pain, but providers did not know how to make these types of recommendations. Patients were very worried about medication side effects, but providers and nurses felt they lacked time to discuss this issue with patients. Interestingly, most of the providers' insecurity centered around learning and following official guidelines for treating pain, an issue that lacked importance for patients. A qualitative study that examined both primary care provider and patient attitudes and experiences using opioids as a treatment for chronic pain found that providers voiced strong reluctance to prescribe this class of medications for older patients because of concerns about causing harm (AP Spitz, personal communication). Patients frequently reported the need for better education regarding the need for and use of these strong pain relievers, but expressed willingness to take an opioid for pain if prescribed.

Within all these qualitative differences between what patients and providers believe about pain treatments appears the general theme of providers' enthusiasm and patients' skepticism. This has been found explicitly in research looking at perceived effectiveness of pain treatments among older adults who require professional help in their activities of daily living: care providers perceived that most of the methods for managing pain were more effective than the patients did [65]. It would not be surprising that those experiencing pain and those observing or hearing about it would have different interpretations of it, but the trend towards providers' more optimistic beliefs about treatment success is noteworthy and important. There may also be gender effects in providers' beliefs about patients' pain: in a study of pain in primary care, female patients found it more difficult to communicate with physicians about pain, and providers seemed to interpret men's pain symptoms more seriously than women's [74].

Patient preferences for pain treatment

The preferences that older patients express about pain treatments match closely with their pain beliefs and expectations, and illustrate some of the barriers to applying existing treatments. Research has clarified both general preferences for treatment and preferences about specific modalities. A qualitative study of older adults with chronic pain in Australia found that they generally wished to be active in their treatment, to make informed choices, and to try new methods [75]. While few strategies appealed uniformly to all the participants, they preferred approaches that could be self-administered and included both physical and cognitive elements. At the same time, some specific strategies were identified as being least preferred, including conventional treatments such as analgesic medications, exercise, and physiotherapy. The key barriers identified to using treatments were cost, access to care, related medical conditions, attitudes of health professionals about pain, lack of communication, and fear of losing independence. Another study of older adults with persistent musculoskeletal pain highlighted the importance of using approaches besides medications, which were considered a treatment of last resort [59]. Incorporating family and friends in the decision-making process was considered to be very important in decision-making about pain, with physicians mentioned as important only when other approaches did not work. This preference for using treatments besides medications and for avoiding discussion with physicians demonstrates again how older adults do not treat chronic pain as purely or primarily a medical problem, a finding that may surprise medical providers.

Research has elicited specific preferences about medications for pain in later life, especially osteoarthritis. Patients have been found to prefer topical treatments such as capsaicin over oral agents, and to

dislike non-selective NSAIDs [76]. COX-2 inhibitors were preferred only if they were reported as being three times as effective as capsaicin and low-cost. Safety seemed to be a key factor in this decision, since all patients switched preferences when offered a safer but less effective treatment option [77]. Side effect severity has been identified as a strong predictor of health state preference [78]. Patients with osteoarthritis pain have shown considerable variety in their willingness to accept risks in exchange for improvements in pain control [79]. About 20% were unwilling to accept any additional risk for reductions in pain, and the remainder were willing to accept some additional risk of serious medical complications (stomach bleed or heart attack/stroke) for an improvement in pain relief. There may be differences in risk acceptance with age, since older patients with osteoarthritis seem to be more willing than younger patients to accept an increased risk of serious side effects for an improvement in pain symptoms [80]. These preferences contrast markedly with observed provider behaviors: of patients presenting for initial primary consultation for symptomatic knee or hip pain, over half were prescribed NSAIDs, and 15% were prescribed a potentially unsafe NSAID [81].

Despite the preferences elicited, patient knowledge about the real mechanisms and risks of medications has been found to be quite low. The majority of patients with osteoarthritis were unaware of any specific adverse effects from COX-2 inhibitors or NSAIDs [76] despite expressing a preference for the former. An examination of patient knowledge about osteoarthritis found that the majority were not able to describe side effects of analgesics, and that less than one-third knew that they could take pain medications prophylactically [13]. As noted earlier, many older adults characterize pain medications as dangerous or addictive [3, 31], which would naturally discourage their use, but it is unclear if improved knowledge about the real safety risks would change preferences.

Key barriers to improving pain management in older adultS

Examining the approaches older adults use to cope with pain, their beliefs about pain and pain treatments, and their preferences regarding specific treatments delineates several key barriers to better pain management of older adults in medical settings. We will discuss those areas with the most relevance to clinical settings, with a particular focus on provider-level barriers.

Provider discomfort

Although there has been little research about how providers experience treating older patients with chronic pain, it seems to be a particularly difficult task [82]. Only 34% of primary care physicians felt comfortable managing patients with chronic non-malignant pain [83]. Education increased their comfort, and seemed to have the greatest effect when pain management skills were taught after rather than during residency training. As mentioned earlier, medical students have been found to become less idealistic about older patients and patients in chronic pain [1]. Physicians appear to find it difficult to communicate about chronic pain, and less than one-third of patients with osteoarthritis reported receiving any information about it from their primary care provider [84]. Providers have difficulty communicating about lifestyle changes and other non-medical approaches to pain [72], and patients wish that they could learn more about topics which their physicians often do not cover [73]. From a shared decision-making perspective, patient–provider interactions about pain show poor communication [71]. The challenges involved in treating and communicating with older adults in pain likely stem from the issues discussed above, and relate to additional barriers described below.

Values and expectancies about pain in aging

The variety of values and expectancies about pain and pain treatments held by both patients and providers constitute significant barriers to effective care. The beliefs that pain is just a part of getting older or that people get used to living with pain are common, and encourage tolerance and stoicism rather than treatment. If patients or providers believe that the condition is intractable or that stoicism is the best approach to dealing with pain, it is unlikely that effective treatments will be sought, recommended, or prescribed. Providers value finding the right diagnosis and medical treatments, but older patients focus more on the subjective experience of pain and its effects on quality of life, and some patients have expressed that medical care from physicians is the last-resort option for dealing with pain. Many patients expect that medical treatments for pain are dangerous and only moderately effective, and that the risks are not worth the benefits. Providers often are more optimistic than patients about the degree to which treatments can ameliorate pain, and they generally consider their evidence-based treatments to be the gold standard. These points of mismatch between provider and patient perspectives may interfere with effective provision of care, especially in the ability to communicate about what causes pain, how it will change over time, what effects it will have, and how one should treat it.

Beliefs about medications

A specific area in which beliefs are integral to the behaviors of both patients and providers is the use of analgesic medications. Oral medications, either prescription or non-prescription, are the most common treatments recommended for older adults with pain, yet they are often described by patients as the least preferred treatments. Patients consistently report taking less medication than recommended, and adhering to analgesics differently than to other medications [31]. Most providers seem to eschew this dilemma, and recommend or prescribe medications in a matter-of-fact manner. Their tacit assumptions about medication-related behaviors are, "If I recommend the pill, the patient will take it." And "If the pill works, the patient will continue to take it." Yet as we have seen, neither of these assumptions holds, and patient behaviors around analgesics are anything but straightforward. Numerous factors predict adherence to medications, and involve a patient's implicit cost-benefit analysis of prognosis, effectiveness, risks, and social appropriateness, as well as other cultural and contextual issues [85, 86].

The topic of adherence to medications is complicated, and low adherence is certainly not limited to analgesic agents, but addressing adherence and medication-related beliefs may be especially important in attempting to improve pain treatments. The following general conclusion about adherence highlights the root of the problem: "The main reason why people do not take their medications as prescribed is not because of failings in patients, doctors, or systems, but because of concerns about the medications themselves. On the whole, the findings point to considerable reluctance to take medicine and a preference to take it as little as possible" [2]. This understanding of medication use is substantially different from the simplistic goal of "finding the right drug to help a patient with a particular kind of pain," and attempting to apply such a purely medical model will likely hinder the dialogue between patients and providers about medications.

Associated conditions

While co-morbidity demands attention in all aspects of geriatric care, pain appears to be associated with several other hard-to-treat conditions. As discussed above, pain and depression commonly occur together, and pain impedes improvements in depression. Depressed patients are a challenge even if they are not in pain, and depression interferes with patients' ability to self-manage medical problems, to initiate and sustain effective treatments, and to become activated. Late-life depression is also very hard to treat in primary care settings, with fewer than one-quarter of depressed older adults showing a significant symptom reduction at 12 months [87]. Given the close link between depression and pain, and the difficulty in separating out psychic from physical pain, it can be very challenging for providers to treat both simultaneously. Similarly, the high prevalence of sleep disturbance among older adults with chronic pain can confound their care. The association between sleep difficulties, pain, poorer self-rated health, poorer physical functioning, and depressive symptoms [38] illustrates the complexity and challenge that older patients with pain present for busy providers. Finally, obesity has been found to be strongly associated with chronic pain among older adults – compared to those with normal weight (BMI 18.5–24.9), older obese subjects (BMI 30–34.9) were twice as likely to report chronic pain, and severely obese (BMI ≥ 35) were more than four times as likely [88]. Weight loss is, like pain control, easy to recommend but hard to accomplish, and patients who are both obese and in pain present a particular dilemma for clinicians, especially if the obesity is considered to be a major factor in the pain. While none of these conditions – pain, depression, sleep problems, or obesity – are entirely intractable in older adults, addressing them necessitates a broad biopsychosocial approach, consideration of the patients' beliefs and expectations, and education about pain, treatment, and risks, all of which are hard to provide in busy clinical settings.

Environmental constraints

There are several specific barriers to effective pain management in older adults which may impact use of treatments. Time conflicts and transportation have been identified as barriers to using exercise and relaxation programs [61]. Cost may hinder some older adults from using specific treatments for chronic pain [75]. Over half of older adults taking analgesic medications have problems opening bottle caps [89]. Cognitive impairments also make it more difficult for patients to self-manage pain [90]. While most of this discussion has addressed cognitive rather than environmental barriers, the ability to start and continue treatments is important as well, and merits careful attention from providers.

How can providers improve pain management?

We attempt to distill the various research findings described here into suggestions for ways to address the primary barriers to effective management of pain in older adults. These are not evidence-based recommendations, but rather follow logically from the previously described findings.

Recognize that pain is poorly treated in older adults, mainly through undertreatment

While there are some cases of medication abuse or dependence, the overwhelming finding of this review is that pain among older adults is "markedly undertreated" [47]. Providers can and should do more to treat pain in older adults – not through standard approaches, many of which are not preferred by patients, but rather by finding better ways of engaging patients in managing their pain. Some of these ways are described below.

Fight myths of pain and aging

This review has documented that both patients and providers can hold distorted ideas about pain and aging. Recognizing and challenging these preconceptions in clinical settings – including those of front-line staff (e.g., nurses aides) and primary care providers (e.g., nurse practitioners and physicians) – is an important first step in initiating and sustaining a dialogue about how best to treat pain. The goals of treating chronic pain in older adults are no different than in younger adults, and providers need not lower their expectations for patients who are older, have cognitive impairments, or suffer from other co-morbidities. Instead, providers who are attentive to treating pain in older adults will frame pain management in a patient-specific context that incorporates the patient's beliefs, expectations, and behaviors around aging, pain, quality of life, mental health, and the risks and benefits of various treatments. It is promising that a previous investigation found that the majority of older adults with pain could be managed successfully in primary care, and did not require treatment in specialty pain clinics [91].

Do not make the final goal "to apply the right evidence-based treatment"

While evidence from research studies is important in assessing the merits of various treatments, our review highlights the gap between evidence, real use, and real-world benefits. What stops treatments from working is not that the treatments are not good enough, but rather that patients are not using them. The factors that hinder use of any treatment have been developed in the research presented here: beliefs and expectations about pain and aging, beliefs and expectations about the treatment, experience from prior treatment trials, material barriers to undertaking certain actions, and aversion to undertake risk. In this light, choosing a good treatment is just the first step, and attention to the other cognitive and behavioral factors constitutes the real work of pain management. Remembering patient preferences may be essential in this process. As demonstrated in one study, giving patients a choice about which interventions to apply, instead of prescribing the one that seems the most evidence-based, produced better outcomes for older adults with pain [92].

Address and treat depression

While depression merits treatment in its own right, the strong association of pain with depression in older adults argues for attentive treatment of mental health symptoms. There is some evidence that treating depression in older adults with pain reduces pain and improves functional status and quality of life [93]. This certainly does not indicate that depression should be treated instead of pain, but rather that depression should not be ignored, and that one should not assume that patients in pain become depressed naturally, as a result of hurting. There are novel approaches to collaborative care for depression and pain together that show significant reductions in pain and moderate reductions in depression [94], and these may be adapted in the future for all older adults with pain.

Elicit and discuss the patient's beliefs and preferences

Our discussion has also emphasized how important beliefs are regarding the ways that patients apply medical treatments and manage their pain. Patients engage in a heterogeneous, complex, and plastic process of coping with pain. Providers can learn about this process by encouraging discourse about the meaning of pain for the patient. This can be accomplished by asking questions such as, "What concerns do you have about your pain?"; "How do you deal with the pain now?"; "What do you think can be done to help your pain?"; "What do you think will happen to the pain in the coming years?"; "What concerns do you have about pain treatments?" Such discussion can start the process of defining goals and finding ways of treating pain that will fit best with a patient's values and preferences.

Involve the family

While families are typically enlisted only in the care of patients with cognitive or functional impairments, there is some evidence that understanding family issues can improve both the assessment and the care of patients with pain. As noted earlier, patients often consider family and friends more important than physicians in making decisions about pain management [59]. There is also evidence that family dyads with beliefs that pain is controllable have less symptom distress and caregiver burden than dyads with beliefs that pain is not controllable [95]. The provider can either ask the family to be directly involved in care decisions around pain, or can solicit the patient's perspectives on this issue through such questions as, "How does your husband/wife cope with your pain?"; "What do your friends and family say about your pain?"; "How does your pain impact your relationship with family and friends?" These strategies would also apply to older adults whose primary caregivers are not family members, including home health aides/attendants and other providers such as geriatric care managers.

Learn about and be able to recommend non-pharmacologic treatments

Providers are very comfortable prescribing medications, but much less so with non-pharmacologic treatments. There is a strong evidence base for many of these strategies, with controlled trials showing the benefits of treatments such as cognitive-behavioral therapy [96], strengthening exercise, aerobic exercise, and water-based exercise [67, 97]. Instead of enumerating all of the available treatments and their indications, we suggest that providers familiarize themselves with various treatment modalities for chronic pain (none of which are specific to older adults), and engage patients in discussions about their use, risks, and benefits. Many pain management programs are offered in diverse community settings such as senior centers and faith-based organizations. The Arthritis Foundation sponsors a diverse array of programs in all 50 states including exercise (e.g., tai chi, aquatic classes) and self-management courses. Providers are encouraged to contact local community senior centers as well as other community-based agencies that provide services to older adults and inquire about the specific types of programs offered and to refer patients when appropriate.

Do not prescribe analgesic medications without discussing first

Our synthesis of medication-related behaviors, beliefs, and preferences revealed it to be a complicated issue. There is no simple solution to limited adherence, but some of the key barriers have been identified in this review. The primary finding, which may seem counter-intuitive to providers, is that most older patients seek to take medications as little as possible. Patients engage in an implicit cost-benefit analysis of necessity versus concerns, and concerns frequently win [86]. While it would be impractical to try to address all of the cognitive factors that determine patient behavior, providers can be aware of some of the key concerns, especially the belief that medications are dangerous or addictive, and that medications should be used only when the pain is at its worst. Providers can easily discuss real medication use in a non-threatening way by, as recommended by Hill and Bird [13], asking a simple question: "How and when are you planning to take this medication?" This is quite different than telling a patient, "This medication will help your pain – take it when you hurt, up to three times a day, and it is safe." Selecting a specific medication requires a full appreciation of the patients' history and co-morbidities (see the American Geriatric Society persistent pain management guidelines), but this is neither the first step (which should be eliciting patients' preferences for treatments and educating them about various pain management options) nor the last step (which should be discussing treatment response, adherence, and beliefs) in engaging patients in managing their pain. There is evidence that programs directed at increasing patient self-efficacy about medications can improve medication adherence [98].

Learn about and be able to communicate medication risks

Analgesics can confer significant risks in all patients, with increased risks in older adults and patients with co-morbidities. The quality of care for osteoarthritis in older adults is particularly suboptimal around medication safety [54]. Managing risk has two aspects, both of which are important. First, providers can both learn and apply updated guidelines so that the medications they prescribe are as safe as possible for patients. Second, providers can discuss a patient's willingness to accept risk on an individual basis in order to determine the treatment that matches best with the patient's preferences. As described earlier, different patients have different levels of tolerance regarding medication risk [79], and may be willing to accept more or less potential harm in exchange for better pain control. Clearly, communicating risk is a difficult endeavor [99]. Providers are therefore encouraged to identify and employ communication strategies that work best for each provider and engage patients in this important discussion.

Consider systematic treatment approaches

A number of programs to treat persistent pain in older adults have been developed, and while there are no large controlled studies, many show promise. While these may be difficult to implement in different care settings, most involve only minimal staff time and specialized training, and little or no equipment. A medication self-management program has been shown to improve adherence [98]. A telephone-based intervention in which nurse educators telephoned patients with pain and psychosocial problems to teach problem-solving and basic pain management skills has demonstrated benefits [6]. A multicomponent physical activity intervention for lower extremity osteoarthritis, "Fit and Strong", has shown promise for pain and physical functioning [101]. Collaborative care treatments for either depression [93] or depression with osteoarthritis pain [94, 102] have been shown to reduce pain and depressive symptoms. An intervention for the management of osteoarthritis in which a practice nurse telephones patients on a monthly basis to discuss adherence and side effects is underway, and results are pending [103]. These programs, which may be the wave of the future in primary care, may exert positive effects because they systematically address some of the key barriers such as knowledge, adherence, and associated conditions, in ways that individual providers cannot.

Resources

A selected list of books and guidelines that focus on the assessment and treatment of pain among older adults

Table 24.1 Pain management resource

Reference		Further details
Books	*Persistent Pain in Older Adults*	Eds. DK Weiner, K Herr, TE Rudy (Springer, 2003); ISBN-13: 978-0826138354
	Managing Pain in the Older Adult	Ed. MP Jansen (Springer, 2008); ISBN-13: 9780826115676
	Pain Management for Older Adults: A Self-Help Guide	Eds. T Hadjistavropoulos and HD Hadjistavropoulos (IASP, 2008); ISBN 978-0-931092-70-1
	Pain in Older Persons: Progress in Pain Research Management	Editors: SJ Gibson and DK Weiner (IASP, 2005); ISBN 978-0-931092-59-6
Guidelines	AGS Guide on the Management of Persistent Pain	www.americangeriatrics.org/education/manage_pers_pain.shtml
	Persistent Pain Management	www.guideline.gov/summary/summary.aspx?ss=15&doc_id=8627&nbr=4807
Other resources	National Arthritis Foundation	www.arthritis.org/
	National Council on Aging's Center for Health Aging	www.healthyagingprograms.org
	National Institute of Senior Centers	www.ncoa.org/content.cfm?sectionID=342
	National Institutes of Health Pain Consortium	http://painconsortium.nih.gov/
	Stanford University Patient Education Research Center	http://patienteducation.stanford.edu/programs
	American Chronic Pain Association	www.theacpa.org
	American Pain Society	www.ampainsoc.org

appears in Table 24.1. In addition, agencies/organizations (and their corresponding websites) that contain both provider and patient-relevant resources and listings that can help to identify local community-based programs that may be relevant for seniors with pain are also shown. Finally, most states have Departments of Aging that can be contacted to learn more about pain-relevant programs offered at local senior centers and other senior service organizations.

Conclusion

Our review has consistently emphasized that patients and providers frequently have misconceptions about pain and aging that can operate as significant barriers to effective pain management. Older adults use a variety of coping strategies to manage their pain, including both pharmacologic and non-pharmacologic interventions. Most of these approaches are characterized as only moderately helpful, indicating the need for new strategies to address this efficacy gap. As importantly, patients' beliefs and expectations regarding pain and pain treatments are often discordant with those held by treating providers. Clinicians

are encouraged to adopt the steps listed above as a means of improving the management of later life pain. We submit that addressing common myths about pain and aging, working proactively with older patients to gain an understanding of their views and expectations regarding pain and associated treatments, educating patients and families about the breadth of treatment options available, and recommending interventions that are concordant with patients' preferences, can yield substantial dividends.

References

1. Griffith CH, III, Wilson JF. The loss of student idealism in the 3rd-year clinical clerkships. *Eval Health Prof* 2001; **24**: 61–71.

2. Pound P, Britten N, Morgan M, *et al.* Resisting medicines: a synthesis of qualitative studies of medicine taking. *Soc Sci Med* 2005; **61**: 133–55.

3. Gignac M, Davis A, Hawker G, *et al.* "What do you expect? You're just getting older": a comparison of perceived osteoarthritis-related and aging-related health experiences in middle- and older-age adults. *Arthritis Rheum* 2006; **55**: 905–12.

4. Gagliese L, Melzack R. Chronic pain in elderly people. *Pain* 1997; **70**: 3–14.

5. Herr KA, Garand L. Assessment and measurement of pain in older adults. *Clin Geriatr Med* 2001; **17**: 457–78, vi.

6. Gureje O, Simon GE, Von Korff M. A cross-national study of the course of persistent pain in primary care. *Pain* 2001; **92**: 195–200.

7. Centers for Disease Control and Prevention, National Center for Health Statistics. Special Feature: Pain. In: Health, United States, 2006 with Chartbook on Trends in the Health of Americans: Centers for Disease Control and Prevention.

8. Gibson SJ, Helme, RD. Age differences in pain perception and report: A review of physiological, psychological, laboratory and clinical studies. *Pain Reviews* 1995; **2**: 111–37.

9. Helme RD, Gibson SJ. The epidemiology of pain in elderly people. *Clin Geriatr Med* 2001; **17**: 417–31, v.

10. Brattberg G, Parker MG, Thorslund M. A longitudinal study of pain: Reported pain from middle age to old age. *Clin J Pain* 1997; **13**: 144–9.

11. Gallagher RM, Verma S, Mossey J. Chronic pain. Sources of late-life pain and risk factors for disability. *Geriatrics* 2000; **55**: 40–44, 47.

12. Appelt CJBC, Siminoff LA, Kwoh CK, Ibrahim SA. Health beliefs related to aging among older male patients with knee and/or hip osteoarthritis. *J Gerontol A: Biol Sci Med Sci* 2007; **62**: 184–90.

13. Hill J, Bird H. Patient knowledge and misconceptions of osteoarthritis assessed by a validated self-completed knowledge questionnaire (PKQ-OA). *Rheumatology (Oxford)* 2006; **46**: 796–800.

14. Keller ML, Leventhal H, Prohaska TR, *et al.* Beliefs about aging and illness in a community sample. *Res Nurs Health* 1989; **12**: 247–55.

15. Weiner DK, Rudy TE, Gaur S. Are all older adults with persistent pain created equal? Preliminary evidence for a multiaxial taxonomy. *Pain Res Manag* 2001; **6**: 133–41.

16. Busse EW. Aging and health. *Rep Natl Forum Hosp Health Aff* 1985: 1–13.

17. Peters TJ, Sanders C, Dieppe P, *et al.* Factors associated with change in pain and disability over time: a community-based prospective observational study of hip and knee osteoarthritis. *Br J Gen Pract* 2005 **55**(512): 205–11.

18. van Dijk GM, Dekker J, Veenhof C, *et al.* Course of functional status and pain in osteoarthritis of the hip or knee: a systematic review of the literature. *Arthritis Rheum* 2006; **55**: 779–85.

19. Sharma L, Cahue S, Song J, *et al.* Physical functioning over three years in knee osteoarthritis: role of psychosocial, local mechanical, and neuromuscular factors. *Arthritis Rheum* 2003; **48**: 3359–70.

20. Rustoen T, Wahl AK, Hanestad BR, *et al.* Age and the experience of chronic pain: differences in health and quality of life among younger, middle-aged, and older adults. *Clin J Pain* 2005; **21**: 513–23.

21. Dawson J, Linsell L, Zondervan K, *et al.* Impact of persistent hip or knee pain on overall health status in elderly people: a longitudinal population study. *Arthritis Rheum* 2005; **53**: 368–74.

22. Salaffi F, Stancati A, Silvestri CA, *et al.* Minimal clinically important changes in chronic musculoskeletal pain intensity measured on a numerical rating scale. *Eur J Pain* 2004; **8**: 283–91.

23. Reid MC, Williams CS, Gill TM. Back pain and decline in lower extremity physical function among community-dwelling older persons. *J Gerontol A Biol Sci Med Sci* 2005; **60**: 793–7.

24. Turk DC, Okifuji A, Scharff L. Chronic pain and depression: role of perceived impact and perceived control in different age cohorts. *Pain* 1995; **61**: 93–101.

25. Bair MJ, Robinson RL, Katon W, *et al.* Depression and pain comorbidity: a literature review. *Arch Intern Med* 2003; **163**: 2433–45.

26. Rosemann T, Backenstrass M, Joest K, *et al.* Predictors of depression in a sample of 1,021 primary care patients with osteoarthritis. *Arthritis Rheum* 2007; **57**: 415–22.

27. Sale JE, Gignac M, Hawker G. The relationship between disease symptoms, life events, coping and treatment, and depression among older adults with osteoarthritis. *J Rheumatol* 2008; **35**: 335–42.

28. Bookwala J, Harralson TL, Parmelee PA. Effects of pain on functioning and well-being in older adults with osteoarthritis of the knee. *Psychol Aging* 2003; **18**: 844–50.

29. Dominick KL, Ahern FM, Gold CH, *et al.* Health-related quality of life and health service use among older adults with osteoarthritis. *Arthritis Rheum* 2004; **51**: 326–31.

30. Gibson SJ, Farrell M. A review of age differences in the neurophysiology of nociception and the perceptual experience of pain. *Clin J Pain* 2004; **20**: 227–39.

31. Sale J, Gignac M, Hawker G. How "bad" does the pain have to be? A qualitative study examining adherence to pain medication in older adults with osteoarthritis. *Arthritis Rheum* 2006; **55**: 272–8.

32. Mossey JM, Gallagher RM. The longitudinal occurrence and impact of comorbid chronic pain

and chronic depression over two years in continuing care retirement community residents. *Pain Med* 2004; **5**: 335–48.

33. Emptage NP, Sturm R, Robinson RL. Depression and comorbid pain as predictors of disability, employment, insurance status, and health care costs. *Psychiatr Serv* 2005; **56**: 468–74.

34. Kenefick AL. Pain treatment and quality of life: reducing depression and improving cognitive impairment. *J Gerontol Nurs* 2004; **30**: 22–9.

35. Thielke SM, Fan MY, Sullivan M, *et al.* Pain limits the effectiveness of collaborative care for depression. *Am J Geriatr Psychiatry* 2007; **15**: 699–707.

36. Mavandadi S, Ten Have TR, Katz IR, *et al.* Effect of depression treatment on depressive symptoms in older adulthood: the moderating role of pain. *J Am Geriatr Soc* 2007; **55**: 202–11.

37. Karp JF, Weiner D, Seligman K, *et al.* Body pain and treatment response in late-life depression. *Am J Geriatr Psychiatry* 2005; **13**: 188–94.

38. Wilcox S, Brenes GA, Levine D, *et al.* Factors related to sleep disturbance in older adults experiencing knee pain or knee pain with radiographic evidence of knee osteoarthritis. *J Am Geriatr Soc* 2000; **48**: 1241–51.

39. Power JD, Perruccio AV, Badley EM. Pain as a mediator of sleep problems in arthritis and other chronic conditions. *Arthritis Rheum* 2005; **53**: 911–9.

40. Yong HH, Gibson SJ, Horne DJ, *et al.* Development of a pain attitudes questionnaire to assess stoicism and cautiousness for possible age differences. *J Gerontol B Psychol Sci Soc Sci* 2001; **56**: P279–84.

41. Leventhal EA, Prohaska TR. Age, symptom interpretation, and health behavior. *J Am Geriatr Soc* 1986; **34**: 185–91.

42. Mechanic D, Angel RJ. Some factors associated with the report and evaluation of back pain. *J Health Soc Behav* 1987; **28**: 131–9.

43. Yates P, Dewar A, Fentiman B. Pain: the views of elderly people living in long-term residential care settings. *J Adv Nurs* 1995; **21**: 667–74.

44. AGS Panel on Persistent Pain. The management of persistent pain in older persons. *J Am Geriatr Soc* 2002; **50**: S205–224.

45. Barry L, Gill T, Kerns R, *et al.* Identification of pain-reduction strategies used by community-dwelling older persons. *J Gerontol A Biol Sci Med Sci* 2005; **60**: 1569–75.

46. Lin JJ, Alfandre D, Moore C. Physician attitudes toward opioid prescribing for patients with persistent noncancer pain. *Clin J Pain* 2007; **23**: 799–803.

47. Pitkala KH, Strandberg TE, Tilvis RS. Management of nonmalignant pain in home-dwelling older people: a population-based survey. *J Am Geriatr Soc* 2002; **50**: 1861–5.

48. Lin EH, Tang L, Katon W, *et al.* Arthritis pain and disability: response to collaborative depression care. *Gen Hosp Psychiatry* 2006; **28**: 482–6.

49. Auret K, Schug SA. Underutilisation of opioids in elderly patients with chronic pain: approaches to correcting the problem. *Drugs Aging* 2005; **22**: 641–54.

50. Hutt E, Pepper GA, Vojir C, *et al.* Assessing the appropriateness of pain medication prescribing practices in nursing homes. *J Am Geriatr Soc* 2006; **54**: 231–9.

51. Won AB, Lapane KL, Vallow S, *et al.* Persistent nonmalignant pain and analgesic prescribing patterns in elderly nursing home residents. *J Am Geriatr Soc* 2004; **52**: 867–74.

52. Kee WG, Middaugh SJ, Redpath S, *et al.* Age as a factor in admission to chronic pain rehabilitation. *Clin J Pain* 1998; **14**: 121–8.

53. Chodosh J, Solomon DH, Roth CP, *et al.* The quality of medical care provided to vulnerable older patients with chronic pain. *J Am Geriatr Soc* 2004; **52**: 756–61.

54. Ganz D, Chang J, Roth C, *et al.* Quality of osteoarthritis care for community-dwelling older adults. *Arthritis Rheum* 2006; **55**: 241–7.

55. Tallon D, Chard J, Dieppe P. Exploring the priorities of patients with osteoarthritis of the knee. *Arthritis Care Res* 2000; **13**: 312–9.

56. Kemp C, Ersek M, Turner J. A descriptive study of older adults with persistent pain: use and perceived effectiveness of pain management strategies [ISRCTN11899548]. *BMC Geriatr* 2005; **5**: 12.

57. Barry L, Kerns R, Guo Z, *et al.* Identification of strategies used to cope with chronic pain in older persons receiving primary care from a Veterans Affairs Medical Center. *J Am Geriatr Soc* 2004; **52**: 950–6.

58. Briggs A, Scott E, Steele K. Impact of osteoarthritis and analgesic treatment on quality of life of an elderly population. *Ann Pharmacother* 1999; **33**: 1154–9.

59. Ross M, Carswell A, Hing M, *et al.* Seniors' decision making about pain management. *J Adv Nurs* 2001; **35**: 442–51.

60. Tse M, Chan B. Knowledge and attitudes in pain management: Hong Kong nurses' perspective. *J Pain Palliat Care Pharmacother* 2004; **18**: 47–58.

61. Austrian J, Kerns R, Reid M. Perceived barriers to trying self-management approaches for chronic pain in older persons. *J Am Geriatr Soc* 2005; **53**: 856–61.

62. Gignac MA, Cott C, Badley EM. Adaptation to disability: applying selective optimization with compensation to the behaviors of older adults with osteoarthritis. *Psychol Aging* 2002; **17**: 520–4.

63. Ersek M, Turner J, Kemp C. Use of the chronic pain coping inventory to assess older adults' pain coping strategies. *J Pain* 2006; **7**: 833–42.

64. Tan G, Jensen MP, Robinson-Whelen S, *et al.* Coping with chronic pain: a comparison of two measures. *Pain* 2001; **90**: 127–33.

65. Blomqvist K, Edberg A. Living with persistent pain: experiences of older people receiving home care. *J Adv Nurs* 2002; **40**: 297–306.

66. Turner J, Ersek M, Kemp C. Self-efficacy for managing pain is associated with disability, depression, and pain coping among retirement community residents with chronic pain. *J Pain* 2005; **6**: 471–9.

67. Zhang W, Moskowitz RW, Nuki G, *et al.* OARSI recommendations for the management of hip and knee osteoarthritis, part I: critical appraisal of existing treatment guidelines and systematic review of current research evidence. *Osteoarthritis Cartilage* 2007; **15**: 981–1000.

68. Hadjistavropoulos H, Shymkiw J. Predicting readiness to self-manage pain. *Clin J Pain* 2007; **23**: 259–66.

69. Goodwin JS, Black SA, Satish S. Aging versus disease: the opinions of older black, Hispanic, and non-Hispanic white Americans about the causes and treatment of common medical conditions. *J Am Geriatr Soc* 1999; **47**: 973–9.

70. Parsons S, Harding G, Breen A, *et al.* The influence of patients' and primary care practitioners' beliefs and expectations about chronic musculoskeletal pain on the process of care: a systematic review of qualitative studies. *Clin J Pain* 2007; **23**: 91–8.

71. Frantsve LM, Kerns RD. Patient-provider interactions in the management of chronic pain: current findings within the context of shared medical decision making. *Pain Med* 2007; **8**: 25–35.

72. Rosemann T, Wensing M, Joest K, *et al.* Problems and needs for improving primary care of osteoarthritis patients: the views of patients, general practitioners and practice nurses. *BMC Musculoskelet Disord* 2006; **7**: 48.

73. Neville C, Fortin PR, Fitzcharles MA, *et al.* The needs of patients with arthritis: the patient's perspective. *Arthritis Care Res* 1999; **12**: 85–95.

74. Birdwell BG, Herbers JE, Kroenke K. Evaluating chest pain. The patient's presentation style alters the physician's diagnostic approach. *Arch Intern Med* 1993; **153**: 1991–5.

75. Lansbury G. Chronic pain management: a qualitative study of elderly people's preferred coping strategies and barriers to management. *Disabil Rehabil* 2000; **22**: 2–14.

76. Fraenkel L, Bogardus ST, Jr, Concato J, *et al.* Treatment options in knee osteoarthritis: the patient's perspective. *Arch Intern Med* 2004; **164**: 1299–1304.

77. Fraenkel L, Wittink DR, Concato J, *et al.* Informed choice and the widespread use of antiinflammatory drugs. *Arthritis Rheum* 2004; **51**: 210–4.

78. Chang J, Kauf TL, Mahajan S, *et al.* Impact of disease severity and gastrointestinal side effects on the health state preferences of patients with osteoarthritis. *Arthritis Rheum* 2005; **52**: 2366–75.

79. Richardson CG, Chalmers A, Llewellyn-Thomas HA, *et al.* Pain relief in osteoarthritis: patients' willingness to risk medication-induced gastrointestinal, cardiovascular, and cerebrovascular complications. *J Rheumatol* 2007; **34**: 1569–75.

80. Ratcliffe J, Buxton M, McGarry T, *et al.* Patients' preferences for characteristics associated with treatments for osteoarthritis. *Rheumatology (Oxford)* 2004; **43**: 337–45.

81. Linsell L, Dawson J, Zondervan K, *et al.* Prospective study of elderly people comparing treatments following first primary care consultation for a symptomatic hip or knee. *Fam Pract* 2005; **22**: 118–25.

82. Davis MP, Srivastava M. Demographics, assessment and management of pain in the elderly. *Drugs Aging* 2003; **20**: 23–57.

83. O'Rorke JE, Chen I, Genao I, *et al.* Physicians' comfort in caring for patients with chronic nonmalignant pain. *Am J Med Sci* 2007; **333**: 93–100.

84. McHugh GA, Luker KA, Campbell M, *et al.* A longitudinal study exploring pain control, treatment and service provision for individuals with end-stage lower limb osteoarthritis. *Rheumatology (Oxford)* 2007; **46**: 631–7.

85. Carr A. Barriers to the effectiveness of any intervention in OA. *Best Pract Res Clin Rheumatol* 2001; **15**: 645–56.

86. Horne R, Weinman J. Predicting treatment adherence: an overview of theoretical models. In *Adherence to Treatment in Medical Conditions*, eds. L B Meyers and K Midence. (Amsterdam: Harwood Academic, 1998).

87. Unutzer J, Katon W, Callahan CM, *et al.* Collaborative care management of late-life depression in the primary care setting: a randomized controlled trial. *JAMA* 2002; **288**: 2836–45.

88. McCarthy LH, Bigal ME, Katz M, *et al.* Chronic pain and obesity in the elderly: Results from the Einstein Aging Study. *J Am Geriatr Soc* 2008; **57**: 115–9.

89. Blenkiron P. The elderly and their medication: understanding and compliance in a family practice. *Postgrad Med J* 1996; **72**: 671–6.

90. Wheeler MS. Pain assessment and management in the patient with mild to moderate cognitive impairment. *Home Healthc Nurse* 2006; **24**: 354–9; quiz 360–1.

91. Kung F, Gibson SJ, Helme RD. Older people with chronic pain; an intervention study comparing pain clinic patients and a community sample. *The Pain Clinic* 2000; **12**: 103–12.

92. Kung F, Gibson S, Helme R. A community-based program that provides free choice of intervention for older people with chronic pain. *J Pain* 2000; **1**: 293–308.

93. Lin EH, Katon W, Von Korff M, *et al.* Effect of improving depression care on pain and functional outcomes among older adults with arthritis: a randomized controlled trial. *JAMA* 2003; **290**: 2428–9.

94. Unutzer J, Hantke M, Powers D, *et al.* Care management for depression and osteoarthritis pain in older primary care patients: a pilot study. *Int J Geriatr Psychiatry* 2008; **23**: 1166–71.

95. Riley-Doucet C. Beliefs about the controllability of pain: congruence between older adults with cancer and their family caregivers. *J Fam Nurs* 2005; **11**: 225–41.

96. Kerns RD, Otis JD, Marcus KS. Cognitive-behavioral therapy for chronic pain in the elderly. *Clin Geriatr Med* 2001; **17**: 503–23, vii.

97. Devos-Comby L, Cronan T, Roesch SC. Do exercise and self-management interventions benefit patients with osteoarthritis of the knee? A metaanalytic review. *J Rheumatol* 2006; **33**: 744–56.

98. Lowe CJ, Raynor DK, Courtney EA, *et al.* Effects of self medication programme on knowledge of drugs and compliance with treatment in elderly patients. *BMJ* 1995; **310**: 1229–31.

99. Moore RA, Derry S, McQuay HJ, *et al.* What do we know about communicating risk? A brief review and suggestion for contextualising serious, but rare, risk, and the example of cox-2 selective and non-selective NSAIDs. *Arthritis Res Ther* **2008**; **10**: R20.

100. Ahles TA, Wasson JH, Seville JL, *et al.* A controlled trial of methods for managing pain in primary care patients with or without co-occurring psychosocial problems. *Ann Fam Med* 2006; **4**: 341–50.

101. Hughes SL, Seymour RB, Campbell R, *et al.* Impact of the fit and strong intervention on older adults with osteoarthritis. *Gerontologist* 2004; **44**: 217–28.

102. Dobscha SK, Corson K, Perrin NA, *et al.* Collaborative care for chronic pain in primary care: a cluster randomaized trail. *JAMA* 2009; **301**(12): 1242–52.

103. Rosemann T, Korner T, Wensing M, *et al.* Rationale, design and conduct of a comprehensive evaluation of a primary care based intervention to improve the quality of life of osteoarthritis patients. The PraxArt-project: a cluster randomized controlled trial [ISRCTN87252339]. *BMC Public Health* 2005; **5**: 77.

Practice, policy, and research
Policy and practice issues in pain management

Samantha Boris-Karpel

Introduction

This chapter considers some of the most salient and pertinent issues in pain management policy and presents the perspectives of various stakeholders and players in the policy debate – including epidemiologists, public health professionals, health administrators, politicians, research scientists, investors, legal scholars, and clinicians.

Policy changes rapidly. And any publication that professes to address "current events" may find itself quickly outdated. With this changing landscape in mind, we have selected to discuss here issues that may provide a historical context that can best help us understand the policy behind pain management.

A population in pain

Ours is a population in pain, and has been described as representing "a medical and social emergency" [1] and a "an immense invisible crisis"[2]. And for the past 50 years, experts in the fields of medicine and epidemiology have been affirming this by documenting the high incidence and prevalence rates of pain in the population. Based on the data, they conclude, that we are, in fact, a public health crisis [1–7]. On average, reports estimate that the global prevalence of chronic pain is currently at 20% – or one in five persons who are likely to suffer from chronic pain [4–10]. Utilizing population pain prevalence data for guidance in resource planning is necessary; however, it can also be a thorny issue. This is because in the body of published prevalence reports, each one may have been generated using a different methodology. Overall, most population estimates of pain prevalence focus exclusively on chronic pain. Nevertheless, some studies do not discriminate between chronic pain and current (possibly acute) pain. Even within surveys that address only chronic pain, however, the operationalization of pain is diverse

(e.g. cancer-related pain, non-malignant chronic pain, widespread pain, neuropathic pain, musculoskeletal pain). Furthermore, these reports survey different types of population samples – from sampling with a focus on particular age groups to sampling with a focus on particular geographic communities.

Examining the estimated prevalence rates of a highly surveyed region of the world, such as Europe, illustrates the effects of methodology on the variability of reports. Overall, the pain prevalence rate estimates from the reported European community samples range from 19% to 53% [4, 9, 11]. The more specified the population and type of pain, the lower the population estimate tends to be. Another often-cited statistic for the continent of Europe estimates that there are currently more than 100 million people living with chronic pain due to a musculoskeletal condition [4, 6]. Note that presenting the data in this way highlights the enormity of the overall numbers. In Australia, 19% of the community suffers from chronic pain, according to the most commonly cited evidence [12]. Meanwhile, 42.2 million or 41.2% of Japanese adults experience musculoskeletal pain, according to a 2005 report, with 9.1 million (8.8%) encountering interference in their daily activities [13]. For Korea, a meta-analysis shows that the reported prevalence estimates of chronic widespread pain range from 7.3% to 14.0% [14]. Again, the reported numbers for different communities vary depending on the study's operationalization of pain, and its health correlates.

For the USA, some pain experts estimate that annually up to 30% of the population is affected by persistent pain [15, 16]. According to Lazarus and Newman [7], the prevalence rate for pain in the USA and Canada is around 24%, a number that falls within the average of estimates. The American Pain Society's "Chronic Pain Survey: Roadblocks to Relief" reports that 9% of the US adult population suffers from "moderate to severe non-cancer related chronic pain," one of the lowest

Behavioral and Psychopharmacologic Pain Management, ed. Michael H. Ebert and Robert D. Kerns. Published by Cambridge University Press. © Cambridge University Press 2011.

estimates available [17]. The likely pain prevalence rate for a general US population sample is estimated to be in the range 13–53%, again varying depending on how pain was defined [18].

To translate the US percentages into population estimates, the 1999 National Pain Survey estimated that "over 75 million Americans suffer serious pain annually: 50 million of those endure serious chronic pain (pain lasting 6 months or more), and another 25 million experience acute pain" [19, 20]. Green reports that the current pain prevalence in the USA is now approaching 100 million and continues to increase [21].

Reports of health service and social service utilization also illuminate an important aspect of the epidemiology of pain. The National Ambulatory Medical Care Surveys (NHAMCS) from 1995 to 1998 show that back pain was the fifth most common reason for an office visit to a physician. It has been estimated that each year 80% of all office visits to a healthcare provider are for "pain-related issues" [22, 23]. A 1998 World Health Organization (WHO) survey estimated that more than 17% of US patients who visit primary care physicians have chronic pain, and that pain medications account for the second largest category of pharmacological prescriptions [11].

In the USA, the estimates vary as to how many persons are currently not being treated for their pain. One of the most widely accepted conservative estimates – that of the Chronic Pain in America study's Chronic Pain Survey: Roadblocks to Relief (1999) estimates that four out of 10 adults with pain are not currently receiving or seeking healthcare for their pain, and that "only one in four of those with pain received adequate treatment" [17]. It is this epidemic of undertreatment of chronic pain that David Morris refers to when he writes that there is an "immense invisible crisis at the center of contemporary life," [2], with the result being poor health, physical suffering, and emotional, social, and financial costs.

The epidemiology of pain can help us better understand how widespread pain suffering is among the population. This, in turn, informs public health measures aimed at alleviating this burden. There are, however, particular concerns when considering epidemiological studies of pain. For one, epidemiological analyses often struggle to measure disparate indicators of pain (i.e. pain duration, location, etiology, severity, impaired functioning) in much the same way as clinical studies struggle with defining their outcome measures (i.e. pain reduction; return to work; restoration of physical

functioning, psychosocial recovery). Measurement considerations of pain duration have particular significance as pain duration has clinical correlations to the degree of suffering, disability, and healthcare costs [24]. For epidemiological surveys, retrospective assessments of pain duration may not be accurate, and so longitudinal studies with frequent measurement points have yielded the most reliable estimates, but these studies are often costly and complex to undertake [25, 26]. Epidemiology also has been utilized as a tool to identify possible risk factors for developing chronic pain [27, 28, 29]. In this way, the approach has helped to identify effective preventive health services as well [30, 31]. Finally, the epidemiological approach has helped to underscore that many persons still remain undertreated or untreated for their pain [26, 32].

With these important contributions at stake, the epidemiological study of pain is still a developing work in progress. For example, epidemiology has been slow to take into account the multidimensional aspects of widespread and multi-site pain. Until recently, epidemiological surveys asked questions in limiting ways that focused on pain in specific anatomical parts, therefore failing to capture the chronic pain prevalence of persons with widespread, multi-site, persistent pain [33].

Furthermore, while there are a number of published reports from epidemiological surveys estimating the pain prevalence rates in the wealthiest regions – the USA, Canada, Europe, Japan, South Korea, and Australia [3, 4, 6, 14, 34, 35] – unfortunately, a body of official pain prevalence estimates for less affluent regions in the Americas, Africa, and Asia does not yet exist. Generally, the lack of pain prevalence data from low-income countries is a probable indicator that these areas are lacking in health service resources. Thus, it is most likely that these poorest areas of the world are significantly lagging in the healthcare and treatment of persons with pain.

The undertreatment of pain is also endemic to the wealthiest nations, however, and there is much data to describe it. The following estimates are amongst the most often cited figures for population-specific undertreatment of pain. Grossman and colleagues report that "70% of those with cancer experience significant pain during their illness, yet in early studies of cancer pain fewer than half received adequate treatment for their pain" [36, 37]. The American Pain Foundation (APF), also cites two studies that showed, respectively, that 24% of nursing home patients with significant pain received no treatment or intervention other than aspirin, and that "41% of nursing home patients who were admitted with moderate to severe pain still had approximately the same level of pain" six months later [38, 39]. While these numbers point to an epidemic of untreated and poorly treated pain, some scholars believe these statistics actually underestimate the true incidence rates of undertreatment

The undertreatment of pain is not always random in the population. Instead undertreatment seems to follow demographic patterns of disparities regarding both the access to, and receipt of, pain management services [40–46]. Later sections of this chapter will consider some of the policy-related issues that contribute to barriers to pain care. In the USA, these barriers disproportionally affect children, older adults, women, people of color, and those with the least financial resources [39–45]. Sadly, the population groups most affected and stymied by barriers to pain care are many of the same groups with the highest prevalence rates of pain. A review of published reports shows that chronic pain prevalence rates are higher in females than in men, and higher in older adults than younger persons, and higher among those who are unemployed and who have not attained a high school diploma or college degree [47]. That the patterns of health and treatment disparities in chronic pain are greatest in the population groups who are most at risk for chronic pain incidences creates a public health crisis.

For public health planning, the projected analyses of future population pain rates are as important as reports of current population pain rates. Due to overall medical and public health advances that bolster lifespan longevity, and contribute to the recovery from disease and injury, as well as the "graying" of the US population (with the cohort of 'baby-boomers' entering their sixth decade), the prevalence rates of chronic pain in the US population are projected to increase significantly [21, 48]. This aging of large population cohorts together with increased life expectancy are expected to be key components in causing an increase in overall chronic diseases as well. With an increase in chronic diseases, there is likely to be a greater increase in chronic pain. In the USA and other wealthy industrialized nations, the twentieth century saw a shift from deaths caused by infectious illness or other injuries that caused death "with certainty and relative rapidity" to causes of death dominated by chronic disease and involving long-term deteriorative co-morbidities [49]. Now, at the dawn of the twenty-first century, it is estimated that 70–80% of persons from the wealthy industrialized nations die

during a long, deteriorative chronic disease process [49, 50].

Indeed, this "immense invincible crisis", this "social and medical emergency" of high rates of pain in the population shows all the signs of growing. On the one hand, advances in research and clinical practice are leading to more effective treatment interventions for pain. However, on the other, the USA is struggling with structural barriers to and costs of pharmacological, behavioral and multidisciplinary interventions for pain. And so, this epidemic of pain has been paralleling a path of "growing pains" for USA and global policy regarding pain management. The following is an overview of policy and practice issues presented within a historical context, with an emphasis on the current state of affairs and the most pressing issues facing the field of pain management.

Pain management comes into its own

Broadly, the history of pain management has influenced, and been influenced by, the changing scientific conceptualizations of anatomy, physiology, and the relationship between the mind and body. Over the past century and a half in the western hemisphere, scientific advances have paralleled military battles and thus have marked milestones in the development of modern pain management as a field of practice [51].

Epistemologically, the "mind-body problem" or the "metaphysical paradox" that is the discourse on the nature of the relationship between the mind and body, has been integral in informing the medicocultural conceptions of pain. The debate between monism, which views the mind and body as one and integrated, and dualism, which posits that the mind and body are discrete and separate entities, has been viewed as a major influence upon the way pain is conceptualized, expressed, reacted to, and treated. In Western culture this debate between monism and dualism entered the historical records around 520BC with many starts and turns along the way. One of the most influential publications to affect this debate and the historical development of pain management was the 1621 publication of Descartes' *Meditations. Meditations* contains Descartes' treatise on mind-body separation. The widespread acceptance of Descartes' treatise marked the domination of dualism in both popular culture, scientific and scholarly study and the emerging medical profession. This dualistic mind/body split contributed to the foundation of the so- called "organic model of pain" [52].

Two hundred years later, this organic model of pain gave rise to the *theory of sensory specificity*, most often credited to Johannes Muller in his 1826 publication on *Specific Nerve Energies*, which posited that all signals for sensation and function ran along observable committed nerve pathways [53, 54]. The theory of sensory specificity posited that a specific receptor stimulates a specific pathway and a specific brain center [55]. The theory of sensory specificity symbiotically supported the discoveries of the "anatomy of nerve pathways and the physiology of nerve impulses," which began in earnest in the late 1800s [55]. The theory of sensory specificity coexisted with the conceptual model of biomedical efficiency in healthcare. This was a reductionist, functional approach that valued hospital-centered interventions that were built upon the foundations of pain medicine: anesthesia and surgery [55]. Prescription medicines such as opioid analgesics and corrective surgeries were seen as the most effective approaches, and medicine was reductionist, functional, invasive, and newly hygienic. As part of this shift in the mid-twentieth century, physiotherapy as a profession in the USA ceased to exist. Pared down and renamed as "physical therapy" it entered the hospital sphere, leaving its other components such as massage therapy outside the field of medical practice. At this time, the "touch therapy" components of nursing practice also became a more marginal aspect of hospital care [56]. It would be another half century later that hospitals began to expand the medical model by providing or endorsing massage therapy and bodywork modalities for pain management and rehabilitation.

In practical opposition to the biomedical model is the biopsychosocial model, a perspective on health that incorporates the psychological and social as well as the biological. Although scholarship on the biopsychosocial model in the Western scientific cannon began to gain momentum at the turn of the twentieth century, it was subaltern to the reigning biomedical model. Indeed, the biomedical model often deemed considerations of the influence of the "mind" (cognitions, emotions) on health and medicine as "unscientific" [57]. It was during World War II, at a time when the scientific culture fell under the influence of the dominating biomedical model that the physician John Bonica began making innovations in pain therapy interventions that eventually led to his 1953 publication *The Management of Pain* [51]. This seminal publication was seen as the birth of a new medical specialty: pain medicine.

Bonica's practice and publication heralded the birth of pain medicine as a medical discipline. Furthermore, Bonica posited pain management as a multidisciplinary endeavor, including anesthesiology, neurology, orthopedics, and psychiatry as integral aspects of the treatment endorsed [58]. Including psychiatry was revolutionary. However, it wouldn't be until Ronald Melzack and Patrick Wall's 1965 publication describing the gate control theory of pain [59], that a paradigm shift would begin to move the practice of pain management away from the reductionist, dualistic biomedical model of pain and towards the more biopsychosocial model that Bonica had endorsed [51, 58, 59]. Melzack and Wall's gate control theory of pain reintroduced the importance of emotions, cognitions, behaviors, and environment in pain. This theory was lauded as the "the end of the reign of the organic model of pain" [52]. With the reacceptance of the biopsychosocial model into the practice of medicine, therapies categorized as "mind-body therapies" – some of which had already existed for millennia in Asia and elsewhere – began to be brought into the fold of Western medicine. The introduction, or reintroduction, of these modalities was first brought in as an allied alternative, labeled "complementary and alternative medicine" or CAM. Then, as the trend towards integration of CAM into allopathic medical practice developed, most CAM approaches were renamed "integrative medicine" (IM). At the same time the evolution of the cognitive-behavioral therapy (CBT) approach to psychological interventions brought in a more health psychology focus on mind-body techniques for physiological relaxation, distraction, and focus which drew much of its practice from medical traditions in Asia. With this development and expansion of CBT in psychology, along with a growing literature publishing supportive CBT efficacy trials, the development of evidence-based psychological approaches to pain management began in earnest.

This shift towards mind-body connection within a more biopsychosocial model caused significant changes in pain management. Rollin Gallagher notes that "historically, the concept of mind-body duality in medicine… has impeded the development of adequate treatments for persistent pain conditions and diseases". For Gallagher, best practices in pain management necessarily take into account the biopsychosocial model. He outlines his best practices proposal as "goal-directed, outcomes-focused biospsychosocial treatment plans that efficiently integrate physical, behavioral, and medical approaches" [60]. Indeed, the current gold standard of best practices for pain management is an interdisciplinary and comprehensive approach to the biopsychosocial mode. The core of this gold standard of interdisciplinary care includes the disciplines of anesthesiology, rheumatology, orthopedics, neurology, nursing, psychology, pharmacology, physical therapy, occupational therapy, and social work.

Nevertheless, this paradigm shift from the biomedical to biopsychosocial model of pain, although praised by many scholars, is still not widespread. Conceptual inconsistencies regarding the exact nature of chronic pain, its etiology, and which treatment is most effective, still run rampant within both medical culture and popular culture [61].

According to Gallagher "most experienced clinicians accept the conceptual validity and the clinical effectiveness of the biopsychosocial model, [but that] implementation may be difficult," and a major –but not insurmountable – problem for the "busy clinician" in implementing the biopsychsocial model is the achievement of "efficiency" [60]. This is to be expected, as the problem of achieving efficiency is often prevalent in any attempts to implement a more comprehensive standard of care in lieu of a more reductionist and one-axial treatment. However it is important to note that research shows this evidence-based interdisciplinary standard of care has the best health outcomes for the patient [62].

Another dimension of chronic pain care with important policy and practice considerations is the nexus of pain management with psychiatric and psychological services. High incidence rates of psychiatric co-morbidities with chronic pain are well-documented [28, 57, 63]. The role of chronic pain in the etiology of psychoemotional distress, and vice-versa, is a hearty area of debate [64–66]. However, what is clear from the literature is that evidence-based psychological and psychiatric treatments (including behavioral and psychopharmacological approaches) are an effective part of providing comprehensive healthcare for chronic pain patients [58]. A universal recommendation comes in no uncertain terms from noted pain manager Robert Gatchel: "all pain management approaches" states Gatchel, ... require a strong mental health component" [57].

The two most common therapeutic missions for chronic pain – (1) to convince the patient that "the pain will not harm them" and (2) to encourage the

patient "to become more active" [15, 67] – are well complemented and reinforced by mental health services. Fully implementing these strategies and encouraging the patient to be proactive in his or her own care are often best facilitated by an interdisciplinary team of providers rather than a single provider carrying this message.

Building competency in the workplace

The interdisciplinary field of pain management is still a young specialty, one that is growing more innovative, effective, common, and accessible. However, the pressures of the undertreated chronic pain epidemic demands further growth in accessibility, flexibility, effectiveness, and quality. Logistically, to fuel further growth in the field of pain management, it is essential to ensure the education and training of a competent workforce in pain treatment approaches and care. In fact in 1986, the US Department of Health and Human Services (HHS) wrote a letter to the Director General of the WHO stating that the major obstacles to pain relief are not in the areas of opioid "regulation and distribution", but rather in the area of "health provider education". The HHS stated that their current efforts are to improve provider education by working with professional organizations, medical schools, local government agencies, and the private sector [68]. Now a quarter century later, the stakeholders are the same, and the need to further invest in training and innovation of the workforce infrastructure continues.

In the domain of medical education, the US Accreditation Council for Graduate Medical Education (ACGME) provides some guidance for building competency within the field of pain medicine. Pain medicine is not a specialty at the residency level, but rather, is structured and accredited as a sub-specialty post-residency fellowship. In its 2007 publication, the ACGME identified six areas of core competencies for all medical training – patient care, medical knowledge, practice-based learning and improvement, interpersonal and communication skills, professionalism, and systems-based practice. Within these areas of core competencies, the ACGME publication outlines the minimum curriculum and experiential requirements for postgraduate medical training in pain medicine for physicians [69]. In an endorsement of the interdisciplinary standard within pain medicine, the ACGME will only accredit post-residency training in pain medicine if

411

the sponsoring institution already has at least two of the following accredited residency programs: anesthesiology, neurology, psychiatry, and physical medicine and rehabilitation. As per their accreditation guidelines, there may not be more than one pain medicine fellowship program within one institution [69].

Despite the ACGME's emphasis on interdisciplinary training, a number of program evaluators have noted that there still are many pain medicine programs that adhere exclusively to a narrow biomedical model while eschewing the more comprehensive biopsychosocial model [70]. Based on efficacy studies, the more ideal pain medicine program would exemplify the more comprehensive and interdisciplinary model. A useful example of a progressive interdisciplinary care program that does embrace the biopsychosocial model is the joint pain care program at the VA Puget Sound and the University of Washington. At that program, Jacobson and colleagues practice what they term "co-disciplinary care," meaning that the anesthesiologists work in partnership with psychologists to treat pain patients. As an academic teaching hospital, the "training reach" of this program is amplified. The program's practice of co-disciplinary care helps their anesthesiology trainees to adopt new skills and interdisciplinary roles that are considered non-traditional for anesthesiologists [70].

The ACGME guidelines only extend to physicians from anesthesiology, neurology, psychiatry, and physical medicine and rehabilitation. There does not yet exist centralized and well-outlined competency standards for other disciplines which participate clinically in pain management. As previously mentioned, outside of pain medicine there are a number of disciplines in which personnel choose to specialize in pain management, such as psychology, physical therapy, occupational therapy, chiropractic, social work, nursing, rheumatology, primary care, pediatrics, chaplaincy, and recreational therapy. However, in acknowledgment of these providers who hail from outside of pain medicine, the field of pain management has sought to improve the pain assessment and pain management competency of generalists and pain care providers from various disciplines. In fact, in the past two decades, outside of pain medicine, program developers and researchers have targeted nursing, primary care, pediatrics, palliative care, geriatrics, and social work for improvements in pain management training [71]. This past decade has seen innovative initiatives created to help providers become more competent in pain

management areas. There has been an increase in in-service trainings, online web-based continuing education trainings, as well as modules added to curriculums of existing clinical training programs [72, 73].

These targeted interventions may also be seen as a response to recent research that found many training programs lacking in the area of pain management [74, 75]. Many studies have found workforce competency and knowledge to still be sub-par for those professionals who do not sub-specialize in pain management, but who serve a clinical population with pain [76–79].

A review of the professional education literature reveals that among all the disciplines, the field of nursing has been the most examined and targeted for competency-building [75, 80, 81]. Reviews of general nursing school curriculums have found an overall paucity of training in pain management techniques for nursing students [75, 80]. In 1995, Zalon reported that an average of 9 hours of nursing training was dedicated to pain, including only 2.9 hours dedicated to non-pharmacological approaches to pain [75]. Since Zalon's report, there have been clear advances made by nurse training programs to include pain management skills; however, there are still specialized areas within pain management that continue to be underemphasized in these training programs. Among these undertaught areas are: nonpharmacological pain management techniques, geriatric pain care, and pediatric pain management techniques [81, 82]. To address these gaps in skills acquisition, additional opportunities to teach pain management techniques should be created for nurse training programs, as well as for continuing education and in-service professional trainings.

Outside of the profession of nursing, studies also have revealed that many other allied health professionals who work in clinical residential settings also lack the knowledge and skill sets important for pain management for older adults [82]. In light of the aging population, many public health advocates, administrators, and clinicians are calling for greater educational outreach and professional training for the non-nursing staff of nursing homes and eldercare facilities.

While these investigations and calls for improvements in training have yielded positive responses, the advancements have been piecemeal, with various small initiatives addressing this global dearth of training. One notable example is MacLaren and colleagues' progressive initiative in which pediatric nurses are trained in evidence-based cognitive-behavioral techniques for pain [82]. Another innovative site of training is the development of two recent web-based pain management courses for healthcare professionals. One program is the fee-based Virginia Commonwealth University (VCU) Chronic Non-Malignant Pain Management Course, developed by Leanne Yanni, that provides continuing education credit and is free for certain healthcare practitioners. The other is the web-based training for VA professionals that provides a tailored professional education program based on the discipline, knowledge base and pain management experience of healthcare professionals [83], (A. Mariano, personal communication, 2009). These innovations in professional training are currently localized, but the expansion of such endeavors would likely make an even larger mark on the field.

This mission for professional enhancement aims to achieve the goal of creating a highly competent and responsive workforce in pain management. Attaining this goal would ultimately provide greater accessibility for patients to higher quality interdisciplinary pain management. This accessibility is an issue of patient rights and, many would argue, human rights. As such, the urgency and necessity of enhancing professional competence can be seen from the perspective of legal liability concerns for responsible and due care.

An example of a policy statement that links stated educational standards directly to issues of legal accountability can be found in the 2004 "Public Policy Statement on the Rights and Responsibilities of Healthcare Professionals in the use of Opioids for the Treatment of Pain." This public policy statement was a consensus document issued by three major professional organizations: the American Academy of Pain Medicine, the American Pain Society (APS), and the American Society of Addiction Medicine [84]. The conclusion of that document enumerates eight recommendations related to the practice of pain medicine. The recommendations emphasize that pain medicine, such as opioids, should be prescribed in a lawful and clinically sound manner. Furthermore, the recommendations delineate discrete interventions for addressing transgressions in the clinical practice of pain management, depending on the intentions and track record of the healthcare provider in question.

The recommendations advocate for two different approaches to clinician error. If the clinician has a history of clinical errors involving opioid prescriptions, and there is evidence of purposeful unethical practice, then the recommendations condone licensing or legal sanction of the offending clinician, as indicated. If the transgressor does not meet that criterion then an educational intervention is suggested.

Educational standards are woven throughout the eight Rights & Responsibilities recommendations. For example, the recommendations emphasize that regulatory reviewers of clinical cases involving opioids themselves have a "requisite level" of knowledge and "understanding" about pain medicine and addiction medicine. The recommendations also indicate that "appropriate education in addiction medicine and pain medicine should be provided as part of the core curriculum at all medical and other provider training schools" [84]. This is a strong statement advocating changes and standards in healthcare curricula and training from the perspective of ethical and legal rights and responsibilities.

And so, within the USA, regulatory agencies, professional organizations, federal healthcare organizations, and private healthcare providers have all been contributing to setting standards for training and creating educational innovations in pain management. Outside of the USA, similar training needs are apparent in other comparable high income countries. And yet, in line with the global patterns of disparity, there are even more severe training needs in lower-income countries. For the poorest nations, both WHO and the International Association for the Study of Pain (IASP) have been leading funders and supporters of professional training programs for pain [85–87]. These training programs are often disease-specific, driven by grants and initiatives to develop skills and competencies in pain care and symptom management for patients with such diseases as advanced cancer, HIV-AIDS, cardiac and renal diseases, and degenerative neurological diseases [87].

Pharmacological standards of care: A delicate balance

In the USA, the practice of opioid prescribing has varied widely, enduring wide swings of the pendulum from the standard of "broad indiscriminate use" at the turn of the twentieth century to a more restrictive standard of practice in the mid-century [88]. Concerning pharmacological approaches to pain, the overriding public health goal of the last three decades has been to "prevent diversion and abuse of prescription controlled substances, while ensuring their availability for legitimate medical use" [89]. Scott Fishman's physician's guide for opioid prescribing presents data on the endemic problem of opioid diversion. Fishman used data from 2005 that shows that:

"More than 10 million Americans were abusing prescriptions drugs, more than the combined number of people using cocaine, heroin, hallucinogens, and inhalants… [and that] the trend of abusing pain relievers is doubling. The CDC reports that prescription opioids are now associated with more drug overdose deaths than cocaine and heroin combined" [90].

Tragically, the stakes are high; and this balance between monitoring and ensuring availability can be difficult to maintain. As mentioned elsewhere in this chapter, the tensions between conservative prescription monitoring and the right and obligation to treat a patient's pain have caused polarizing reactions among regulatory agencies, public health professionals, clinicians, addiction specialists, and patients' rights advocates. One area that has been rife with controversy has been "prescription monitoring programs" (PMPs), or "prescription drug monitoring programs" (PDMPs). Overseen by the federal Drug Enforcement Administration (DEA), these programs are legislated at the state level. Per state, PMPs vary in structure, stakeholders, and administrative prescription requisites. Prescription monitoring programs implement such monitoring activities as requiring mandatory multiple-copy forms for some prescription medications and creating Internet databases on patient prescription history. Currently, about 32 US states have operational PMPs, and 6 others have passed the necessary legislation to implement a program [91]. It is likely that more states will soon begin to implement these programs as well. Some prescribing clinicians have lauded the establishment of state-wide PMPs as a grand step toward assisting prescribers with information to help them make clinically sound decisions and avoid inadvertently prescribing to patients who are illicitly misusing prescription opioids and/or misrepresenting their prescription history [92, 93]. Among those advocating for more government oversight is Laxmaiah Manchikanti, a CEO of the American Society of Interventional Pain Physicians. Manchikanti, citing the variation across the country from state to state, writes that the current prescription monitoring programs are "ineffective and incoherent." Manchikanti argues for the funding of the National All Schedules Prescription Reporting Act of 2005 instead of continuing to fund the current piecemeal-style program overseen by the DEA [93]. In contrast, many prescribing clinicians feel that the increased oversight of the Government ultimately infringes on prescribers' ability to make clinical and ethical decisions, and

negatively affects patient care [94–101]. Arthur Lipman writes that "the federal law that created the DEA specifically precludes the agency from interfering with medical practice, but the agency's actions are not always consistent with that proscription" [98]. Lipman and others dispute the DEA's interpretation of federal law in which the DEA criminalizes the act of preparing multiple prescriptions for a Category II medication for a single patient, on the same day, with instructions to fill each prescription on different dates [98].

As the technology of prescription monitoring advances, new oversight issues may emerge, just as others may become more resolved or accepted. Advances in technology and knowledge have also created new approaches to analgesic pharmacology. The older standard of "monopharmacy," the treatment of pain symptoms with one medication, has been eclipsed by the popular approaches of "rational polypharmacy" for patients with moderate to severe pain. Rational polypharmacy entails co-pharmacotherapy, or the integration of two or more pharmacological agents to treat pain symptoms. The combinations, doses, and time-release characteristics must be carefully considered, and medications are chosen in the hope of minimizing break-through pain episodes. By integrating these different medications that are metabolized differently, the hope is to also minimize the patient's tolerance to the drugs, obviating or slowing down the need to increase dosage [102–104]. While rational polypharmacy may make analgesic pharmacology ultimately more effective for an individual patient, the approach also makes the practice of prescribing pain medication even more complicated and delicate, as more medications translate into higher risk of drug interactions and side effects [105]. The advent of a rational polypharmacy approach to pain management highlights the need for specialized pain management training among prescribing clinicians [88, 103–105]. This is especially true for prescribers outside of pain medicine, such as primary care professionals who, over the past decade, have been increasingly prescribing opioids for their patients' pain [88].

Globally, another opioid-related public health issue is the limited access that most of the population in low- and middle-income countries have to opioid medications. The WHO and its USA-based collaborating center, the Pain & Policy Studies Group (PPSG), and the IASP have all been involved in establishing resources to help ensure opioid availability in geographic areas of need. These collaborators have activated a wide range of methods for widening access to pharmacological pain care. Principal among these methods is the identification of public health professionals from these areas of need to collaborate with healthcare infrastructure enhancements. Areas that have been enhanced for greater accessibility include the local pain pharmacy resources and epidemiological and public health resources to aid in the analysis indicators of opioid need and consumption. These initiatives aim to ultimately enhance and better organize access to pharmacological policy information and resources at the local and national levels [105].

The public policy playing field: legislatures, regulating bodies, committees, collaborating centers, societies, boards, and facilities

Within the US government, there are many federal and state agencies that have had a hand in pain management policy. Furthermore, non-governmental organizations have been active participants, too: creating, advocating for, and monitoring pain care policies. Two oversight organizations that generate and monitor standards are the ACGME and the Joint Commission on Accreditation of Healthcare Organizations (JCAHO). The ACGME is responsible for the accreditation of postdoctoral medical training programs within the USA. The Joint Commission is an accreditation agency comprised of individuals from both the public and private medical sector to develop, establish, and maintain standards of care for both public and private participating clinical health facilities in the USA. As such, the roles that these two centralized organizations have in establishing standards of education and standards of care for pain management are potentially transformative.

National, local, and international non-governmental organizations have also been active stakeholders and agents in influencing clinical policies, research policies, and public health policy in pain management. For example, recently in the USA, 125 non-governmental organizations signed a consensus statement in support of the National Pain Policy Act of 2009, which is still waiting to be voted on by the US House of Representatives [107]. Depending on the organization, the administrators may be paid or volunteers, and the stakeholders and operating bases of the organizations are as varied as their mission statements. Some organizations are free-standing and not affiliated with research, clinical, or academic institutions; others are branches of, or programs under the aegis of, larger institutions. Some sectors of these organizations act as mostly professional societies whose varied functions are akin to professional guilds for health specialists. Prominent examples include the American Society of Interventional Pain Physicians, the American Society of Anesthesiologists, and the American Academy of Pain Management. These societies also have a role in oversight of specialized clinical practice.

The APS, on the other hand, is a professional and research organization that is distinct in that it is highly interdisciplinary (incorporating nursing, social work, psychology, chiropractic, and physical therapy along with pain medicine, for example). As such, it also functions as an interdisciplinary professional forum. The Mayday Fund is also interdisciplinary and focuses on forwarding multidisciplinary pain research. Another segment of notable organizations act as patient advocacy groups which are open to the general public as well as health professionals. Prominent examples of this category are the APF, the American Chronic Pain Association, the American Council for Headache Education, the National Headache Foundation, the National Foundation for the Treatment of Pain, the Arthritis Foundation, and the National Chronic Pain Outreach Association.

Internationally, the largest and most well-known organization is the International Association for the Study of Pain. The IASP is non-governmental and multinational and has many chapters around the world. In addition to being a research and academic organization, it is also considered a global leader in public health advocacy for pain management.

Finally, any consideration of international public health issues must include a review of the largest public multinational enterprise: the United Nations (UN) and its health agency, the World Health Organization (WHO). The WHO has been involved with pain care in "three overlapping areas: the promotion and dissemination of guidelines on pain management, advocacy of improved access to opioid analgesics, and national programs of palliative care and pain relief" [108]. In 2004, the IASP and WHO cosponsored a "Global Day Against Pain", with the theme "Pain Relief should be a human right". Now leaders in pain management advocacy are asking the UN to consider establishing an "International Year of Pain Management" [108]. There is much work to be done and there is a need for creativity in future initiatives, conventions, and public awareness campaigns. Public–private partnerships have been lauded as the wave of the future of public health initiatives [109, 110]; perhaps more multi-national, public-private partnerships for pain will be created.

Ethics: Pain management as a human right

Recent forums have been conducted on the topic of ethical guidelines for the treatment of pain, and there have been several published proposals on this subject [108, 111–117]. However, while there are publications that propose suggested guidelines, there currently exist no official standards of professional ethical practices specific to the practice of pain management [113]. Currently, each specialist who works within the pain management field may be guided by these umbrella proposals and also by the published standards of their respective specialty. Mary Lou Taylor likens this to "fitting general standards to a very specific setting," an enterprise fraught with complexities considering the interdisciplinary aspect of pain management, the nascent aspect of the field as a discipline (less than 60 years old), and the emerging challenges that are specific to the field [113].

Fueling the ethics debate is an understanding of the human costs of untreated or mismanaged pain. As Gilson and colleagues write, aptly and hauntingly: "the costs of pain, both emotional and financial can be enormous... unrelieved severe pain can limit a person's functioning and sometimes even destroy the will to live" [118].

The undertreatment of pain has been documented in persons who are receiving medical care within the healthcare system, as well as in persons who are not seeking healthcare. Among healthcare-seeking persons, evidence of undertreatment pervades, in care of both outpatients and inpatients. In 1973, Marks and Sachar published a historic study that revealed that 73% of inpatients, hospitalized for medical reasons, had experienced undertreated "moderate-to-severe pain" [119, 120]. The Marks and Sachar study further investigated the clinical practices that lead to such a poor pain treatment outcome. The results showed that attending medical staff had poor knowledge of "appropriate analgesic use and made incorrect decisions regarding the treatment of pain" [119, 120]. Pasero and McCaffery report that 30 years later, "recent research [still concludes] that providers today have many of the same weaknesses [as

outlined in the Marks and Sachar study] and that pain continues to be undertreated" [119].

The framing of pain management interventions as a fundamental human right has gained strength in recent years; and this increased traction has been credited to the involvement of patients, consumers, and grassroots advocacy groups. Prominent organizations such as the APS, the APF and the IASP have also utilized this concept of pain management as a human right. In Brennan, Carr, and Cousins' analysis on the factors contributing to the "marginalization of pain management as a priority" they include the "biomedical model of disease [that focuses] on pathophysiology rather than quality of life," along with other "cultural, societal, religious, and political attitudes." When pain management is not viewed as a human right, theorized outcomes are the undertreatment of patients in pain, a low prioritization of funding for pain management practice and research, and a moral acceptance of torture [108].

The formulation of a governmentally recognized human right as a gateway for legal rights is a public policy and constitutional law discipline unto itself. Ethical and legal statements concerning the human right to pain care encompass the fields of medicine, public health, law, and ethics. As previously stated in this chapter, the standard of pain management is interdisciplinary, involving numerous specialty fields. In addition, within pain management there are considered to be four pain care categories, one for each of these pain presentations, respectively: (1) acute pain; (2) cancer-related pain; (3) non-malignant chronic pain, and (4) end-of-life care. As such, when considering proposals for statutory codes regarding pain management, the specific issues from any one of these pain care categories may affect the policy issues within the others. This diversity and specificity of pain care needs makes the drafting of pain care policy even more far-reaching and complex.

Policy issues around end-of-life care are particularly controversial, touching upon deep cultural, spiritual, and legal sensibilities. Moreover, the specific policy debates surrounding end-of-life care have wide-reaching ramifications that may potentially affect the development of pain management policy and practice as a whole. In a pointed critique of the standards of care in end-of-life pain management, Imhof and Kaskie decry "the "continued undertreatment of pain...[that has still] not been resolved through increased public awareness, the issuance of clinical guidelines for providers, or organizational commitments" [121]. They offer that the path towards resolution of this "substantive public health problem" of undertreatment would be most effective by enacting state legislation. However, Stephen Arons' writes in his constitutional law essay that such an endeavor would be unlikely and difficult, suggesting that the establishment of a legal right to palliative care appears unattainable. Any consideration of legal codification regarding end-of-life care "would be a complex matter," as it is inextricably tied to such complicated ethical debates as euthanasia and refusal of treatment [111].

While the US Supreme Court has failed to recognize a federal constitutional right to pain relief, there has been more legislative activity, at the state-level, concerning patient's rights [108, 111, 122]. Brennan and colleagues further highlight legislative activity and strides towards codifying patient's rights being made in other parts of the globe. In 1994, as part of its Medical Treatment Act, Australia instituted an "explicit statutory statement of the right to pain relief," that is, compared to other extralegal declarations, both "unambiguous and legally enforceable" [108]. Among several clauses designed to protect patient's rights, it states "a health professional shall pay due regard to the patient's account of his or her level of pain and suffering" [108]. In another advance for pain care advocates who utilize a human rights framework, the European Federation of the International Association of the Study of Pain Chapters (EFIC) has recently submitted a "declaration to the European Parliament [of the European Union] proposing that chronic non-cancer pain is a 'disease in its own right' that warrants increased attention" [108].

Law enforcement and statutory protection for medical prescribers

It is important to consider the functional and jurisprudential distinctions between laws (including statutes, acts, and regulations) that are "rules of conduct with binding legal force" and guidelines that are "official policy statement[s] which do not have the force of law" [118, 123]. There are three levels of legality: (1) laws, (2) regulations, and (3) guidelines/position statements [124]. Laws are found in federal, or state-level, acts, statutes, or codes. Regulations usually add additional enforceable boundaries to laws. For pain management issues, an example of federal regulations may be found in the Code of Federal Regulations (CFR) that gives oversight to the DEA to monitor the exchange of controlled substances. On the state-level, regulations are found in state-licensing boards for health professionals. Regulations have the force of law, be it civil

sanctions or professional sanctions. Guidelines do not have the force of law, although they are often used in the context of litigation to establish the framework of civil and criminal lawsuits. Kara Fermani published a critique of a malpractice lawsuit in which the plaintiff's attorney instructed the jury to consider that the physician-defendant's "duty to the patient was mandated" by the practice guidelines of the American Society of Anesthesiologists (ASA) [125]. While the jury eventually ruled in favor of the defendant, Fermani points out that, had they not, this would have set a "dangerous precedent", for while guidelines "may represent the standard of care in many cases, they remain guidelines, not mandates… there are those clinical scenarios [in which] deviation from the guidelines is appropriate" [125].

Guidelines and advisories fall into the category of "practice parameters," which are distinct from "standards." Practice parameters do not carry the same imperatives as standards of care. They are not mandatory and often are considered debatable. They are used to "serve as a clinical tool to guide the practitioner in decision-making"; by contrast, "standard of care" is a "medicolegal term" since a failure to maintain a standard of care that results in harm to a patient may result in legal liability [129].

In the USA, the dynamics of legal protection from prosecution of pain medicine prescribers is played out in the dynamic balance of power between the federal reach of laws and each state's own legislation. In fact, on the state level, the protective statutes have arisen from the state medical boards. Their purposes are to offer protection to prescribers of "controlled substances … given in the course of treatment of a person for 'intractable pain'" [108].

While state-level medical boards are one of the most active areas in which policy change occurs, medical boards do not solely act within the individual state level. In fact, the Federation of State Medical Boards (FSMB) has issued a few iterations of a federal-level "model policies," or "model guidelines," which address prescriptions practices for pain management. The first "model policy" was adopted by the FSMB in 1998, and the second one in 2004 [126, 127]. According to the Pain Policy Study Group, more than 20 states have adopted at least some of the 1998 version of these model guidelines. There is still much diversity in state-level policy and enforcement, via laws, clinical licensing and accreditation [89]. Although the latest guidelines (2004) do include updated pain evaluation criteria, both iterations of these guidelines have a less interdisciplinary view of pain management and focus instead on a pharmacological approach that addresses prescription practices in pain management.

Another major player in USA national policy is the JCAHO, which inspects and accredits clinical institutions based on a centralized criterion. In 2001, the Joint Commission included pain-management-specific criteria in its standards, requiring that hospitals apply "appropriate pain assessment, [pain] management, and patient education [regarding pain and pain management]"[128]. These criteria help to create basic professional and institutional standards; however, how clinical settings meet these standards is still individually variable. In 2003, the Joint Commission published a guide with a decidedly more interdisciplinary and comprehensive approach to pain management [129]. In addition to pharmacological approaches to pain management, the guidelines also recommend the incorporation of evidence-based "non-pharmacological treatments" such as behavioral techniques, and "complementary and alternative therapies" with a focus on evidence-based acupuncture. Overall, the Joint Commission accreditation criteria are quite general in the area of pain management. Even so, these 2003 guidelines have been utilized by individual hospitals and health care institutions as one way of employing a best practices model. These institutions then document the ways in which they have interpreted the general standards of care into specific practices and striven for their best quality of therapeutic interventions [128].

"Opiophobia": An unfriendly regulatory environment?

The National Foundation for the Treatment of Pain (NFTP) published a list of "talking points" for its campaign for public awareness of pain. Among the information included in the public campaign was the following oft cited statistic: that one out of every 1400 physicians in the United States gets criminally prosecuted for prescribing pain medication. In the view of the Foundation, the treatment of pain in America is in a "downward spiral", due to physician fear of prosecution for treating pain [130]. In her constitutional law essay on pain management, Amy Dilcher writes that "opiophobia is the fear that the use of narcotics causes a drug addiction and drug abuse, and consequently is a factor that creates a barrier to pain management"; she points out, however, that, "for centuries, the medical profession has utilized opium [and its derivatives]… to treat pain… [but that]

opioids did not become a target of federal regulation [in the USA]… until the early 1900s" [132]. "As a consequence of self-protective regulatory restraint, patients may be suffering needlessly simply because the regulatory environment is unfriendly to aggressive pain management" [131]. Dilcher's overall thesis is that the well-documented undertreatment of pain in the USA is due in large part to fear of prosecution and censure.

It is often a confusing landscape that providers must navigate, one that propagates fear of prosecution and censure. US federal and state policies on the medical use of controlled substances are often at odds with each other. State-level statutory policy on the medical use of controlled substances is manifested in the oversight and policy of state congressional laws and state licensing boards.

In addition to this overlap between US federal mandates and state-level mandates, there is also some overlap between federal agencies that have mandates to oversee medical use of controlled substances. These agencies are: the US Attorney General's Office, the DEA, the National Institute on Drug Abuse, the Department of Health and Human Services, and its sub-branch, the Food and Drug Administration (FDA) [131].

While Dilcher applauds some legislative activity on the state-level and the creation of state-specific "intractable pain therapy acts [IPTAs]," she writes that "efforts to improve the pain management problem have been piecemeal and have consequently failed to achieve an improvement in the management of pain….A comprehensive public policy that addresses the multiple barriers is needed to address the inadequate management of pain in America." She also enumerates four areas for policy and program implementation: investigations and enforcement, healthcare facility inspection requirements, reimbursement, and education [131].

Quite markedly, however, not all pain care advocating voices are in unison. While many advocates and scholars who focus on the epidemic of undertreatment in pain care do report on the phenomenon of "undermedication", others argue the opposite point. An example of this is Charles Lucas and colleagues, who called for more "balance" in academic reporting so that gross clinical errors in "overmedication" are reported and highlighted in clinical policy debates as well [132]. The authors' stance is that there has been an "excessive [public and academic] emphasis on undermedication at the same time ignoring overmedication." This area of debate draws in issues related to ethics, legislation, clinical practice, research, and funding.

Elsewhere, Robert Kerns has editorialized that "no other issue in the field of pain management is more controversial than the appropriateness of prescribing opioid medications for non-cancer pain." He summarized the debate by observing "the lack of provider knowledge about appropriate use of these medications as well as dogmatic, stigmatizing, and ill-informed attitudes and beliefs about chronic opioid therapy may represent additional barriers to appropriate pain care and safe use of opioid medications" [133].

Pioneering legislation

In 2003, during the 108th session of congress, US Representative Micheal Rogers (R-MI) and Representative Grace Napolitano (D-CA) proposed a bill called the National Pain Care Act of 2003. It directed the President of the USA "to convene a White House Conference on Pain Care." It directed the Secretary of Health and Human Services "to establish a National Center for Pain and Palliative Care Research at the National Institutes of Health (NIH) to discuss the translation of pain research results into health services delivery, including mental health services to people experiencing chronic pain and those needing end-of-life care" and "to establish and implement a national campaign to provide information to the public on responsible pain management, related symptom management, and palliative care." It further outlines new standards of care regarding pain management for the governmental health insurance programs of Medicare and TRICARE (for the military). It also would have amended federal law to direct the Secretary of Veterans Affairs, along with the Secretaries of Defense, Transportation, and Health and Human Services, "to develop and implement a palliative pain care initiative in all health care facilities of the uniformed services,… and in all health care facilities of the Department of Veterans Affairs" and "to discuss the translation of pain research results into health services delivery, including mental health services to people experiencing chronic pain and those needing end-of-life care" [134].That same year another bill, Conquering Pain Act of 2003 (H.R. 2507/S. 1278) – was proposed by Darlene Hooley (D-OR) and Ron Wyden (D-OR). These bills contained "broad provisions related to the development of guidelines for the treatment of pain and Internet access to them by providers, quality improvement education projects, pain coverage quality evaluation and information, and family support networks in and insurance coverage of pain and symptom management" [135].

These bills failed to be voted on in both the House and the Senate before the congressional session expired, and so they never became law. In 2005, the National Pain Care Policy Act was reintroduced as a bill for the 109th session of congress as H.R. 1020, sponsored again by Representative Mike Rogers. After again failing to become law, it was reintroduced once more in 2008 as the house bill H.R. 2994 by Representative Lois Capps (D-CA), and the senate bill S. 3387, by Senator Orrin Hatch (R-UT) and Senator Christopher Dodd (D-CT), for the 110th session of congress. In a repeat of the 108th congressional session outcome, these bills failed to become ratified into law before the 110th congressional session [136, 137]. Finally, provisions for pain management related to the military and Veterans Affairs were passed in 2008, not as components of the National Pain Care Policy Act, but as components of two separate bills which focused on the healthcare of military personnel and veterans. These two bills are the Veterans Mental Health and Other Care Improvements Act of 2008, proposed as S. 2162 and sponsored by Senator Daniel Akaka (D-HI) and The Military Pain Care Act, proposed as the bill H.R. 5465, proposed by Representative David Loebsack (D-IA) [138, 139]. The Veterans Mental Health and Other Care Improvements Act of 2008, which is now a law, requires that there be a pain care program, for all VA inpatient facilities. As mandated, this program must include acute pain care and management to prevent long-term chronic pain disability. It also must include long-term mental health and substance abuse care. The mandate requires an interdisciplinary pain treatment approach to existing inpatient facilities. It also increases the mandate for VA research on pain and expands programs on staff education regarding pain assessment and treatment. The Military Pain Care Act, as part of S. 3001, the National Defense Authorization Act, directs the Department of Defense to implement a pain management initiative in all military health facilities for both active and retired military personnel and their dependents. This directive promotes both specialty pain medicine and interdisciplinary pain management. The act also mandates that these facilities conduct ongoing assessments to ensure that patients are receiving sufficient pain management services.

Most recently, for civilian health care, bill H.R. 756, sponsored by Representative Lois Capps and Representative Michael Rogers, has been forwarded by the House Committee on Energy and Commerce and is on the congressional agenda to receive a house-wide vote [140]. If passed by the house, it would move to the senate for a vote. This bill upholds the directives that the original 2003 National Health Care Policy bill proposed, minus the provisions for the military and veterans and creates a Pain Consortium and Pain Conference at the National Institutes of Health (NIH) to promote research on pain treatment and etiologies of pain. The bill also provides for "comprehensive pain care education and training" for all healthcare professionals, as well as the creation of "a national public awareness campaign on pain management" [140].

At the state level, the California Business and Professional Code (2001) has been cited as a best practice model of legislation. The legislation's three legal directives were unprecedented in the USA [26, 108, 141]. Among its provisions, the code makes it legally imperative that any healthcare provider who refused to prescribe opioid analgesics to a patient with intractable pain must inform the patient that there are other healthcare providers who specialize in pain management [108, 141]. The code also stipulates that continuing education in pain management and end-of-life care be mandatory for physicians in the state. Finally, the code requires that the California Medical Board create a protocol for investigating and acting upon complaints of the undertreatment of pain, and that a report of this activity be submitted annually to the government for state congressional approval [108, 141]. Encouraged by the government of California's statutory involvement in pain management practice and standards, advocates for more state regulation of pain management standards are pushing for similar legislation in the other states. The Commonwealth of Massachusetts is another state with a public policy pain initiative that brings together legislators, clinicians, public health professionals, and grassroots activists by using public hearings and media relations to compose diverse interdisciplinary subcommittees for stakeholders and constituents [141].

And so, where are we now with regards to state regulatory practices? Most recently, Gilson, Joranson, and Maurer of the University of Wisconsin Pain and Policy Studies Group, part of a WHO collaborating center, published a report that included a pilot examination of all state regulatory policies towards prescribers. Their conclusions were that these state laws "contained a number of outdated medical concepts and prescribing restrictions and did not contain key elements of law that can make pain management a priority for licensed medical practitioners" [118]. It is quite evident that the

most vocal advocates in the pain medication debate, from each side of the issue, are not resting on their laurels – instead they are calling for more work to be done. A commonality between the debating parties is that each side is seeking to highlight that we, as a society, are still very much in the early developmental stages of public policy, public awareness, and public debate on pain management issues.

The "other" pain management debate: medical marijuana

Marijuana has been illegal in the USA since the first quarter of the twentieth century. The debate that has emerged regarding the medicinal use of marijuana has stood alone and apart from the overall debate determining the codification of opioid/opiate usage. Perhaps due to historical, cultural, and legal reasons, considerations of medical marijuana have been marginalized in the overall discussion around pharmacological approaches to pain management. In fact, most publications by pain organizations and pain management scholars do not make reference to the debate around the criminalization of medicinal marijuana. In 2005, the Harvard Law Review published a 23-page report discussing "the substantive due process implications of prohibitions on medical marijuana", which was written, conveniently, by "Anonymous" [143]. The confidentiality of the author's identity may be seen as another sign of this marginalization and stigma surrounding medical marijuana advocacy. Another aspect of marginalization, critics argue, is that scientific research into the efficacy and effectiveness of medicinal marijuana is being stifled by US government regulations which have rendered marijuana research difficult to undertake for legal and financial reasons [144].

While the reference to medical marijuana has been minimized in the context of efficacy research, and the legalization advocacy movement has not entered into the mainstream pain policy debate – still, the existence of marijuana has not been fully ignored within the discourse of pain management providers. In fact, it is commonly mentioned as a verboten entity listed in opioid agreements, in which the signing patient must promise to abstain from abusing and using illicit substances (such as marijuana) while being treated with legally prescribed opioids under the medical care of the provider.

There may be a shift occurring, however. Since 1996, when the state of California passed Proposition 215 into law, aiming to decriminalize medical marijuana, the movement to legalize marijuana use for medicinal purposes has gained traction. Nevertheless, this 1996 California law creates a legislative and clinical paradox as it runs counter to federal law, which prohibits clinicians from even recommending that their in-pain patients try marijuana [143, 145]. Legal preemption dictates that when two laws are in conflict, such as state and federal laws, the stricter law prevails. However, preemption will also tend to side with federal over state when two laws are in conflict. To add to the legislative contradictions, there have been subsequent legal rulings regarding medicinal marijuana, including those by the US Supreme Court, that have effectively side-stepped the default mechanism of preemption [146]. Of course, this is not completely novel; legal conundrums (especially between state and federal statutes) plague other contested areas of pain management as well. However, medical marijuana has, perhaps, the quickest evolving and most "complex legal framework" of all the contested pharmacological approaches to pain [146].

Increasingly, within the law literature, legal analysts and scholars have been evoking the human rights rationale toward the legalization of medical marijuana. The right to medical treatment with marijuana has been equated with a right to health and posited as not only a question of ameliorating suffering, but rather a life or death issue for some patients [143]. With the movement to legalize marijuana gaining more credibility in the medical community, it is likely that the law and the debate will continue to shift and evolve over the next few years [146].

Footing the bill: The costs of chronic pain and chronic pain management

As stated by Gilson, "The costs of pain, both emotional and financial can be enormous" [118]. Chronic pain takes a toll on the individual suffering from the pain. There are multiple facets to the costs incurred: physical, psychological, social, and financial. Families may suffer as well, and the toll is often felt on a larger social and organizational level. These societal tolls include increased healthcare costs, a thriving illicit drug trade, disability claims, workforce absenteeism, and lowered production rates.

With the many costs of chronic pain, cost-effective analysis of chronic pain treatments can be difficult to compare with each other, especially if the analyses have operationalized "success" or "improvement"

differently. Was the treatment goal a reduction in pain severity on a particular subjective measure? Was it resumption of activities or return to work? Was success measured from a multi-dimensional perspective that took into account physical, social, psychological, and occupational functioning?

Nevertheless, despite some of these inconsistencies, researchers have compiled meta-analyses of various efficacy studies. These analyses help to compare the financial costs and specific outcome measures of treatment efficacy (such as return to work and reported pain improvement). These studies have also been important in forwarding the interdisciplinary model of pain management as a highly effective evidence-based approach.

While "conventional" or "unidimensional" approaches to pain management may include physical therapy along with pharmacological and surgical interventions, a "multidimensional" approach emphasizes the physical, psychosocial, and behavioral components of pain. A multidisciplinary pain center (MPC), then, may include non-pharmacologic approaches such as cognitive-behavioral therapy along with physical therapy, occupational therapy, nursing, and pain medicine. A 1993 meta-analysis of 65 studies evaluating MPCs found these treatments to be more effective at reducing back pain than back surgery is [62]. Despite the fact that this and many other studies have found MPC treatments more effective than surgical interventions at helping patients return to work and increasing their activity levels [62, 147, 148], surgical intervention, especially back surgery, is still considered the "gold standard of treatment" by some clinicians and many healthcare insurance companies. Due to this perception, surgical interventions for chronic pain are more likely to be reimbursed by health insurance organizations rather than the evidence-based MPC approach. Opioid therapy is also more likely than MPC approaches to be covered by health insurance organizations, even though recent randomized control trials (the gold standard of efficacy studies) have found that opioid therapy is not highly effective for long-term use for chronic pain [149, 150]. It seems that the reimbursement policies are not in line with the empirical research on treatment efficacy.

On the cost side of the cost-effective equation, Okifuji et al. [62] present the following data. They estimated that 10 years ago, in the USA, over $125 billion dollars were spent annually on chronic pain management. The costs for 2009, then, would be even greater. By

1999 standards, the following are the estimated costs of different treatment approaches. Funding treatment at an MPC averages around $8100 per patient. Treatment by "conventional" modalities (pain medicine and physical therapy) would average around $26 000 per patient. Surgical intervention for chronic pain would average around $15 000 for treatment. Therefore, based on these numbers, MPC approaches have the highest efficacy for the lowest cost.

It would seem that MPCs could be the silver bullet of chronic pain management. However, while early efficacy studies and trends in improving healthcare service sparked the flourishing of MPC in the 1970s and 1980s, there has been little growth since then. Main & Spanswick wrote that the 1990s saw an expansion of pain treatment centers, but the expansion was "chaotic … entrepreneurial" and despite the 1997 publication of the IASPs of "desirable characteristics" of pain management programs, the quality varied [151]. While MPCs are cost-effective, their interdisciplinary nature and complex perspective on pain can make them complex to run. Plus, costs for the multiple health professionals all at one time may seem burdensome to consumers and health insurance organizations. The bulk costs "upfront" may be one of the factors deterring insurance companies from favoring these treatments, or funding them at all. Okifuji and colleagues pointed out that in two decades there has not been much growth of multidisciplinary pain clinics. They cite Modell's estimate that in 1977 there were around 327 MPCs in the USA while in 1996 the APS estimated that there are 352 MPCs – an increase of only 25 [152, 153]. This growth-rate is considered stymied compared to the increasing needs and numbers of chronic pain patients. Along with the paucity of new clinics, the closing of existing programs may be contributing to this slow growth-rate.

It is quite telling, perhaps, that up-to-date data on the number of pain clinics and type of established pain clinic operations (i.e., multidisciplinary versus singular modality) are not readily available. This problem plagues the data for pain clinics in the USA, as well as for pain clinics abroad. Recent authoritative texts such as the 2001 edition of *Bonica's Management for Pain* and Main and Spanswick's *Pain Management: An Interdisciplinary Approach*, utilize data from 1979 and 1985 as the latest documentation on overall pain clinic numbers and descriptors [58, 151]. And so, in comparing the 1985 international data to the 1985 US estimates, one can see that multidisciplinary comprehensive pain care centers were a rarity abroad. According to Brena's data, Europe had one-quarter the number of multidisciplinary comprehensive pain clinics as the USA, while Canada, Asia and Australia/New Zealand each had about one-tenth of the number of multidisciplinary comprehensive pain clinics as compared with the USA. In this 1985 report, Brena reported only one multidisciplinary comprehensive pain clinic for all of Latin America, and the data for Africa were not available [58, 151, 154].

Clinical best practices: Pain management, assessment, quality improvement and admission criteria

The treatment of an invisible symptom, like pain, relies heavily on clinical measurement and assessment. Clinicians must assess how to incorporate function, emotion, and quality of life in pain assessments. Strides in pain measurement have incorporated function, emotion, and quality of life into multidimensional assessments such as the 1975 McGill Pain Questionnaire, the 1985 West Haven-Yale Multidimensional Pain Inventory (WHYMPI), and the 2002 Multidimensional Affect and Pain Survey (MAPS) [155–157]. The McGill, WHYMPI, and MAPS all assess qualitative and quantitative perceptions of pain and dysfunction. All three gather information on global mood and affect as well as pain-specific affects and states (i.e., pain catastrophizing).

These pain assessments are crucial in creating treatment plans. However, they are also indispensable as quality indicators within a larger quality improvement evaluation. As Gordon notes in his assessment of the state of the field in program enhancement and healthcare improvement for pain management: "Efforts to improve the quality of pain management must move beyond assessment and communication of pain to implementation and evaluation of improvements in pain treatment that are timely, safe, evidence based, and multimodal" [158].

A best practice example of "moving beyond assessment and communication" for quality improvement comes from Pasero and McCaffery's comfort–function model of pain management program improvement. In their model, the authors stress goal-setting, accountability, reviews, collaborative feedback, and collaborative treatment meetings for two major goals: comfort, i.e., an alleviation of pain severity, and function, i.e., increased functionality or activity [120]. One benefit of establishing a measurable comfort–function goal for each patient is that this may help to prevent the clinician's own personal biases from adversely affecting the treatment of pain. The patient-reported pain assessment and stated goal may help to avoid clinical prejudices reported in the research literature. For example, the authors cite research that showed that "nurses are likely to allow their personal opinions on the intensity of a patient's pain, and not the patient's rating of it, to determine their choice of analgesic dose" [120]. Furthermore, by using measurable and individualized comfort–function goals, there is increased accountability on the part of providers to strive to reach these stated goals for each patient. Pasero and McCaffery's model also encourages the use of "staff in-services and meetings [as] ideal times to discuss the use of the comfort–function goals, identify and solve pain problems unique to each care unit, and develop ways to improve pain management at the institutional level" [120].

In quality improvement, another best practice component is the aspect of longitudinal process and assessment. In reporting on their successes in implementing a longitudinal quality improvement project for pain management in post-operative patients, Meissner and colleagues recommend two strategies [159]. First, "a continuous quality improvement process" should be established, one that would include "frequent assessments of process and outcome parameters, regular benchmarking and implementation of feedback mechanisms" [159]. Second, based on the successes they have had in meeting their outcome and process parameters (i.e., lower pain ratings and pain intensity reports from patients), the authors recommend implementing a quality improvement process for pain management:

> "...Changes in [the] organization of medical management and multidisciplinary teamwork seem to be more important than medical or technical aspects... Transparency and multidisciplinary teamwork as well as benchmarking and prompt feedback mechanisms seem to be key elements of the successful implementation of a quality management initiative" [159].

While Meissner's group posits the idea of "multidisciplinary teamwork", the benchmarks utilized in their program improvement study are quite pharmacologically focused and do not include metrics associated with a more interdisciplinary approach that might integrate additional behavioral techniques.

It seems that the adherence to stated benchmarks and continuous review are two hallmarks of success in quality improvement for pain management. Gordon and colleagues observe that "although there are no perfect measures of quality, longitudinal data support the validity of a core set of indicators that could be used to obtain benchmark data for quality improvement in pain management in the hospital setting." [160].

Best practices: Case studies

Who gets accepted into a given pain treatment program and why? The answer depends entirely on the particular program, with admission criteria to pain treatment programs varying widely. Clinical standards and guidelines in this area are important because admission criteria act as gateways to care when so many go untreated. One program held up by the Joint Commission as a best practice model of admission criteria is the Georgia Comprehensive Sickle Cell Center [130]. The center's approach is a rather simple one; it has the following pain-related requisites for admission: a "failure to be pain free after 8 hours of outpatient treatment," and a "return for further therapy within 48 hours of previous inpatient or outpatient treatment of a pain episode." Furthermore, patients presenting with sickle-cell specific symptomology are brought in for treatment [129]. Theirs is a simple and straightforward method that has proven effective in maintaining accessibility and underscoring the importance of treatment.

Admissions criteria for comprehensive pain management treatment programs are site specific and as such differ widely and may be sensitive to change over time. In addition, quite often third-party payers' organizations have their own criteria for considering comprehensive pain management for identified chronic pain sufferers, while at the same time each private and public clinical setting may also have their own unique criteria. How selective are pain management programs currently? Recent data surveying the field over the past five years have not yet been published. In 1987, it was reported that on average, pain management programs accepted one-third of all of their applicants as patients, a paucity of information being available on the characteristics of patients who are getting rejected from these programs [161]. Unfortunately, this gap in information still exists.

The following case studies are presented as applied best practice models of an interdisciplinary and comprehensive initiative drawn from the Department of Veteran Affairs, Veterans Health Administration (VA), whose clinics have been in the vanguard of comprehensive pain management clinics for several reasons. One factor is likely the VA mission statement, which calls for prioritizing the most evidence-based treatment among treatment options. Another factor is likely the cost-benefit analysis of patient care that takes into account and often prioritizes long-term outcomes over short-term ones. In other words, a care facility that treats patients for the span of their lives is likely to be an environment that is more favorable to valuing higher financial cost of therapy (in this case, for comprehensive interdisciplinary pain management) if the end result is a greater health outcome in the *long-term*, rather than lower cost financial investment in the short-term but poorer health outcome in the long-term (as research suggests is the case with pharmacologic therapy only).

In response to widespread and long-term neglect of pain assessment in clinical practice, especially primary care, the APS began to promote the conceptualization of pain as "the fifth vital sign". Then in 1999, concept promotion became policy when the VA established an initiative to include pain measurement in the measurement of vital signs, declaring it officially the "fifth vital sign" in clinical care [162]. It was heralded as a "first step in what will be a long-term process to make pain management a routine part of patient care.... The VA project has the potential to transform pain management nationwide" [163]. Schuster emphasizes the VA's influence, pointing out that, in addition to treating close to four million patients, the VA "is the country's largest trainer of health care practitioners... Approximately half of all medical students... rotate through the VA medical system, which creates an opportunity to improve medical education around pain management" [163].

Pain as the fifth vital sign is part of a larger VA initiative, the "National Pain Management Strategy." The VA National Pain Management strategy was first implemented in 1998 and has been held up internationally as a best practice model because of its documented successes and continuous process design that has led to "rapid improvement" in comprehensive care [164–166]. Part of this strategy has been a collaboration with the Institute of Healthcare Improvement (IHI) to employ the " 'break-through series' model for rapid change in a healthcare system" [165]. As stated, the VHA National Pain Management Strategy's goal is "to develop a comprehensive, multicultural, integrated, system-wide approach to pain management that reduces pain for veterans with acute and chronic pain associated with a wide range of illnesses, including terminal illness" [165]. Its specific objectives are to optimize care in a way that

is interdisciplinary, multimodal and involves patients and families as active participants while providing for clinician preparation and systemic feedback and evaluation [164–166]. Its organizational structure includes committees and points of contact at the national level, regional level, facility level and even the caregiver levels. The VA National Pain Management Strategy Coordinating Committee (NPMSCC) also coordinates multiple interdisciplinary work groups that focus on, among other things, clinical guidelines, pharmacy, outcome measurement, research, and education.

In a 2003 report, Cleeland and colleagues reported from a survey of "collaborative data" over a 6-month time period that included data averaging between 20 and 40 facilities per goal and objective assessment [166]. The results showed significant improvement over all the target goals and objectives. Generally, screening for pain was up, the prevalence of severe pain was reduced, and documentation of a pain management plan and patient education were increased. It is important to note, that these data, as an aggregate set, reflects systemic and organizational changes, "rather than individual-specific measures." Such promising improvements are not evident in every facility in the VA, and more work needs to be done across the system.

With an eye on system improvement, in 2005, Mularski and colleagues did a survey of one singular outpatient general medical clinic in the VA system for the purpose of assessing the effects of the VA National Pain Management Strategy for improved pain care [168]. The authors found that instead of the adoption and implementation of the comprehensive collaborative system, the most evident change was a significant increase in screenings for pain. As such, the survey of this one site was disappointing and the results indicated that "routinely measuring pain as the 5th vital sign did not increase the quality of pain management". The results highlight how the lack of comprehensive follow-up, feedback, and collaboration can lead to substandard health outcomes even when pain severity is being duly documented [167].

As a best practice model, this VA National Pain Management Strategy has been compared favorably to strategies in Australia, Canada, and France [164]. Likewise, it seems that the critical lessons reported would be applicable to healthcare settings not just beyond the VA system, but beyond the USA.

Two site-specific best practice models within the VA are the Chronic Pain Rehabilitation Program (CPRP) at the James A. Haley VA Hospital in Tampa,

Florida, and the Comprehensive Pain Management Center (CPMC) at the VA Connecticut Healthcare System in West Haven, Connecticut. These clinics are within the vanguard of best practices for interdisciplinary and comprehensive pain management clinics, and both incorporate comprehensive pain assessment, interdisciplinary collaboration, and pharmacologic and non-pharmacologic treatment plans.

The VA's CPRP is a model of an extensive care unit encompassing inpatient and outpatient care. As such, it demonstrates how advanced and comprehensive pain care can be when there has been a substantial investment into the funding of such a program. On the other end of the spectrum, the VA's CPMC is more limited in scope, serving an outpatient population only. However, despite its more modest ambitions, the CPMC serves as a model of how hospitals and clinics can reorganize their pain care to create a comprehensive interdisciplinary center, even with restricted financial budgets.

The APS recently named the CPRP in Tampa a Clinical Center for Excellence in Clinical Care [168]. The CPRP in Tampa has a dedicated pain rehabilitation inpatient center and rehabilitation outpatient clinic. As part of the admission screening, each patient is evaluated, with clinicians considering "physiological, psychological, situational, adaptive, and restorative factors" [169].

The profile of the patient candidate for CPRP is as follows:

> "They must be motivated for treatment and willing to terminate the use of opioid analgesics and muscle relaxants for pain control. In general, past participants in the program have had very long-standing pain, are moderately to severely disabled, have numerous concurrent medical or emotional problems, and have been heavy consumers of medical resources." [169].

In addition to meeting the criteria for Veterans' health services, prospective participants for their program should have already had "non-cancer chronic pain of at least three to six months duration which has been refractory to standard therapy."

Patients with significant histories of substance abuse must complete "appropriate substance abuse treatment" and "attain a minimum of three months of abstinence from substances to be considered for admission." Furthermore, patients with very unstable physical or emotional states would be excluded from the inpatient rehabilitation program, as would those patients who are significantly limited in their abilities to engage in activities of daily living. However,

the CPRP may, ultimately, refer these patients to the outpatient pain rehabilitation clinic or they to a physical medicine rehabilitation program in which less physical activity is required [169, 170].

The VA Connecticut Healthcare System is in the process of innovating its system of pain management for outpatients. The program, the CPMC, is a model of how to create low-cost interdisciplinary care. In the initial visit to the clinic, patients rotate through individual evaluations by multiple providers: a doctoral-level physical therapist, a neurologist, an anesthesiologist, a pain medicine APRN, and a clinical health psychologist. Immediately after the evaluations are complete, the providers gather together for clinical rounds to collaborate on a treatment plan and recommendations for the patient. Other disciplines may also attend these rounds and participate; most often providers from substance abuse, psychiatry, chiropractic, infectious disease, and chaplaincy contribute to discussions of how to optimize an individual patient's care. Finally, the CPMC offers patient education on pain management and has begun an initiative to expand its patient education on pain management into a workshop series for other members of the VA community. The in-person consultation-evaluations, interdisciplinary pain rounds, and patient education module are all conducted within half a day.

Research trends

In 2000, in what many hoped would be an auspicious milestone for the field, the United States Congress and President Clinton signed a legal proclamation "that declared the 10-year period that began January 1, 2001, as the Decade of Pain Control and Research" [171]. Per this proclamation, it was anticipated that the NIH, which funds around one-third of all biomedical research in the USA, would be greatly increasing its allocation of funds to pain research [172].

Since the Decade of Pain Control and Research was proclaimed. the APS has called for pain management advocacy groups and scholarly societies to push for a comprehensive pain research agenda within governmental agencies and to also further partner with private non-governmental entities for research funding such as insurance and managed care organizations.

However, despite these calls for action from the pain management community, five years later, in a bold and timely focus-article from the *Journal of Pain*, Bradshaw and colleagues exposed the surprising and disappointing reality of NIH funding trends for pain research from 2003 to 2007 [172]. With the hope of providing more transparency around biomedical funding activities, Bradshaw and colleagues developed a methodology for tracking patterns in NIH funding. The authors note that the NIH has experienced "unprecedented reduction in its customary annual budgets increases" during the years 2003–2007, despite the hopeful 2000 proclamation. In fact, apart from slight increases in funding for projects related to nausea and dyspnea (which can be classified as pain-related studies), there has been an overall *reduction* in the numbers of grants and funding for pain research. This decline in funding "exceeds the reduction in the total NIH budget": in 2003, total NIH spending for pain research, be it clinical or basic science, was at less than 1% of its overall spending [172]. However, as the authors' analyses show, overall spending in pain research has declined even further since then, falling from 0.78% in 2004 to 0.61% in 2007 [172]. In an article inviting interested parties to become involved in legislative advocacy, Mitchell Max reported that pain research advocates have taken the Bradshaw *et al.* report and presented it to key legislators of the US Congress in the hopes of affecting appropriations reports for the coming year [173].

In February 2009, the US Congress passed a stimulus package that included an additional $10 billion of funding for the NIH. Within the NIH this has not been publicly earmarked, and so at press time it is unknown what these funds will be used for. In the meantime, the latest iteration of the National Pain Care Policy Act, passed by the House of Representatives for the 111th session of congress (HR 756), and waiting to be presented to the Senate, "includes a provision calling for pain research at NIH. If that bill becomes law, presumably additional funding for research will be provided" [84]. The authors call for more than increases and "changes to the budget" to address this funding deficit for pain research. Specifically, they call for "additional measures... to be taken by NIH to improve the chances of funding for meritorious applications proposing research on pain" [84].

Conclusion

Globally, the epidemic of both cancer- and non-cancer-related chronic pain is only worsening. Considering that our healthcare system is not adequately addressing our current needs, it is worrisome that, in the coming years, due to a shift in morbidity rates, the population's pain prevalence is expected to increase. This shift, due to the aging population and the rise of chronic disease prevalence, brings the suffering of chronic morbidities to the fore and highlights the need for palliative care and pain management.

Perhaps the same population and morbidity dynamics that are exacerbating this severe public health crisis of pain undertreatment will be the same dynamics that push policy towards prioritizing pain management and working towards better solutions. Metzger and Kaplan point out that the last 10 years have seen brisk change and improvements in palliative end-of-life care [174]. Perhaps the changes set in motion by the palliative healthcare movements, which were launched to better ensure less suffering in the dying, may indeed help all pain patients with less suffering as they live their lives. There may be many advocacy and policy avenues to help pain patients receive and participate in the type of care that can give them their lives back. As this chapter contends, an interdisciplinary approach that offers behavioral interventions in addition to pharmacological approaches may be the best for helping pain patients reclaim their lives.

Current clinical evidence indicates that pain treatment at an MPC "is consistently most effective for most outcomes" [143]. As a corollary, "the nature of MPC programs suggests strongly that evaluation... should be multidimensional, longitudinal, and should reflect the clinical, economic, and humanistic results of care" [143]. However costs associated with MPC treatment present a challenge for managed care organizations and other third-party payers. This is one of the major challenges of care and infrastructure growth.

The dynamics of pain management public policy reveal some of the most important features of the field and practice of pain care, some which continue to be battlegrounds of debate. Among these features of field and practice are: the slow shift to a recognition and conceptualization of pain as a biopsychosocial entity; the interdisciplinary nature of contemporary pain management; the relatively recent creation of the field of pain management, in its modern form; the jurisprudential and substance abuse issues related to the use of controlled substances for pain relief; and the serious public health crisis of pain undertreatment.

In its 2003 guide for clinical leaders, the Joint Commission emphasized another feature of pain management: "What makes the area of pain control so fascinating and sets it apart from other areas of health care is that at its core lies the subjective experience of diverse populations" [129]. This makes pain, the fifth vital sign, a unique phenomenon in clinical practice. Indeed, history of pain management policy and its accompanying issues are unique in the development of healthcare and public health policy. And so it may be that as pain management policy develops to more fully meet the needs of patients, it will move above and beyond the precedents of existing health policy as we know it.

Acknowledgments

The author wishes to extend her gratitude to Jared B. Katz, Jane Weinstein Brandes, Brook Moshan Gesser, and Abby Sher for all of their support – editorial and otherwise.

References

1. Wilson PR. Multidisciplinary ... transdisciplinary ... monodisciplinary ... where are we going? *Clin J Pain* 1996; **12**: 253–4.

2. Morris DB. *The Culture of Pain* (Berkeley: The University of California Press, 1991).

3. Blyth FM, March LM, Brnabic AJ, Cousins MJ. Chronic pain and frequent use of health care. *Pain* 2004; **111**: 51–8.

4. Breivik H, Collett B, Ventafridda V, Cohen R, Gallacher D. Survey of chronic pain in Europe: prevalence, impact on daily life, and treatment. *Eur J Pain* 2006; **10**: 287–333.

5. Elliott AM, Smith BH, Penny KI, Smith WC, Chambers WA. The epidemiology of chronic pain in the community. *Lancet* 1999; **354**: 1248–52.

6. Gerdle B, Bjork J, Henriksson C, Bengtsson A. Prevalence of current and chronic pain and their influences upon work and healthcare-seeking: a population study. *J Rheumatol* 2004; **31**: 1399–1406.

7. Lazarus H, Neumann C. Assessing undertreatment of pain: the patients' perspectives. *J Pharm Care Pain Symptom Control* 2001; **9**: 5–34.

8. Breivik H, Hattori S, Moulin DE. *Prevalence and impact of chronic pain: a systematic review of epidemiologic studies on chronic pain*. Paper presented at the International Association for the Study of Pain (IASP) 11th World Congress on Pain, Sydney, Australia. 2005.

9. Andersson HI, Ejlertsson G, Leden I, Rosenberg C. Chronic pain in a geographically defined general population: studies of differences in age, gender, social class, and pain localization. *Clin J Pain* 1993; **9**: 174–82.

10. Deyo RA, Mirza SK, Martin BI. Back pain prevalence and visit rates: estimates from U.S. national surveys, 2002. *Spine (Phila Pa 1976)* 2006; **31**: 2724–7.

11. Gureje O, Von Korff M, Simon GE, Gater R. Persistent pain and well-being: a World Health Organization study in primary care. *JAMA* 1998; **280**: 147–51.

12. Blyth FM, March LM, Brnabic AJ, *et al.* Chronic pain in Australia: a prevalence study. *Pain* 2001; **89**: 127–34.

13. Suka M, Yoshida K. Musculoskeletal pain in Japan: prevalence and interference with daily activities. *Mod Rheumatol* 2005; **15**: 41–7.

14. Kim SH, Bae GR, Lim HS. Prevalence and risk factors of fibromyalgia syndrome and chronic widespread pain in two communities in Korea – First report in Korean. *J Korean Rheum Assoc* 2006; **13**: 18–25.

15. Bonica JJ, Loeser JD. History of pain concepts and therapies. In *Bonica's Management of Pain*, eds. JD Loeser, SH Butler, CR Chapman, DC Turk. (Philadelphia: Lippincott, Williams, Wilkins, 2000), pp. 3–16.

16. Kerns RD, Thorn BE, Dixon KE. Psychological treatments for persistent pain: an introduction. *J Clin Psychol* 2006; **62**: 1327–31.

17. Roper Starch Worldwide Inc. *Chronic Pain in America: Roadblocks to Relief*: A study conducted by Roper Starch Worldwide for American Academy of Pain Medicine, American Pain Society and Janssen Pharmaceutica, 1999; www.ampainsoc.org/links/roadblocks/

18. Porreca F, Schug SA, Bellamy N. Challenging perception in chronic pain. *CME 2006*, 2006; www.medscape.com/viewprogram/4952

19. Fishman SM, Gallagher RM, Carr DB, Sullivan LW. The case for pain medicine. *Pain Med* 2004; **5**: 281–6.

20. Painter FM. *1999 National Pain Survey – Executive Summary, conducted for Ortho-McNeil Pharmaceutical*, 2009; http://chiro.org/LINKS/FULL/1999_National_Pain_Survey.shtml Accessed October 2009.

21. Green CR. The healthcare bubble through the lens of pain research, practice, and policy: advice for the new President and Congress. *J Pain* 2008; **9**: 1071–3.

22. Kerns RD, Otis J, Rosenberg R, Reid MC. Veterans' reports of pain and associations with ratings of health, health-risk behaviors, affective distress, and use of the healthcare system. *J Rehabil Res Dev* 2003; **40**: 371–9.

23. Woodwell DA. *National Ambulatory Medical Care Survey: 1998 Summary. Advance data from vital and health statistics; no. 315. Hyattsville, Maryland: National*

Center for Health Statistics, 2000; /www.cdc.gov/nchs/data/ad/ad315.pdf

24. LeResche L, Von Korff M. Epidemiology of chronic pain. In *Handbook of Pain Syndromes: Biopsychosocial Perspectives*, eds. AR Block, EF Kremer and E Fernandez. (Mahwah, NJ: Lawrence Erlbaum Associates, Inc., 1998), pp. 3–22.

25. Elliott AM, Smith BH, Chambers WA. Measuring the severity of chronic pain: a research perspective. *Expert Rev Neurother* 2003; **3**: 581–90.

26. Rashiq S, Schopflocher D, Taenzer P. (eds.). *Chronic Pain: A Health Policy Perspective* (Weinheim: Wiley-VCH Verlag GmbH Co. KGaA, 2008).

27. Smith BH, Macfarlane GJ, Torrance N. Epidemiology of chronic pain, from the laboratory to the bus stop: time to add understanding of biological mechanisms to the study of risk factors in population-based research? *Pain* 2007; **127**: 5–10.

28. Tunks ER, Crook J, Weir R. Epidemiology of chronic pain with psychological comorbidity: prevalence, risk, course, and prognosis. *Can J Psychiatry* 2008; **53**: 224–34.

29. Tunks ER, Weir R, Crook J. Epidemiologic perspective on chronic pain treatment. *Can J Psychiatry* 2008; **53**: 235–42.

30. Deer TR. Challenges in establishing the epidemiology of adverse events associated with interventional therapies for chronic pain. *Pain Med* 2008; **9**(Suppl 1): S2–S4.

31. Verhaak PF, Kerssens JJ, Dekker J, Sorbi MJ, Bensing JM. Prevalence of chronic benign pain disorder among adults: a review of the literature. *Pain* 1998; **77**: 231–9.

32. Ospina M, Harstall C. *Prevalence of chronic pain: an overview. Alberta Heritage Foundation for Medical Research, Health Technology Assessment. Report no. 28*, 2002. www.ihe.ca/documents/prevalence_chronic_pain.pdf

33. Hadler NM. *Worried Sick: A Prescription for Health in an Overtreated America* (Chapel Hill: University of North Carolina Press, 2008).

34. Helme RD, Gibson SJ. Pain in the elderly. In *Progress in Pain Research and Management: Proceedings of the 8th World Congress on Pain*, eds. TS Jensen, JA Turner, Z Wiesenfeld-Hallin. (Seattle Washington: IASP Press, 1997), pp. 919–44.

35. Kitahara M, Kojima KK, Ohmura A. Efficacy of interdisciplinary treatment for chronic nonmalignant pain patients in Japan. *Clin J Pain* 2006; **22**: 647–55.

36. Grossman SA, Sheidler VR, Swedeen K, Mucenski J, Piantadosi S. Correlation of patient and caregiver ratings of cancer pain. *J Pain Symptom Manage* 1991; **6**: 53–7.

37. Von Roenn JH, Cleeland CS, Gonin R, Hatfield AK, Pandya KJ. Physician attitudes and practice in cancer pain management. A survey from the Eastern Cooperative Oncology Group. *Ann Intern Med* 1993; **119**: 121–6.

38. Bernabei R, Gambassi G, Lapane K, *et al.* Management of pain in elderly patients with cancer. SAGE Study Group. Systematic Assessment of Geriatric Drug Use via Epidemiology. *JAMA* 1998; **279**: 1877–82.

39. Teno JM, Weitzen S, Wetle T, Mor V. Persistent pain in nursing home residents. *Jama* 2001; **285**: 2081.

40. Anderson KO, Richman SP, Hurley J, *et al.* Cancer pain management among underserved minority outpatients: perceived needs and barriers to optimal control. *Cancer* 2002; **94**: 2295–304.

41. Baker TA, Green CR. Intrarace differences among black and white Americans presenting for chronic pain management: the influence of age, physical health, and psychosocial factors. *Pain Med* 2005; **6**: 29–38.

42. Green CR. Racial and ethnic disparities in the quality of pain care: The anesthesiologist's call to action. *Anesthesiology* 2007; **106**: 6–8.

43. Edwards RR, Doleys DM, Fillingim RB, Lowery D. Ethnic differences in pain tolerance: clinical implications in a chronic pain population. *Psychosom Med* 2001; **63**: 316–23.

44. Green CR, Ndao-Brumblay SK, West B, Washington T. Differences in prescription opioid analgesic availability: comparing minority and white pharmacies across Michigan. *J Pain* 2005; **6**: 689–99.

45. Green C, Todd KH, Lebovits A, Francis M. Disparities in pain: ethical issues. *Pain Med* 2006; **7**: 530–3.

46. Ndao-Brumblay SK, Green CR. Racial differences in the physical and psychosocial health among black and white women with chronic pain. *J Natl Med Assoc* 2005; **97**: 1369–77.

47. Ruehlman LS, Karoly P, Newton C, Aiken LS. The development and preliminary validation of the Profile of Chronic Pain: Extended Assessment Battery. *Pain* 2005; **118**: 380–9.

48. Gatchel RJ, Okifuji A. Evidence-based scientific data documenting the treatment and cost-effectiveness of comprehensive pain programs for chronic nonmalignant pain. *J Pain* 2006; **7**: 779–93.

49. Stillion JM. Understanding the end of life: an overview. In *Psychosocial Issues Near the End of Life: A Resource for Professional Care Providers,* eds. JL Werth Jr. and D Blevins. (Washington DC: APA, 2005), pp. 11–26.

50. Lunney JR, Lynn J, Foley DJ, Lipson S, Guralnik JM. Patterns of functional decline at the end of life. *JAMA* 2003; **289**: 2387–92.

51. Meldrum ML. A capsule history of pain management. *JAMA* 2003; **290**: 2470–5.

52. Meyer C. Making sense of pain. *Minnesota Medicine.* 2001; www.mmaonline.net/Publications/MnMed2001/July/Meyer.html

53. Lü G, Li Q, Meng Z, Liu X. Can we be aware of both visceral and somatic sensations via a single neuronal pathway? *Chinese Sci Bull* 2002; **47**: 1940–5.

54. Norrsell U, Finger S, Lajonchere C. Cutaneous sensory spots and the "law of specific nerve energies": history and development of ideas. *Brain Res Bull* 1999; **48**: 457–65.

55. Ogoke BA. *The History of Pain Management as a Discipline,* 2008; www.northernpainmanagement.com/history.html. Accessed February 2009.

56. Dreeben O. *Introduction to Physical Therapy for Physical Therapist Assistants* (Boston: Jones Bartlett Publishers, Inc., 2006).

57. Gatchel RJ. Comorbidity of chronic pain and mental health disorders: the biopsychosocial perspective. *Am Psychol* 2004; **59**: 795–805.

58. Loeser JD, Turk DC. Multidisciplinary pain management. In *Bonica's Management of Pain,* 3rd edn., eds. JD Loeser, SH Butler, CR Chapman and DC Turk, (Philadelphia: Lippincott, 2001), pp. 2069–79.

59. Melzack R, Wall PD. Pain mechanisms: a new theory. *Science* 1965; **150**: 971–9.

60. Gallagher RM. Pain science and rational polypharmacy: an historical perspective. *Am J Phys Med Rehabil* 2005; **84**(3 Suppl): S1–3.

61. Boris-Karpel SM. *Measuring and Examining Correlates of Attitudes Towards Mind-body Connectivity in the Pain Experience.* (New York: Teachers College Columbia University, 2008).

62. Okifuji A, Turk DC, Kalauokalani D. Clinical outcome and economic evaluation of multidisciplinary pain centers. In *Handbook of Pain Syndromes. Biopsychosocial perspectives,* eds. AR Block, EF Kremer, E Fernande. (Mahway, NJ: Laurence Erlbaum Associates Publishers, 1999), pp. 87–98.

63. Rush AJ, Polatin P, Gatchel RJ. Depression and chronic low back pain: establishing priorities in treatment. *Spine* 2000; **25**: 2566–71.

64. Fishbain AD, Cutler BA, Rosomoff HL, Rosomoff RS. Pain facilities: a review of their effectiveness and referral selection criteria. *Curr Pain Headache Rep* 1997; 1: 107–16.

65. Karoly P, Ruehlman LS. Motivational implications of pain: chronicity, psychological distress, and work goal construal in a national sample of adults. *Health Psychol* 1996; **15**: 383–90.

66. Lackner JM, Gurtman MB. Pain catastrophizing and interpersonal problems: a circumplex analysis of the communal coping model. *Pain* 2004; **110**: 597–604.

67. Loeser JD. Economic implications of pain management. *Acta Anaesthesiol Scand* 1999; **43**: 957–9.

68. Macdonald DI. Letters supporting WHO and the Wisconsin initiative for improving cancer pain management. *J Pain Symptom Manage* 1986; 1: 182–3.

69. Accreditation Council for Medical Education. *ACGME Program Requirements for Graduate Medical Education in Pain Medicine.* 2007; www.acgme.org/acWebsite/downloads/RRC_progReq/sh_multiPainPR707.pdf Accessed March 2009.

70. Jacobson L, Mariano AJ, Chabal C, Chaney EF. Beyond the needle: expanding the role of anesthesiologists in the management of chronic non-malignant pain. *Anesthesiology* 1997; **87**: 1210–8.

71. Aronoff GN, McAlary PW. Organization and Personnel Functions in the Pain Clinic. In *The Multidisciplinary Pain Center: Organization and Personnel Functions for Pain Management,* ed. JN Ghia. (Boston: Kluwer Academic, 1998), pp. 21–43.

72. Mitka M. "Virtual textbook" on pain developed: effort seeks to remedy gap in medical education. *JAMA* 2003; **290**: 2395.

73. Vadivelu N, Kombo N, Hines RL. The urgent need for pain management training. *Acad Med* 2009; **84**: 408.

74. Leo RJ, Pristach CA, Streltzer J. Incorporating pain management training into the psychiatry residency curriculum. *Acad Psychiatry* 2003; **27**: 1–11.

75. Zalon ML. Pain management instruction in nursing curricula. *J Nurs Educ* 1995; **34**: 262–7.

76. Clarke EB, French B, Bilodeau ML, *et al.* Pain management knowledge, attitudes and clinical practice: the impact of nurses' characteristics and education. *J Pain Symptom Manage* 1996; **11**: 18–31.

77. Glajchen M, Bookbinder M. Knowledge and perceived competence of home care nurses in pain management: a national survey. *J Pain Symptom Manage* 2001; **21**: 307–16.

78. Laborde EB, Texidor MS. Knowledge and attitudes toward chronic pain management among home health

care nurses. *Home Health Care Manag Pract* 1996; **9**: 73–7.

79. McCaffery M, Ferrell BR. Opioids and pain management: what do nurses know? *Nursing* 1999; **29**: 48–52.

80. Maclaren JE, Cohen LL. Teaching behavioral pain management to healthcare professionals: a systematic review of research in training programs. *J Pain* 2005; **6**: 481–92.

81. Salanterä S, Lauri S, Salmi TT, Helenius H. Nurses' knowledge about pharmacological and nonpharmacological pain management in children. *J Pain Symptom Manage* 1999; **18**: 289–99.

82. Weiner DK, Turner GH, Hennon JG, Perera S, Hartmann S. The state of chronic pain education in geriatric medicine fellowship training programs: results of a national survey. *J Am Geriatr Soc* 2005; **53**: 1798–1805.

83. Yanni LM. *Virginia Commonwealth University (VCU) Chronic Non-Malignant Pain Management Course*, 2009; www.paineducation.vcu.edu. Accessed March 2009.

84. American Academy of Pain Medicine, The American Pain Society, The American Society of Addiction Medicine. *Public Policy Statement on the Rights and Responsibilities of Healthcare Professionals in the Use of Opioids for the Treatment of Pain*, 2004; www.ampainsoc.org/advocacy/rights.htm. Accessed February 2009.

85. Joranson DE, Rajagopal MR, Gilson AM. Improving access to opioid analgesics for palliative care in India. *J Pain Symptom Manage* 2002; **24**: 152–9.

86. International Association for the Study of Pain. *History of IASP* 2009; hwww.iasp-pain.org/AM/Template.cfm?Section=History1&Template=/CM/HTMLDisplay.cfm&ContentID=1609. Accessed March 2009.

87. Maddocks I. Palliative care education in the developing countries. *J Pain Palliat Care Pharmacother* 2003; **17**: 211–21.

88. Sinatra R. Opioid analgesics in primary care: challenges and new advances in the management of noncancer pain. *J Am Board Fam Med* 2006; **19**: 165–77.

89. Joranson DE, Carrow GM, Ryan KM, *et al.* Pain management and prescription monitoring. *J Pain Symptom Manage* 2002; **23**: 231–8.

90. Fishman SM. *Responsible Opioid Prescribing: A physician's guide.* (Washington DC: Federation of State Medical Boards, Waterford Life Sciences, 2007).

91. IJIS Institute. PMP Committee Phase II PMIX Pilot Project Survey of State Prescription Monitoring Programs, 2007; http://www.kms.ijis.org/db/share/public/PMIX/ijis_pmix_survey_ta_report_20070204.pdf.

92. Brushwood DB. Maximizing the value of electronic prescription monitoring programs. *J Law Med Ethics* 2003; **31**: 41–54.

93. Manchikanti L. National drug control policy and prescription drug abuse: facts and fallacies. *Pain Physician* 2007; **10**: 399–424.

94. Bolen J. DEA and Schedule II "Do Not Fill Prescriptions" – Disappointing Enforcement Activity. *Pain Med* 2006; **7**: 80–5.

95. Covington E. DEA and pain practitioners: common goals, adversarial stance? *Pain Med* 2006; **7**: 75–5.

96. Fishman SM. The DEA and pain medicine. *Pain Med* 2006; **7**: 71.

97. Heit HA. Healthcare professionals and the DEA: trying to get back in balance. *Pain Med* 2006; **7**: 72–4.

98. Lipman AG. Does the DEA truly seek balance in pain medicine? A chronology of confusion that impedes good patient care. *J Pain Palliat Care Pharmacother* 2005; **19**: 7–9.

99. Passik SD. Pain management misstatements: ceiling effects, red and yellow flags. *Pain Med* 2006; **7**: 76–7.

100. Rich BA. Of smoke, mirrors, and passive-aggressive behaviors. *Pain Med* 2006; **7**: 78–9.

101. Rowe W. Pain, the DEA, and the impact on patients. *Pain Med* 2006; **7**: 86–6.

102. Fine PG. The evolving and important role of anesthesiology in palliative care. *Anesth Analg* 2005; **100**: 183–8.

103. Kingsbury SJ, Yi D, Simpson GM. Psychopharmacology: rational and irrational polypharmacy. *Psychiatr Serv* 2001; **52**: 1033–6.

104. Zacharoff, K. *The Role of Rational Polypharmacy in Pain Management*, 2008; www.painedu.org/articles_timely.asp?ArticleNumber=17. Accessed February 2009.

105. Driver LC. Managing cancer pain: practical principles and pearls for pragmatic polypharmacy. *Clin J Pain* 2008; **24** Suppl 10: S1–2.

106. Joranson DE, Ryan KM. Ensuring opioid availability: methods and resources. *J Pain Symptom Manage* 2007; **33**: 527–32.

107. American Pain Foundation. *Consensus Statement Supporting the National Pain Care Policy Act of 2009 (HR 756/S.660)*, 2009; www.painfoundation.org/take-action/natl-efforts/consensus-statement.html. Accessed March 2009.

108. Brennan F, Carr DB, Cousins M. Pain management: a fundamental human right. *Anesth Analg* 2007; **105**: 205–21.

109. Kickbusch I. Responding to the health society. *Health Promot Int* 2007; **22**: 89–91.

110. Kickbusch I, Payne L. Twenty-first century health promotion: the public health revolution meets the wellness revolution. *Health Promot Int* 2007; **18**; 275–8.

111. Arons S. Palliative Care in the US Health Care System: Constitutional right or criminal act? *West New Engl Law J Rev* 2007; **29**: 309–56.

112. Fields HL. *Core Curriculum for Professional Education in Pain* 2nd edn. (Seattle: IASP Press, 1995).

113. Taylor ML. Ethical issues for psychologists in pain management. *Pain, Med* 2001; **2**: 147–54.

114. Blacksher E. Hearing from pain: using ethics to reframe, prevent, and resolve the problem of unrelieved pain. *Pain Med* 2001; **2**: 169–75.

115. Cousins MJ, Brennan F, Carr DB. Pain relief: a universal human right. *Pain* 2004; **112**: 1–4.

116. Vasudevan SV. Commentary: empower and educate patients diagnosed with chronic nonmalignant pain. *J Pain* 2005; **6**: 10–11.

117. Lebovits A. The ethical implications of racial disparities in pain: are some of us more equal? *Pain Med* 2001; **6**: 3–4.

118. Gilson AM, Joranson DE, Maurer MA. Improving state pain policies: recent progress and continuing opportunities. *CA Cancer J Clin* 2007; **57**: 341–53.

119. Marks RM, Sachar EJ. Undertreatment of medical inpatients with narcotic analgesics. *Ann Intern Med* 1973; **78**: 173–81.

120. Pasero C, McCaffery M. Comfort-function goals: a way to establish accountability for pain relief. *Am J Nurs* 2004; **104**: 77–8, 81.

121. Imhof S, Kaskie B. How can we make the pain go away? Public policies to manage pain at the end of life. *Gerontologist* 2008; **48**: 423–31.

122. Weinman BP. LeTourneau Award. Freedom from pain. Establishing a constitutional right to pain relief. *J Leg Med* 2003; **24**: 495–539.

123. Pain Policy Study Group. *Pain Policy Glossary,* 2009; www.medsch.wisc.edu/painpolicy/glossary.htm. Accessed February 2009.

124. Bolen J. Ethical issues in the treatment of chronic non-malignant pain: a focus on the legal side. *Pain Pract* 2008; **18**: S1–8.

125. Liang BA, Fermani K. "Standards" of anesthesia: law and ASA guidelines. *J Clin Anesth* 2008; **20**: 393–6.

126. Federation of State Medical Boards. *Model Policy for the Use of Controlled Substances for the Treatment*

of Pain. 2004; www.fsmb.org/pdf/2004_grpol_Controlled_Substances.pdf. Accessed March 2009.

127. Federation of State Medical Boards. *Development of the Model Policy for the Use of Controlled Substances for the Treatment of Pain.* 2009; www.fsmb.org/grpol_pain_policy_resource_center.html. Accessed March 2009.

128. Joint Commission on Accreditation of Healthcare Organizations *Pain Standards for 2001*, 2001; www.jcaho.gov/. Accessed February 2009.

129. Joint Commission on Accreditation of Healthcare Organizations. *Pain Standards for 2003*, 2003; www.jcaho.gov/. Accessed February 2009.

130. National Foundation for the Treatment of Pain. *National Pain Awareness Campaign.* 2003; www.paincare.org/pain_awareness/index.html. Accessed February 2009.

131. Dilcher AJ. Damned if they do, damned if they don't: the need for a comprehensive public policy to address the inadequate management of pain. *Ann Health Law* 2004; **13**: 81–144.

132. Lucas CE, Vlahos AL, Ledgerwood AM. Kindness kills: the negative impact of pain as the fifth vital sign. *J Am Coll Surg* 2007; **205**: 101–7.

133. Kerns RD. Research on pain and pain management in Veterans Health Administration: promoting improved pain care for veterans through science and scholarship. *J Rehabil Res Dev* 2007; **44**: vii–x.

134. The National Pain Care Act of 2003, H.R. 1863, House of Representatives, 108th Cong., 1st Sess.(2003a).

135. Conquering Pain Act of 2003, H.R. 2507, House of Representatives, 108th Cong., 1st Sess.(2003b).

136. The National Pain Care Policy Act of 2005, H.R. 1020, House of Representatives, 109th Cong., 1st Sess. (2005).

137. National Pain Care Policy Act of 2008, H.R. 2994, House of Representatives, 110th Cong., 1st Sess. (2008).

138. Veterans' Mental Health and Other Care Improvements Act of 2008, S. 2162, Senate, 110th Cong., 1st Sess.(2008).

139. Military Pain Care Act of 2008, H.R. 5465, House of Representatives, 110th Cong., 1st Sess.(2008).

140. National Pain Care Policy Act of 2009, H.R. 756, House of Representatives, 111th Cong., 1st Sess. (2009).

141. Charatan F. New law requires doctors to learn care of the dying. *BMJ* 2001; **323**: 1088.

142. Lande S, Kulich R. (eds.). *Managed Care and Pain.* (Glenview, Illinois: American Pain Society, 2000).

143. Anonymous. Last resorts and fundamental rights: the substantive due process implications of prohibitions on medical marijuana. *Harvard Law Rev* 2005; **118**: 1985–2006.

144. Krisberg K. Court decision on medical marijuana use worries patient advocates. *Nations Health* 2005; **35**: 14.

145. Pacula RL, Chriqui JF, Reichmann DA, Terry-McElrath YM. State medical marijuana laws: understanding the laws and their limitations. *J Public Health Policy* 2002; **23**: 413–39.

146. Seamon MJ, Fass JA, Maniscalco-Feichtl M, Abu-Shraie NA. Medical marijuana and the developing role of the pharmacist. *Am J Health Syst Pharm* 2007; **64**: 1037–44.

147. Flor H, Fydrich T, Turk, DC. Efficacy of multidisciplinary pain centers: A meta-analytic review. *Pain* 1992; **49**: 221–30.

148. Wiesel SW, Feffer HL, Rothman RH. Industrial low-back pain. A prospective evaluation of a standardized diagnostic and treatment protocol. *Spine* 1984; **9**: 199–203.

149. Ballantyne JC, Shin NS. Efficacy of opioids for chronic pain: a review of the evidence. *Clin J Pain* 2008; **24**: 469–78.

150. Martell BA, O'Connor PG, Kerns RD, *et al.* Systematic review: opioid treatment for chronic back pain: prevalence, efficacy, and association with addiction. *Ann Intern Med 2007*; **146**: 116–27.

151. Main, CJ, Spanswick CC. The origins and development of modern pain management programmes. In *Pain Management*, eds. CJ Main and CC Spanswick. (Edinburgh: Churchill Livingstone, 2000), pp. 107–14.

152. American Pain Society. *1996 Pain Facilities Directory.* (Glenview, IL, 1996).

153. Modell J. *Directory of Pain Clinics* (Oak Ridge, TN: American Soceity of Anesthesiologists, 1977).

154. Brena SF. Pain control facilities: patterns of operation and problems of organization in the USA. *Clin Anesthesiol* 1985; **3**: 183–95.

155. Clark WC, Yang JC, Tsui SL, Ng KF, Bennett Clark S. Unidimensional pain rating scales: a multidimensional affect and pain survey (MAPS) analysis of what they really measure. *Pain* 2002; **98**: 241–7.

156. Kerns RD, Turk DC, Rudy TE. The West Haven-Yale Multidimensional Pain Inventory (WHYMPI). *Pain* 1985; **23**: 345–56.

157. Melzack R. The McGill Pain Questionnaire: major properties and scoring methods. *Pain* 1975; **1**: 277–99.

158. Gordon DB, Dahl JL, Miaskowski C, *et al.* American Pain Society recommendations for improving the quality of acute and cancer pain management: American Pain Society Quality of Care Task Force. *Arch Intern Med* 2005; **165**: 1574–80.

159. Meissner W, Ullrich K, Zwacka S. Benchmarking as a tool of continuous quality improvement in postoperative pain management. *Eur J Anaesthesiol* 2006; **23**: 142–8.

160. Gordon DB, Pellino TA, Miaskowski C, *et al.* A 10-year review of quality improvement monitoring in pain management: recommendations for standardized outcome measures. *Pain Manag Nurs* 2002; **3**: 116–30.

161. Osterweis, M, Kleinman, A, Mechanic, D. (eds.). *Pain and Disability: Clinical, Behavioral, and Public Policy Perspectives* (Washington DC: National Academy Press, 1987).

162. Lynn J, Schuster JL, Wilkinson A, Simon LN. *Improving Care for the End of Life: A sourcebook for health care managers and clinicians*, 2nd edn. (New York: Oxford University Press, 2007).

163. Schuster JL. Veterans Health Administration's addition of pain as a fifth vital sign may have far-reaching effects, 1999; www.mywhatever.com/cifwriter/content/19/abcd617.html. Accessed June 2010,

164. Dobkin PL, Boothroyd L. Organizing health services for patients with chronic pain: when there is a will there is a way. *Pain Medicine.* 2008; **9**: 881–9.

165. Kerns RD, Craine M. Pain management improvement strategies in the Veteran's Health Administration. *APS Bulletin* 2003; **13**: 5.

166. Cleeland CS, Reyes-Gibby CC, Schall M, *et al.* Rapid improvement in pain management: The Veterans Health Administration and the Institute for Healthcare Improvement Collaborative. *Clin J Pain*, 2003; **19**: 298–305.

167. Mularski, RA, White-Chu F, Overbay D, Miller L, Asch SM, Ganzini L. Measuring pain as the 5th vital sign does not improve quality of pain management. *J Gen Intern Med* 2006; **21**: 607–12.

168. American Pain Society. APS Press Room: American Pain Society Announces Recipients of Clinical Centers of Excellence in Pain Management Awards. 2007; www.ampainsoc.org/press/2007/041207.htm

169. Corsini, E. (Interviewer) & Walker, R. (Interviewee). (2006b). *US War Veterans and Pain #2* [Interview transcript]. Retrieved from Pain.EDu.org Spotlight Interviews web site: www.painedu.org/spotlight.asp?spotlightNumber=31&UserID=0

170. Corsini, E. (Interviewer) & Walker, R. (Interviewee). (2006a). *US War Veterans and Pain #1* [Interview transcript]. Retrieved from Pain EDu.org Spotlight Interviews web site: www.painedu.org/spotlight. asp?spotlightNumber=30&UserID=0

171. Loeser JD. The decade of pain control and research, 2003; www.ampainsoc.org/pub/bulletin/may03/article1.htm. Accessed June 2010.

172. Bradshaw DH, Empy C, Davis P, *et al*. Trends in funding for research on pain: A report on the National Institutes of Health Grant Awards Over the Years 2003 to 2007. *J Pain 2008*; **9**: 1077–7.e1078.

173. Max MB. Addressing the decline in NIH pain research funding. *J Pain 2008*; **9**: 1074–6.

174. Metzger M, Kaplan KO. *Transforming Death in America: A State of the Nation Report* (Washington, DC: Last Acts, 2001).

Practice, policy, and research

Diversity and disparities in pain management

26

Carmen R. Green and Alexandra S. Bullough

Introduction

The US is rapidly aging and diversifying to become the most multi-ethnic, multi-racial, and multi-generational nation ever seen in history (Figures 26.1–4) [1–4]. By 2030, non-white racial and ethnic groups (e.g., African Americans, Hispanics, and Native Americans) as well as women will constitute a majority of the American population (figure 4). The World Health Organization (WHO) defines health as a state of complete physical, social, and emotional well-being and not merely the absence of disease and infirmities [5, 6]. In an increasingly diverse society, socio-demographic factors (i.e., age, race, ethnicity, gender, and class) will play a significant role in determining health and well-being [7–9]. These socio-demographic factors not only affect health status but also significantly influence the quality of healthcare [10]. However, the literature discussing global disparities in health and the healthcare experience for underserved and potentially vulnerable populations such as racial and ethnic minorities, women, elderly, and impoverished individuals has rarely addressed the quality of pain care or the impact pain has on overall health and well-being [11–21].

To date the health and healthcare disparities literature has primarily focused on a few disease states such as cardiovascular disease, cancer, diabetes, osteoarthritis, and obesity [22–27]. Although they are extremely common chronic diseases, it is important to note that they are all also associated with acute, chronic, or cancer pain. The challenge is that both the medical and public health communities tend to view pain as a symptom rather than as a disease state with unique sequelae significantly impacting an individuals physical, social, emotional, and economic health and well-being [28]. The relative omission of pain, chronic pain, and disparities in pain care is particularly problematic considering the socio-economic implications associated with

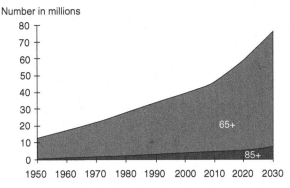

Figure 26.1 1999 US Census projections (millions). Source: Health, United States, 1999 and US Bureau of the Census With permission from the US Census Bureau.

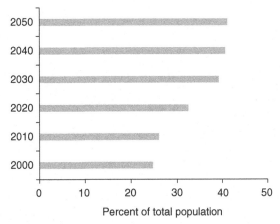

Figure 26.2 Projected population growth, adults ≥ 65. Source: US Census Bureau, 2004. Projected Population Change in the USA, by Age and Sex: 2000 to 2050. www.census.gov/ population/www/projections/usinterimproj/natprojtab02b.pdf Internet Release Date: March 18, 2004.

Behavioral and Psychopharmacologic Pain Management, ed. Michael H. Ebert and Robert D. Kerns. Published by Cambridge University Press. © Cambridge University Press 2011.

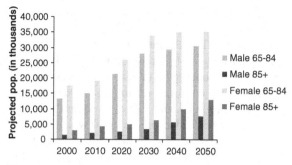

Figure 26.3 Gender and aging.
Source: US Census Bureau, 2004. Projected Population of the USA, by Age and Sex: 2000 to 2050. www.census.gov/population/www/projections/usinterimproj/natprojtab02a.pdf Internet Release Date: March 18, 2004.

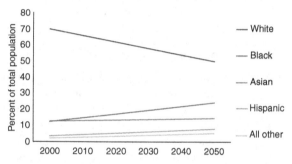

Figure 26.4 Projected population growth, by race.
Source: US Census Bureau, 2004. Projected Population Change in the USA, by Race and Hispanic Origin: 2000 to 2050. http://www.census.gov/population/www/projections/usinterimproj/natprojtab01b.pdf Internet Release Date: March 18, 2004.

pain in terms of disability and healthcare utilization [2, 29]. This is an important consideration since the scientific literature provides ample evidence for pain being the third largest global health problem [30–33]. In addition, differences in the pain experience based upon these socio-demographic factors show minorities, women, the elderly, and the impoverished are at increased risk for poor assessment and treatment of their pain complaints [34–36]. Nonetheless, most health professionals do not consider the role socio-demographic factors have when evaluating and treating their patients.

Overall, pain is a significant national and global public health problem issue causing tremendous suffering and disability [37–40]. People with chronic pain often experience concomitant depression, anxiety, post-traumatic stress disorder (PTSD), sleep disturbance, fatigue, and decreased physical functioning [11, 13, 41–44]. Pain may also lead an individual to withdraw from

their societal roles leading to impaired family and work relationships while also diminishing health and quality of life (QOL) [42, 46–49]. Consistent with emerging policy discussions positioning pain relief as a human rights issue, this chapter will highlight literature supporting pain's impact on overall health and well-being while providing support for its appropriate assessment and treatment. It also provides information on pain as a quality of care issue. Background information serves as a platform for discussing the role race, ethnicity, age, gender, and class have on pain care for an increasingly aging and diversifying society. Lastly, this chapter will focus on disparities in pain assessment and treatment, access to quality pain care, and clinician variability in pain management decision-making.

Why do healthcare disparities matter?

The importance of health and healthcare disparities has attracted attention from all branches of government and at the local, state, and federal level [22, 26]. Several federal agencies have addressed the inequality of health and healthcare across a full spectrum of disease states and treatments. The National Institutes of Health (NIH) was one of the first federal agencies to define health disparities as a "difference in incidence, prevalence, mortality and burden of disease and other adverse health conditions" [50]. The Institute of Medicine (IOM) of the National Academy of Sciences defined healthcare disparities as racial or ethnic differences in the quality of healthcare that are not due to access related factors, clinical needs, preferences, or appropriateness of interventions. Implicit in all definitions is disadvantage and increased disease burden for those impacted [51].

The Legislative Branch of the US government has attempted to address health and healthcare disparities. The US Congress charged the IOM to assess healthcare inequities and disparities in the delivery of healthcare services. The resulting IOM report, *Unequal treatment and unequal burdens: Racial and ethnic disparities in healthcare*, confirmed disparities through the healthcare system, for acute and chronic conditions, and clinician variability [22, 26, 52]. Although the IOM report viewed pain management as one of the clinical areas where disparities exist, the discussions regarding pain were limited to a few pages and were directed at acute and cancer pain only. Yet, there is literature documenting variability and disparities in pain care based upon race, ethnicity, and gender across several painful conditions (e.g., osteoarthritis, sickle cell anemia, fibromyalgia, lupus), types of pain (i.e., acute, cancer, and chronic pain), and treatment settings (e.g., ambulatory, inpatient) [3, 53–68]. In general, minority patients (i.e., African Americans, Hispanics, Native Americans), lower socio-economic status individuals, and women (regardless of age) receive lesser quality pain care when compared to Caucasian men [35]. Despite much being written about disparities and clinician variability in decision-making based upon patient gender, the IOM did not specifically address gender related disparities in these reports. Instead they concluded that these disparities persisted regardless of age, sex, and socio-economic status (SES) [26]. Regardless, legislation designed to address health and healthcare disparities has just begun to focus on pain while proposing new legislation and policy designed to understand, reduce, and eliminate disparities in pain care (e.g., the National Pain Care Policy Act of 2007; H.R. 2994).

Overall, the Executive Branch through the Department of Health and Human Services has sponsored many research initiatives and spent millions of dollars attempting to understand, reduce, and eliminate health disparities [69]. Surprisingly, there is a lack of attention to pain in general and disparate pain care in particular. Pain is also missing from other well publicized public health agendas designed to improve the nation's colloquial health related quality of life [70–73]. Federal agencies, e.g., NIH, Agency of Health Research and Quality (AHRQ), Centers for Disease Control (CDC), have acknowledged health disparities and inequities while setting goals toward eliminating racial and ethnic disparities in health status and healthcare [74, 75]. Yet, these same agencies have not addressed the differential impact pain has on minorities, vulnerable populations, and the underserved in terms of their health and well-being. An emerging literature has begun to highlight differences in pain perception as well as disparities in pain care for racial and ethnic minorities for all types of pain (i.e., acute, chronic, and cancer pain) and across all settings (i.e., inpatient and outpatient settings), although less than 1% of NIH research dollars are directed at primary pain research [35, 76–79].

The Judicial Branch of the US government has also contributed to the disparities discussion through their rulings on affirmative action as a means to ensure diversity. In the US Supreme Court case *Grutter v. Bollinger*, the Supreme Court narrowly ruled (5:4) that the University of Michigan may consider socio-demographic factors, specifically race and ethnicity, as a factor in admission to the University of Michigan's law school.[1] The US Supreme Court further ruled that the University of Michigan's law school did not violate the constitutional rights of non-minority applicants by doing so. The corporate sector (e.g., Ford motor company), the military, and former President of the USA Gerald Ford provided amicus briefs which stated that creating a "critical mass" of racial and ethnic diversity was in the best interest of the students, school, university, and the nation. Beyond ensuring that race and ethnicity can be used as one of many factors in selecting students for admission to the law school, the ruling impacts women and socio-economically disadvantaged individuals while having far reaching implications for health professional schools and healthcare disparities as the USA ages and increasingly diversifies.

Why diversity is important?

Overall, the literature supports that increasing diversity yields improved educational experiences for all students and health professionals during their training as well as for their patients [80]. Yet, African Americans, Hispanics, and Native Americans are significantly underrepresented in medicine and the health professions [81]. However, underrepresented minority physicians are more likely to serve the medically underserved and racial and ethnic minority populations. Both racial and gender congruence is also an important consideration for patient care [60]. Given a choice, racial and ethnic minority patients and women are more likely to choose a physician with the same race, ethnicity, or gender. Overall, women physicians spend more time with their patients than their male counterparts leading to more positive discussions, explanations, rapport, and emotional support [82, 83]. In pediatrics, doctor visits with women pediatricians were 29% longer than those with men [82]. Women provided more encouragement, reassurance, and communication during the physical examination, and obtained more information from children when compared to their male counterparts. Particularly compelling are data suggesting that parents were more satisfied and children also

---

[1] A comprehensive review of the history, documents, and arguments associated with the University of Michigan cases is provided at: www.oyez.org/cases/2000–2009/2002/2002_02_241/.

communicated more with women physicians [81]. The result is improved physician–patient communication, greater patient satisfaction, better healthcare quality, and the potential to diminish disparities for an increasingly diverse population [84].

According to the Bureau of Labor Statistics, the participation rates of women and minorities in the labor force will continue to increase [85]. Women will make up nearly half of the total labor force and the majority of medical students [86]. Many health professional groups have worked tirelessly to increase the preparation and status of underrepresented minorities, women, and socio-economically disadvantaged individuals into the health professions [80]. In contrast, the representation of racial and ethnic minorities within medicine (especially academic medicine) and all health professions is significantly less than their representation in the general population. The cost of higher education remains a significant barrier to increasing the diversity of graduates from health professional schools. In addition, underrepresented minority and low-income students have increased educational debt upon graduation. Recent state and federal constraints have contributed to reductions in governmental aid. Considering the recent economic downturn and increasing financial insecurity, the potential for barriers to obtaining educational loans has increased.

The IOM has also addressed the importance of diversity in the report, *In the nation's compelling interest: Ensuring diversity in the healthcare workforce* [80]. The IOM's report provided support for diversity in general as well as for a diverse workforce in reducing and eliminating disparities in health and healthcare. However, their work supporting the importance of diversity primarily focused on the importance and challenges of diversifying the health professions pipeline. Nonetheless, several IOM report intrinsically supported the importance of cultural awareness, sensitivity, and competence while providing evidence that diversity in healthcare represents a critical underpinning for improving healthcare quality [4, 22, 25, 80]. This is in contrast with resident-physician reports that they were ill prepared to provide cross-cultural care [87].

There are many benefits to diversity such as increasing team creativity and communication [88]. An article in Harvard Business Review reports that minorities provide additional leadership by their leadership and community service [89]. For instance, in academics and professional societies, minorities and women are disproportionately asked to provide scientific service

(e.g., serving on committees, mentoring) that are often unrecognized but are extremely important to the institution's mission [89]. Thus, a clear statement about the value of diversity during health professional educational programs and within continuing education programs should be incorporated to reflect the diversity within our health professional schools and professional societies to reflect the increasing diversity of the patient populations served and new colleagues. Also required is additional research designed to evaluate the effectiveness of pipeline programs in reducing and eliminating health and healthcare disparities.

The impact of pain on overall health and well-being

The medical advantages yielding increased longevity and quality of life for most Caucasians have not been uniformly applied. More specifically, there have been many advances in the treatment modalites available and guidelines to improve pain assessment and measurement. Yet, they have not been uniformly implemented. Nearly 100 million Americans have pain with minorities, women, the elderly, and lower SES individuals disproportionately experiencing increased pain severity and disability [90–93]. As the prevalence of pain increases worldwide, there are many potentially devastating socio-economic and health ramifications for both the individual and society. Currently, pain leads to over 700 million lost workdays and greater than $60 billion in healthcare expenditures annually in the USA [30, 31, 94–96]. Americans spend an additional $40 billion annually on chronic pain medications and aides [93, 97]. Chronic pain remains the most frequent cause of disability in the US and is the second leading cause for all physician visits [97]. Indeed without necessary improvements in the quality of chronic pain management, the increasing prevalence of chronic pain will have devastating socio-economic and health ramifications as our society ages and diversifies.

Thirty to fifty percent of elderly Americans currently live with pain. The presence of pain in the elderly interferes with successful aging and their ability to independently navigate their environments [93]. Elderly people living with chronic pain often avoid social activities for fear that they will not be able to meet their engagements resulting in social isolation [93]. When compared to Caucasian elders, racial and ethnic minority elders are more likely to rate their health as poor while also reporting increased pain and disability

[35, 45, 61, 62]. Considering the impact of accelerated aging in racial and ethnic minorities, pain may further worsen health in this population. Thus, those already at the most risk for poor assessment and treatment – impoverished and racial and ethnic minority elders – are particularly vulnerable to diminished health when they have pain. Yet, few studies have described the impact of chronic pain on health in ethnically diverse individuals across the life span.

The chronic pain experiences of vulnerable and underserved people have not been well described. In a series of studies using 7000 African American and Caucasian men and women with chronic pain across the life span, important and persistent differences were found in health based upon race and ethnicity [98]. Overall, African Americans reported significantly more co-morbidities, higher pain scores, increased pain severity, more suffering, and less control of pain than Caucasians across the life span, regardless of gender. African Americans also reported increased physical disability, i.e., impairment in activities of daily living due to pain (e.g., sexual, self-care, occupation, family life), and more problems with sleep (i.e., difficulty falling asleep, difficulty staying asleep). Regardless of age and gender, emotional health was also severely impacted by chronic pain in African Americans. They were significantly more depressed (moderate to severe depression) and had more symptoms consistent with PTSD and anxiety than Caucasians. These findings may reflect poor assessment, inadequate treatment, over-reporting differences or some combination of all of the above. However, most individuals with mental health disorders do not receive treatment while racial and ethnic minorities and socio-economically disadvantaged individuals are often more reluctant to seek treatment than Caucasians. Thus, it follows that the adverse sequelae associated with pain are more likely to decrease their overall health and well-being while further diminishing their quality of life.

Pain assessment

An extensive literature documents the benefits of optimizing pain management. The Agency for Health Research and Quality [formerly the Agency for Healthcare Policy and Research (AHCPR)] sponsored the development of guidelines for pain assessment and treatment for several common conditions e.g., acute pain, chronic low back pain, and cancer pain [100–103]. In addition, several professional societies have developed guidelines for managing pain [104]. An important limitation is that few guidelines specifically address the differential impact pain has on racial and ethnic minorities, women, and the socio-economically disadvantaged individual [100]. Despite these guidelines designed to improve the quality of pain care in the US, 40% of people in the US reported significant acute post-operative pain following surgery and 70% of people die with unrelieved pain worldwide [101]. There is also clear evidence that underserved and vulnerable populations suffer disproportionately more unrelieved pain regardless of pain etiology from all types of pain than Caucasians. Thus, a significant pain care gap exists.

The cornerstone to quality care is pain assessment [10]. Optimizing pain assessment can be problematic since pain is a subjective experience, and there are no objective measures. The pain experience varies substantially at the individual level while being influenced by sex, hormones, age, and culture [105, 106]. Patients with the same disease activity may report differences in pain intensity and its impact on their lives. Both racial and ethnic minorities and women respond differently to a painful stimulus than Caucasian men. Race, increasing age, and female gender may substantially increase the risk for physical and psychological impairment and disability due to pain [35]. In addition, clinician assessment of a patient's pain is also subjective and often discordant with the patient's pain report [57]. These are important considerations since elderly people, racial and ethnic minorities, and women, often report increased pain and sequelae while being at increased risk for poor assessment and under-treatment of their pain complaints.

Overall, the advancements in technology allowing an individual to survive significant and life-threatening trauma that would have previously ended in death a decade ago may now be associated with persistent and chronic pain [13]. Thus, the epidemiology of pain is changing. Beyond racial and gender differences in the pain experience, intra-race differences also exist [107]. For instance, contrary to what is expected, younger African Americans and Caucasians experience more morbidity and disability than their elderly counterparts with chronic pain suggesting potential differences in coping and a generation gap in pain.

How race and ethnicity, gender, and age influence pain management seeking behavior is unknown. What is known is that there is disturbing variability in how the pain complaints of racial and ethnic minorities, the elderly, women, and impoverished individuals are assessed and managed [55, 59, 61, 62]. As previously mentioned, although the gold standard for pain assessment is patient report, clinician estimates of a patient's pain intensity are often lower than the patient's report [93]. Complementing or complicating the process is patient behavior, communication styles, clinician–patient communication, and stereotyping. There are often differences in the way the elderly, women, racial and ethnic minorities communicate their pain experiences regardless of socio-economic status [93]. These communication difficulties are especially problematic if there is also a language barrier. These differences increase the likelihood of miscommunication and poor communication as well as the pain complaints being discounted, especially when the patient's gender, race, or ethnicity is not the same as their clinician's [107]. In addition, most measures used to assess pain lack cultural and linguistic sensitivity and fail to take into account the patient's literacy, in general, and health literacy, in particular.

Biological, physiological, and social mechanisms may explain differences in vulnerability to pain. Differences in pain-learning, culturally imposed factors, pain care beliefs, and gender and social roles may predispose certain individuals toward actions that exacerbate rather than minimize threats to pain. There is wide variability in responses to experimental pain models with differences in pain response attributed to race, ethnicity, gender, disease, age, culture, socio-economic status, past experiences, response bias, and experimental setting [78, 109]. However, the ability to correlate experimental pain differences to the clinical pain syndromes is unclear.

Disability, depression, and pain intensity issues often complicate chronic pain assessment and management. In a study evaluating race, age, and gender influences among black and white clusters of chronic pain patients (i.e., chronic pain syndrome, good pain control, and disability with mild pain syndrome), important racial and age-related variability in pain symptom severity when patients presented with similar physical, emotional, and pain characteristics were revealed [99]. Overall, these findings show racial and ethnic minorities experience more disease burden than their Caucasian counterparts.

The major and most important building block for quality pain care and physician pain management decision-making is optimizing pain assessment. Yet, this is a neglected topic in most medical, nursing, dental, and pharmacy school curricula, further leading to suboptimal pain assessment and treatment [39, 55, 59, 61, 63, 110]. A study in Michigan revealed nearly 30% of physicians reported they had not received any medical school, residency, or continuing medical education directed at assessing and managing pain [55, 59, 61, 62, 111]. Thus, it is not surprising that physicians and healthcare professionals are ill-equipped to assess and treat pain. In addition, clinician knowledge and education, healthcare system factors, trust, legal factors, and clinician variability in decision-making influences how well pain is assessed and treated.

Racial and ethnic minorities are at risk for poor pain assessment [34, 112]. Todd's studies in the emergency department revealed a two-fold difference in the ability to receive analgesics based upon patient ethnicity in patients with isolated long bone fractures [111]. The majority of Hispanics (55%) with isolated femoral shaft, tibia, fibula, or humerus fractures received no analgesics while 74% of Caucasians with similar injuries received analgesics. Pain assessment appears to be the most likely mediator for the physician decision-making as well as severity of illness. In a 1994 follow-up study, Todd found no differences in pain assessment when patients had less severe bone trauma [113]. Schulman's study using black and white actors presenting with similar acute chest pain complaints found women and racial and ethnic minorities received lesser quality care for their chest pain complaints [114]. Bernabei's study of black and white elderly nursing home residents with cancer found that blacks were less likely to have their pain score assessed and documented in their medical charts [115]. Blacks were also 63% more likely than whites to receive no pain medications. Even when they reported daily pain (40%), 25% received no analgesics whatsoever. Sickle cell anemia is often considered the *sine que non* for disparities in pain care [34, 113]. The sickle cell patient (often a racial or ethnic minority) presenting to the Emergency Department with acute pain is where the healthcare provider-patient interaction can be challenging and fraught with the potential for racial stereotyping, mistrust, and problematic physician–patient communication. Patients with sickle cell anemia (and their families) provide compelling stories documenting poor pain assessment and inadequate pain care during acute pain crises and for the chronic pain that often follows. However, Ng found that, although ethnic minorities were prescribed less opioid analgesics for their pain via patient-controlled analgesia following similar orthopedic procedures than whites, the amount patients self administered did not differ based upon race [116]. These findings suggest physician variability in prescribing analgesics.

Patient barriers, perceptions, and attitudes

Several patient related-barriers prevent optimal pain assessment. While health insurance coverage provides access to medical care it does not ensure equal health or healthcare delivery [117, 118]. Racial and ethnic minorities are also more likely to be uninsured or underinsured. Not having health insurance, a physician, or a usual source of medical care hinders access to quality pain care. Individuals without health insurance coverage or a primary care physician are more likely to use emergency departments for care and have less access to specialty care. Even when minorities have a primary care physician and health insurance, they may experience more difficulty in securing referrals to specialty physicians from their primary care physician. Since there is a close association between race, ethnicity, and income, rising co-pays for healthcare services tend to impact racial and ethnic minorities disproportionately more than whites. These findings are consistent with literature reporting blacks having increased difficulty paying for healthcare and chronic pain being a major problem, despite having insurance and access to a tertiary care pain center [119]. Overall, racial and ethnic minorities have less access to pain management specialists, receive less pain medication, and are at risk for under-treatment of their pain complaints while also having an increased disease burden for many co-morbid conditions associated with pain, e.g., diabetes, cancer.

Patient coping styles, attitudes, and experiences may influence their healthcare preferences, information seeking, and decision-making [119]. For instance, passive coping and catastrophizing is detrimental to successfully coping with a pain problem [120]. Overall, blacks with chronic pain report significantly more suffering due to pain, less ability to control their pain symptoms, and more impairment in their sleep due to pain than whites regardless of age or gender [44, 121]. There are also differences based upon age with older blacks reporting more ability to cope with pain than younger blacks, younger whites, and older whites [45]. John Henryism (i.e., a pattern of high output active coping characterized by working harder against a potentially insurmountable obstacle) is associated with hypertension and bodily pain in blacks

[122–124]. This coping style is consistent with the attitudes and beliefs of some minorities where blacks with chronic pain tend to believe race and ethnicity affected the healthcare and pain care they received. They also believed good patients avoid talking about pain, and pain medications could not really control pain [119]. These findings point to differences in trust and problematic communication while begging the question whether the origin of these perceptions and attitudes is due to their previous healthcare experiences. Thus, differences in social support, coping styles, and attitudes may contribute to how an individual experiences and lives with pain.

Variability in accessing and treating pain

Although pain is ubiquitous, healthcare providers are not knowledgeable or satisfied with the pain care they provide. Physicians express confidence in their pain management with little knowledge and varying goals for pain relief based upon the type of pain [55, 59, 61, 62]. Physicians report lower goals and less satisfaction with their chronic pain management while providing lesser quality pain care when compared to acute and cancer pain. This is an important consideration since the physicians reported seeing a higher percentage of chronic pain patients. Race, age, gender, and class seem to play a role in how physicians make their decisions for similar pain problems. The inability to receive chronic pain complaints contributes to sub-optimal care. An analysis of the workers' compensation system revealed racial and ethnic minorities were twice as likely to be disabled 6 months following occupational back injuries than Caucasians [125]. Altogether these findings suggest treatment disparities lead to increased disability.

Sub-optimal pain management leads to poorer health status and quality of life. In a chronic pain sample, blacks believed they should have been referred to a pain center sooner, reported decreased access to healthcare overall, and believed ethnicity influenced pain care [119]. Several studies show minorities with cancer pain received significantly less potent analgesics than those recommended by the WHO [3, 58, 64]. In settings with predominant minority patients, the majority were under treated using WHO standards. Anderson showed physicians under estimated pain severity for the majority of the Hispanic and black patients [3, 58, 64]. Overall, racial and ethnic minority patients reported more pain, less pain relief, and were less likely to be adequately assessed for all types of pain and in all settings than Caucasian patients. Physician gender and race also affect pain management decision-making [57, 63, 67, 126]. Male primary care physicians prescribed more pain medicine to their male patients than to their female patients. Regardless of pain type, the literature continues to suggest women and minorities receive lesser quality pain care and thus, it is not surprising disparities in health and healthcare persist.

Despite increased efforts to improve cultural competency by incorporating cultural competency training into the curriculum of most US medical schools, residents completing their final year of residency training often feel they were unprepared to deal with diverse patients [87]. A large proportion of residents reported they received little or no cross-cultural training. They felt unprepared to treat patients with religious beliefs that were not Western, who do not trust in the US health system, who have religious beliefs that may affect treatment, who use complementary or alternative medicines, or who are new immigrants. Thus, although cultural competency is part of the medical school curriculum, translating the principles of cultural competence into clinical practice is much more problematic.

Racial and ethnic minorities face additional barriers to adequate pain management. Pharmacies located in minority neighborhoods were less likely to carry opioid analgesics than those in non-minority neighborhoods [127, 128]. Thus, poor pain assessment, inadequate pain treatment, and decreased ability to obtain pain medications (even when medications are prescribed) complicate quality pain management for all racial and ethnic minority persons, in particular, thereby impairing their overall health and well-being. Even at higher incomes, whites have increased access to specialty care (including pain care and pharmacies) in their local communities than minorities.

Conclusion

Pain profoundly affects morbidity, mortality, quality of life, and healthcare expenditures. The potential implications of poorly treated pain are devastating for the individual and the fincancial cost to society is staggering. Therefore, ensuring optimal pain management is critically important from a public health perspective. There is evidence that pain (especially chronic pain) has unique health implications based

upon race and ethnicity, gender, age, and class that are often overlooked. Longitudinal and prospective studies examining the long-term effects of pain on overall health and well-being in an ethnically diverse population are necessary. Appropriate cultural and linguistic interventions must be developed to ensure quality pain assessment and management such that racial and ethnic disparities in pain care are reduced and eliminated. The role of healthcare provider variability in pain management decision-making as well as healthcare system factors must be examined. In a climate where there is increasing attention regarding patient safety, inadequate pain assessment and treatment must also be viewed as a quality of care issue. By improving pain care in the underserved and most vulnerable populations, the quality of pain care will be improved for all [44]. Overall, adequate pain relief is a human rights and social justice issue and there remains much more to do to improve the quality of pain care for all [44].

Acknowledgments

The author wishes to thank the Michigan-Pain Outcomes Study Team (M-POST) for their inspiration and ongoing support.

References

1. Centers for Disease Control and Prevention, The Merck Company Foundation. *The State of Aging and Health in America 2007* (Whitehouse, NJ: The Merck Company Foundation, 2007).

2. Farrell MJ. Pain and aging. *Am Pain Soc Bulletin* 2000; **10**: 8–12.

3. Anderson GF, Hussey PS. Population aging: A comparison among industrialized countries. *Health Affairs (Millwood)* 2000; **19**: 191–203.

4. Institute of Medicine. *Retooling for an Aging America: Building the Health Care Workforce* (Washington, DC: The National Academies Press, 2001).

5. Breslow L. A quantitative approach to the World Health Organization definition of health: Physical, mental and social well-being. *Int J Epidemiol* 1972; **1**: 347–55.

6. Pearl JD. Cancer pain management: Still a public health issue. *Am Soc Anesthesiol Newsletter* 1998; **62**: 18–20.

7. Helme R, Gibson S. Pain in older people. In *Epidemiology of Pain*, ed. IK Crombie. (Seattle: IASP Press, 1999), pp. 103–121.

8. Mayberry RM, Mili F, Vaid I, *et al. Racial and Ethnic Differences in Access to Medical Care: A synthesis of the*

literature (The Henry J. Kaiser Family Foundation, Morehouse Medical Treatment Effectiveness Center (MMEDTEC), 1999).

9. Mayberry RM, Mili F, Ofili E. Racial and ethnic differences in access to medical care. *Med Care Res Rev* 2000; **57**(Suppl 1): 108–45.

10. Institute of Medicine. *Crossing the Quality Chasm: A new health system for the 21st century* (Washington, DC: National Academy Press, 2001).

11. Crombie IK, Davies HT, Macrae WA. The epidemiology of chronic pain: Time for new directions. *Pain* 1994; **57**: 1–3.

12. LeResche L. Gender differences in pain: Epidemiologic perspectives. *Pain Forum* 1995; **4**: 228–30.

13. Crombie IK, Croft PR, Linton SJ, LeResche L, VonKorff M. *Epidemiology of Pain* (Seattle: IASP Press, 1999).

14. Gallagher RM. Primary care and pain medicine. A community solution to the public health problem of chronic pain. *Med Clin North Am* 1999; **83**: 555–83.

15. Gallagher RM, Verma S. Managing pain and comorbid depression: A public health challenge. *Semin Clin Neuropsychiatry* 1999; **4**: 203–20.

16. LeResche L. Gender considerations in the epidemiology of chronic pain. In *Epidemiology of Pain*, eds. IK Crombie, PR Croft, SJ Linton, L LeResche, M VonKorff. (Seattle: IASP Press, 1999), pp. 43–51.

17. IASP Special Interest Group on Sex, Gender, and Pain. *Sex, Gender, and Pain*, Vol. 10, eds. JSI Mogil, RG Fillingim. (Siena, Italy: IASP Press, 2000).

18. LeResche L. *Epidemiologic Perspectives on Sex Differences in Pain*, Vol. 17 (Seattle: International Association of the Study of Pain, 2000).

19. Fishman SM, Gallagher RM, Carr DB, Sullivan LW. The case for pain medicine. *Pain Med* 2004; **5**: 281–6.

20. Whelan CT, Jin L, Meltzer D. Pain and satisfaction with pain control in hospitalized medical patients: No such thing as low risk. *Arch Intern Med* 2004; **164**: 175–80.

21. Fuentes M, Hart-Johnson T, Green CR. The association among neighborhood socioeconmic status, race and chronic pain in black and white older adults. *J Natl Med Assoc* 2007; **99**: 1160–9.

22. Institute of Medicine. *The Unequal Burden of Cancer: An Assessment of NIH Research and Programs for Ethnic Minorities and the Medically Underserved.* (Washington, DC: National Academy Press, 1999).

23. Baquet CR, Hammond C, Commiskey P, Brooks S, Mullins CD. Health disparities research – a model for conducting research on cancer disparities: characterization and reduction. *J Assoc for Acad Minor Phys* 2002; **13**: 33–40.

24. Egede LE, Zheng D, Simpson K. Comorbid depression is associated with increased health care use and expenditures in individuals with diabetes. *Diabetes Care* 2002; **25**: 464–70.

25. Institute of Medicine. *Goal to Eliminate Health Care Disparities: Guidance for the National Healthcare Disparities Report* (Washington, DC: National Academies Press, 2002).

26. Institute of Medicine. *Unequal Treatment: Confronting Racial and Ethnic Disparities in Health Care* (Washington, DC: The National Academies Press, 2002).

27. Caldwell J, Hart-Johnson T, Green CR. Body mass index and quality of life: Examining blacks and whites with chronic pain. *J Pain.* 2009; **10**: 60–7.

28. Stewart WF, Ricci JA, Chee E, Morganstein D, Lipton R. Lost productive time and cost due to common pain conditions in the US workforce. *JAMA* 2003; **290**: 2443–54.

29. Green CR. The healthcare bubble through the lens of pain research, practice, and policy: Advice to the New President and Congress. Editorial. *J Pain* 2008; **9**: 1071–3.

30. Ferrell BR, Dean GE. Ethical issues in pain management at home. *J Palliat Care* 1994; **10**: 67–72.

31. Ferrell BR, Griffith H. Cost issues related to pain management: Report from the cancer pain panel of the agency for health care policy and research. *J Pain Symptom Manage* 1994; **9**: 221–34.

32. Gunn CC. Chronic pain: Time for epidemiology. *J R Soc Med* 1996; **89**: 479–80.

33. Moore R, Brodsgarrd I. *Cross Cultural Investigations of Pain Epidemiology of Pain* (Seattle: International Association for the Study of Pain, 1999).

34. Bonham VL. Race, Ethnicity, and pain treatment: Striving to understand the causes and solutions to the disparities in pain treatment. *J Law Med Ethics* 2001; **29**: 52–68.

35. Green CR, Anderson KO, Baker TA, *et al.* The unequal burden of pain: Confronting racial and ethnic disparities in pain. *Pain Med* 2003; **4**: 277–94.

36. Green CR, Tait RC, Gallagher RM. Introduction. The unequal burden of pain: disparities and differences. *Pain Med* 2005; **6**: 1–2.

37. Cleeland CS. The impact of pain on the patient with cancer. *Cancer* 1984; **54**(11 Suppl): 2635–41.

38. Gibson S, Kart, B, Corran, TM, Farrell, MJ, Helme, RD. Pain in older persons. *Disabil Rehabil* 1994; **16**: 127–39.

39. IASP Task Force on Professional Education. Core Curriculum for Professional Education in Pain, ed. HL Fields. (Seattle: IASP Press, 1995).

40. Skevington SM. Investigating the relationship between pain and discomfort and quality of life, using the WHOQOL. *Pain* 1998; **76**: 395–406.

41. Scher AI, Stewart WF, Lipton RB. Epidemiology of migraine and headache: A meta-analytic approach. In *Epidemiology of Pain*, ed. IK Crombie. (Seattle: IASP Press, 1999), pp. 159–70.

42. Kulich RJ, Mencher P, Bertrand C, Maciewicz R. Comorbidity of post-traumatic stress disorder and chronic pain: Implications for clinical and forensic assessment. *Curr Rev Pain* 2000; **4**: 36–48.

43. Schmader KE. Epidemiology and impact on quality of life of postherpetic neuralgia and painful diabetic neuropathy. *Clin J Pain* 2002; **18**: 350–4.

44. Green C, Todd KH, Lebovits A, Francis M. Disparities in pain: Ethical issues. *Pain Med* 2006; **7**: 530–3.

45. Green CR, Baker TA, Smith EM, Sato Y. The effect of race in older adults presenting for chronic pain management: A comparative study of black and white Americans. *J Pain* 2003; **4**: 82–90.

46. Feine JS, Lund JP. An assessment of the efficacy of physical therapy and physical modalities for the control of chronic musculoskeletal pain. *Pain* 1997; **71**: 5–23.

47. Menefee LA, Frank ED, Doghramji K, *et al.* Self-reported sleep quality and quality of life for individuals with chronic pain conditions. *Clin J Pain* 2000; **16**: 290–7.

48. Call-Schmidt TA, Richardson SJ. Prevalence of sleep disturbance and its relationship to pain in adults with chronic pain. *Pain Manag Nurs* 2003; **4**: 124–133.

49. Buchwald D, Goldberg J, Noonan C, *et al.* Relationship between post-traumatic stress disorder and pain in two American Indian tribes. *Pain Med* 2005; **6**: 72–9.

50. NIH. *NIH State-of-the-Science Conference on Symptom Management in Cancer: Pain, Depression, and Fatigue.* (National Institutes of Health, Bethesda, Maryland, 2002) pp. 1–80.

51. Sohler N, Walmsley PJ, Lubetkin E, Geiger HJ. *Equal Treatment: An Annotated Bibliography of Studies on Race and Ethnic Disparities in Healthcare, Their Cause, and Related Issues* (New York: Physicians for Human Rights, 2003).

52. Smedley BD. Expanding the frame of understanding health disparities: From a focus on health systems to social and economic systems. *Health Educ Behav* 2006; **33**: 538–41.

53. Lurie N, Margolis KL, McGovern PG, Mink PJ, Slater JS. Why do patients of female physicians have higher rates of breast and cervical cancer screening? *J Gen Intern Med* 1997; **12**: 34–43.

54. Todd KH, Deaton C, D' Adamo AP, Goe L. Ethnicity and analgesic practice. *Ann Emerg Med* 2000; **35**: 11–16.

55. Green CR, Wheeler JR, Marchant B, LaPorte F, Guerrero E. Analysis of the physician variable in pain management. *Pain Med* 2001; **2**: 317–27.

56. Green CR, Hart-Johnson T. The adequacy of chronic pain management prior to presenting at a tertiary care pain center: the role of patient socio-demographic characteristics. *J Pain* 2010; **11**(8): 746–54.

57. Weisse CS, Sorum PC, Sanders KN, Syat BL. Do gender and race affect decisions about pain management? *J Gen Intern Med* 2001; **16**: 211–17.

58. Anderson KO, Richman SP, Hurley J, *et al.* Cancer pain management among underserved minority outpatients: Perceived needs and barriers to optimal control. *Cancer* 2002; **94**: 2295–304.

59. Green CR, Wheeler JR, LaPorte F, Marchant B, Guerrero E. How well is chronic pain managed? Who does it well? *Pain Med* 2002; **3**: 56–65.

60. Lurie N. Addressing health disparities: Where should we start? *Health Serv Res* 2002; **37**: 1125–7.

61. Green CR, Wheeler JR. Physician variability in the management of acute postoperative and cancer pain: A quantitative analysis of the Michigan Experience. *Pain Med* 2003; **4**: 8–20.

62. Green CR, Wheeler JR, LaPorte F. Clinical decision making in pain management: Contributions of physician and patient characteristics to variations in practice. *J Pain* 2003; **4**: 29–39.

63. Weisse CS, Sorum PC, Dominguez RE. The influence of gender and race on physicians' pain management decisions. *J Pain* 2003; **4**: 505–10.

64. Anderson KO, Mendoza TR, Payne R, *et al.* Pain education for underserved minority cancer patients: A randomized controlled trial. *J Clin Oncol* 2004; **22**: 4918–25.

65. Lurie N. Health disparities – less talk, more action. *N Engl J Med* 2005; **353**: 727–9.

66. Lurie N, Jung M, Lavizzo-Mourey R. Disparities and quality improvement: Federal policy levers. *Health Aff* 2005; **24**: 354–64.

67. Weisse CS, Foster KK, Fisher EA. The influence of experimenter gender and race on pain reporting: Does racial or gender concordance matter? *Pain Med* 2005; **6**: 80–7.

68. Todd KH, Green C, Bonham VL, Jr, Haywood C, Jr, Ivy E. Sickle cell disease related pain: Crisis and conflict. *J Pain* 2006; **7**: 453–8.

69. US Department of Health and Human Services. *Healthy People 2010: Understanding and Improving Health* (Washington, DC: Department of Health and Human Services, Government Printing Offices, 2000).

70. Agency for Healthcare Research and Quality. *Reducing Ethnic and Racial Inequities in Health Care: AHRQ Resources for Research*. AHRQ Publication No. 02-P009. Rockville, MD: Agency for Healthcare Research and Quality, December 2001.

71. Agency for Healthcare Research and Quality. *National Healthcare Disparities Report*. 2004a. Rockville, MD: Agency for Healthcare Research and Quality, 2004.

72. Agency for Healthcare Research and Quality. *National Healthcare Quality Report*. 2004b. Rockville, MD: Agency for Healthcare Research and Quality, 2004.

73. Agency for Healthcare Research and Quality. *Health Care for Minority Women*. AHRQ Publication No. 06-P017. Rockville, MD: Agency for Healthcare Research and Quality, June 2006.

74. Nerenz DR, Bonham VL, Green-Weir R, Joseph C, Gunter M. Eliminating racial/ethnic disparities in health care: Can health plans generate reports? *Health Aff (Millwood)* 2002; **21**: 259–63.

75. Frist WH. Shattuck Lecture: Health care in the 21st Century. *N Engl J Med* 2005; **352**: 267–72.

76. Fillingim RB, Edwards RR, Powell T. The relationship of sex and clinical pain to experimental pain responses. *Pain* 1999; **83**: 419–25.

77. Fillingim RB. Sex, gender, and pain: Women and men really are different. *Curr Rev Pain* 2000; **4**: 24–30.

78. Edwards CL, Fillingim RB, Keefe F. Race, ethnicity and pain. *Pain* 2001; **94**: 133–7.

79. Bradshaw DH, Nakamura Y, Chapman CR. National Institutes of Health Grant awards for pain, nausea, and dyspnea research: An assessment of funding patterns in 2003. *J Pain* 2005; **6**: 275–6.

80. Institute of Medicine. *In the Nation's Compelling Interest–Ensuring Diversity in the Health Care Workforce*. (Washington, DC: National Academy of Sciences, 2004).

81. Thomas-Goering J, Green CR. Diversity and disparities in health and health care: Why it matters to anesthesiology. *Adv Anesth* 2006; **24**: 149–61.

82. Hall J, Irish J, Roter DL, Ehrlich C, Miller L. Gender in medical encounters: An analysis of physician and patient communication in a primary care setting. *Health Psychol* 1994; **13**: 384–92.

83. Elderkin-Thompson V, Waitzkin H. Differences in clinical communication by gender. *J Gen Intern Med* 1999; **14**: 112–21.

84. Comstock LM, Hooper EM, Goodwin JM, Goodwin JS. Physician behaviors that correlate with patient satisfaction. *J Med Educ* 1982; **57**: 105–12.

85. Bureau of Labor Statistics. Women's share of labor force to edge higher by 2008. *OCCUP Outlook Q* 1999: 33–8.

86. American Association of Medical Colleges. *Women in US Academic Medicine Statistics and Medical School Benchmarking*, 2004–2005.

87. Weissman JS, Betancourt J, Campbell EG, *et al.* Resident physicians' preparedness to provide cross-cultural care. *JAMA* 2005; **294**: 1058–67.

88. American College of Physicians. Racial and ethnic disparities in healthcare: A position paper of the American College of Physicians. *J Natl Med Assoc* 2004; **96**: 1178–84.

89. Hewlett SA, Luce CB, West C. Leadership in your midst: Tapping the hidden strengths of minority executives. *Harv Bus Rev* 2005; **83**: 74–82, 166.

90. Pilowsky I, Crettenden I, Townley M. Sleep disturbance in pain clinic patients. *Pain* 1985; **23**: 27–33.

91. Flor H, Turk DC, Scholz OB. Impact of chronic pain on the spouse: Marital, emotional and physical consequences. *J Psychosom Res* 1987; **31**: 63–71.

92. Schlenk EA, Erlen JA, Dunbar-Jacob J, *et al.* Health-related quality of life in chronic disorders: A comparison across studies using the MOS SF-36. *Qual Life Res* 1998; **7**: 57–65.

93. Levitt SH, Kempen PM. Managing pain in elderly patients. *JAMA* 1999; **281**: 605; discussion 606.

94. Ferrell BR, Jacox A, Miaskowski C, Paice JA, Hester NO. Cancer pain guidelines: Now that we have them, what do we do? *Oncol Nurs Forum* 1994; **21**: 1229–31.

95. Ferrell BR, Rhiner M. Managing cancer pain – a three-step approach. *Nursing* 1994; **24**: 57–9.

96. Ferrell BR, Rhiner M, Shapiro B, Strause L. The family experience of cancer pain management in children. *Cancer Pract* 1994; **2**: 441–6.

97. Canine C. Pain, profit, and sweet relief. *Worth* March 1997; 79–157.

98. Ndao-Brumblay SK, Green CR. Racial differences in the physical and psychosocial health among black and white women with chronic pain. *J Natl Med Assoc* 2005; **97**: 1369–77.

99. Green CR, Ndao-Brumblay SK, Nagrant AM, Baker TA, Rothman E. Race, age, and gender influences among clusters of African American and White patients with chronic pain. *J Pain* 2004; **5**: 171–82.

100. Payne R. Pain management in sickle cell disease. Rationale and techniques. *Ann NY Acad Sci* 1989; **565**: 189–206.

101. Carr DB, Jacox A, Chapman CR. *Acute Pain Management: Operative or Medical 100. Procedures and Trauma: Clinical Practice* Guideline No. 1. Rockville, MD: U.S. Public Health Service, Agency for Health Care Policy and Research, 1992.

102. Carr DB, Miaskowski C, Dedrick SC, Williams GR. Management of perioperative pain in hospitalized patients: A national survey. *J Clin Anesth* 1998;**10**: 77–85.

103. Carr TD, Lemanek KL, Armstrong FD. Pain and fear ratings: Clinical implications of age and gender differences. *J Pain Symptom Manage* 1998; **15**: 305–13.

104. Rose VL. Guidelines from the American Geriatric Society target management of chronic pain in older persons. *Am Fam Physician* 1998; **58**: 1213–14, 1217.

105. Edwards R, Augustson EM, Fillingim R. Sex-specific effects of pain-related anxiety on adjustment to chronic pain. *Clin J Pain* 2000; **16**: 46–53.

106. Fillingim RB, Edwards RR, Powell T. Sex-dependent effects of reported familial pain history on recent pain complaints and experimental pain responses. *Pain* 2000; **86**: 87–94.

107. Baker TA, Green CR. Intrarace differences among black and white americans presenting for chronic pain management: The influence of age, physical health, and psychosocial factors. *Pain Med* 2005; **6**: 29–38.

108. Green CR. Unequal burdens and unheard voices: Whose pain? Whose narratives? In *Narrative, Pain, and Suffering, Progress in Pain Research and Management.* DB Carr, JD Loeser, DB Morris, eds. (Seattle: IASP Press, 2005).

109. Fillingim RB. *Sex, Gender and Pain: A Biopsychosocial Framework*, Vol. 17 (Seattle: International Association for the Study of Pain Press, 2000).

110. IASP Task Force on Professional Education. Postoperative Pain. *Core Curriculum for Professional Education in Pain*, ed. HL Fields (Seattle: IASP Press, 1995) pp. 99–101.

111. Todd K, Samaroo N, Hoffman J. Ethnicity as a risk factor in inadequate emergency department analgesia. *JAMA* 1993; **269**: 1537–9.

112. Anderson KO, Green CR, Payne R. Racial and ethnic disparities in pain: causes and consequences of unequal care. *J Pain* 2009; **10**(12): 1187–204.

113. Todd KH, Lee T, Hoffman JR. The effect of ethnicity on physician estimates of pain severity in patients with isolated extremity trauma. *JAMA* 1994; **271**: 925–8.

114. Schulman KA, Berlin JA, Harless W, *et al.* The effect of race and sex on physicians' recommendations for cardiac catheterization. *N Engl J Med* 1999; **340**: 618–26.

115. Bernabei R, Gambassi G, Lapane K, *et al.* Management of pain in elderly patients with cancer. SAGE Study Group. Systematic Assessment of Geriatric Drug Use via Epidemiology. *JAMA* 1998; **279**: 1877–82.

116. Ng B, Dimsdale JE, Rollnik JD, Shapiro H. The effect of ethnicity on prescriptions for patient-controlled analgesia for post-operative pain. *Pain* 1996; **66**: 9–12.

117. Institute of Medicine. *Coverage Matters: Insurance and Health Care* (Washington, DC: National Academy Press, 2001).

118. Institute of Medicine. *Care Without Coverage: Too Little, Too Late* (Washington, DC: National Academy Press, 2002).

119. Green CR, Baker TA, Ndao-Brumblay SK. Patient attitudes regarding healthcare utilization and referral: A descriptive comparison in African- and Caucasian Americans with chronic pain. *J Natl Med Assoc* 2004; **96**: 31–42.

120. Roth RS, Geisser ME, Bates R. The relation of post-traumatic stress symptoms to depression and pain in patients with accident-related chronic pain. *J Pain* 2008; **9**: 588–96.

121. McCracken LM, Matthews AK, Tang TS, Cuba SL. A comparison of blacks and whites seeking treatment for chronic pain. *Clin J Pain* 2001; **17**: 249–55.

122. James SA, Hartnett SA, Kalsbeek WD. John Henryism and blood pressure differences among black men. *J Behav Med* 1983; **6**: 259–78.

123. James SA, Strogatz DS, Wing SB, Ramsey DL. Socioeconomic status, John Henryism, and hypertension in blacks and whites. *Am J Epidemiol* 1987; **126**: 664–73.

124. James SA, Keenan NL, Strogatz DS. Socioeconomic status, John Henryism and blood pressure in black adults: The Pitt County Study. *Am J Epidemiol* 1992; **135**: 59–67.

125. Tait RC, Chibnall JT. Factor structure of the pain disability index in workers, compensation claimants with low back injuries. *Arch Phys Med Rehabil* 2005; **86**: 1141–6.

126. Levy S, Dowling P, Boult L, Monroe A, McQuade W. The effect of physician and patient gender on preventive medicine practices in patients older than fifty. *Fam Med* 1992; **24**: 58–61.

127. Morrison RS, Wallenstein S, Natale DK, Senzel RS, Huang LL. "We don't carry that" – failure of pharmacies in predominantly nonwhite neighborhoods to stock opioid analgesics. *N Engl J Med* 2000; **342**: 1023–6.

128. Green CR, Ndao-Brumblay SK, West B, Washington T. Differences in prescription opioid analgesic availability: Comparing minority and white pharmacies across Michigan. *J Pain* 2005; **6**: 689–99.

Practice, policy, and research

Directions in pain research: Contemporary questions and methods

David A. Williams and Daniel J. Clauw

In 2000, the United States government passed into law a provision declaring the 10-year period 2001–2010 the Decade of Pain Control and Research. In 2010, at the end of this decade, many of the obstacles for delivering evidence-based methods of controlling pain still remained [1] and federal support for pain research is diminishing rather than growing [2, 3]. While camps of investigators are each making respectable inroads towards understanding pain, there is no over-arching agenda or roadmap guiding the future of pain research as a discipline. This chapter attempts to identify several broad topics where meaningful advancements could be made in order to more fully address the needs of individuals suffering from pain. These are as follows: (1) to better understand the neurobiological underpinnings of pain so as to use this information to move towards a mechanistic understanding of pain and personalized analgesia, (2) to enhance the validity and sensitivity of current methods of assessing pain and chronic illness, (3) to enhance the capacity to train junior investigators in emerging methods for studying pain such as techniques in neuroimaging and novel clinical trial designs, (4) to gain a better understanding of the factors responsible for some individuals transitioning from an acute pain condition to one that is chronic, and (5) to identify novel methods of moving evidence-based pain interventions into clinical practice.

Looking forward by learning from our past

A brief look at the history of pain research helps to provide a perspective for understanding how we have arrived at our current understanding of pain and reveals how pedagogical biases about the nature of pain shapes the availability of interventions and a society's ability to treat chronic pain effectively. Hopefully the next generation of pain research will successfully dismantle poorly working paradigms from the past and break new ground aligned more fully with evidence.

Pain has been a recognized part of the human experience for thousands of years. Some of the earliest writings about pain date back to 2600 BC [4]. Early notions about pain considered it to be the product of evil magic or demons that entered the body though its openings (e.g., wounds). The pain that was experienced was not considered to come from the body itself; but rather from the activity of the evil spirits within the body. Relief from the pain was therefore left to interventionists with expertise in removing demons (e.g., sorcerers and shamen) who believed that spirits left the body through bodily fluids (e.g., vomiting, sneezing, urinating, sweating, bleeding). Healers would therefore encourage the flow of bodily fluids using a variety of means [5, 6].

Greek and Roman societies developed new ideas about the nature and origin of sensation that involved nerves for both movement and sensation. Theories on pain were advanced by thinkers such as Hippocrates and Plato who viewed pain as being attributable to natural body processes rather than the supernatural [5, 6]. Such ideas were short-lived however for as the Roman Empire fell so did a focus on the physiological basis of pain perception.

During the Middle Ages (e.g., between the sixth century and the Renaissance period), much of the Western world was under the control of the church. Christian societies were notorious for imbuing pain with religious meaning [7, 8]. During the Middle Ages, pain was thought to be God's punishment to humanity for Adam's original sin. Thus, bodily defects, painful illnesses, and death were attributed to the will of God. Interference with the will of God was not encouraged and as such, interventions aimed at relieving pain were less common than in previous eras.

Behavioral and Psychopharmacologic Pain Management, ed. Michael H. Ebert and Robert D. Kerns. Published by Cambridge University Press. © Cambridge University Press 2011.

The Renaissance and Classical periods resurrected ideas from a thousand years earlier suggesting that the brain and spinal cord worked together to produce sensations of pain. During this period, pain fell under the purview of medicine and physicians began using opium and sherry to control it. The medical emphasis, however, was not to eradicate pain; but rather to use it in a controlled manner to stir vital healing forces. Interventions that produced great pain were thought to be the most powerful and effective. Thus, interventions that "stirred" weak or dormant vital forces in the body were desirable and considered necessary for the promotion of healing [8].

It was not until the eighteenth and nineteenth centuries that pain relief became viewed as a societal good. Surgeons capable of performing procedures quickly, with as little pain as possible, became valued and were considered to be the most skilled. The introduction of surgical anesthesia, however, changed how the western world thought about pain. The intrigue surrounding anesthesia and narcotic analgesics to eliminate acute pain from injuries and medical procedures produced a false confidence that the pathophysiology of pain was largely understood. Such false confidence contributed to the belief that pain, resistant to conventional treatment, was a psychiatric illness [8].

The bifurcation of pain into physical vs. psychological or real vs. fabricated is perhaps the greatest misstep early clinicians made in trying to understand pain. This bifurcation artificially cleaved from consideration the important role of the mind in mediating the perception of pain and for many years fractured the study of pain into the physiological and psychological.

In 1965, the introduction of the gate control theory of pain provided a neurobiological model that helped to reunite the mind and the body and explained how clinical pain reports could be inconsistent with observable physical damage [9]. This theory ascribed important roles for learning, behavior, cognition, and affect in the perception of pain and as such, opened the door for professional disciplines other than physicians to play important roles in the study of pain. In 1972 John Bonica held the first international meeting of scientists interested in the study of pain. This meeting evolved into the International Association for the Study of Pain (IASP) an international organization with numerous country-specific chapters such as the American Pain Society in the USA, each espousing the importance of an interdisciplinary perspective on pain. Thus today, pain is thought to be an integrated subjective personal experience involving nociception, affect and cognition. There is a strong sense in the USA and the world at large that pain needs to be treated aggressively when possible [10] and should be considered a disorder worthy of treatment in its own right [11]. With chronic pain still affecting between 15 and 20% of adults [12, 13], there remains a societal mandate to continue to advance our understanding of pain and to move our best treatments into the clinical arena. The remainder of this chapter examines a research agenda containing some of the more promising avenues of research for accomplishing this objective.

Using genetics and other methods to develop a mechanistic understanding of the pain in each individual, to achieve personalized analgesia

Pain sensitivity is thought to be partially heritable, a finding first identified in rodents by several independent laboratories [14, 15]. In humans, twin studies provided some of the first evidence that pain sensitivity might be inherited in a variety of pain conditions including low back pain [16], dysmenorrheal pain [17] and irritable bowel syndrome [18]. These studies suggest that up to 50% of the variability in pain can be attributable to genetic influences and that of that 50%, a quarter of the variance is likely attributable to structural pathology with the remaining three-quarters being attributable to genetic influences on central pain processing [19].

The heritability of pain sensitivity does not suggest that some individuals are sensitive to pain while others are not; rather, there is great variability in pain sensitivity within any given sample of humans [20]. For a specific individual, pain sensitivity may be related to a genetically determined "set point" of sensitivity, which influences pain perception to a far greater extent than how much inflammation or damage can be identified in peripheral tissues. Chronic pain may therefore be a partially heritable disease with specific bodily locations being less relevant than an individual's genetically determined set point for pain sensitivity.

A number of genes appear to be responsible for determining this "set point" of pain sensitivity. Evidence now supports genes such as catechol-O-methyltranferase (COMT) and GTP cyclohydrolase 1 (GCH1) to be amongst many that exert significant control over human pain perception [21–23, 93].

COMT is one of the more heavily researched candidate genes related to pain sensitivity. COMT codes for one of the enzymes that degrades noradrenaline and dopamine. In rats, inhibition of COMT results in a profound increase in pain threshold (e.g., being less sensitive to pain) [24]. Zubieta was the first to show that COMT affected human pain sensitivity, demonstrating that those who were homozygous for the Met158Val allele were more pain sensitive than heterozygotes, and that this effect was partly mediated via mu opioid receptors [25]. While some investigators have failed to find an association between COMT and pain sensitivity [26], Diatchenko et al. found that by adding synonymous single nucleotide polymorphisms (SNPs) to their analysis, the use of haplotype analyses could identify three subsets of individuals termed "low pain sensitivity" (36.5% frequency) – these individuals were more sensitive to pain and exhibited rapid metabolism of noradrenaline, "average pain sensitivity" (48.7% frequency), and "high pain sensitivity" (10.7%) – these individuals were least sensitive to pain and exhibited the slowest catabolic rate of noradrenaline [23]. More recent work suggests that in animal models, pain amplification associated with low COMT activity may also be mediated through B2-adrenergic and B3-adrenergic receptor mechanisms [27].

Even in conditions with known structural deformities COMT appears to exert considerable influence over pain perception [28]. Within a large osteoarthritis database a very weak association was found between the degree of osteoarthritis deformity of the knee or hip and pain [29]. However, in this database individuals with the 158-Met COMT variant had nearly a three-fold higher risk ($p = 0.02$) of having pain as compared to those with the other genotype variants. This effect was fully driven by the women in the sample. Female carriers of the Met158Val allele were 4.9 times more likely to have pain (95% CI: 1.6–14.8; $p = 0.005$), even though radiographic damage to the hip was present in each genotype group. This gender difference is not surprising as COMT is believed to be inducible by estrogen.

A second candidate gene known to be heavily involved in human pain sensitivity is GCH1. This gene codes for an enzyme that limits the synthesis of tetrahydrobiopterin, which is essential to the production of catacholamines, serotonin, and nitric oxide. Heightened efficiency of GCH1 would be expected to be associated with more limited production of noradrenaline and serotonin and thus heightened pain perception. Combinations of SNPs in the study of GCH1 have identified a pain-protective haplotype (15% frequency) where individuals possessing this uncommon variant were less sensitive to painful stimuli [21, 23].

Most who study the genetics of pain believe that there will be scores of genes that play some role in pain and sensory sensitivity, and that this information will be very useful clinically in selecting treatment for a given individual. For example, if an individual is identified as having fibromyalgia (FM) or another heightened central pain transmission state, genetic testing may identify that the patient displays the COMT high pain sensitivity haplotype, and this patient may respond better to drugs that affect catecholaminergic function. Conversely, another patient with a polymorphism in a gene involving glutamate breakdown might respond better to a drug that modulates glutamatergic activity. As genome-wide association studies become more affordable, researchers will have a greater ability to identify genetic variances responsible for set-points as well as genotypes associated with affective vulnerability that may in part drive the transition from an acute pain state into one that is more chronic. For example, individuals with genetic predisposition for heightened pain or affect may need supplemental preparation (e.g., coping resources, behavioral interventions or additional medications) prior to or following surgery.

Genetic testing represents only one part of the diagnostics that will allow us to personalize analgesia. Due to the extensive changes that can occur to sensory processing systems with stress and other factors, epigenetic and other post-transcriptional changes lead to variations in pain processing that cannot be predicted simply with genetic testing. Functional tests of relevant pain and sensory processing systems need to be developed and validated for use in clinical practice. Such tools would allow us to identify patients with diffuse hyperalgesia/allodynia, global sensory sensitivity, central sensitization, and the absence of descending analgesia, which like genetic information, would inform the choice of appropriate analgesic strategies.

Looking to the mechanism rather then to the regional diagnosis has been helpful in gaining insight into a number of chronic pain conditions. For example, hyperalgesia and/or allodynia in both clinical sites as well as "neutral" sites has been identified for a number of chronic pain conditions including irritable bowel syndrome, temporomandibular syndrome, tension headache, idiopathic low back pain, tension headache, and vulvodynia [30–38] suggesting a diffuse central (rather than regional) etiology of these conditions.

Within studies of chronic pain conditions, there is a widely distributed range of hyperalgesia/allodynia. Since a distribution exists for hyperalgesia/allodynia and this phenomenon is not present in all individuals diagnosed with chronic pain (but rather subsets), it might be possible to differentiate those individuals with primary peripheral or nociceptive pain syndromes (e.g., osteoarthritis) from those who have more prominent features associated with widespread hyperalgesia.

Until very recently, there were no studies that examined whether the hyperalgesia "caused" the pain in these "central pain syndromes," or occurred because of the presence of central pain. Diatchenko and colleagues performed a longitudinal study of 202 young pain-free women, and followed them for 2 years, with the outcome of interest being those women who developed new onset of temporomandibular disorder (TMD) [23]. Fifteen individuals developed TMD over the course of this study, and an individual's central pain threshold at baseline (i.e. while asymptomatic, at the beginning of the study) was a strong predictor of the development of TMD [39]. Moreover, these investigators showed that polymorphisms in COMT predicted both the individual's baseline pain sensitivity, as well as the risk of developing TMD [23, 39]. These data are consistent with the Zubieta studies showing that the COMT polymorphisms predicted pain threshold (as measured both by experimental pain testing and functional neuroimaging) in healthy normal individuals [25].

In addition to genetics and experimental evoked pain measurement, other tests have been developed and validated to probe specific molecular mechanisms for heightened pain states. The two best examples are (1) testing for wind-up and temporal summation when looking for evidence of NMDA-receptor mediated central sensitization, and (2) performing descending noxious inhibitory control (DNIC) testing to assess the integrity of descending analgesic activity in both opioidergic and serotonergic/noradrenergic pathways [40, 41].

The DNIC test has been shown to be consistently abnormal in subsets of both FM and irritable bowel syndrome patients [41, 43, 44], and has been shown to predict the development of post-operative pain [45]. In FM, there are ample data that suggest that the attenuated descending analgesic activity is due to a specific deficiency in serotonergic/noradrenergic activity, given the complementary descending analgesic pathway in humans, the opiodergic pathway, appears to be intact and/or even hyperfunctional [46, 47]. Thus assessing the integrity of DNIC might identify a group of individuals who have attenuated serotinergic/noradrenergic function, and who might preferentially respond to drugs that raise these neurotransmitters.

Similarly, a number of chronic pain states have been shown to be characterized by increased temporal summation, or "wind-up," on experimental pain testing [48, 49]. Since this phenomenon is felt to be due to increases of glutamate and substance P at the level of the spinal cord, identifying individuals who display this phenomenon might identify a subset of individuals with central pain who respond to drugs that decrease the release or activity of these neurotransmitters [50].

Finally, both pain threshold and the integrity of descending analgesic systems can also be corroborated by functional MRI (fMRI). Pressure pain threshold is accurately measured via fMRI in both normal individuals and in disease states, and our group has recently found that in longitudinal studies, fMRI changes over time in parallel with changes in both spontaneous pain and experimental pain in FM [51–53]. We and others have also demonstrated a reduction in stimulus-induced activity in the brainstem in FM patients that we feel parallels the defective serotonergic/noradrenergic analgesia [54, 55]. Thus fMRI confirmation of the presence or absence of activity in the brainstem could also be used as a tool to personalize analgesia.

The utility of these methods is all predicated upon educating clinicians that pain occurs not only because of damage or inflammation in the region of the body experiencing pain. It will be increasingly important to educate clinicians to adopt diagnostic and treatment strategies that incorporate a more mechanistic understanding of the pain in individual patients, acknowledging that different underlying mechanisms require differing treatment strategies.

Figure 27.1 provides a suggested mechanistic characterization scheme for chronic pain patients. In this scheme, pain is considered to be nociceptive (because there is an appropriate inflammatory or mechanical stimulus in the periphery), neuropathic, or non-nociceptive (i.e. "central pain"). In general, conditions such as osteoarthritis, rheumatoid arthritis, and cancer pain are considered prototypical nociceptive pain syndromes. However, certain individuals with these conditions may have elements of non-nociceptive pain, thus accounting for the fact that there is sometimes a mismatch between the degree of joint space damage, inflammation, extent of metastatic disease, and the amount of pain an individual experiences. At the other end of this mechanistic continuum are "central" pain conditions. Conditions that are primarily due

Peripheral (nociceptive)	Neuropathic	Central (non-nociceptive)

▪ Primarily due to inflammation or mechanical damage in periphery
▪ NSAID, opioid responsive
▪ Responds to procedures
▪ Behavioral factors minor
▪ Examples
  ▪ Osteoarthritis
  ▪ Rheumatoid arthritis
  ▪ Cancer pain
	▪ Damage or entrapment of peripheral nerves
	▪ Responds to both peripheral and central pharmacological therapy
		▪ Primarily due to a central disturbance in pain processing
		▪ Tricyclic, neuroactive compounds most effective
		▪ Behavioral factors more prominent
		▪ Examples
		  ▪ Fibromyalgia
		  ▪ Irritable bowel syndrome
		  ▪ Tension headache
		  ▪ Idiopathic low back pain

Figure 27.1 Mechanistic characterization of pain

to disturbances in pain and sensory processing at the level of the spinal cord or brain may need to be treated with different classes of drug and non-drug therapies. Neuropathic pain has elements of both peripheral and central pain and tends to respond to both types of treatments.

Individuals with central pain occurring in isolation (as in fibromyalgia), or in combination with neuropathic or nociceptive pain can be identified both by clinical symptoms, as well as with other types of testing. For example, individuals with "central" pain are more likely to have more episodes of pain over their lifetime, and more widespread pain [56]. They are also more likely to have somatic symptoms other than pain, such as fatigue, insomnia, memory difficulties, and dysfunction of visceral organs (e.g., irritable bowel, interstitial cystitis). They may be more likely to feel their pain in muscles than in other structures, and to have pain in regions such as the thoracic region that do not commonly develop arthritis.

Advances in patient reported outcomes measurement

Currently, there is no machine or sensor capable of directly measuring the conscious perception of pain. Building such a device would be difficult given that the conscious experience of pain in humans is a final product arising from an integrated processing of sensory, affective, and cognitive/evaluative cortical events [52]. While it is important to assess the symptom of pain in chronic pain conditions, there are also many other health-related concerns that contribute to the well-being of such patients. Currently there are several large-scale initiatives each attempting to identify domains of

relevance beyond pain intensity that impact the lives of individuals with pain.

The Outcomes Measures in Rheumatology (OMERACT) organization has helped to resolve problems in outcomes measurement by establishing core data sets that should be collected and reported in clinical trials involving rheumatological conditions [57]. One task force within OMERACT has focused upon domains of relevance to fibromyalgia (FM) a chronic pain condition. The work of this group suggests that in addition to pain, the assessment of FM should include the measurement of patient global impression of well-being, fatigue, functional status, sleep, mood, tenderness/stiffness, and problems with concentration/memory (i.e. dyscognition) [58] in order to properly capture the impact of an intervention and assess the well-being of the patient.

The Initiative on Methods, Measurement, and Pain Assessment in Clinical Trials (IMMPACT) is a second organization focused upon identifying the domains that should be assessed in research involving chronic pain. This group identifies four core areas for assessment: (1) pain intensity, (2) physical functioning, (3) emotional functioning, and (4) overall improvement/well-being [59]. The remarkable agreement between these two independent organizations focused upon assessment in painful conditions provides confidence that assessment of pain intensity alone is largely insufficient for chronic pain populations.

A third organization showing similar agreement with OMERACT and IMMPACT is the World Health Organization, International Classification of Functioning Disability and Health initiative (WHO-ICF) [60]. The WHO-ICF developed a domain categorization coding system that identifies the relevant domains of functional status for medical illnesses in general. This large system can be broken down into core sets for specific illnesses. Currently there are several core sets of relevance to chronic pain. These include: chronic low back pain, musculoskeletal pain, chronic wide-spread pain, and rheumatological conditions [61–65]. When used, this coding system helps to identify relevant domains of functional limitations for different diseases/conditions and then provides a code (much like an ICD code) that identifies the areas of functioning that are affected by the condition.

While IMMPACT, OMERACT, and WHO-ICF offer guidance as to the domains of relevance for chronic pain conditions, the assessment of those domains must be done with valid assessment tools. Often assessment measures are developed and validated for specific clinical populations which were never intended for use in different patient groups. With the recognition that many domains need to be assessed in individuals with chronic pain comes the challenge of assessing these multiple domains with validity and without creating tremendous patient burden (i.e. filling out many questionnaires).

One large scale project to develop brief, yet valid assessments of multiple domains of quality of life is an NIH Roadmap initiative known as PROMIS (Patient-Reported Outcomes Measurement Information System). In the development of PROMIS, each domain was defined generically and then patient reported outcome items were developed, linked, and calibrated to those specific domain definitions using analytic techniques from item response theory. These calibrations, based upon large samples of well-characterized individuals, facilitates the use of computer-adaptive testing, which selects only those items from an item bank that provide relevant information for a given individual. PROMIS can be used clinically or for research purposes for the efficient and generic measurement of patient reported outcomes (PROs) across a wide range of chronic diseases and dimensions [66]. The benefit of this system is the ability to assess multiple domains using fewer items (i.e. less patient burden) with greater precision (i.e. increased power for clinical trials with fewer subjects). While PROMIS was established for the general assessment of chronic illnesses; greater precision can be attained when the item banks are further developed for use with specific illnesses.

The future of outcomes assessment and patient characterization for phenotyping studies is likely to rely heavily upon the current work in progress by the above organizations. These organizations are making a large investment in needed methodological revisions and advances that will serve medical research in general, but that will have relevance to the field of pain research specifically. Future large-scale pain research initiatives should be certain to leverage the diligence and rigor that has gone into the resources being developed by these organizations.

Training the next generation of pain researchers

Historically pain-specific research has been conducted by a relatively small group of researchers from the fields of anesthesiology, psychology, neurology, neuroscience, dentistry, and nursing. Such insular training has limited the breadth of perspectives, methods, and analytic interpretations brought to bear on the academic challenges of pain research. Additional training for junior investigators now entering the field in methods such as neuroimaging techniques and novel experimental clinical research designs could greatly enhance the progress of pain research.

Functional neuroimaging

Functional MRI, positron emission tomography (PET), and proton spectroscopy (H-MRS) are all techniques that can be used to non-invasively assess pain processing in individuals. To date, these techniques have helped to corroborate pain report with cortical activity and to document unique cortical activation patterns associated with pathological states such as hyperalgesia and allodynia [55]. While fMRI can be used to examine changes in blood flow in certain brain regions when pain stimuli are applied (i.e. the BOLD signal), newer techniques such as functional connectivity, resting state analyses, voxel-based morphometry, and arterial spin labeling can be derived from fMRI sequences and can give complementary information about the connection between brain regions, absolute (rather than relative) quantification of blood flow, and information regarding brain structure [67, 68].

While various fMRI techniques generally give information about *what* is happening in the brain, other neuroimaging techniques can help tell *why*, by measuring the levels of certain neurotransmitters involved in pain transmission. For example, PET has been used to examine opioidergic and dopaminergic activity in chronic pain states, whereas H-MRS can measure non-specific metabolites that are indicative of neuronal activity, as well as specific neurotransmitters involved in pain transmission such as glutamate and GABA [47, 69, 70].

These imaging techniques are now being used by the pharmacological industry in the evaluation of analgesic drug development, and could eventually be used to more accurately diagnose unique characteristics of pain that a given individual is experiencing. The ability to quantify cortical activity associated with the integrated pain signature [52] permits more sensitive evaluation of pain processing when assessing the merits of novel compounds. For example, the enhanced sensitivity of these techniques allows the use of smaller sample sizes in Phase IIa proof-of-concept studies with potential analgesic compounds [71]. Use of such techniques in clinical trials have the added potential to save tremendous amounts of time and money in helping to make early and accurate "go-no-go" decisions prior to investing enormous financial resources in large clinical trials in order to learn whether a compound is efficacious.

Novel approaches to clinical trials

Randomized controlled trials (RCTs) have long been considered the gold standard against which to evaluate the merits of an intervention. Recently, the RCT has received challenges and criticism for being too narrow in its design to address all potentially relevant clinical research questions. Alternative designs are rapidly emerging and pain researchers need to be aware of these alternative designs so as to be informed about which designs would be best to use in addressing specific clinical questions.

The RCT seeks to reduce variability in a study by controlling and equating (by randomization) as many sources of variance as possible except for the one variable that the investigator wants to manipulate (i.e. the treatment). This design is ideal for (1) understanding whether a treatment elicits a specific effect, (2) understanding how a given intervention works when many other contributing factors are controlled, or (3) establishing support for the efficacy of an intervention. Disappointingly, the RCT rarely reflects the real world – which is not highly controlled, which does not screen out patients by inclusion and exclusion criteria, which does not blind patients or clinicians to the care actually being administered – and can be extremely costly

when implemented in a scientifically rigorous manner. To address questions such as how does this intervention work in the real world, or how does this intervention work in combination with other complementary interventions (e.g., pharmacological interventions along with cognitive-behavioral therapy for pain), an alternative class of effectiveness designs might be considered. One such design is the practice-based evidence for clinical practice improvement design (PBE-CPI) [72].

PBE-CPI relies heavily upon the broad multi-dimensional characterization of each patient (see related section above on advances in patient characterization). It is likely that patients will differ in their responses to treatment(s) and experience improvements along a variety of dimensions of well-being, not just the primary outcome variable of a study. The efficient assessment of multiple outcomes, more general hypotheses about improvement, and the assessment of multiple mediator and moderator variables help to differentiate these designs from more traditional RCTs. In addition, these designs utilize minimal patient selection criteria and use statistical correction for differences between groups of patients rather than relying on the imposed artificiality of randomization. The advantages of these designs are related to the ability to conduct these studies in collaborative practice networks, at lower cost than RCTs, and the ability to identify small incremental benefits associated with interventions delivered in combination – reflective of real world clinical practice.

Another design variant that deviates from the RCT are adaptive designs. Adaptive trial design allows use of information gathered during the initial period of the clinical study to modify subsequent periods of the trial without undermining the validity and integrity of the trial. The information could be data collected from other concurrent studies, emerging literature, or data collected from within the study itself. Such considerations may lead to changes in the study endpoint, recalculating and amending sample sizes, re-evaluation of the control groups, or even alteration of the key assessments required to confirm the methodological and/or statistical hypotheses stated in the initial study protocol. This flexibility in clinical trials could improve the quality, speed, and efficiency of decision making in understanding and treating pain. The adaptive trial design approach may have particular advantages in small population studies, as well as in exploratory studies. Adaptive design appears to be best suited for dose escalation trials [73] and for Phase III trials where sample re-estimation may be required [74]. While not without its critics, these designs suffer more from uninformed misapplication than from limitations in methodology. Education and consensus about how and when to properly use these designs could greatly benefit the field of pain research [75].

A third design variant that could have application in studies of pain is a propensity score matching design [76]. Many institutions have implemented databases and registries in which large amounts of data have been collected over many years on a routine basis. These databases are rarely used to answer *a priori* hypothesis-driven questions and lack the ability to be randomized for group comparisons given the inherent serial manner by which registries are populated. If comparisons between groups of patients are desired from such databases (e.g., average pain level in OA pain vs. FM pain) it is likely that there will be numerous uncontrolled confounding variables (e.g., inherent age differences in the samples, sex differences). These group differences would need to be controlled for statistically by methods such as matching or stratification. With increasing numbers of confounding variables (which is likely on a very large databases) sample size concerns become relevant. An alternative design is to control a large number of covariates through the use of a propensity score. In this example, the propensity score would be the probability of being in the OA group or the FM group based upon the various covariates needing to be controlled. The propensity score is derived through methods of regression (often logistic) and each individual in the registry is assigned their own propensity score. Matching algorithms can then use the propensity score to match OA cases with FM cases thus resulting in a balanced matched case-control dataset based on propensity score, which will be a subset of the larger registry database. Specific outcomes of interest can then be compared while being assured that the many covariates are equivalently distributed.

Understanding the transition from acute to chronic pain

Pain that is unresponsive to traditional pain interventions has often been attributed to psychogenic factors [8]. Early investigations into the factors responsible for the transition of acute pain into chronicity tended to support this notion. For example, a number of reports identified depression, anxiety, and personality disorders to be commonly associated with persistent pain [77–82]. One of the more heavily studied predictors of the transition of acute to chronic pain was the presence of a personality disorder. Personality disorders are characterized by a persistent constellation of behaviors and inner experiences that are associated with problematic functioning. The prevalence of personality disorders in the general adult population is estimated at between 5–15% [83]; but in pain populations personality disorders are seen at much higher rates, e.g., 58.4% [84]; 51%, [85]. Current approaches to psychiatric diagnostics identifies 10 personality disorders and has grouped them into 3 clusters: "odd or eccentric" (i.e. Cluster A: schizoid, schizotypal, paranoid personality disorders), "dramatic emotional, or erratic" (i.e. Cluster B: histrionic, borderline, narcissistic, antisocial personality disorders), and "anxious or fearful" (i.e. Cluster C: avoidant, dependent, obsessive-compulsive personality disorders). In one study of patients with chronic low back pain, 44% had Cluster A disorders, 31% Cluster B disorders, and 25% Cluster C disorders [85]. In longitudinal prediction studies, the presence of any personality disorder has been found to be an important predictor of which patients will transition from acute to chronic pain [77, 79, 80].

More recent work from psychophysiological and genetic studies, suggests that there are many more potential predictors of who will transition from acute to chronic pain (see earlier section) An individual's susceptibility to chronic pain is highly variable and once pain has become chronic, changes (neurobiological and behavioral) may have occurred that cannot be easily reversed. The lack of well-defined phenotypes that reflect not only the psychiatric status but also the cellular, molecular, genetic, psychosocial, cognitive, and behavioral changes occurring within individuals as they transition to chronic pain has been a major barrier in the development of personalized approaches to pain intervention.

It is critical that research efforts move toward more personalized approaches to pain treatment both in the recommendations for interventions and in the approaches used in the prevention of acute to chronic transition. Importantly, there needs to be a more balanced understanding of the benefits offered by analgesics in the traditional treatment of acute pain, with the benefits of psychosocial interventions used in combination with analgesics to address the complexities of chronic pain, which include diminished functional status and other affective/behavioral influences on pain.

Moving evidence-based interventions into practice

Currently, 20% of physician visits are related to pain complaints [86] with billions of dollars of the US economy being consumed by treatment costs, lost productivity, and disability associated with pain [87]. Given the magnitude of suffering and the cost associated with pain, it is remarkable that the current practice of chronic pain medicine has changed little in the past three decades. With the exception of a few new compounds, chronic pain management consists largely of legacy approaches with little differentiation in practice being based upon the type of pain or characteristics of the individual patient. For example, a comparison of healthcare utilization between 33 000 individuals with FM and 33 000 general medical patients found that individuals with FM were prescribed four times the amount of opioids as general medical patients [88], and this is in spite of the fact that there is no evidence from RCTs that the pain of FM is opioid-responsive.

Given the need for effective interventions, it is unfortunate that some of the most efficacious evidence-based approaches for chronic pain (i.e. behaviorally-based or multidisciplinary-based interventions) are just as inaccessible today as they were 10–20 years ago. The challenge facing clinicians and patients alike is the need to ensure that practitioners are educated in the latest models of pain and perhaps most importantly, ensuring that the economic incentives for delivering pain treatments are consistent with evidence-based approaches.

There is strong evidence that non-pharmacological interventions such as cognitive-behavioral therapy (CBT) can improve pain and function in a variety of chronic pain conditions [89–91]. Non-pharmacological interventions however are less commonly used in pain management despite efficacy and relatively lower cost [1]. The reasons behind the failure to integrate non-pharmacological interventions into more routine care are varied. While physicians have ready access to information about pharmacological agents through industry marketing or through continuing medical educational courses, non-pharmacological interventions rarely get disseminated beyond academic forums, do not have marketing behind them, and are more likely to be published in non-medical journals. Thus physician awareness is a potential pitfall limiting the integration of non-pharmacological approaches to pain management. If a clinician is aware of these complementary interventions, he/she is likely to have difficulty locating a qualified practitioner of the intervention. Cognitive-behavioral therapy for pain is quite different from CBT for depression, anxiety, or even diabetes management. Additional training in behavioral medicine or pain medicine beyond the applications of CBT in mental health settings is recommended when searching for a qualified provider. Locating such providers, particularly in rural settings, is likely to be a challenge to the average clinician. Patients with pain may also be unaware of the important role that they need to play in pain management and as such, may prefer the simplicity of a pill, device, or procedure even though these interventions have limits to their efficacy. Taking all of these factors into account, even the savviest clinician and the most informed patient may still not be able to put together the right combination of evidenced-based pharmacological and non-pharmacological interventions due to barriers imposed by third party payers. Financial barriers to integrated evidence-based pain management are perhaps the greatest challenges facing chronic pain management today. While evidence for combination treatment is strong and studies have shown clinical benefits and cost-effectiveness for multi-disciplinary care routine, access to these treatment combinations remains limited [1]. Research dollars might be better placed in tearing down barriers to using the efficacious treatments we already possess; rather than spending $ millions on the next compound that reduces subjective pain report by another fraction of a % point on a visual analogue scale.

Knowing that some of the non-pharmacological interventions possess strong evidence for efficacy, new modes of delivering these services into the practice setting need to be explored and evaluated. Options for managing chronic pain in the context of primary care are limited. Clinicians need additional options that facilitate moving effective behavioral and self-management strategies into the hands of clinicians and their patients.

The provision of standardized educational self-management resources has demonstrated effectiveness in the management of numerous medical conditions (e.g., diabetes, cancer, brain injury, and cardiovascular problems), has strong evidence of patient satisfaction, and is particularly beneficial for reaching out to provide healthcare in rural settings when modified to function on a telehealth platform [92]. Such resources developed for pain management would provide the primary care physician with access to standardized evidence-based information that can be shared with patients, possess the name-recognition of originating with specialists in the field familiar with non-pharmacological interventions, and could be used by the clinician along with their own standard approach to pain care. This is not to say that there will not be a subset of patients who will require more intensive specialty pain clinic care, but a sizable number of individuals are capable of benefiting from standardized instruction in behavioral self-management skills under the recommendation of their trusted physician.

At the University of Michigan and in conjunction with the Avera Research Institute in Sioux Falls, SD, a clinical trial of standardized web-based educational materials targeting the multimodal management of FM in rural clinical practices is underway. This low-cost intervention is added to standard pharmacological management in order to gain better improvement in both pain and functional status in this condition. This intervention augments existing clinical practices and reaches a rural population of individuals with pain who might never have access to the non-pharmacological elements of care found in larger tertiary care centers.

Conclusion

Even though there have been many neuroscience research methodologies such as genetics and functional neuroimaging that have revolutionized our ability to study pain; we are just beginning to understand the neurophysiological processes that underlie pain and sensory transmission. The challenge in clinical practice is to determine how to use this knowledge to personalize analgesia. The diagnosis of pain in the future will undoubtedly involve much less looking for the peripheral cause of pain using traditional diagnostics, but rather begin using standardized evoked pain testing, genetic analysis, and functional neuroimaging. Then insights as to neural mechanisms operating within a given individual can better identify targets of care. Similarly, treatments will move from the over-use of longstanding classes of drugs that have limited overall efficacy (e.g., opioids and NSAIDs), and greater use of drugs that alter the levels of neurotransmitters that help to create an individual's set point of pain and sensory sensitivity. Similarly, promising techniques such as neurostimulatory therapies that can non-invasively (e.g., transcranial magnetic or electrical stimulation) or invasively (e.g., vagal nerve stimulation, spinal cord stimulation, deep brain stimulation) reduce pain by altering neurotransmission are likely to lead to more effective pain control. These "high-tech" therapies will need to be augmented by finding ways to integrate education, CBT, and exercise programs in routine clinical care, to create patient-centered "disease management" models of care rather than our current care systems. As these advances occur we will need to appropriately train a new generation of clinician-scientists that can translate these advances into routine clinical care.

References

1. Turk DC. Clinical effectiveness and cost-effectiveness of treatments for patients with chronic pain. *ClinJ Pain* 2002; **18**: 355–65.

2. Bradshaw DH, Empy C, Davis P, *et al.* Trends in funding for research on pain: a report on the national institutes of health grant awards over the years 2003 to 2007. *J Pain* 2008; **9**: 1077–87.

3. Green CR. The healthcare bubble through the lens of pain research, practice, and policy: advice for the new President and Congress. *J Pain* 2008; **9**: 1071–3.

4. Bonica JJ. History of pain concepts and theories. In *The Management of Pain,* eds. JJ Bonica, JD Loeser, CR Chapman, WE Fordyce. (Philadelphia: Lea Febiger, 1990), pp. 2–17.

5. Rey R. *History of Pain* (Paris: Editions la Découverte, 1993).

6. Clipper SE. A brief history of pain *Office of Communications and Public Relations, NINDS/NIH,* 2008; www.ninds.nih.gov/disorders/chronic_pain/detail_chronic_pain.htm#140513084; [accessed May 2010].

7. Morris DB. *The Culture of Pain* (Berkley, CA: University of California Press, 1994).

8. Meldrum ML. A capsule history of pain management. *JAMA* 2003; **290**: 2470–5.

9. Melzack R, Wall PD. Pain mechanisms: a new theory. *Science* 1965; **150**: 971–9.

10. Brennan F, Carr DB, Cousins M. Pain management: a fundamental human right. *Anesth Analg* 2007; **105**: 205–21.

11. Liebeskind JC. Pain can kill. *Pain* 1991; **44**: 3–4.

12. Breivik H, Collett B, Ventafridda V, Cohen R, Gallacher D. Survey of chronic pain in Europe: prevalence, impact on daily life, and treatment. *Eur J Pain* 2006; **10**: 287–333.

13. Verhaak PF, Kerssens JJ, Dekker J, Sorbi MJ, Bensing JM. Prevalence of chronic benign pain disorder among adults: a review of the literature. *Pain* 1998; **77**: 231–9.

14. Mogil JS, Wilson SG, Bon K, *et al*. Heritability of nociception I: responses of 11 inbred mouse strains on 12 measures of nociception. *Pain* 1999; **80**: 67–82.

15. Devor M, Raber P. Heritability of symptoms in an experimental model of neuropathic pain. *Pain* 1990; **42**: 51–67.

16. Bengtsson B, Thorson J. Back pain: a study of twins. *Acta Genet Med Gemellol (Roma)*, 1991; **40**: 83–90.

17. Treloar SA, Martin NG, Heath AC. Longitudinal genetic analysis of menstrual flow, pain, and limitation in a sample of Australian twins. *Behav Genet* 1998; **28**: 107–16.

18. Morris-Yates A, Talley NJ, Boyce PM, Nandurkar S, Andrews G. Evidence of a genetic contribution to functional bowel disorder. *Am J Gastroenterol* 1998; **93**: 1311–7.

19. Battie MC, Videman T, Levalahti E, Gill K, Kaprio J. Heritability of low back pain and the role of disc degeneration. *Pain* 2007; **131**: 272–80.

20. Mogil JS, Yu L, Basbaum AI. Pain genes: natural variation and transgenic mutants. *Annu Rev Neurosci* 2000; **23**: 777–811.

21. Tegeder I, Costigan M, Griffin RS, *et al*. GTP cyclohydrolase and tetrahydrobiopterin regulate pain sensitivity and persistence. *Nat Med* 2006; **12**: 1269–77.

22. Amaya F, Wang H, Costigan M, *et al*. The voltage-gated sodium channel Na(v)1.9 is an effector of peripheral inflammatory pain hypersensitivity. *J Neurosci* 2006; **26**: 12852–60.

23. Diatchenko L, Slade GD, Nackley AG, *et al*. Genetic basis for individual variations in pain perception and the development of a chronic pain condition. *Hum Mol Genet* 2005; **14**: 135–43.

24. Nackley AG, Shabalina SA, Tchivileva IE, *et al*. Human catechol-O-methyltransferase haplotypes modulate protein expression by altering mRNA secondary structure. *Science* 2006; **314**: 1930–3.

25. Zubieta, JK, Heitzeg, MM, Smith, YR, *et al*. COMT val158met genotype affects mu-opioid neurotransmitter responses to a pain stressor. *Science* 2003, **299**, 1240–3.

26. Armero P, Muriel C, Santos J, *et al*. COMT (Val158Met) polymorphism is not associated to neuropathic pain in a Spanish population. *Eur J Pain*, 2005; **9**: 229–32.

27. Nackley AG, Tan KS, Fecho K, *et al*. Catechol-O-methyltransferase inhibition increases pain sensitivity through activation of both beta2- and beta3-adrenergic receptors. *Pain* 2007; **128**: 199–208.

28. Clauw DJ, Witter J. Thinking outside the joint. *Arthritis Rheumatism* 2009; **60**: 321–4.

29. van Meurs JB, Uitterlinden AG, Stolk L, *et al*. A functional polymorphism in the catechol-O-methyltransferase gene is associated with osteoarthritis-related pain. *Arthritis Rheum* 2009; **60**: 628–9.

30. Teders SJ, Blanchard EB, Andrasik F, *et al*. Relaxation training for tension headache: comparative efficacy and cost-effectiveness of a minimal therapist contact versus a therapist-delivered procedure. *Behav Ther* 1984; **15**: 59–70.

31. Wilder-Smith OH, Tassonyi E, Arendt-Nielsen L. Preoperative back pain is associated with diverse manifestations of central neuroplasticity. *Pain* 2002; **97**: 189–94.

32. Kashima K, Rahman OI, Sakoda S, Shiba R. Increased pain sensitivity of the upper extremities of TMD patients with myalgia to experimentally-evoked noxious stimulation: possibility of worsened endogenous opioid systems. *Cranio* 1999; **17**: 241–6.

33. Maixner W, Fillingim R, Booker D, Sigurdsson A. Sensitivity of patients with painful temporomandibular disorders to experimentally evoked pain. *Pain* 1995; **63**: 341–51.

34. Leffler AS, Hansson P, Kosek E. Somatosensory perception in a remote pain-free area and function of diffuse noxious inhibitory controls (DNIC) in patients suffering from long-term trapezius myalgia. *Eur J Pain* 2002; **6**: 149–59.

35. Whitehead WE, Holtkotter B, Enck P, *et al*. Tolerance for rectosigmoid distention in irritable bowel syndrome. *Gastroenterology* 1990; **98**: 1187–92.

36. Gibson SJ, Littlejohn GO, Gorman MM, Helme RD, Granges G. Altered heat pain thresholds and cerebral event-related potentials following painful CO_2 laser stimulation in subjects with fibromyalgia syndrome. *Pain* 1994; **58**: 185–93.

37. Kosek E, Ekholm J, Hansson P. Increased pressure pain sensibility in fibromyalgia patients is located deep to the skin but not restricted to muscle tissue [published erratum appears in *Pain* 1996; **64**: 605]. *Pain* 1995; **63**: 335–9.

38. Giesecke J, Reed BD, Haefner HK, *et al*. Quantitative sensory testing in vulvodynia patients and increased peripheral pressure pain sensitivity. *Obstet Gynecol* 2004; **104**: 126–33.

39. Diatchenko L, Nackley AG, Slade GD, *et al*. Catechol-O-methyltransferase gene polymorphisms are associated with multiple pain-evoking stimuli. *Pain* 2006; **125**: 216–24.

40. Le Bars D, Villanueva L, Bouhassira D, Willer JC. Diffuse noxious inhibitory controls (DNIC) in animals and in man. *Patol Fiziol Eksp Ter* 1992; 55–65.

41. Price DD, Mao J, Frenk H, Mayer DJ. The N-methyl-D-aspartate receptor antagonist dextromethorphan selectively reduces temporal summation of second pain in man. *Pain* 1994; **59**: 165–74.

42. Wilder-Smith CH, Robert-Yap J. Abnormal endogenous pain modulation and somatic and visceral hypersensitivity in female patients with irritable bowel syndrome. *World J Gastroenterol* 2007; **13**: 3699–704.

43. Kosek E, Hansson P. Modulatory influence on somatosensory perception from vibration and heterotopic noxious conditioning stimulation (HNCS) in fibromyalgia patients and healthy subjects. *Pain* 1997; **70**: 41–51.

44. Julien N, Goffaux P, Arsenault P, Marchand S. Widespread pain in fibromyalgia is related to a deficit of endogenous pain inhibition. *Pain* 2005; **114**: 295–302.

45. Yarnitsky D, Crispel Y, Eisenberg E, *et al.* Prediction of chronic post-operative pain: pre-operative DNIC testing identifies patients at risk. *Pain* 2008; **138**: 22–8.

46. Baraniuk JN, Whalen G, Cunningham J, Clauw DJ. Cerebrospinal fluid levels of opioid peptides in fibromyalgia and chronic low back pain. *BMC Musculoskelet Disord* 2004; **5**: 48

47. Harris RE, Clauw DJ, Scott DJ, *et al.* Decreased central mu-opioid receptor availability in fibromyalgia. *J Neurosci* 2007; **27**: 10000–6.

48. Staud R, Vierck CJ, Mauderli AP, Martin AD, Price DD. Effect of exercise on temporal summation of second pain (wind-up) in patients with fibromyalgia syndrome. *Arthritis Rheum* 1999; **42**: S342.

49. Arendt-Nielsen L, Graven-Nielsen T. Central sensitization in fibromyalgia and other musculoskeletal disorders. *Curr Pain Headache Rep*, 2003; **7**: 355–61.

50. Xu XJ, Dalsgaard CJ, Wiesenfeld-Hallin Z. Spinal substance P and N-methyl-D-aspartate receptors are coactivated in the induction of central sensitization of the nociceptive flexor reflex. *Neuroscience* 1992; **51**: 641–8.

51. Coghill RC, Sang CN, Maisog JM, Iadarola MJ. Pain intensity processing within the human brain: a bilateral, distributed mechanism. *J Neurophysiol* 1999; **82**: 1934–43.

52. Tracey I, Mantyh PW. The cerebral signature for pain perception and its modulation. *Neuron* 2007; **55**: 377–91.

53. Gracely RH, Petzke F, Wolf JM, Clauw DJ. Functional magnetic resonance imaging evidence of augmented pain processing in fibromyalgia. *Arthritis Rheum* 2002; **46**: 1333–43.

54. Cook DB, Lange G, Ciccone DS, *et al.* Functional imaging of pain in patients with primary fibromyalgia. *J Rheumatol* 2004; **31**: 364–378.

55. Tracey I. Imaging pain. *Br J Anaesth* 2008; **101**: 32–9.

56. Clauw DJ. Fibromyalgia: update on mechanisms and management. *J Clin Rheumatol* 2007; **13**: 102–9.

57. Tugwell P, Boers M, Brooks P, *et al.* OMERACT: an international initiative to improve outcome measurement in rheumatology. *Trials* 2007; **8**: 38.

58. Mease PJ, Arnold LM, Crofford LJ, *et al.* Identifying the clinical domains of fibromyalgia: contributions from clinician and patient Delphi exercises. *Arthritis Rheum* 2008; **59**: 952–60.

59. Dworkin RH, Turk DC, Wyrwich KW, *et al.* Interpreting the clinical importance of treatment outcomes in chronic pain clinical trials: IMMPACT recommendations. *J Pain* 2008; **9**: 105–21.

60. World Health Organization. *International Classification of Functioning, Disability and Health* (Geneva, 2001).

61. Weigl M, Cieza A, Cantista P, Reinhardt JD, Stucki G. Determinants of disability in chronic musculoskeletal health conditions: a literature review. *Eur J Phys Rehabil Med* 2008; **44**: 67–79.

62. Stucki G, Boonen A, Tugwell P, Cieza A, Boers M. The World Health Organisation International Classification of Functioning, Disability and Health: a conceptual model and interface for the OMERACT process. *J Rheumatol* 2007; **34**: 600–6.

63. Cieza A, Stucki G, Weigl M, *et al.* ICF Core Sets for Chronic Widespread Pain. *J Rehabil Med Suppl* 2004; **44**: 63–8.

64. Prodinger B, Cieza A, Williams DA, *et al.* Measuring health in patients with fibromyalgia: content comparison of questionnaires based on the International Classification of Functioning, Disability and Health. *Arthritis Rheum* 2008; **59**: 650–8.

65. Schwarzkopf SR, Ewert T, Dreinhofer KE, Cieza A, Stucki G. Towards an ICF Core Set for chronic musculoskeletal conditions: commonalities across ICF Core Sets for osteoarthritis, rheumatoid arthritis, osteoporosis, low back pain and chronic widespread pain. *Clin Rheumatol* 2008; **27**: 1355–61.

66. Fries JF, Bruce B, Cella D. The promise of PROMIS: using item response theory to improve assessment of patient-reported outcomes. *Clin Exp Rheumatol* 2005; **23**: S53–S57.

67. Apkarian AV, Bushnell MC, Treede RD, Zubieta JK. Human brain mechanisms of pain perception and regulation in health and disease. *Eur J Pain* 2005; **9**: 463–84.

68. Pattinson KT, Mitsis GD, Harvey AK, *et al.* Determination of the human brainstem respiratory control network and its cortical connections in vivo using functional and structural imaging. *Neuroimage* 2009; **44**: 295–305.

69. Wood PB, Schweinhardt P, Jaeger E, *et al.* Fibromyalgia patients show an abnormal dopamine response to pain. *Eur J Neurosci* 2007; **25**: 3576–82.

70. Zubieta, JK, Smith, YR, Bueller, JA, *et al.* Regional mu opioid receptor regulation of sensory and affective dimensions of pain. *Science* 2001; **293**: 311–5.

71. Schweinhardt P, Bountra C, Tracey I. Pharmacological FMRI in the development of new analgesic compounds. *NMR Biomed* 2006; **19**: 702–11.

72. Horn SD, Gassaway J. Practice-based evidence study design for comparative effectiveness research. *Med Care* 2007; **45**: S50–S57.

73. Bretz F, Hsu J, Pinheiro J, Liu Y. Dose finding – a challenge in statistics. *Biom J* 2008; **50**: 480–504.

74. Gao P, Ware JH, Mehta C. Sample size re-estimation for adaptive sequential design in clinical trials. *J Biopharm Stat* 2008; **18**: 1184–96.

75. Coffey CS, Kairalla JA. Adaptive clinical trials: progress and challenges. *Drugs RD* 2008; **9**: 229–242.

76. Reeve BB, Smith AW, Arora NK, Hays RD. Reducing bias in cancer research: application of propensity score matching. *Health Care FinancRev* 2008; **29**: 69–80.

77. Gatchel RJ, Polatin PB, Kinney RK. Predicting outcome of chronic back pain using clinical predictors of psychopathology: a prospective analysis. *Health Psychol* 1995; **14**: 415–20.

78. Gatchel RJ. Psychological disorders and chronic pain: cause-and-effect relationships. In *Psychological Approaches to Pain Management: a practitioner's handbook* eds. DC Turk RJ Gatchel. (New York: Guilford Press, 1996), pp. 33–52.

79. Gatchel RJ, Polatin PB, Mayer T. The dominant role of psychosocial risk factors in the development of chronic low back pain disability. *Spine* 1995; **20**: 2702–9.

80. Gatchel RJ. The significance of personality disorders in the chronic pain population. *Pain Forum* 1997; **6**: 12–15.

81. Large RG. The psychiatrist and the chronic pain patient: 172 anecdotes. *Pain* 1980; **9**: 253–63.

82. Merskey H. Chronic pain and psychiatric illness. In *The Managemenet of Pain,* 2nd edn., ed. JJ Bonica. (Philadelphia: Lea Febiger, 1990), pp. 320–7.

83. American Psychiatric Association *Diagnostic and Statistical Manual of Mental Disorders*, 4th edn. (Washington, DC: American Psychiatric Press, 1994).

84. Fishbain DA, Goldberg M, Meagher BR, Steele R, Rosomoff H. Male and female chronic pain patients categorized by DSM-III psychiatric diagnostic criteria. *Pain* 1986; **26**: 181–97.

85. Polatin PB, Kinney RK, Gatchel RJ, Lillo E, Mayer T. Psychiatric illness and chronic low-back pain. The mind and the spine – which goes first? *Spine* 1993; **18**: 66–71.

86. Schappert SM. National Ambulatory Medical Care Survey: 1992 summary. *Adv Data* 1994 Aug 18; 1–20.

87. Stewart WF, Ricci JA, Chee E, Morganstein D, Lipton R. Lost productive time and cost due to common pain conditions in the US workforce. *JAMA* 2003; **290**: 2443–54.

88. Berger A, Dukes E, Martin S, Edelsberg J, Oster G. Characteristics and healthcare costs of patients with fibromyalgia syndrome. *Int J ClinPract* 2007; **61**: 1498–1508.

89. Goldenberg DL, Burckhardt C, Crofford L. Management of fibromyalgia syndrome. *JAMA* 2004; **292**: 2388–2395.

90. Hoffman BM, Papas RK, Chatkoff DK, Kerns RD. Meta-analysis of psychological interventions for chronic low back pain. *Health Psychol* 2007; **26**: 1–9.

91. Morley S, Eccleston C, Williams A. Systematic review and meta-analysis of randomized controlled trials of cognitive behaviour therapy and behaviour therapy for chronic pain in adults, excluding headache. *Pain* 1999; **80**: 1–13.

92. Whitten P, Sypher BD. Evolution of telemedicine from an applied communication perspective in the United States. *Telemed J E Health* 2006; **12**: 590–600.

93. Diatchenko L, Nackley AG, Tchivileva IE, Shabalina SA, Maixner W. Genetic architecture of human pain perception. *Trends Genet* 2007; **23**: 605–13.

Practice, policy, and research

Ethics and pain management

Ingra Schellenberg and Mark D. Sullivan

Introduction

Over the past two decades, untreated pain has been increasingly recognized as a public health concern by medical professionals [1] and the general public [2]. The primary focus of this concern has been on the treatment of pain from cancer, and especially on pain management at the end-of-life. There are signs that this is changing. In December 2001, the American Medical Association (AMA), the Joint Commission on Accreditation of Healthcare Organizations (JCAHO), and the National Commission on Quality Assurance (NCQA) began a 2-year initiative to "improve the quality and consistency of pain management" focusing on pain from back problems, arthritis and cancer [3]. In 2002, pain management was ranked as "the most challenging standard for behavioral healthcare organizations" by the JCAHO [4].

The provision of pain relief poses a unique ethical challenge relative to other medical treatments. While helping to relieve patients' pain seems an obvious good, the most common treatment for pain is opioids. Almost all medical treatments carry unwanted side effects, but there is increasing debate about the use of opioids to treat chronic non-malignant pain [5] as opioids present serious risks and may burden patients more than their presenting complaint. Moreover, these risks are extremely difficult to quantify. Pain management thus requires care to avoid *both* undertreatment and overtreatment of pain. Clinicians have to strike a complicated balance of providing pain relief without worsening overall patient well-being. Some experts are championing broad use of opioids as an expression of patients' "right to pain relief" [6] and others warning us that long-term opioid therapy provides net harm to our patients [7]. However, we are generally unsure about how to extend the ethos of palliative care to the problem of non-malignant pain [8]. We are also

not convinced that the invocation of a "right to pain relief" is the best bioethical strategy to help clinicians or patients navigate the moral complexity of pain management. We will present some of the key arguments in favor of appeal to a "right to pain relief" and then our reservations about this position.

In this chapter, we will first summarize several dominant conceptions and definitions of pain, as well as some foundational values for various responses to pain. We will then present a brief history of pain management in America as it has unfolded in government initiatives and medical practices, and attempt to show how the different definitions of pain and ethical values have shaped this history. In particular, we will examine how the idea of a right to pain relief was introduced as a guide about how best to respond to pain. In our view, the appeal to patients' rights expresses significant moral insights, but there are also serious limitations to this approach.

Meanings and definitions of pain

In the last several decades, a tremendous change has taken place among Western healthcare providers about the meaning of pain. Earlier, pain was seen primarily as a symptom of a more fundamental health problem such as injury or disease. As a symptom of injury or disease, pain was acknowledged, but not granted primary importance. The diagnosis and treatment of the underlying disease held the center-stage. The view was that clinicians should aim to cure the underlying pathology and pain would take care of itself. However, the clinical dominance of disease over pain is not as marked as it once was. Now, many argue that pain merits treatment in its own right, independent of whatever disease may or may not underlie it [9].

Given that clinicians now acknowledge the importance of treating pain itself, a working definition of pain

Behavioral and Psychopharmacologic Pain Management, ed. Michael H. Ebert and Robert D. Kerns. Published by Cambridge University Press. © Cambridge University Press 2011.

is crucial. But this quest for clear definition is complicated by the inherently felt aspect of pain, which makes it an essentially subjective experience. What pain *feels like* to its sufferer is not available to observers. One way to interpret this inescapable subjectivity of pain is to say that pain is ultimately private. The ultimate privacy of pain worries many clinicians, who fear being misled by patients exaggerating pain or reporting pain that does not exist. This fear becomes pressing for many in light of the addictive properties of many pain treatments. Patients seeking long-term opioid therapy, especially without serious or progressive disease, are regarded with suspicion. As one primary care colleague of ours puts it: "We don't want to provide opioids for patients who claim to have pain in their bodies, but really have pain in their soul."

It might be thought that defining pain carefully – in a way that makes it clear when someone is or is not in pain – might circumvent this worry. Two such proposals are physiological and behavioral definitions of pain. Physiological definitions assert that pain is simply some third-person observable physiological event, and variants of these materialistic definitions have been endorsed by clinicians and philosophers. Specific proposals include, for example, various neuronal activities, like A delta- and c-fiber firing. The attractiveness of this proposal for medicine is obvious, as it would allow clinicians to circumvent the fear of being misled. Clinicians often prefer to work with objective phenomena, like blood tests, because they are measurable from a third-person perspective. If pain just *is* some neuronal activity, then objective tests can be devised for that activity, and the clinician can be sure that a patient who claims to be in pain really *is* in pain.

Unfortunately, this definition of pain simply leaves out too many cases where we are truly confident that the person is experiencing pain, despite our inability to locate the pain or the cause of the pain through some objective test. Pain is a highly complex physiological and psychological phenomenon, and there is no single objective event found in every case of pain. Some might hope that it would be possible to create a disjunctive criteria set of physiological signs for pain, e.g., either c-fiber firing or thalamic and anterior cingulate activation. There have been great hopes that functional neuroimaging may sort out subjective variability in pain experience. A recent scientific paper on pain neuroimaging concluded: "By identifying objective neural correlates of subjective differences, these findings validate the utility of introspection and

subjective reporting as a means of communicating a first-person experience" [10]. But the latest evidence indicates that a dispersed and variable set of brain sites are activated during pain experience, so we do not have even a disjunctive collection of signs that capture every instance of pain [11].

A second proposal is that pain is necessarily linked to certain third-person observable behaviors (e.g., wincing, avoidance). Again, this proposal has the advantage of being third-person accessible, but here, too, there is tremendous variance in pain behaviors between individuals and between cultures. It is thus impossible to capture every instance of pain with a finite list of necessary and sufficient pain behaviors. It is also not possible to judge whether pain behaviors are "exaggerated" on purely scientific grounds by comparing pain intensity with pain behavior. Some reference to cultural norms of appropriate behavior is necessary [12].

In light of these challenges in developing physiological or behavioral definitions of pain, the International Association for the Study of Pain (IASP) has proposed a purely subjective definition of pain, wholly dependent on patient reports: "An unpleasant sensory and emotional experience associated with actual or potential tissue damage, or described in terms of such damage" [13]. This proposal is unacceptable to some, as it seems to abandon the effort to gain third-person legitimacy for patient pain reports [14].

In our view, a third-person accessible definition of pain is not needed to deal with most clinical pain challenges. We would like to point out that, despite pain's inherent subjectivity, there are essential public features of pain that we use when we learn about pain from our parents [15]. Clinicians can often find public physiological and behavioral markers that give confidence that someone is in pain, although they do not add up to necessary and sufficient conditions for identifying pain. A large body of research has shown that both pain expression and experience are shaped by social factors that are shared within a community [16]. Although we cannot really feel each other's pain as we can both watch the same sunset, we typically do know when someone is experiencing pain. It is, as Ludwig Wittgenstein reminded us, distinctly uncomfortable to be in the presence of someone in severe pain [17]. In our view, clinicians do not need to worry about the specter of systematic patient deception about pain, even if clinically the definition of pain is ultimately grounded in subjective patient reports. In particular, clinicians need to keep in mind that deception about pain is more common in settings like emergency departments or urgent care clinics, where there is not an enduring clinician–patient relationship, than in primary care clinics [18].

Values in pain management

Before presenting some of the history of opioid policy, we would like to offer some preliminary remarks about two core – and sometimes opposing – values that we think have been and continue to be important influences on governmental and medical responses to opioids use: safety and freedom. In general, governments have obligations to protect citizens from various dangers, as well as obligations to respect civil liberties. The American government's involvement in the manufacturing, distribution, and consumption of narcotics, opiates and opioids highlights efforts to honor one or the other of these two values. Early in the history of narcotics consumption in America, the government left citizens complete freedom to make, sell, and consume these drugs as they saw fit. Through the twentieth century, this position has been dramatically reversed, leading to stringent government control of narcotics generally, and opioids specifically. There is an interesting set of questions that arise about why the American government became so concerned to prevent and manage opioid use. We will not be pursuing these issues here, but some writers have speculated that these worries were driven by several different cultural forces (e.g., disapproval of addiction or pleasure, obsession with work and efficiency, fear of loss of control, fear of immigrant groups associated with drug use) [19].

American governmental involvement in control of opioid consumption to prevent addiction seems to be at odds with the background presumption in America that citizens should be free to take risks that only affect themselves. America has come to treat substances with abuse potential in two very different ways. Those that are associated with crime, other antisocial behavior, and disfavored immigrant groups (e.g., heroin, marijuana) have been outlawed. Addictive substances not associated with antisocial behavior or its threat (e.g., nicotine) have remained legal. Alcohol was briefly moved from the legal to the illegal category, but was too popular and deeply engrained in our culture to remain there. However, the "War on Drugs" remains official government policy, with its focus recently shifted to prescription drugs [15].

A slightly different story can be seen in the history of medical practice and the use of opioids. Patients' rights to control their own bodies are balanced in medical practice against the physician obligation to protect their patients from harm. In the case of opioid use, this obligation has most often been interpreted to require physicians to protect their patients from iatrogenic "physician-caused" addiction, as well as to protect them from the potentially lethal side effects of various opioids. This was understood as the dominant medical obligation from the early twentieth century into the 1970s [20].

This valuing of patient safety puts medical obligation at odds with patient freedom. The valuing of freedom in medicine has typically been interpreted in America to mean that physicians have an obligation to respect their patients' autonomy. In practice, this means that physicians are not allowed to impose their own value judgments on patients' medical decision-making. Instead, the assumption is that patients know their own values and are typically the best judges about what course of treatment to pursue. But when physicians focus on patient safety and addiction prevention, patients' freedom and their requests for opioid therapy can be pushed to the wayside. Generally, a focus on patient safety has led to restricting access of patients to opioids. The valuing of patient safety, however, can also be interpreted to require physicians to relieve their patients' pain. This was the argument of John Liebeskind's famous article, "Pain can kill" [21]. According to this view, opioids are the tool that best allows this physician obligation to promote patient safety to be met. However, most clinicians and most governmental agencies do not interpret patient safety as including relief of the patient's suffering. This is an interesting position worth examining, but is beyond our scope in this chapter.

History of pain management

Let us now turn to an overview of the historical initiatives and practices that demonstrate these values at work. In this brief section, we will primarily be discussing American history, but similar interactions between government legislation of opioids and medical practice regarding pain can be found in most Western nations. At the end of the nineteenth century in America, the government was not usually involved in regulation of the manufacture or distribution of ingestible substances. The first federal legislation that constrained such substances was the Biologics Control Act (1902) that demanded oversight of vaccine production. Prior to this act, there were only a few patchy state laws related to food and drugs [22]. Narcotics generally, and opiates in particular, were not substances that raised concern, and freedom to consume these substances prevailed. Medicines were seen as good if they made a person feel good [23] and tonics that contained various narcotics, including opiate derivatives, were sold without oversight.

As these tonics became increasingly common, however, worries arose about the safety of their ingredients, as well as their addictive properties, both within the government and the medical community. The Harrison Narcotic Act of 1914 was the legislative result of the merging of those concerns. It provided the first restrictions on the manufacture and distribution of narcotics (including opiates), and made access to narcotics dependent on physicians' prescriptions [24]. Shortly after the Act came into effect, the courts also ruled that physicians could not distribute narcotics to addicts. This established a dynamic that has lasted until now, of physicians being concerned about potential prosecution for providing patients with narcotics, including opiates and opioids.

The Harrison Narcotic Act was supplemented over the next 60 years with various legislative updates. The medical community tacitly endorsed its underlying value of safety by maintaining an active concern with illicit drug use and iatrogenic addiction. Due to concern about protecting patients, most clinicians prescribed narcotics very sparingly, even to post-surgery patients [24] and patients with terminal conditions, in order to prevent addiction. For example, in an important textbook on cancer from 1952, the author described the possibility of a patient with terminal cancer becoming addicted to opiates as a "hideous spectacle" and urged that physicians only provide minimal pain relief at the end of life in order to ensure that their patients did not become addicts in their last days [25].

These concerns with addiction became more pronounced in late 1960s America, during Richard Nixon's presidency. Several commentators believe that this issue became especially pressing at this time due to the appearance of drug use and addiction among the counterculture and veterans of the war in Vietnam. In 1971, Nixon declared a "War on Drugs" [26], thereby setting the tone for how these substances would be often be viewed by the American government and broader culture until today. Nixon's administration argued the value of safety, not only to keep people safe from becoming addicts, but to keep society at large safe from the antisocial actions of addicts. Nixon's administration oversaw the creation of the Drug Enforcement Agency (DEA), and the creation of the current system of classification of drugs into five "schedules" with Schedule I drugs being declared highly addictive and having no

medical use and Schedule V drugs having low potential for addiction and having accepted medical uses. The opioid medications considered most effective in pain relief were classified as Schedule II or III (where they remain today). This subjected them – and the physicians who prescribe them – to considerable attention and regulation by the DEA.

During this same time, physicians caring for dying patients began to push against these restrictions on access to opioids. Initially, this resistance was likely not motivated by a strong shift toward valuing patient freedom and respect for autonomy. Instead, it was likely primarily motivated by a commitment to beneficence, and concern to provide better patient care. Much of this globally influential work initially took place in Britain, in the form of the modern hospice movement started by Cicely Saunders and Robert Twycross, both of whom cared for patients who were at the end of their lives. In providing this care, both became frustrated with the nearly exclusive medical focus on curative efforts, and the associated neglect of the comfort of dying patients [27]. For these early advocates of the hospice movement, there was moral outrage about the reasons used to justify the restrictions on opioid access (e.g., fear about addiction or diversion) for patients who were literally on their deathbeds.

As the palliative care work inspired by Saunders and Twycross extended from dying patients to patients with cancer pain, and eventually non-cancer pain, pain increasingly became a clinical phenomenon of interest in itself. In America, this increased attention to pain was linked in bioethics and legal decisions to greater insistence on respecting patients' autonomy and treatment choices. Both of these shifts have encountered resistance among clinicians, but the trend is definitely toward their adoption. These shifts have coalesced into the call for a "right to pain relief." But it is not clear to us that all these different populations of patients experiencing pain should be addressed though a single right to pain relief. We will discuss these concerns later in the chapter.

Greater support for patient autonomy in the arena of pain relief was opposed by shifts in the legal and political culture of the American 1980s. Failure of the war on illicit drugs as well as continued political concern about drug addiction led the DEA to focus on prescription drugs, and potential prosecutions of prescribers of scheduled drugs [28]. The DEA became concerned with the possibility of "diversion," where prescribers become suppliers of opioids to people who go on to sell those drugs on the street. New standards of record keeping and patient management were imposed, and the threat of criminal prosecution of physicians became more substantial. Thus, there is currently a tension between government policies regarding opioid use and clinical ideals in pain management. We will explore the ramifications of this tension in the next section.

Bad justifications that lead to undertreatment

The current dominant framework for moral obligation in the arena of pain relief is captured by the phrase "right to pain relief." Advocates of a patient's "right to pain relief" often invoke it to counteract what they see as inadequate support for or illegitimate interference in a patient's access to pain treatments. These advocates typically believe that undertreatment of pain is a greater problem than overtreatment, and cite studies to back up this view. Indeed the phrase – right to pain relief – implicitly denies that overtreatment is a serious concern. While we will ultimately argue that overtreatment can still be a problem and that physicians rightly strive to avoid it, let us first discuss the problem of undertreatment. Physicians have at times unreasonably limited access to pain medication, and this problem merits examination.

Proponents of a "right to pain relief" have argued that physicians are resistant to providing adequate pain relief for bad reasons. Ben Rich characterizes these bad reasons as: (1) ignorance; (2) indifference; and (3) fear [29]. While we do not endorse Rich's ultimate argument, we find these three categories useful for characterizing problems in pain management. Let us first discuss the problem of ignorance. For Rich, one reason patients receive inadequate pain treatment is that many physicians are poorly informed about current best practice standards in the arena of pain management. Uses and recommended doses for various medications have changed dramatically in recent years and not all clinicians have kept up. This is, we agree, a bad reason for a patient to experience pain, one that all clinicians have an obligation to fight against, by supporting education in pain management for themselves and colleagues.

According to Rich, clinician indifference to patients' pain also interferes with patients receiving adequate pain relief. This is a claim that many clinicians may resist. But as we discussed earlier, the focus on pain as worthy of specific clinical attention is a change from recent medical tradition. For many decades, pain was understood "merely" as a symptom of some other,

more significant underlying health problem. While this understanding may have helped clinicians to assiduously seek the cause of a patient's pain underlying pathological condition, it also led to illegitimate lack of concern with patients' pain. Moreover, in cases of pain without further underlying disease (e.g., fibromyalgia, non-specific low back pain), thinking of a patient's pain exclusively as a symptom can be an impediment to good care. While it is no longer accepted that pain is not clinically significant in its own right, no doubt some amount of the view that pain is only important as a symptom of some other health problem still lingers. And to the extent that it does, the result may be what Rich ultimately labels "indifference." In our view, this is indeed a bad reason for not providing pain relief, and clinicians should work to ensure that they are truly engaging with their patients' pain in itself.

The final bad reason for inadequate pain treatment Rich considers is fear, which he characterizes as "exaggerated concerns about addiction, adverse side effects and regulatory scrutiny" [29]. We will consider this last issue – regulatory scrutiny – first. As we discussed earlier, in America, the DEA's placement of many pain-relieving drugs in restrictive classes has opened the door to the prosecution of physicians who provide these controlled medications to patients in ways that the DEA considers careless. This prosecution is not limited to medical malpractice, but has included criminal prosecutions for drug diversion. In addition, state medical boards have also developed regulations regarding the prescription of opioids, largely due to worries about iatrogenic addiction, and have initiated disciplinary proceedings against physicians who have not adhered to the regulations, even when those regulations contradict best practice standards recommended by pain specialists [30]. These prosecutions have led to physician caution in prescribing these medications. We would like to make clear that we think worry about such prosecution is a legitimate concern for physicians [31].

But – and this is an important caveat – we also believe that physicians may *not* use fear of such prosecution to justify sweeping denial of adequate pain management to their patients. The law in America in fact allows physicians great latitude in using schedule II and III drugs, and physicians have an obligation to their patients to understand what is permitted and to act within *actual* constraints, not imagined ones. In fact, for physicians concerned about the legal ramifications of their prescribing practices, it is significant to note that there have recently been successful cases brought against physicians for *undertreatment* of pain [30]. Of course, the ambiguity of recognized indications for chronic pain treatment contributes to physicians' hesitations to prescribe opioids in the presence of even a remote possibility of legal sanctions. We are sympathetic to hesitation in some cases, but for a clinician to withhold medically indicated medication because the clinician has some vague idea that he she could run into legal problems for doing so is not acceptable. Like many other areas of medicine, clinicians treating pain not only have an obligation to be informed about the current best practices but also to be informed about the true state of the law.

As a final note, it is important to keep in mind that the same bad reasons that lead to physician undertreatment of pain – ignorance, indifference, and fear – are also endorsed by patients, which leads them to underreport their pain experiences [32]. Elderly patients in particular may be ignorant about what pain relief is possible. They may also take their pain to be unimportant in its own right, and they may be fearful about government scrutiny of the consumption of opioids. In the same way that clinicians must guard against their own tendencies to adopt these worrisome attitudes, they must assist their patients in avoiding these pitfalls as well.

The right to pain relief

As the palliative care movement has gained support (since the early days of Saunders' and Twycross' work), there has also been an increased support for the provision of pain relief in acute cases. In 1992, the first clinical practice guidelines for acute pain management were issued by the Agency for Healthcare Research and Quality. This, in turn, has led to a growing demand to provide more pain relief more generally. In 1995, the American Pain Society called for the adoption of pain as the "fifth vital sign." This was followed, in 1998, by the Veterans Health Administration developing a National Pain Management Strategy and, in 2001, by JCAHO developing pain management standards, which included the right to appropriate assessment and management of pain. These initiatives culminated in the Global Day Against Pain (October 11, 2004) during which the World Health Organization, the IASP and the European Federation of IASP Chapters declared that "the relief of pain should be a human right."

The concept of pain relief as a human right is derived from the United Nation's 1966 International Covenant on Economic, Social and Cultural Rights "right to the highest attainable standard of health" [33]. The aim of the proponents of this right to pain relief

is to: (1) improve relief of all forms of pain to permit optimal quality of life and productivity; (2) include a right to pain relief in constitutions; (3) enact statutory requirements for education of health professionals about pain relief; and (4) promote opioid deregulation and affordability.

Most of these goals are clearly laudable. We certainly support (1) and (3) and offer a qualified endorsement of (4) – but we are not convinced that invoking a "right to pain relief" is necessary to achieve these goals. While motivated by noble goals, we think that a single "right to pain relief" is ill considered for a number of reasons. It encourages over-simplification of the nature of pain relief, especially for chronic non-cancer pain. It also minimizes the serious side effects of some pain treatments, most particularly long-term opioid use. Pain is strongly influenced by social and psychological factors, as well as purely physiological events. Thus, physiological pain is not separable from a more holistic conception of suffering. No clinician committed to relieving a patient's pain can afford to do so without engagement with these multiple other factors associated with suffering, and opioids are not always helpful in this project.

In light of the many barriers to adequate pain relief, we can appreciate how a "right to pain relief" has become such a powerful commitment among many clinicians concerned to provide adequate pain relief for their patients. Both government policies and pervasive but unacknowledged medical commitments have worked in concert to prevent many patients from having access to medical interventions that might help to relieve their pain. As we have argued, many of these barriers are illegitimate, and clinicians have aspired to respond to them with a claim on patients' behalf that would end this problem. In this climate, the claim arose that patients had a right to pain relief. So understood, the "right to pain relief" is often characterized as an antidote for the laws, which are seen as curtailing physicians' abilities to adequately prescribe pain-relieving medications, especially opioids [34]. And the "right to pain relief" is invoked to encourage physicians to abandon what are seen as out-dated and immoral attitudes towards their patients' pain.

Striking the balance

The significance of patient populations and locus of pain treatment

What is crucial to notice, however, is that most of the arguments that patients have a right to pain relief have been motivated by examination of cases where patients were dying. While we accept that a "right to pain relief" has considerable force in such cases, we are not convinced that the justification of this ideal with this patient population can be easily carried over to justify a similar claim for other patient populations. We think that there are several questions about the pain experiences in different patient populations that are relevant to the ethical challenges in the provision of pain relief: What are the sources of the pain? Where is this pain relief normally pursued? What are the trade-offs involved? We will consider these questions in the case of four patient populations: patients at the end of life, patients with acute or post-operative pain, patients with cancer pain and patients with chronic pain.

First, we'll consider pain at the end of life. Its causes include disease-related tissue, nerve damage, and organ failure, as well as psychological and spiritual suffering. Pain relief in these situations is typically administered either within a medical setting or under the umbrella of hospice care in the home. Once it is clear that the patient is at the end of life, the trade-offs involved in administering opioids are importantly effected. There are no longer substantial commitments to providing life-prolonging care, and pain relief rises in importance because the underlying disease cannot be stopped. So while opioid use at the end of life can still affect a patient's physiology and psychology in negative ways, these negative effects are often substantially outweighed by the commitment to easing pain in the time that immediately precedes death. In our view, a patient's right to pain relief at the end of life is unqualified – if pain medication is requested, we believe clinicians should provide it. This view appears now to be the dominant view. While there are still cases of patients having uncontrolled pain at the end of their lives, the consensus among medical practitioners now seems to be that these cases are a failure of good medical care.

Of course, worries have arisen in these cases about the possibility of opioid use hastening death. Typically, these worries have been circumnavigated by appealing to the "doctrine of double effect" – that is, the clinician's intentions underlying the prescription of these medications is purely to ease pain (i.e. the intended effect), and hastening death (i.e. the unintended, double, effect) is simply a wholly unavoidable side effect of this legitimate therapeutic goal. While there are important concerns about the validity of this argument, it is important to note that while the US Supreme Court has

not recognized a right to die, it has expressed support for a constitutional right to "adequate palliative care" and urged states not to obstruct it, notably in the decisions rendered in *Washington v. Glucksberg* and *Vacco v. Quill*, which we believe is consistent with our commitment to the unfettered access to opioids for terminally ill patients.

The second patient population to consider is patients with acute pain and/or post-operative pain. In these cases, the pain is caused primarily by tissue or nerve damage, but can sometimes possibly be affected by psychological and spiritual suffering. The pain treatment is typically initiated within medical setting, and may continue outside the clinic, but only for a circumscribed period of time. Unlike patients at the end of life, the trade-offs of good pain relief for these patients are the traditional medical risks to life and safety. Because pain in these contexts usually responds to traditional medical treatments such as repair and medication, and typically the course of pain for these patients is relatively clear early on, balancing these trade-offs is often not that problematic. Moreover, the balancing has gotten easier, as better data have been developed that show that fears about iatrogenic addiction in this patient population have historically been overstated.

Because of these factors, we believe (as with patients at the end of life) that there should be a strong presumption in favor of providing these patients with the pain relief they request. It looks like there are still problems in providing this patient population with adequate pain relief (e.g., the IASP estimates that 50% of post-operative and trauma patients have severe to intolerable pain), and we support efforts of clinicians to eliminating non-medically-indicated barriers to pain relief. Of course, the focus on providing pain relief should not be used to discount the serious side effects of opioids, and care must be taken to minimize the very real increased risks of mortality and morbidity that come with high opioid doses [35].

A third patient population that has received significant attention in the literature about the ethics of pain management has been cancer patients. Historically, pain in cancer patients has been grappled with as part of the discussion about pain management at the end of life. Now, of course, that is no longer the case. Some cancer patients are now a better fit in the category of patients with acute and/or post-operative pain – short-term, primarily tissue/nerve damage-related, pain experienced in the hospital. But more commonly, these successfully treated cancer patients are now part of a much larger group of patients who experience chronic pain without progressive disease. This is the final, and most vexing, patient population we would like to consider.

The causes of pain in this patient population are varied, and sometimes unknown, but often psychological and spiritual issues are highly significant. For these patients, their pain does not have a short (anticipated) time-horizon, their pain occurs outside of a healthcare institution, and their pain treatment must be offered on an outpatient basis, independent of frequent medical oversight. And in the assessment of trade-offs, it is often difficult to be confident about where the benefits and burdens lie in offering opioids for pain management. Often, chronic pain does not respond straightforwardly to any standard pain management strategies, nor is there likely to be a straightforward, finite, anticipated course of the pain. These patients' diseases are not expected to be terminal, so their pain management strategies have to be integrated into their broader life goals. It is with this population that we have reservations about appealing to a right to pain relief to guide clinical pain management.

The central claim that motivates our position is that patients *should* not have analgesia as their sole or primary goal. Desperate patients may state that pain relief is their only goal. But if they can be encouraged to look beyond their immediate sense of crisis, most patients will acknowledge that pain relief must be part of their broader set of life goals. Relief from pain is a good in itself, but it is significant to patients because pain relief would allow them to do other things. Pain relief does not always increase the capacity to do other things. In the most extreme cases, analgesia is only possible with a total loss of consciousness. But even in less extreme cases, opioids negatively affect and limit patients' physiological and mental capacities, including those needed for e.g., discharging their professional responsibilities, pursuing other pleasurable activities, and participating in meaningful relationships.

For terminally ill patients, for acutely ill, or post-operative patients, balancing off these considerations is typically uncomplicated, for the reasons we discussed above. But for chronic pain patients who are integrating opioid consumption into their daily lives with relatively little medical oversight, it is a serious challenge for clinicians to offer them assistance that takes their total, long-term well being into consideration – not just short-term pain relief goals.

Saying that patients have a "right to pain relief" does not facilitate this task. Patients in pain do not always appreciate the grave long-term risks associated with opioid use. We are extremely sympathetic to their requests for pain relief. But the obligation to take patients' pain, and the pleas for relief, seriously, does not entail that the physician should simply keep the prescription pad at the ready. Physicians are in a position to know what their patients may not – that there is such a thing as *too much* pain relief. Conveying this troubling fact to patients, and developing with them a treatment plan that is sensitive to this worry, is extremely difficult. Creating a climate where clinicians and patients alike view pain relief as a right only makes it harder.

There is a battle being waged in the realm of pain management. On the one side are people calling for greater access to opioids, characterized in our view by the call for recognition of a right to pain relief. On the other side is resistance to widespread use of opioids, typically primarily motivated by fears about addiction. Our analysis, we hope, shows that neither side in this struggle is wholly right or wrong. Moreover, we believe that framing the clinical struggles associated with pain management in this way obscures the true challenge – that of balancing the deep moral obligation of medicine to alleviate pain and suffering against the commensurate obligation to be very cautious in providing therapies that offer powerful short-term benefits but that also carry real risks of long-term harm to overall patient well-being.

Conclusion

We hope we have shown in this chapter that pain has indeed been historically neglected in favor of a fairly exclusive focus on disease. For us, this means that increased attention to pain is appropriate and important. We also believe, however, that there are two important problems with the call for a "right to pain relief." First, this call ignores the diversity of clinical pain populations and their associated treatment settings – in our view, these setting significantly shape how a pain treatment should be pursued. Second, the claim that there is a right to pain relief implicitly casts the harm of unrelieved pain as a lack of access by an individual with pain to a clinical service. But there are several problems with this implicit assumption. For one, it overestimates the role of clinical services and underestimates the role of the patient in shaping both the pain he/she experiences and the relief that is possible. Further, this assumption neglects too many other considerations, including the harm associated with pain treatments, as well as the other life goals and facets of patients' well-being that must be balanced against pain relief.

References

1. Jacox A, Carr DB, Payne R. New clinical-practice guidelines for the management of pain in patients with cancer. *N Engl J Med* 1994; **330**: 651–5.

2. Bostrom M. Summary of the Mayday Fund Survey: public attitudes about pain and analgesics. *J Pain Symptom Manage* 1997; **13**: 166–8.

3. American Medical Association. *AMA, JCAHO and NCQA to focus on measuring effectiveness of appropriate pain management: Joint Commission on Acccreditation of Healthcare Organizations*; Press Release Dec. 17, 2001.

4. Joint Commission Resources. *How to Meet the Most Challenging Joint Commission Requirements for Behavioral Health Care* (Oakbrook Terrace, IL: Joint Commission Resources, 2006).

5. Mitka M. Experts debate widening use of opioid drugs for chronic nonmalignant pain. *JAMA* 2003; **289**: 2347–8.

6. Lipman AG. Pain as a human right: the 2004 Global Day Against Pain. *J Pain Palliat Care Pharmacother* 2005; **19**: 85–100.

7. Wittgenstein L. *Philosophical Investigations* (New York: Macmillan, 1953).

8. Sullivan M, Ferrell B. Ethical challenges in the management of chronic nonmalignant pain: negotiating through the cloud of doubt. *J Pain* 2005; **6**: 2–9.

9. Merskey H. Logic, truth and language in concepts of pain. *Qual Life Res.* 1994; **3** Suppl 1: S69–76.

10. Coghill RC, McHaffie JG, Yen YF. Neural correlates of interindividual differences in the subjective experience of pain. *Proc Natl Acad Sci USA* 2003; **100**: 8538–42.

11. Moisset X, Bouhassira D. Brain imaging of neuropathic pain. *Neuroimage.* 2007; **37** Suppl 1: S80–88.

12. Sullivan M. Exaggerated pain behavior: by what standard? *Clin J Pain* 2004; **20**: 433–9.

13. IASP Task Force on Taxomony. *Classification of Chronic Pain* (Seattle: IASP Press, 1994).

14. Apkarian AV, Baliki MN, Geha PY. Towards a theory of chronic pain. *Prog Neurobiol* 2009; **87**: 81–97.

15. Fine G. *Review of the Drug Enforcement Administration's Investigations of the Diversion of Controlled Pharmaceuticals* 2002. I-2002–010.

16. Von Korff M, Deyo RA. Potent opioids for chronic musculoskeletal pain: flying blind? *Pain* 2004; **109**: 207–9.

17. de CWAC, Craig KD. A science of pain expression? *Pain* 2006; **125**: 202–3.

18. McCaffery M, Grimm MA, Pasero C, Ferrell B, Uman GC. On the meaning of "drug seeking". *Pain Manag Nurs* 2005; **6**: 122–36.

19. Musto DF. The mystery of addiction. *Lancet* 1999; **354** Suppl: SIV1.

20. Wasan AD, Correll DJ, Kissin I, O' Shea S, Jamison RN. Iatrogenic addiction in patients treated for acute or subacute pain: a systematic review. *J Opioid Manag* 2006; **2**: 16–22.

21. Liebeskind JC. Pain can kill. *Pain.* 1991; **44**: 3–4.

22. Po A. Too much, too little, or none at all: dealing with substandard and fake drugs. *Lancet* 2001; **357**: 1904.

23. Acker C. Take as directed: the dilemmas of regulating addictive analegics and other psychoactive drugs. In *Opioids and Pain Relief: A Historical Perspective (Progress in Pain Research and Management, Vol. 25)*, ed. M. Meldrum. (Seattle: IASP Press, 2003).

24. Loeser J. Opiophobia and opiophyllia. *Opioids and Pain Relief: A Historical Perspective (Progress in Pain Research and Management, Vol. 25)*, ed. M. Meldrum. (Seattle: IASP Press, 2003).

25. Meldrum M. The property of euphoria: research and the cancer patient. In *Opioids and Pain Relief: A Historical Perspective (Progress in Pain Research and Management, Vol. 25)*, ed. M. Meldrum. (Seattle: IASP Press, 2003).

26. Ballantyne J. Medical use of opioids: what drives the debate? A brief commentary. *European J Pain Suppl* 2008; **2**: 67–8.

27. Clark D. Rise and demise of the Brompton cocktail. In *Opioids and Pain Relief: A Historical Perspective (Progress in Pain Research and Management, Vol. 25)*, ed. M. Meldrum. (Seattle: IASP Press, 2003).

28. US General Accounting Office. *Department of Justice: Status of Achieving Key Outcomes and Addressing Major Management Challenges: U.S. General Accounting Office*; 2001. GAO-01-729.

29. Rich BA. Moral conundrums in the courtroom: reflections on a decade in the culture of pain. *Camb Q Healthc Ethics* 2002; **11**: 180–90.

30. Rich BA. Overcoming legal barriers to competent and compassionate pain relief for patients with chronic nonmalignant pain. *APS Bulletin* Vol **15**; 2005.

31. Goldenbaum DM, Christopher M, Gallagher RM, *et al.* Physicians charged with opioid analgesic-prescribing offenses. *Pain Med* 2008; **9**: 737–47.

32. Dahl J. The state cancer pain initiative movement in the United States: successes and challenges. In *Opioids and Pain Relief: A Historical Perspective (Progress in Pain Research and Management, Vol. 25)*, ed. M. Meldrum. (Seattle: IASP Press, 2003).

33. Office of the High Commissioner for Human Rights. *United Nation's International Covenant on Economic, Social and Cultural Rights (ICESCR)*; 1966.

34. Weinman BP. 2003 LeTourneau Award. Freedom from pain. establishing a constitutional right to pain relief. *J Leg Med* 2003; **24**: 495–539.

35. Taylor S, Voytovich AE, Kozol RA. Has the pendulum swung too far in postoperative pain control? *Am J Surg* 2003; **186**: 472–5.

Practice, policy, and research

Realizing the promise of optimal pain care: What does the future hold?

Robert D. Kerns and Michael H. Ebert

Pain and behavioral medicine: The coming of age of the biopsychosocial model

Even a cursory review of the table of contents for the book may arouse an awareness of the broad scope of the psychosocial dimension of the field of pain and pain management. The importance of the psychosocial context for the field is readily apparent by personal reflection on one's own experiences with pain. Appreciation of the covert, subjective, and idiosyncratic experience of pain is entirely consistent with the central place that the psychosocial dimension has assumed in the core conceptual framework for scientific inquiry and practice in the field.

The biopsychosocial model, as articulated by George Engle and others, highlights the inextricable and reciprocating relationships among health and illness, behavior, and the social context [1, 2]. This perspective emphasizes the critical need to examine multiple levels of the organism (e.g., molecular, organ, person, family) in order to fully appreciate the nature of the problem, its contributors, and its impacts. The model similarly recognizes that components of the system are hierarchically ordered, that components are themselves comprised of multiple subcomponents, and that each component is part of a larger whole. Furthermore, intervention targeting any one component or level of the system necessarily results in changes in other components or levels. The biopsychosocial framework supersedes more simplistic, reductionistic, and unidimensional biomedical models that are consistent with historical and limited mind-body dualistic notions of disease.

Of course, many of the clinical implications of the biopsychosocial model are recognized as being particularly difficult to implement in the present healthcare system. Such is the case for research and educational efforts informed by the model, as well. The model encourages what to some seems to be an unwieldy and even unrealistic requirement of conducting a comprehensive evaluation across multiple levels of analysis in order develop a truly integrated treatment plan. Proponents of the model argue for investment in resources and innovation in this process in order to accrue its potential health benefits.

Relationship among healthcare providers, patients, and families are also emphasized by the model. In fact, Engel suggested that the failure to appreciate the nature of provider–patient interactions is a critical flaw of the current healthcare system and the practice of medicine [2]. The study of such interactions is made even more complex when considering the broader context of multidisciplinary healthcare delivery systems and models of chronic, longitudinal care, and care coordination.

As the field of pain management has embraced the biopsychosocial perspective it can be argued that it has served a pioneering role in the broader field of behavioral medicine [3]. The accepted definition of behavioral medicine as "an *interdisciplinary* field concerned with the development and integration of behavioral *and* biomedical science knowledge and techniques relevant to health and illness and the application of this knowledge and these techniques to prevention, diagnosis, treatment and rehabilitation" is entirely consistent with present day pain management [4]. The impact has been felt across clinical practice, research, and educational settings, particularly with regard to its truly interdisciplinary nature. Explicit attention to the experience of pain itself as a multidimensional phenomenon, the increasing attention to pain and its multiple common medical and psychiatric co-morbidities, and the recognition of the importance of a multimodal approach to intervention is entirely consistent with the

Behavioral and Psychopharmacologic Pain Management, ed. Michael H. Ebert and Robert D. Kerns. Published by Cambridge University Press. © Cambridge University Press 2011.

biopsychosocial framework. In many ways, the increasing emphasis on pain "management" as opposed to treatment or cure is symbolic of a more sophisticated understanding of health and illness, adjustment and adaptation, and health-related quality of life as continua rather than static states of being.

Application of the biospsychosocial model

The chapters by Dennis Turk and colleagues and June Dahl open this text with a detailed discussion of the biopsychosocial framework and its explicit role in defining the practice of pain management. As they note, accepted definitions of pain emphasize the multidimensional nature of pain and specifically highlight interactions between biological and psychological systems. According to the International Association for the Study of Pain, pain is "An unpleasant sensory and emotional experience associated with actual or potential tissue damage or described in terms of such damage" [4]. It is accepted as a complex perceptual experience involving all domains of persons' lives, and multidimensional and multidisciplinary approaches to pain assessment and management that attend to concomitant changes in physical and emotional functioning and overall quality of life, in addition to pain, per se, are increasingly accepted as key components of optimal pain care.

An ever expanding empirical literature continues to inform sophisticated understanding of key psychological and behavioral factors that reliably influence the perpetuation, if not the development, of pain and pain related disability. Early work focused on personality factors – such as having a predisposition towards denying emotional and/or interpersonal distress, being overly preoccupied with somatic symptoms, or displaying features associated with a "depression-prone" personality such as pessimism – that were hypothesized to be associated with pain severity and the persistence of pain over time [6, 7]. Laboratory and clinical studies on relationships between pain and affect continues to be a primary focus of investigation [8]. Operant behavioral theory has been influential in emphasizing the role of social learning in the experience of pain [9]. Specifically, the model has played an important heuristic role in informing research that has identified the role of social contingencies (e.g., expressions of sympathy from family members and friends, disability payments, prescription medications) for overt expressions of pain, termed "pain behaviors" (e.g., verbal and paraverbal expressions of pain, visits to doctors, avoidance of work-related activities and social responsibilities) [10–12]. Turk's cognitive-behavioral perspective played an important role in encouraging research that led to the identification of cognitive factors strongly and reliably positively associated with pain severity and disability [13]. Among factors that have the strongest empirical support are such constructs as pain catastrophizing [14], fear avoidance [15], low self-efficacy and lack of perceived control [16, 17] and passive pain coping [18].

The biopsychosocial model of pain and pain management is not without its critics, however. Although the validity of the model is generally recognized, its application in clinical settings remains challenging. Conduct of a comprehensive pain assessment informed by the model is virtually impossible in busy primary care and family practice settings due to time limitations, costs, as well as expertise. Development of an integrated treatment plan informed by a comprehensive assessment is one thing, but enactment of the plan represents a burden on the healthcare system and patients alike. The need for efficiency in the application of the model is quite apparent.

Psychological and psychiatric influences on the assessment and management of pain

Assessment of pain begins with respect for each person's reports of his or her pain experience and always circles back to these reports when attempting to determine the effectiveness of interventions targeting pain relief. The chapters in section two of this text detail strategies designed to quantify and measure the experience of pain and pain-related interference with functioning, emotional well-being, and quality of life. These chapters highlight each of the core domains of pain outcome assessment asserted by the Initiative on Methods, Measurement, and Pain Assessment in Clinical Trials (IMMPACT) consensus group and serve to emphasize the importance of assessing the broader multidimensional experience of pain in clinical settings [19]. These chapters further highlight significant advances on the clinical assessment front, including the proliferation of an extensive array of psychometrically sound assessment strategies including semi-structured interviews, questionnaires and inventories, diaries, behavioral observation methods, psychophysiological methods, and strategies for assessing the family context.

Continued efforts to develop assessment methods that can be quickly and reliably employed in busy practice settings may be critical to the continued application of systematic pain assessment in clinical settings. The "Pain as the 5th Vital Sign" initiative promulgated by the Joint Commission, that is, the use of a single pain numeric rating scale to screen for the presence and intensity of pain, currently serves as the sole approach to pain assessment that has found its way into routine clinical practice [20]. Although this approach has certainly helped draw clinician's attention to pain, its obvious limitations leave clinicians without an efficient way of quantifying pain's broader impacts on physical and emotional functioning and quality of life, and perhaps most importantly, without an easy way to reassess the effectiveness of a pain intervention. Current work that employs computer adaptive testing to develop more efficient approaches to capturing the broader domains of the pain experience hold promise in this regard [21].

Section three of this text offers a comprehensive look at the broad array of pharmacological and non-pharmacological approaches to pain treatment that are currently available. Advances in the domain of pharmacological treatment have led to recommendations for employing algorithmic, rational polypharmacy to optimally treat complex chronic pain conditions that are not responsive to single pain medications [22]. These approaches further take into account an appreciation of important medical and psychiatric co-morbidities and the need to consider a variety of individual difference factors in developing a pharmacological treatment plan. Of course, the chapter by Smith and Argoff on opioid therapy discusses the central role that this class of medications has assumed in the clinician's armamentarium in efforts to promote optimal pain control. As the controversy over the increasing use of opioids for the management of chronic non-cancer pain continues, explicit attention to the safe prescribing of these medications to protect both patients and the broader public from harm will be critical.

As early as the late 1960s, data began to emerge that supported the effectiveness of psychological interventions for persistent pain, either in the context of multidisciplinary pain programs or in isolation of other interventions. A range of specific psychological interventions have considerable support for their efficacy including cognitive-behavioral interventions, as well as self-regulatory interventions such as relaxation training, hypnosis, and biofeedback. Research

has documented the benefits of various psychological interventions for such pain conditions as headache [23], low back [24], and arthritis [25], among many others. One particularly influential meta-analysis of the cost-effectiveness of multidisciplinary pain care, published by Flor and her colleagues, documented the benefits of such programs on pain and functioning, including return to work [26]. A recent line of investigation has begun to focus on identification of predictors of change during pain treatment, the process of change, and the potential to improve outcomes through a process of matching individual characteristics with different treatments [27–29].

The chapters in section three were selected to highlight some of the most common psychological interventions for chronic pain including operant-behavioral treatment, cognitive-behavioral therapy, and family therapy. The chapter by Tan and colleagues on Complementary and Alternative Modalities represents an explicit acknowledgement of the growing interest in these approaches and the emerging data supporting their efficacy. The chapter by Pence and colleagues draws attention to the large and continually growing psychological literature on pain and cognition and on the construct of coping, more specifically. Advances in this domain will almost certainly continue to drive refinements in psychological interventions to improve their effectiveness and widespread adoption as alternatives to traditional medical approaches to pain care. Finally, the focus on treatment approaches that integrate pharmacological and non-pharmacological approaches is particularly well described in the chapter by Leo. Of note is a quite recent publication by Kurt Kroenke and colleagues in which a treatment approach that combined optimized antidepressant therapy and brief pain self-management therapy resulted in clinically meaningful improvements in both depression and pain severity for persons with these commonly co-occurring conditions [30]. We can expect to continue to see the proliferation of innovative and integrative treatments as investigators and clinicians work side by side to address the challenges of managing complex co-morbid health conditions.

Section four of this text begins with specific consideration of the "bread and butter" of the practice of pain medicine, namely the management of common painful conditions including diseases of the spine, other musculoskeletal conditions, arthritis, neuropathic pain disorders, and headache. Written by experts in the field, these chapters emphasize the diagnostic and management challenges and provide a thorough consideration of state-of-the-art approaches to address these challenges. A second set of chapters in this section discuss the management of pain experienced by persons known to be particularly vulnerable to undertreatment of pain, namely persons with terminal cancer and other life-ending disorders, children and adolescents, the elderly, and racial and ethnic minorities. Excellent contributions by leaders in the field represent a call for improvement for meeting the pain care needs of those most likely to require special attention and care.

The chapters preceding this concluding chapter serve as a similar challenge to the future leaders of the field of pain management. Boris-Karpel provides a particularly comprehensive and compelling review of the history of the field and the current policy challenges that demand our collective attention. The final two chapters in this section provide equally thoughtful discussions of the future of scientific inquiry and ethical discourse that provides an important context for thinking about the future of the field. A recent published review of the field of translational pain research serves to further characterize trends in our field [31]. And, not surprisingly, as the debate about the "right to pain management" continues to heat up in western cultures, the ethical, legal, regulatory, and political contexts of the field of pain management will require practitioners in the field to pay close attention to these discussions and their implications.

The field of pain management: Promise and challenges

The field of pain management has evidenced remarkable changes in the past several years. These changes promise to advance care for millions of persons to promote optimal pain control and improve functioning and quality of life in a range of clinical and everyday settings. Favorable legislation, regulation, and policy informed by sound expert opinion and cultural influences, and a sense of a moral imperative have promoted and sustained these advances in pain care. Many advances in the field of pain management have been informed by an increasingly sophisticated and comprehensive biopsychosocial model of pain that has relatively direct implications for care of the person with pain. Theory-driven research is on the rise with greater attention to research with transparent implications for changes in practice and policy [31]. The

drive for improved clinical methods for the assessment and management of pain has led to calls for increased funding across the domains of basic laboratory science, clinical science, rehabilitation, and health services research [32]. Education and training programs for pain medicine physicians, nurses, and associated health professionals have blossomed to keep pace with the demand for competent healthcare professionals with a specific expertise related to pain management. The role of a better informed community of patients, family members, and advocates cannot be understated in promoting improved pain care.

Despite these advances and promise of improved pain care, there remain enormous challenges to assuring access to appropriate pain treatment for all. Inequities of access to optimal pain care abound. The advantages of access to competent healthcare providers, analgesic medications, and other tools of effective pain management afforded to many in parts of the world are largely unavailable in underdeveloped regions of the world. Even in the USA, significant disparities in pain care exist leaving many vulnerable segments of our society, including the very young and old, persons of color, persons living in rural and geographically isolated regions, those with stigmatized medical and psychiatric conditions, and even women, suffering needless pain.

On the legal, ethical, and policy fronts, numerous dilemmas and seeming paradoxes appear to further threaten the sustainability of recent advances. As an increasing number of governments assert that pain management is a human right, an uncertain operationalization of this dictum remains. Does this right include access to opioid medication, for example, even as public health concerns about diversion and addiction are on the rise? Where is the balance between providers' interests in protecting personal and public safety and patients' rights to effective pain management? And as concerns grow about the safety profiles and unintended adverse side effects of analgesic medications, what can be done to ensure that access to these medications for persons with pain is not diminished in the service of protecting others from unintended adverse effects?

The challenges for promoting optimal pain care sometimes seem almost insurmountable in the current climate, at least in the USA and other Western societies. Perhaps no more perplexing is the apparent disconnect between the widely accepted biopsychosocial model of pain and data supporting a multidisciplinary and multimodal approach to pain assessment and treatment and trends in the field of pain management that appear to be more consistent with largely unsupported unidimensional, reductionistic, biomedical models. In the recent past, many have decried the diminishing number of multidisciplinary pain centers that some have hailed as the gold standard for pain care, while observing the rapid rise of interventional pain medicine techniques and procedures that often lack empirical support. As evidence mounts that non-pharmacological interventions for pain, including psychological interventions, structured exercise, and other rehabilitation approaches, are efficacious, insurance coverage for these interventions is often unavailable. Although it appears that a balance in opioid prescribing is in the wings, it is clear that these medications too often are prescribed inappropriately and without attention to commonly accepted safety practices even as evidence supporting their efficacy, at least for chronic, non-cancer pain, is lacking. It is clear that considerable work must continue on multiple fronts to ensure that the term evidence-based pain care does not ring hollow.

A similar discordance between an increasing appreciation and acceptance of the need for more pain research and the reality of the funding scene is apparent, at least in the USA. Despite the designation of the US Congress of the Decade of Pain Control and Research, funding in the NIH for pain-relevant research has apparently declined in recent years [32]. Despite apparent funding limitations, pain researchers continue to make important discoveries that have rapidly transformed our understanding of previously perplexing and common painful conditions including fibromyalgia, complex regional pain syndrome, diabetic peripheral neuropathic pain, and even low back pain. These advances have yielded new medications and other pharmacological and non-pharmacological approaches that have improved the lives of many. Unfortunately, the translation of the evidence into practice has been less than optimal. More attention to translational research and the need to improve processes for rapid and sustained dissemination of evidence is clear [31].

Building capacity for optimal pain care

In many ways the opportunities and challenges of the field converge on the importance of enhancing our capacity for graduate, postgraduate, and life-long education and training of pain scientists and providers in order to build our collective capacity for improving pain care. It is widely appreciated that medical, nursing, and associated health professional training programs have failed to provide an appropriate emphasis on even the basic principles of pain and pain management. The discordance between the prevalence and costs of untreated pain and attention paid to the assessment and management of pain in our educational programs is simply astounding and hard to understand. The result is a healthcare provider workforce that is ill-prepared to care for persons with even common pain conditions. Not surprisingly, primary care and family medicine physicians, for example, report that management of chronic pain is by far their most frustrating problem, far surpassing their experience in caring for persons with complex psychiatric conditions [33]. Without an increased focus on training a competent provider workforce in the management of pain, the realization of improved pain care informed by scientific advances and favorable policy and legislation will remain a distant hope.

It is in this context that the present text was conceived. As expectations for education and training of physician pain specialists were broadened by the Accreditation Council of Graduate Medical Education (ACGME) to incorporate an explicit multidimensional and multidisciplinary perspective, a significant gap in the available literature on the behavioral and psychopharmacological approaches to pain care was identified. The current text was explicitly designed to fill a noted gap by offering a single source text that provides a comprehensive and state-of-the-art consideration of the biopsychosocial perspective on pain and pain management with the pain medicine specialist in mind. It is expected that the text will serve as an important resource for the generalist and other medical specialists as well as for nurses and associated health professionals, as well.

The challenges of building a healthcare provider workforce with the competencies necessary for the management of pain appear to be large and growing. It is increasingly apparent that the access to optimal pain care will require the expanded competencies of virtually all healthcare professionals, not just the proliferation of board certified pain medicine specialists. It seems apparent that the success of this endeavor will include at least a two-pronged approach that targets existing practitioners and encourages continuing education to enhance pain management competencies *and* targets physicians in training to the field of pain medicine and associated healthcare trainees to develop specific expertise in the domain of pain management.

It is not surprising that the American Pain Society (APS), for example, has developed an extensive educational initiative targeting both practitioners and trainees. The APS provides a broad array of continuing medical educational (CME) offerings including an annual scientific meeting with numerous CME opportunities, its own scientific journal, the *Journal of Pain*, and newsletters, and its website even offers formal CMEs for successful completion of an online course on pain management available at its website (www.ampainsoc.org). Another important initiative within the APS and its several collaborating partners is a focus on the development and dissemination of evidence-based practice guidelines and similar practice recommendations. Several years ago the APS, in partnership with industry, began to sponsor an innovative two-day seminar targeting medical residents and other professionals who are potentially interested in advanced education and training in pain management. The course has emerged as a unique opportunity for trainees to learn from and interact with leading experts in the field. But these and other organizational efforts continue to fall far short in meeting the needs of society, and continuing efforts to support the more widespread integration of education and training related to pain management into the rubric of healthcare professional training is critical.

It appears that a particularly daunting challenge in the development of a competent pain management workforce is the field's central aspiration to be defined as a multidisciplinary field that is true to a biopsychosocial model. Multiple forces appear to work against this stated objective, including discipline specific educational models and programs that represent the mainstay of current healthcare professional training. Current trends in healthcare reimbursement have been noted to be almost entirely inconsistent with multidisciplinary functioning and multimodal treatment. The pharmaceutical industry and its well-financed marketing divisions clearly fosters the medicalization of pain management and reinforces consumers' views that pain management is synonymous with the use of pain medications. Twenty-five years after the publication of the seminal review of the effectiveness of multidisciplinary pain centers by Herta Flor and her colleagues, the promise of routine access to such programs for the management of complex chronic pain conditions represents little more than an illusion. It seems clear that a substantial shift in incentives that are consistent with a commitment to interdisciplinary and chronic disease models of pain management will be necessary to reverse the current trends. The recent changes in the ACGME criteria for education and training programs and for credentialing pain medicine specialists are important steps in this direction.

References

1. Engel GL. The clinical application of the biopsychosocial model. *Am J Psychiatry* 1980; **137**: 535–44.

2. Engel G. The need for a new medical model: A challenge for biomedicine. *Science.* 1977; **196**: 129–36.

3. Frantsve LM, Kerns RD, Desan P, Sledge WH. Behavioral medicine. In *Psychiatry*, Vol. 2, 3rd edn. eds. A Tasman, J Kay, J Lieberman, MB First and M Maj. (Chichester: John Wiley and Sons, 2008), pp. 2027–46.

4. Schwartz GE, Weiss SM. Behavioral medicine revisited: An amended definition. *J Behav Med* 1978; **1**: 249–51.

5. Merskey H. Pain terms: A list with definitions and notes on usage. *Pain* 1979; **6**: 249–52.

6. Blumer D, Heilbronn M. Chronic pain as a variant of depressive disease: The pain-prone personality. *J Nerv Ment Dis* 1982; **170**: 381–94.

7. Gentry W, Shows W, Thomas M. Chronic low back pain: A psychological profile. *Psychosomatics* 1974; **15**: 174–7.

8. Fernandez E, Kerns R, eds. Anxiety, depression and anger: Core components of negative affect in medical populations. In *The SAGE Handbook of Personality Theory and Testing: Volume 1: Personality Theories and Models*, eds. G Boyle, D Matthews and D Saklofske. (London: Sage, 2008).

9. Fordyce W. *Behavioral Methods for Chronic Pain and Illness* (St. Louis, MO: Mosby; 1976).

10. Leonard M, Cano A, Johansen A. Chronic pain in a couples context: A review and integration of theoretical models and empirical evidence. *J Pain* 2006; **7**: 377–90.

11. Romano J, Turner J, Jensen M, *et al.* Chronic pain patient-spouse behavioral interactions predict pain disability. *Pain* 1995; **63**: 353–60.

12. Weiss L, Kerns R. Patterns of pain relevant social interactions. *Int J Beh Med* 1995; **2**: 157–71.

13. Turk DC, Meichembaum DM, Genest M. *Pain and Behavioral Medicine: A Cognitive Behavioral Perspective* (New York: Guildford, 1983).

14. Turner J, Aaron L. Pain-related catastrophizing: What is it? *Clin J Pain* 2001; **17**: 65–71.

15. Vlaeyen J, Linton S. Fear avoidance and its consequences in chronic musculoskeletal pain: A state of the art. *Pain*. 2000; **85**: 317–22.

16. Arnstein P, Caudill M, Mandle C, Norris A, Beasley R. Self-efficacy as a mediator of the relationship between these psychological, behavioral, and social variables and the experience of pain and disability. Strategies for the reliable assessment of pain intensity, disability and depression in chronic pain patients. *Pain* 1999; **80**: 483–91.

17. Litt M. Self-efficacy and perceived control: Cognitive mediators of pain tolerance. *J Pers Soc Psych* 1988; **54**: 149–60.

18. McCracken L, Eccleston C. Coping or acceptance: What to do about chronic pain? *Pain* 2003; **105**: 197–204.

19. Turk DC, Dworkin RH, Allen N, Bellamy N *et al.* Core outcome domains for pain clinical trials: IMMPACT recommendations. *Pain* 2003; **106**: 337–45.

20. Kerns RD, Wasse L, Ryan B, Drake A, Booss J. Pain as the 5th Vital Sign Toolkit. V.2. Washington, DC: Veterans Health Administration.

21. Ware JE, Bjorner JB, Kosinski M. Practical implications of item response theory and computer adaptive testing: A brief summary of ongoing studies of widely used headache impact scales. *Med Care* 2000; **38**: II73–82.

22. Fishbain DA. Polypharmacy treatment approaches to psychiatric and somatic comorbidities of chronic pain. *Am J Phys Med Rehab* 2005; **84**: 556–63.

23. Holroyd K, O' Donnell F, Stensland M, *et al.* Management of chronic tension-type headache with tricyclic antidepressant medication, stress management, and their combination. *JAMA* 2001; **285**: 2208–15.

24. Hoffman BM PR, Chatkoff DK, Kerns RD. Meta-analysis of psychological interventions for chronic low back pain. *Health Psychol* 2007; **26**: 10–12.

25. Keefe F, Smith S, Buffington A, *et al.* Recent advances and future directions in the biopsychosocial assessment and treatment of arthritis. *J Consult Clin Psychol* 2002; **70**: 459–62.

26. Flor H, Fydrich, T, Turk, DC. Efficacy of multidisciplinary pain treatment centers: A meta-analytic review. *Pain* 1992; **49**: 221–30.

27. Kerns RD, Habib S. A critical review of the pain readiness to change model. *J Pain* 2004; **5**: 357–67.

28. Kerns RD, Jensen MP, Nielsen WR. Motivational issues in pain self-management. *Proceedings of the 11th World Congress on Pain*, eds. H Flor, E Kelso and JO Dostrovsky. (IASP Press: Seattle, 2006), pp. 555–66.

29. Turk D, Okifuji A. Psychological factors in chronic pain: Evolution and revolution. *J Consult Clin Psycho* 2002; **70**: 678–90.

30. Kroenke K, Bair MJ, Damush TM, *et al.* Optimized antidepressant treatment and pain self-management in primary care patients with depression and musculoskeletal pain. *JAMA* 2009; **301**: 2099–110.

31. Mao J. Translational pain research: Achievements and challenges. *J Pain* 2009; **10**: 1001–11.

32. Bradshaw DH, Empy C, Davis P, *et al.* Trends in funding for research on pain: A report on the National Institutes of Health grant awards over the years 2003–2007. *J Pain* 2008; **9**: 1077–87.

33. Marcus DA. *Chronic Pain: A primary care guide to practical management*, 2nd edn. (New York: Springer, 2009).

Index

Printed in the United States
By Bookmasters